# HOUGH'S
# Cardiorespiratory Care

For Elsevier

*Senior Content Strategist:* Rita Demetriou-Swanwick
*Content Development Specialists:* Joanna Collett and Katie Golsby
*Project Manager:* Joanna Souch
*Designer/Design Direction:* Margaret Reid
*Illustration Manager:* Karen Giacomucci
*Illustrator:* MPS North America, LLC

**Fifth Edition**

# HOUGH'S

# Cardiorespiratory Care

*an evidence-based, problem-solving approach*

## Alexandra Hough MSc, MCSP, DipTP
Respiratory physiotherapist and freelance lecturer

ELSEVIER

Edinburgh   London   New York   Oxford   Philadelphia   St Louis   Sydney   Toronto   2018

# ELSEVIER

First edition © Chapman and Hall 1991
Second edition © Nelson Thornes 1996
Third edition © Cengage Learning 2001
Fourth edition © Cengage Learning 2014
Fifth edition © Elsevier Limited 2018

ISBN 978-0-7020-7184-3
eBook ISBN 978-0-7020-7527-8

**Notices**

Practitioners and researchers must always rely on their own experience and knowledge in evaluating and using any information, methods, compounds or experiments described herein. Because of rapid advances in the medical sciences, in particular, independent verification of diagnoses and drug dosages should be made. To the fullest extent of the law, no responsibility is assumed by Elsevier, authors, editors or contributors for any injury and/or damage to persons or property as a matter of products liability, negligence or otherwise, or from any use or operation of any methods, products, instructions, or ideas contained in the material herein.

**ELSEVIER** your source for books,
journals and multimedia
in the health sciences

**www.elsevierhealth.com**

  Working together
to grow libraries in
developing countries

www.elsevier.com • www.bookaid.org

The
publisher's
policy is to use
**paper manufactured
from sustainable forests**

Printed in Italy

# CONTENTS

v

The book is dedicated to Veronica Bastow,
who has contributed much to humane and thoughtful respiratory care.

*Good facts make good ethics.*

***Ashwal, 2013***

Cardiorespiratory care is an immensely satisfying branch of physiotherapy. It challenges our intellect, exploits our handling skills and employs our humanity to the full. The specialty is both art and science, but not an exact science. Effectiveness depends on problem-solving, which requires evidence-based information, provided here in the form of 5000 online references.

Clinicians, students and educationists also expect integration of theory and practice, explanations that are physiologically sound, and exact detail of technique. This book is written for such readers and for those who question traditional assumptions. Clinical reasoning boxes in the text facilitate critical thinking, and case studies at the end of each chapter aid problem-solving.

Each problem and disease also has a comprehensive list of validated outcome measures. Clarity is assisted by glossary terms highlighted throughout.

The accompanying website contains full references, a bibliography, and appendices which include links and guidelines for professionals, handouts for patients and extra case studies.

Problem-solving requires thinking rather than experience, hence the book is suited to physiotherapists from student level to accomplished practitioner, whether they work in acute or chronic settings, as well as specialist respiratory nurses. The clinician will find here the opportunity to achieve clarity of thought and develop mastery in respiratory care.

The fifth edition includes invaluable contributions from specialists Alison Draper, Jo Sharp, Kath Ronchetti and David McWilliams.

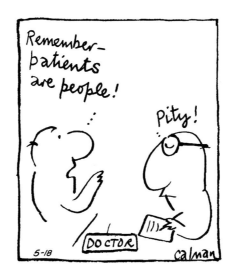

# ACKNOWLEDGEMENTS

Profound thanks to the patients who have taught me much over the years. I am also indebted to Paula Agostini and Anne Canby for their clinical expertise, Jodee Tame for her expert eye and my editor Katie Golsby for her patience and acumen.

# CONTRIBUTORS LIST

**Alison Draper, MCSP, MSc, Cert HE**
Lecturer in Physiotherapy,
School of Health Sciences,
University of Liverpool,
Liverpool, UK

**Tammy Lea, BSc**
Senior Physiotherapist,
Queen Elizabeth Hospital,
Birmingham, UK

**David McWilliams, BSc, MSc**
Consultant Physiotherapist,
Critical Care,
Queen Elizabeth Hospital,
Birmingham, UK

**Paul Ritson, MSc, MCSP**
Clinical Specialist Physiotherapist in
    Paediatric Critical Care,
Alder Hey Children's NHS Foundation
    Trust,
Liverpool, UK

**Kath Ronchetti, BSc (Hons) MCSP**
Highly Specialist Paediatric
    Respiratory Physiotherapist,
Noah's Ark Children's Hospital for
    Wales,
Cardiff, UK

**Jo Sharp, MCSP, MSc, MEd, Cert HE**
Senior Lecturer in Physiotherapy,
School of Health Sciences,
University of Liverpool,
Liverpool, UK

# ABOUT THE AUTHOR

Alexandra Hough is a physiotherapy lecturer. She has taught in the Bahamas, Canada, Chile, Denmark, Gibraltar, Greece, Ireland, Israel, Malta, Oman, Portugal, Singapore, South Africa and around the UK. When not teaching, she works clinically in Eastbourne. She has also worked with torture survivors who have developed hyperventilation syndrome. Her website www.alexhough.com provides updated lists of references by topic.

The author's royalties go to www.reprieve.org.uk.

1

# Physiological Basis of Clinical Practice

## DEFENCE

*Imagine wearing your insides on the outside.*
**British Lung Foundation**

The lung is an 'outdoor' organ that has to interact with the environment while facilitating ventilation. It is the body's primary route of infection (Waterer 2012). Every day, 500 million alveoli in the adult lungs (West 2016, p. 2) allow a surface area the size of a tennis court to be exposed to a volume of air and pollutants that could fill a swimming pool (Hanley & Tyler 1987). It is only by means of a sophisticated biological barrier that the body does not succumb to this onslaught.

Defence against the outside world is based on a network of reflexes, filters, secretions and specialized cells. Physiotherapists treat patients whose defences are breached when the nose is bypassed by mouth-breathing or an artificial airway, cilia are damaged by smoking or disease, and cough inhibited by pain or weakness.

1

## Nose

The nasal passages are the gatekeeper of the respiratory tract, providing the first line of defence by means of:
• sensing suspicious smells
• sneezing in response to irritating substances
• filtering large particles
• insulating against swings in temperature and humidity

## Oral Cavity

Between the lips and the junction of the hard and soft palates, there are over 700 species of microbe, whose purpose is to support the immune system (Gupta 2011). They are harmful only if they reach sites to which they do not normally have access, with most hospital-acquired pneumonias being caused by endotracheal tubes or nebulizers (Guggenbichler et al. 2011).

## Pharynx

The pathways for air and food converge in the pharynx. When a person chews, breathing continues through the nose, but during swallowing the pharynx can only deal with food and the airway is closed off.

The **nasopharynx** exposes inspired and expired gas to a large surface area of highly vascular, moist mucous membrane, delivering warmth and humidity to the inspiratory breath and recovering a third of it on the expiratory breath (Richards et al. 1996). Its lymphoid tissue protects against inhaled antigens (Sepahi & Salinas 2016).

The **oropharynx** extends from the mouth to the tonsils. The tonsils are lymphoid tissue that defend against foreign pathogens. Surgical removal of tonsils and adenoids renders children more vulnerable to passive smoking (Chen et al. 1998).

The **hypopharynx** is responsible for the tricky process of swallowing, for which 56 muscles are required to ensure airway protection while giving food the right of way (Higashijima 2010).

The epiglottis is a leaflike lid which snaps shut over the larynx during swallowing to prevent aspiration into the trachea. The functions of the larynx are primarily to elevate during swallowing to protect the airway, secondarily to stabilize the transition between inhalation and exhalation (p. 6), and only as an afterthought to provide speech.

Cortical, subcortical and brainstem neural control centres help coordinate breathing and swallowing and ensure that swallowing is followed by exhalation, which further helps to prevent aspiration. This tight respiratory–swallowing coupling is compromised by neurological impairment or hypercapnia (Nishino 2012).

## Airways

Inhaled irritant particles increase bronchoconstrictor tone to narrow the airways. This is normally protective, but becomes exaggerated and counterproductive in asthma, when it is called bronchospasm.

Other particles are trapped on a layer of sticky mucus lining the airways from the nasopharynx to the terminal bronchi. This mucous blanket is gripped from underneath by tiny hooks on the tips of hairlike cilia attached to the epithelium. These move ~100 mL mucus per day up to the throat, from where it is swallowed or expectorated (Dickson et al. 2016). This 'mucociliary escalator' can cleanse the lungs in 20 min, moving particles at an average 1–2 cm/min, most rapidly in the trachea and decreasing with each airway generation as the total cross section widens (Morris & Afifi 2010, p. 163).

The cilia beat in a 'sol' layer of watery fluid, reaching up to penetrate the 'gel' layer of mucus, hooking onto it with the onward stroke and diving beneath it into the sol layer on the recovery stroke at 20 beats/s (Fig. 1.1). Balanced systemic hydration keeps the fluid in the sol layer the same height as the cilia. If the sol layer is too deep or the cilia length shortened by smoking (Leopold 2013), the hooks cannot reach the mucus. If the sol layer is too shallow, as in cystic fibrosis, mucus clogs up the delicate cilia. Systemic hydration is relevant to the gel layer because water constitutes 95% of respiratory mucus and helps maintain mucociliary clearance (Nakagawa et al. 2004).

Other protective functions of the mucus are insulating, antibacterial action, and preventing the patient from drying out (Button & Boucher 2008). Moisture in inspired air helps maintain optimum ciliary beat frequency and acts as a buffer against extremes of temperature because water requires four times more energy to change temperature than air (Williams et al. 1996).

This finely coordinated mechanism is compromised by smoking, disease, age (Fig. 1.2), immobility, hypoxia, inflammation, dehydration and prolonged coughing, which narrow the airways (Wanner et al. 1996).

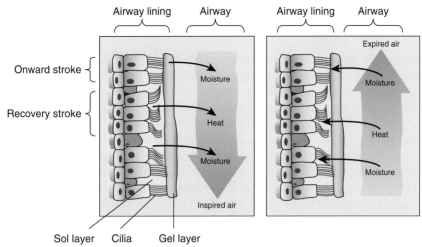

FIGURE 1.1 The humidifying effects of nose breathing on inspiration (left) and expiration. (Modified from Why Humidification is Vital, Fisher & Paykel.)

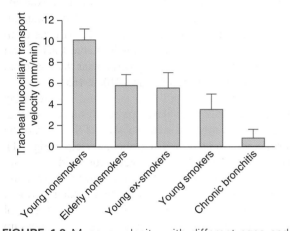

FIGURE 1.2 Mucous velocity with different ages and conditions. (From Wanner et al. 1996.)

ing the cilia (Kinnamon 2011). Traffic pollution evades many of these defences and has been linked to cardiorespiratory disease as well as impaired brain development in the young and cognitive decline in elders (Clifford et al. 2016).

Inflammatory responses in the airway defend against injury, infection and irritation by cells such as neutrophils and eosinophils. Failure to remove an inflammatory stimulus can lead to chronic inflammation, resulting in tissue injury caused by high numbers of these cells, which is the basis of several chronic inflammatory cardiorespiratory diseases (Robb et al. 2016).

> **KEY POINT**
>
> Optimizing systemic hydration should be the first intervention for people with sputum retention.

An extra function of the sol layer is its antimicrobial property, without which inhaled bacteria could double in number every 20 min. Failure to clear excess mucus may disable this chemical shield. An extra function of the gel layer is to engulf particles as well as carry them along on its surface (Knowles & Boucher 2002).

Airway epithelial cells contain pattern recognition receptors, which warn downstream immune cells of approaching bacteria. Further protection is afforded by some interesting taste bud cells that have relocated to the airway and respond to noxious particles by stimulat-

## Cough

*A cough is only as effective as the deep breath preceding it.*

**Sobush 2008**

The cough is a forced expulsive manoeuvre against a closed glottis and is the body's strongest physiological reflex. It has been known to fracture brittle ribs, cause a pneumothorax in an elderly male (O'Beirne et al. 2016) and in extremis rupture the diaphragm (Reper et al.

2012). More usually, it can cause stress incontinence (Luginbuehl et al. 2016), bronchospasm and sometimes exhaustion.

The protective function of coughing is to expel secretions and debris when mucociliary clearance is damaged, as in bronchiectasis, or overwhelmed, as with some chest infections. Like swallowing and belching, it is subject to higher cortical control, either as cough inhibition or a voluntary cough.

A reflex cough occurs if irritants stimulate inflammatory, chemical, mechanical or thermal receptors. These are located in the pleura, upper airways and, unexpectedly, the external auditory canal (Polverino 2012), as those who have Arnold's nerve cough reflex (Ryan et al. 2014) know when they clean their ears. In the airways, the receptors are most sensitive at the glottis and carina. Vagal afferents then transmit the messages to the brainstem, and the phrenic and spinal motor nerves transmit impulses to the respiratory musculature. Stimulation of the pharynx causes a gag rather than a cough.

A cough comprises:

- a deep inspiration to near total lung capacity;
- snapping shut of the glottis (which requires intact bulbar function);
- a short pause to allow distribution of air past secretions;
- sharp contraction of the expiratory muscles to create intrathoracic pressures of at least 100 mmHg;
- sudden opening of the epiglottis, exploding the trapped gas outwards at up to 800 km/h (Polverino 2012).

The resulting shear force overcomes viscous, frictional and gravitational resistance so that secretions are cleared from the upper airway, while deeper secretions are squeezed from the lower airway (Pitts et al. 2013).

Coughing is accompanied by violent swings in pleural pressure, which cause dynamic airway compression (p. 7). This is initiated in the trachea during the cough and extends peripherally as lung volume decreases, ensuring that the full length of the tracheobronchial tree is involved. The airways normally reopen with a subsequent deep breath, but for people unable to take a deep breath, they stay closed for lengthy periods. Coughing may be inhibited by pain, and the mechanism is less efficient in some people with obstructive airways disease if they have poor expiratory flow or airways that collapse on expiration. It is weakened with neurological

disease or if the glottis is bypassed by intubation or tracheostomy.

## Other Defences

Pollutants that manage to reach the alveoli are met with scavenger macrophages and proteolytic enzymes that would be powerful enough to destroy the alveoli themselves if it were not for the presence of an inhibitor from the liver called $\alpha_1$-antitrypsin, lack of which causes $\alpha_1$-antitrypsin deficiency (p. 73) and predisposes to HIV (human immunodeficiency virus) (Ferreira et al. 2014). Pathogens that survive this still have to overcome a barrage of inflammation, the main culprits being traffic pollution and tobacco (Jang et al. 2016). Asbestos particles circumvent all these defences because of their peculiar shape. The surface area of the lungs is decreased by up to 90% in advanced destructive diseases such as emphysema and pulmonary fibrosis, and the resulting concentration of microbes may explain the increased bacterial burden in these patients (Dickson et al. 2016).

The function of the wafer-thin alveolar–capillary membrane is to allow efficient gas exchange, but this also allows carbon monoxide and chemical warfare to cause their mischief.

The entire blood volume passes through the lungs, which help detoxify foreign substances that have made it into the circulation. The pulmonary circulation also performs a range of metabolic functions and acts as a filter to help protect the systemic arterial system, particularly the coronary and cerebral circulations, from blood clots, fat cells, detached cancer cells, gas bubbles and other debris. Extracorporeal support systems such as cardiopulmonary bypass (p. 464) include a filter to perform some of these functions.

## CONTROL

*Breathing is the basic rhythm of life.*

***Hippocrates***

Breathing is under triple control: metabolic, emotional and voluntary (Guyenet 2014). Metabolic control is exquisitely sensitive and pH in the blood is maintained within precise limits despite unpredictable demands. Carbon dioxide ($CO_2$) and oxygen are also controlled, but less tightly.

The respiratory centres comprise clusters of neurons in the pons and medulla, which receive and integrate stimuli from the rib cage, lungs, chemoreceptors and cortex. They then discharge impulses to the respiratory muscles, triggering contraction. They also perceive and respond to posture, coughing, hiccupping, defaecating, stepping into a cold shower and the lactic acid produced by intense exercise (de Souza 2010). Respiratory control occurs at a subconscious level but can be overridden by breathing exercises and modified by positive emotions such as pleasure, love and relief, or negative emotions such as panic, pain and anxiety (Ramirez 2014). These emotional and voluntary aspects of control facilitate the modulation of breathing as an intervention for anxiety (Paulus 2013).

The control of breathing is also affected by some pathological states:

- Several neurodegenerative diseases demonstrate impaired ventilation as the first sign (Urfy & Suarez 2014).
- Chronic obstructive pulmonary disease (COPD) shows less precise control over breathing during sleep and exercise (Dempsey 2002), and some patients have an altered chemoreceptor response, becoming dependent on low oxygen levels (hypoxic respiratory drive) rather than the more usual high $CO_2$ levels (hypercapnic respiratory drive) as a stimulus to breathe (Craig 2017).

Respiratory plasticity enables adjustments to normal physiological changes such as sleep, altitude, aging and pregnancy (Terada & Mitchell 2011). Respiratory and cardiovascular control systems are coupled reciprocally (Dick et al. 2014), e.g. 'fear bradycardia' can be a response to threatened respiratory dysfunction (Paulus 2013).

Sighing is a homeostatic resetting mechanism that reduces cortical excitation and mitigates stress, while maintaining lung compliance and gas exchange (Vaschillo et al. 2015). It is shared with most mammals and linked to emotions via the amygdala and hypothalamus (Ramirez 2014).

Yawning is controlled by the hypothalamus and is thought to relate to thermoregulation of the brain. Boredom and the evening are associated with higher brain temperature. Contagious yawning appears to have evolved in order to coordinate vigilance in budgerigars (Gallup et al. 2015), and has even been considered a prerequisite for a belief in God (Walusinski 2015).

# MECHANICS

*'The mechanics of respiration play a significant role in posture and stabilization of the spine'.*
**Dimitriadis 2016**

## The Respiratory Muscles

The lungs are attached to each other medially by their roots, but do not directly touch any muscle. The chest wall comprises the rib cage and diaphragm, which are expandable. The diaphragm contracts downwards against the abdominal contents, which are themselves incompressible but can push out the abdominal wall, and the pelvic bowl, which is rigid. Other respiratory muscles extend from the mastoid process, tongue and nose to the pubic symphysis.

The diaphragm is the only skeletal muscle vital to life and provides the power for the respiratory pump. It also combines with the abdominal muscles to assist the heart by providing a 'circulatory pump' (Uva et al. 2016).

### Inspiration

The diaphragm, the seat of the soul according to the ancient Greeks, is a dome-shaped sheet of muscle on which the upright lungs rest, separated by the pleura. It is innervated from C3–C5 via the phrenic nerves and generates 70% of tidal volume. Attached to the bottom of the rib cage, it separates two compartments of markedly different densities, the thorax and abdomen.

At rest, or if paralysed or ruptured, the diaphragm extends upwards almost to nipple level (Fig. 1.3). Contraction flattens it, pressing down against the fulcrum of the abdominal contents, displacing the abdominal viscera by 5–7 cm, protruding the abdominal wall (unless prevented by tight clothing or will power) and levering the lower rib cage outwards in a bucket handle action, causing expansion of the lower chest. Displacement of the diaphragm creates negative intrathoracic pressure, which sucks air into the lungs.

Muscles assisting this process are:

- the external intercostals, which stabilize the chest wall so that diaphragmatic contraction can create these pressure changes;
- the scalenes which stabilize the upper rib cage to prevent it being pulled downwards;
- pharyngeal muscles, which prevent collapse of the upper airway from the negative pressure.

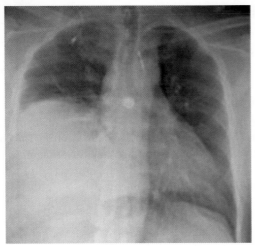

**FIGURE 1.3** Paralysed right hemidiaphragm due to phrenic nerve palsy. (From Casado-Arroyo et al. 2013.)

These and other accessory muscles become major inspiratory muscles when there is increased work of breathing (WOB) such as with airflow obstruction or exercise.

During unsupported upper limb activity, intercostal and accessory muscles are obliged to stabilize the torso, forcing the diaphragm to take a greater load. People with COPD may find daily activities daunting because of the sustained arm movements required, especially in standing when the diaphragm also contributes to postural stability. The benefits of Tai Chi may stem from optimizing the interaction between breathing and postural control (Holmes et al. 2016).

The diaphragm's role in core stability is by controlling intraabdominal pressure and reducing stress on the spine through cooperative action with the abdominal and pelvic floor muscles (Noh et al. 2014). The postural functions of the respiratory muscles have led to links between increased WOB and impaired balance (David et al. 2012), between diaphragm fatigue and recurrent back pain (Janssens et al. 2013) and between limited chest excursion and chronic low back pain, the latter responding to thoracic mobilizations and breathing exercises (Babina et al. 2016).

### Expiration

The transition between inhalation and exhalation is smoothed by a brake on expiratory flow caused by airflow resistance, especially at the larynx, and by continued low-grade diaphragmatic activity during early expiration (Mondal et al. 2016). When the larynx is bypassed by intubation, positive end-expiratory pressure (PEEP) is applied to the airway to support this function, thus avoiding fatigue of the diaphragm during exhalation. This function of the larynx is called 'physiological PEEP'.

Normal exhalation is largely passive, lung elastic recoil providing the driving force. This recoil is created firstly by surface tension acting throughout the vast gas/liquid interface lining the alveoli, and secondly by elasticity of the lung tissue, which has been stretched during inspiration. Elastic recoil is reduced at low lung volumes, like a slack elastic band, and in emphysema because of damaged alveolar septa.

Active expiration becomes stronger with speech, exercise, coughing, giving birth and obstructive airways disease. Abdominal, internal intercostal and pelvic floor muscles may then be recruited to augment passive recoil. Latissimus dorsi is enlisted during singing, and in COPD during forced exhalation, which may explain the benefit found by some patients from joining a choir (Watson et al. 2012).

Speech is created when the expiratory column of air is interrupted by vibrating vocal cords, which break it into sound waves. The sound is then modified by the oropharynx, nasopharynx and oral cavity. A person with COPD may have a weak voice because of inability to generate sufficient expiratory pressure, and a person with neurological disease may have poor articulation because of weakness of the oropharyngeal musculature.

Respiratory muscle dysfunction can occur with COPD, thoracic deformity, critical illness or neurological disease (Gea 2012).

**PRACTICE TIP**

Drop your pen, then pick it up. Did you hold your breath? This illustrates the postural work of the diaphragm.

### Pressures

**Alveolar pressure**: pressure inside the lung.
**Pleural (intrapleural/intrathoracic) pressure**: pressure in the pleural space.
  Pressure equivalents:
- 1 mmHg = 1.36 cmH$_2$O
- 1 kPa = 7.5 mmHg
- 1 torr = 1 mmHg

Alveolar pressure is negative on inspiration and slightly positive on expiration. Pleural pressure is negative to keep the lungs open, achieved by inward pull from lung elastic recoil and outward pull from rib cage recoil. Outward recoil is assisted by the pumping out of pleural fluid via the lymphatics, leading to a total negative pleural pressure of about $-6$ cmH$_2$O, modulated by the breathing pattern (Negrini 2013). Inward and outward forces are in equilibrium at the end of a quiet exhalation, this resting lung volume being termed the functional residual capacity (FRC). Outward recoil assists inspiration, especially from low lung volumes.

These pressures are disturbed by:
- a large pneumothorax, which neutralizes pleural pressure so that the lung's inward pull is unopposed and it shrivels inwards;
- emphysema, which reduces lung elastic recoil so that the outward pull of the chest wall is less opposed and the lung hyperinflates;
- lung resection, leading to reduced compliance due to disturbed pleuro-pulmonary fluid balance (Salito et al. 2015).

Increasing expiratory pressure by coughing or forceful expiration can only generate extra flow in theearly stages because, as airways narrow and frictional resistance increases, pleural pressure exceeds airway pressure and compresses the airways. This 'dynamic airway compression' occurs at about 40 cmH$_2$O (De Beer 2013), presaging the effort-independent portion of the flow-volume relationship (see Fig. 2.33) and can make forceful coughing counterproductive for people with obstructive airways disease.

## Resistance

> **Resistance** = force that must be overcome during breathing
> $$= \frac{\text{pressure change}}{\text{flow change}}$$

### Airflow resistance

Resistance to airflow is caused by friction, which is created in the airways when gas slides against the walls over itself. Airflow resistance therefore depends on the speed of airflow and calibre of the airway.

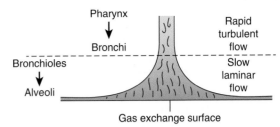
FIGURE 1.4 Increase in total cross section of the airways as they divide, creating less frictional resistance as airflow becomes more laminar and streamline.

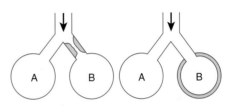
FIGURE 1.5 Left – both alveoli are normal, but the airway supplying alveolus B shows airflow obstruction, which is causing frictional resistance to airflow. Right – both airways are normal, but alveolus B shows reduced compliance caused by a thickened alveolar–capillary membrane, increasing elastic resistance.

Peripheral airflow resistance is low because at the level of the terminal bronchioles the large number of small airways creates a wide total cross-sectional area of 180 cm$^2$, causing laminar flow. The total cross section reduces to 2.5 cm$^2$ in the trachea, where there is higher resistance, creating turbulent and disorganized airflow (Fig. 1.4). Fig. 1.5 shows increased resistance due to airflow obstruction.

Frictional resistance must also be overcome in the chest and abdomen as organs are displaced by the moving lung.

### Elastic resistance

Lung tissue, alveolar surface liquid and the chest wall contribute to elastic resistance, which is increased by conditions such as lung fibrosis (Fig. 1.5), pulmonary oedema, rib cage deformity, obesity or a slumped posture.

## Compliance

$$\text{Compliance} = \frac{\text{volume change}}{\text{pressure change}}$$

Compliance reflects the willingness of the lungs to distend, and elastance the willingness to return to their resting position. Compliance is represented by the relationship between volume and pressure, i.e. how much pressure (work of breathing) is required to expand the lungs. This relationship is curved rather than linear due to a variation in the WOB at different lung volumes (Fig. 1.6).

The lung is least compliant, i.e. stiffest, at either extreme of lung volume, so that it is difficult to inflate alveoli that are closed or hyperinflate those that are fully inflated. Clinical reasoning indicates that prevention of atelectasis would therefore be more sensible than treating it once it has occurred.

### PRACTICE TIP

Blow up a balloon and feel your work of breathing at low, mid and high volumes.

Compliance is lower on inspiration, i.e. it is harder to breathe in than out, due mostly to alveolar fluid surface tension. This process is known as hysteresis and is demonstrated by the pressure–volume loop (Fig. 1.7).

Alveoli are vulnerable to injury at excessively high or low volume, and mechanical ventilation (MV) aims to avoid either extreme, especially in patients with damaged lungs.

The contribution of airways to compliance relates to their calibre, resistance being increased and compliance decreased if airways are narrowed by bronchospasm, oedema, the collapsing airways of emphysema, and sometimes secretions in the large airways where there is greater overall resistance and less collateral ventilation.

The surface tension of alveolar fluid is partially counteracted by surfactant, a constituent in the fluid that acts like detergent, preventing the alveolar walls sticking together and preventing small alveoli collapsing and emptying their contents into large alveoli.

### PRACTICE TIP

Pour some water into a small plastic bag, empty it and then pull the bag open. The forces of surface tension are what make this difficult. Repeat after adding a few drops of washing-up liquid.

The contribution of extrapulmonary structures to compliance relates to the ease with which the chest wall can be pushed away on inspiration. Kyphoscoliosis or a distended abdomen reduce compliance.

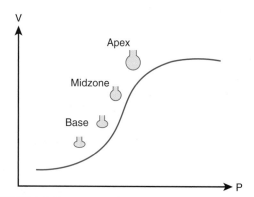

FIGURE 1.6 Pressure–volume (compliance) curve indicating reduced compliance at either extreme of lung volume. The symbols represent alveolar size at different volumes. *V*, lung volume; *P*, pressure, i.e. work to expand the lung.

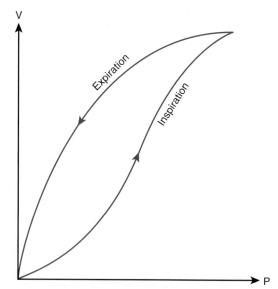

FIGURE 1.7 Pressure–volume loop showing how expiration requires less effort, i.e. less pressure *(P)* for the same change in volume *(V)*, than inspiration.

**Static compliance** is measured during a breath-hold so that equilibrium is achieved between alveolar pressure and mouth pressure, alveoli being filled to a volume determined by their regional compliance. **Dynamic compliance** is measured during breathing. It normally approximates static compliance, but may be less in diseased lungs if regional variations in compliance and resistance mean that alveolar filling is not completed during inspiration.

## Work of Breathing

Work is done during inspiration to overcome the resistive and elastic forces of airways, lungs and chest wall. This work can be defined in two ways:

- the pressure required to move a volume of gas, i.e. transpulmonary pressure × tidal volume;
- oxygen consumed by the respiratory muscles, i.e. the oxygen cost of breathing.

Elastic resistance contributes 80% of the WOB and airflow resistance the remaining 20%. Relative contributions to airflow resistance are:

- nasal passages: 50%
- larynx: 25%
- trachea to eighth generation: 20%
- peripheral airways: 5% (Eriksson 1996)

Normally, breathing is surprisingly efficient, helped by fluid coating the moving surfaces of the pleura, assuring a tight lung–chest wall coupling and allowing lung volume to faithfully follow changes in chest wall volume during the respiratory cycle (Negrini 2013). The pleural cavity however does not appear to be essential: people who have had a pleurectomy, and elephants (West 2001), have no functioning pleura but are able to breathe happily. However, it is handy for thoracic surgeons who would have difficulty if the lung was attached directly to the chest wall.

A change in alveolar pressure of only 1 cmH$_2$O is usually enough for airflow (Negrini 2013) and WOB uses just 2%–5% of total oxygen consumption at rest, but this may be increased to 40% in people with obstructive airways disease (Cairo 2012, p. 194).

Deep breathing increases the work performed against elastic resistance, while rapid breathing increases the work against airways resistance. Most patients find the right balance, but some need breathing re-education to find the optimal breathing pattern to minimize their WOB.

### Inspiratory muscle fatigue

Fatigue reduces the capacity to develop force in response to a load. When acute, it is usually reversible by rest. It can be due to failure of any of the links in the chain of command from brain to muscle. Failure within the central nervous system is called central fatigue and failure at the neuromuscular junction or in the muscle is called peripheral fatigue.

The diaphragm differs from other skeletal muscle in that it has to provide a lifetime of sustained action against elastic and resistive loads rather than irregular action against inertial loads. It is equipped for this by its relative resistance to fatigue and its large reserve so that only during coughing is it fully activated (Mantilla et al. 2014), and by the unusual way in which perfusion increases during contraction (Anzueto 1992). Fatigue occurs if energy demand exceeds supply, as when WOB is increased by airflow obstruction, or when the ability of the respiratory muscles to contract efficiently is impaired by hyperinflation, scoliosis or a flail chest.

Fatigue serves a protective function to avoid depletion of enzymes. Procedures that force patients to overuse fatigued muscles can cause muscle damage (Kallet 2011), which is most likely to occur when weaning patients from MV.

### Inspiratory muscle weakness

Weakness is failure to generate sufficient force in an otherwise fresh muscle. It is not reversible by rest, but is treated by addressing the cause and encouraging activity. Weakness of the respiratory muscles may be caused by:

- neuromuscular disorder
- disuse atrophy
- malnutrition
- hypoxia, hypercapnia or acidosis
- low calcium, potassium or phosphate levels
- steroids
- inflammation, as occurs with COPD, sepsis or multisystem failure

Weakness predisposes a muscle to fatigue. Fatigue differs from weakness in that a normal muscle can become fatigued if faced with excess WOB. Fatigue and weakness often coexist, especially in respiratory failure or during weaning from MV. The clinical features of fatigue and weakness are similar (pp. 37–38). Both are experienced as breathlessness.

# VENTILATION

*We breathe to ventilate and ventilate to respire.*

**Tobin 1991**

---

**Respiration**: (1) exchange of gases between the environment and tissue cells, by external respiration at alveolar–capillary level and internal respiration at capillary–tissue level; (2) regulation of the acid–base, metabolic and defence functions of the respiratory system.

**Ventilation**: gas movement between the outside and the alveoli, i.e. inspiration and expiration (the terms ventilation and respiration are sometimes used interchangeably).

**Breathing**: the process by which the respiratory pump creates ventilation.

**Minute ventilation** or **minute volume ($\dot{V}_E$)**: amount of gas breathed per minute, i.e. tidal volume × respiratory rate (RR).

**Tidal volume ($V_T$)**: volume of air inhaled and exhaled at each breath.

**Alveolar ventilation**: (tidal volume – physiologic dead space) × RR.

---

A healthy spontaneously breathing adult maintains an approximate $\dot{V}_E$ of 5–9 L, moving a $V_T$ of 450–600 mL with a respiratory rate (RR) of 10–15 breaths/min.

Gas that moves in and out of the lungs is made up of:

- alveolar ventilation, which is the fresh air that gets into alveoli and participates in gas exchange, defined above;
- dead space ventilation ($V_D$), which does not contribute to gas exchange.

Most dead space is **anatomical** (Fig. 1.8), which is air in the conducting passages that does not reach the alveoli, i.e. that which is last in and first out. It comprises one-third of $V_T$ in a human, more in a giraffe. **Alveolar** $V_D$, representing air that reaches the alveoli but does not get into the blood, is minimal in normal lungs. The sum of anatomical and alveolar $V_D$ is called **physiological** $V_D$. The presence of $V_D$ is one reason why it is more efficient to increase $\dot{V}_E$ by breathing deeper than by breathing faster, although this varies with lung compliance. Dead space is most usefully expressed in relation to tidal volume ($V_D/V_T$) and is normally 30% of $V_T$ (Gott & Dolling 2013).

Ventilation is not distributed evenly in the lungs (Fig. 1.9). In healthy lungs, most of the tidal volume is directed to dependent lung (Wettstein et al. 2014), with two exceptions:

1. In the upright position, alveoli in upper regions are more inflated, but mostly with $V_D$ gas. Gas travels more easily at first to the open spaces of these non-dependent regions, but they are rapidly filled and gas then travels to the dependent regions below. Alveoli

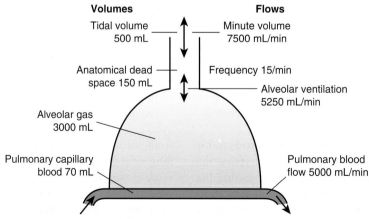

**Volumes**

Tidal volume 500 mL

Anatomical dead space 150 mL

Alveolar gas 3000 mL

Pulmonary capillary blood 70 mL

**Flows**

Minute volume 7500 mL/min

Frequency 15/min

Alveolar ventilation 5250 mL/min

Pulmonary blood flow 5000 mL/min

**FIGURE 1.8** Average volumes and flows of gas and blood in the lungs. *Frequency* = average breaths per minute. (From West 2016.)

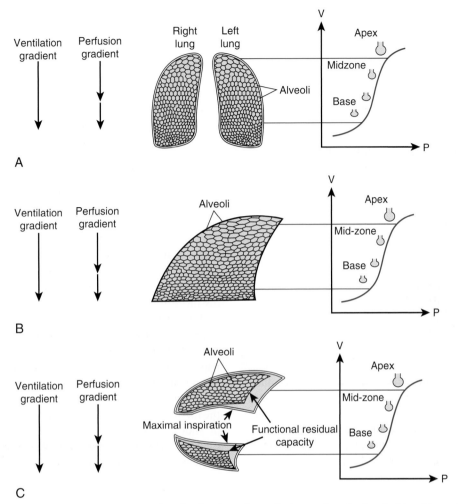

**FIGURE 1.9** Effect of gravity on the distribution of ventilation and perfusion (left), with position of alveoli on compliance curves (right). (A) Upright lungs in a healthy young nonobese person, showing slight downward ventilation gradient and strong downward perfusion gradient. (B) In supine, pressure from the abdominal contents stretches the dependent portion of the diaphragm, compressing dependent alveoli but facilitating more efficient diaphragm contraction. (C) Side-lying allows greater volume change in the dependent lung due to pressure from the abdominal contents stretching this side of the diaphragm. *P*, Pressure required to expand lung; *V*, lung volume.

in dependent regions are partially compressed by the weight of the lungs, heavy with blood, above and around them. They therefore have more potential to expand, i.e. they are more compliant, allowing greater ventilation with fresh gas. This reasoning carries through to whatever position a young adult is in. At the same time, if alveoli are collapsed or compressed,

e.g. if the patient is slumped in a chair, they will be lower on the compliance curve (see Fig. 1.6) and less easy to inflate.

2. In side-lying, fresh gas arriving in the lower lung provides a greater contribution to gas exchange, but the upper lung is more expanded and therefore responds earlier to deep breathing exercises for

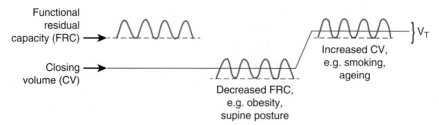

**FIGURE 1.10** Factors that shift tidal breathing into the closing volume range, leading to airway closure in the lung bases during quiet breathing. $V_T$, Tidal volume.

increasing lung volume. For patients with atelectasis, therefore, and indeed for most clinical problems, patients are placed with the affected lung on top (p. 185).

However, unlike the perfusion gradient, the ventilation gradient is only slight and responds to minor fluctuations, so that:

- It is reversed in elderly people, who have a higher closing volume (Fig. 1.10), early airway closure and alveolar collapse in dependent regions during expiration (Wettstein et al. 2014). Most patients are elderly.
- It is reversed in obese people, young children (Wettstein et al. 2014), those on some modes of MV, those who spend time in slumped positions without taking deep breaths, and in young children.
- Prone facilitates a more evenly distributed tidal volume, partly by reversing the ventilation gradient (Kallet 2015).

---

**PRACTICE TIP**

Auscultate a colleague's lungs in standing, sitting, slumped sitting, supine, side-lying and prone.

---

If airways are obstructed, ventilation can continue through collateral channels. These are unimportant in normal lungs and ventilating through them is less efficient than using the main airways because airflow resistance is 50 times greater. This difference is eliminated in emphysema, when collateral ventilation promotes more homogeneous ventilation (Cetti et al. 2006).

Normal breathing creates a $V_T$ of one-tenth the vital capacity, but oscillations in $V_T$ and involuntary sighs every 5–10 min help prevent alveolar collapse. Patients who are drowsy or sedated lose this mechanism.

## DIFFUSION

The wide total cross section of the peripheral airways means that airflow here essentially ceases, and gas movement from the respiratory bronchioles to the alveoli continues by gaseous diffusion. In the alveoli, oxygen dissolves in alveolar fluid and is driven across the alveolar–capillary membrane by the partial pressure difference, with $CO_2$ coming the other way. The alveolar–capillary membrane is 50 times thinner than airmail paper (Weibel 2013) or, for readers too young to remember airmail paper, 0.2–0.3 µm, which means that lung hyperinflation can compromise the barrier function of the membrane (West 2016, p. 7). It comprises two sheets of endothelium held together by wisps of connective tissue support. It is semipermeable, preventing plasma proteins and water leaking into alveoli but allowing gas exchange. Oxygen tension is equalized in one-third of the time that the blood takes to pass each alveolus, while $CO_2$ dissolves 20 times more quickly (Wagner 2015).

Impaired diffusion across the membrane does not play a major role in gas exchange abnormalities except sometimes during exercise or in people with severe interstitial lung diseases (Wagner 2015), or when sepsis causes high cardiac output and shortened transit times (Townsend & Webster 2000).

## PERFUSION

*No other capillaries in the body are shielded from the outside environment by such a minute amount of tissue.*

***West 2013***

The lungs have a dual circulation. The high-pressure (100 mmHg) **bronchial** circulation, from the aorta, supplies the lung tissue itself but is not essential to survival, as shown after lung transplantation when the bronchial vessels are tied. However, the lungs are awash with blood from the dominant low-pressure (~15 mmHg) **pulmonary** circulation, which bathes the surfaces of the alveoli so that gas exchange can occur (West 2013). The pulmonary vasculature is equivalent to 7000 km of capillaries (Denison 1996), which can act as a blood reservoir in case of need such as during haemorrhage.

The pulmonary circulation can respond to changes in flow with little change in pressure, reducing resistance by dilating, recruiting closed capillaries or shifting blood to the systemic circulation.

The effect of gravity on the low-pressure pulmonary circulation is to create a perfusion gradient with more blood in dependent regions (see Fig. 1.9). This is steeper than the ventilation gradient because of the density of blood. The perfusion gradient is represented by zones (West 2016, p. 51):

- Zone I is in the upper nondependent lung, where alveolar pressure exceeds pulmonary arterial pressure so that capillaries are squashed and no blood flows.
- Zone II is in the middle, where pulmonary arterial pressure exceeds alveolar pressure, which in turn exceeds venous pressure.
- Zone III is in dependent lung, where venous pressure exceeds alveolar pressure.

Zone I in health is small or nonexistent. However, if hypovolaemic shock reduces arterial pressure, or MV increases alveolar pressure, Zone I becomes significant. MV also pushes blood downwards (p. 449) and the pressure of this blood may lead to airway closure in Zone III.

In addition, perfusion is affected by:

- lung volume, e.g. the vessels are stretched in the hyperinflated state;
- disease, e.g. alveolar destruction in emphysema causes disruption of both perfusion and ventilation;
- position, e.g. in prone, perfusion is more uniform than supine (Nyren 1999) and better matched with ventilation (Henderson et al. 2013).

## VENTILATION/PERFUSION RATIO

It is no good having a well-ventilated alveolus if it is not supplied with blood, nor a well-perfused alveolus that is not ventilated. Fresh air and blood need to be in the same place at the same time for gas exchange to occur. The matching of these two is expressed as the ratio of alveolar ventilation to perfusion ($\dot{V}_A/\dot{Q}$).

$\dot{V}_A/\dot{Q}$ matching is assisted by the mixing of expired and inspired gases through the common dead space (Glenny et al. 2013), but a degree of $\dot{V}_A/\dot{Q}$ mismatch is normal because of dissonance between ventilation and perfusion gradients, the lung bases receiving 18 times more blood and 3.5 times more gas than the apices in the upright lung (Thomas 1997).

Pathological $\dot{V}_A/\dot{Q}$ mismatch is due to a high or low ratio. A high ratio occurs when the alveoli are ventilated but perfusion is impaired so the oxygen cannot reach the blood, causing increased dead space. For example, pulmonary vasculopathy in heart failure increases dead space and causes breathlessness during exercise (Kee et al. 2016). A low $\dot{V}_A/\dot{Q}$ ratio occurs when lung units are perfused but not adequately ventilated, which is the condition most frequently dealt with by physiotherapists. This creates a **shunt**, defined as the fraction of cardiac output that is not exposed to gas exchange in the lung. A shunt over 20% limits the utility of oxygen therapy because added oxygen cannot reach the shunted blood. The shunt is measured by comparing arterial and mixed venous blood (p. 471), expressed as a percentage of cardiac output. A small shunt is normal because part of the bronchial circulation mingles with pulmonary venous drainage. The mixing of shunted venous blood with oxygenated blood is known as **venous admixture**, which is normally 5% of cardiac output (Takala 2007).

Systemic hypoxia stimulates selective vasodilation to assist perfusion of vital tissues. Pulmonary hypoxia stimulates the opposite response: if a fall in alveolar oxygen tension is detected, an ingenious mechanism called **hypoxic vasoconstriction** helps maintain gas exchange by constricting capillaries adjacent to these alveoli (Fig. 1.11), thus limiting wasted perfusion and improving $\dot{V}_A/\dot{Q}$ match (Craig 2017). When the lung bases are affected, e.g. in pulmonary oedema, obesity (Pedoto 2012) or the early stages of COPD, local shutdown of vessels forces blood to the better-ventilated upper regions, shown radiologically as enhanced vascular markings towards the apices, or 'upper lobe diversion' (see Fig. 4.3). Hypoxic vasoconstriction becomes counterproductive when alveolar hypoxia occurs throughout the lung, as occurs in advanced COPD, leading to generalized vasoconstriction and pulmonary hypertension.

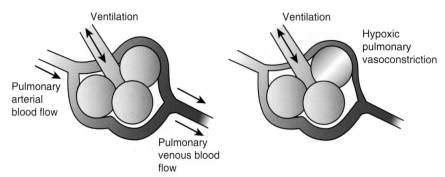

**FIGURE 1.11** Hypoxic pulmonary vasoconstriction. Left: normal alveolar ventilation and perfusion. Right: ↓ ventilation in alveolus (grey) leading to reduced perfusion. (From Dhillon 2012.)

## ARTERIAL BLOOD GASES

**PO₂**: partial pressure or tension of oxygen, i.e. its concentration

**PaO₂**: partial pressure of oxygen in arterial blood, i.e. oxygen dissolved in plasma; normal 11–14 kPa or 82.5–105 mmHg

**SaO₂**: extent to which haemoglobin in arterial blood is saturated with oxygen, i.e. capacity of blood to transport oxygen; normal 95%–98%

**SpO₂**: as above, but described in terms of measurement by pulse oximetry (the distinction is rarely important and normal values are the same)

**Haemoglobin** (Hb): molecule in erythrocytes that binds to and transports oxygen and some $CO_2$ around the body

**PaCO₂**: partial pressure of $CO_2$ in arterial blood; basis of respiratory acid–base balance; normal 4.7–6.0 kPa or 35–45 mmHg

**FiO₂**: fraction (concentration) of inspired oxygen

| TABLE 1.1 **Relationship between oxygen saturation and tension in arterial blood under normal conditions** | | |
|---|---|---|
| **SaO₂ (%)** | **PaO₂ (kPa)** | **PaO₂ (mmHg)** |
| 97 | 12.7–14.0 | 95–105 |
| 94 | 9.3–10.0 | 70–75 |
| 92 | 8.9–9.7 | 67–73 |
| 90 | 7.7–8.3 | 58–62 |
| 87 | 6.9–7.7 | 52–58 |
| 84 | 6.1–6.9 | 46–52 |

Arterial blood gas (ABG) analysis identifies if breathing is effective by giving an indication of gas exchange, ventilation and acid–base status. Readings should be related to the FiO₂ and previous values.

Arterial blood samples are taken either from an indwelling arterial catheter or by intermittent puncture of the radial artery. Local anaesthesia for this procedure is stipulated in the UK Guidelines (BTS 2008) because the pain of a needle going through the arterial wall is greater than puncturing a vein (McKeever et al. 2016), sometimes causing either hyperventilation or apnoea, which can invalidate the results (Lee 2012). This 'significant morbidity' can also be prevented by local anaesthetic cream (p. 300), gels, ice packs or pain-free jet injections (McSwain et al. 2015). Ultrasound guidance increases success (Gu et al. 2016).

Table 1.1 relates the different measurements of arterial oxygenation.

**PaO₂** describes the 2% of oxygen that is dissolved in plasma, and reflects the pressure needed to push oxygen from blood into tissue cells. **SaO₂** describes the 98% of oxygen that is bound to haemoglobin (Hb) for transport. Neither of these gives a measure of oxygenation at tissue level. Also, resting levels do not reflect oxygenation during exercise, nor predict nocturnal oxygenation. **Oxygen content** describes the total amount of oxygen carried in blood, and incorporates PaO₂, SaO₂ and Hb. In practice, oxygen content is assumed from PaO₂ or SpO₂.

Gas exchange entails:
- oxygen dissolving in alveolar lining fluid;
- diffusion of oxygen through the alveolar–capillary membrane into plasma;
- oxygen binding to Hb for transport around the body;

- at its destination, oxygen from Hb dissolving back into plasma;
- diffusion of oxygen across the capillary wall and delivery to the tissues.

The reverse happens to $CO_2$ but it slips back and forth with ease. The movement of $CO_2$ traditionally does not come under the term 'gas exchange'.

## Oxygen Dissociation Curve

The relationship between $SaO_2$ and $PaO_2$ is not direct but expressed by the oxygen dissociation curve (Fig. 1.12). Its S shape illustrates the protective mechanisms that function in both health and disease.

### Upper flat portion of the curve

At the plateau of the curve, the combining of oxygen with Hb is favoured by a high $PO_2$, and its stability is not unduly disturbed by changes in $PaO_2$. In health,

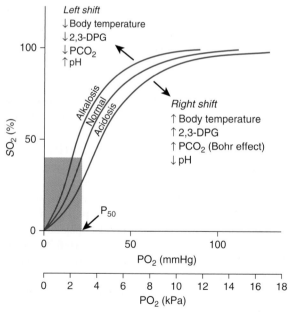

**FIGURE 1.12** Oxygen dissociation curve relating oxygen saturation to oxygen tension. 2,3-DPG is an enzyme in red blood cells that increases in chronic hypoxaemia and allows easier unloading of $O_2$ to hypoxic tissues. $P_{50}$ is the $PaO_2$ at which Hb is 50% saturated and is the most sensitive indicator of a shift in the curve, a high value suggesting poor affinity of Hb for $O_2$. The shaded area represents critical tissue hypoxia.

this encourages loading of oxygen in the high $PO_2$ environment of the lung, and discourages unloading of oxygen before blood reaches the capillary bed. In disease, there can be a significant change in $PaO_2$, e.g. a reduction to 10.7 kPa (80 mmHg), with little change in $SaO_2$.

### Steep portion of the curve

The dissociation of Hb becomes proportionately greater as $PO_2$ falls, so that small changes in $PaO_2$ greatly affect $SaO_2$. In health, this means that Hb can offload quantities of oxygen at cellular level while maintaining oxygen tension in the blood. In disease, large amounts of oxygen can be unloaded when tissues are hypoxic. A $PaO_2$ <7.3 kPa (55 mmHg) tips the patient onto a slippery slope whereby further small drops in $PaO_2$ result in tissue hypoxia.

### Shift of the curve

Another singular way in which the body responds to need is to adjust the affinity of Hb for oxygen, as reflected by a shift of the curve. A right shift means that Hb unloads oxygen more easily at a given $PO_2$. In health, this occurs during exercise, when active muscle generates heat and makes blood hypercapnic and acidic. In disease, this occurs with fever and when tissues need extra oxygen. A left shift occurs when Hb holds tightly onto its oxygen, as with hyperventilation, hypometabolism or a cold environment. Pink ears and noses on frosty mornings are due to the reluctance of Hb to unload oxygen.

## Hypoxaemia and Hypoxia
### Hypoxaemia

Hypoxaemia is reduced oxygen in arterial blood, defined as $PaO_2$ <8 kPa (60 mmHg) or $SaO_2$ <90%. Causes are:
- low $\dot{V}_A/\dot{Q}$ ratio or wasted perfusion ($\uparrow$ shunt)
- high $\dot{V}_A/\dot{Q}$ ratio or wasted ventilation ($\uparrow$ dead space)
- hypoventilation
- diffusion abnormality
- $\downarrow FiO_2$

**Low $\dot{V}_A/\dot{Q}$** occurs when blood is shunted through consolidated, collapsed or damaged lung without seeing any oxygen, somewhat attenuated by hypoxic vasoconstriction. **High $\dot{V}_A/\dot{Q}$** occurs, for example, when a pulmonary embolus blocks perfusion, thus increasing alveolar dead space and causing $\dot{V}_A/\dot{Q}$ mismatch at the other end of the spectrum (Fig. 1.13).

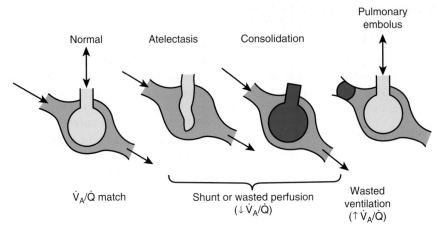

**FIGURE 1.13** Alveoli and surrounding capillary network, showing how impaired ventilation or perfusion upsets $\dot{V}_A/\dot{Q}$ matching.

**Hypoventilation** can be caused by respiratory depression (e.g. from oversedation), respiratory muscle weakness (e.g. with neuromuscular disease), or sometimes with COPD if patients chronically hypoventilate in order to rest the diaphragm (p. 76).

**Diffusion** abnormalities occur in disorders such as pulmonary oedema or fibrosing alveolitis, when a thickened alveolar–capillary membrane increases the $PAO_2$–$PaO_2$ gradient.

↓ **$FiO_2$** is due to inadequate oxygen therapy, high altitude or fire entrapment.

## Hypoxia

The term hypoxia is sometimes used interchangeably with hypoxaemia but it means oxygen deficit at tissue level, when demand exceeds supply, leading to anaerobic metabolism once $PaO_2$ reaches 4.5 kPa (33.8 mmHg) (Townsend & Webster 2000). It is more relevant to body function than hypoxaemia but more difficult to measure.

**Hypoxaemic** hypoxia occurs when hypoxia is caused by hypoxaemia. **Anaemic** hypoxia is when Hb levels are reduced or abnormal Hb cannot carry enough oxygen. **Ischaemic** hypoxia indicates impaired oxygen transport, e.g. haemorrhage, myocardial infarct or peripheral arterial disease. **Histotoxic** hypoxia occurs when cells cannot extract or utilize oxygen, e.g. following cyanide poisoning or in septic shock (Busl & Greer 2016).

## Effects of hypoxaemia and hypoxia

Acute hypoxaemia induces vasodilation of the peripheral vascular beds, increasing cardiac output in an attempt to improve oxygen delivery. Chronic hypoxaemia thickens blood and may strain the right heart (see Fig. 3.5) and even transient hypoxaemia may shorten life (Criner 2013). Cardiac arrhythmias may occur when $SaO_2$ drops below 80%.

Hypoxia leads acutely to tachycardia (Critchley et al. 2015) and chronically to muscle atrophy (D'Hulst et al. 2016). It progressively causes the following:
- $PaO_2$ <7.3 kPa (55 mmHg): memory defect (due to the sensitivity of the hippocampus), impaired judgement;
- <5.3 kPa (40 mmHg): tissue damage;
- <4 kPa (30 mmHg): unconsciousness;
- <2.7 kPa (20 mmHg): death, except in migrating geese and hibernating turtles (Nikinmaa 2013).

The brain is the first organ to be affected, followed by the gut lining. The kidney is also sensitive to hypoxia and manifests its distress more obviously, reducing urine output and increasing potassium, creatinine and urea levels.

Chronic hypoxia leads to increased oxygen utilization and reduced energy-demanding processes (Cummins & Keogh 2016).

## Hypercapnia

Despite large variations in the metabolic production of $CO_2$, $PaCO_2$ is normally kept constant (Guyenet 2014).

## TABLE 1.2  Clinical features of hypoxaemia and hypercapnia

| Hypoxaemia | Hypercapnia |
|---|---|
| Cyanosis | Flapping tremor of hands |
| | ↑ RR |
| | ↑ HR |
| Peripheral vasoconstriction | Peripheral vasodilation, leading to warm hands and headache |
| | Respiratory muscle weakness |
| Arrhythmias or bradycardia | Bradycardia |
| Restlessness → confusion → coma | Drowsiness → hallucinations → coma |

*HR*, Heart rate; *RR*, respiratory rate.

However, hypoventilation causes hypercapnia (↑ $PaCO_2$), leading to respiratory acidosis or compensated metabolic alkalosis. An acutely rising $PaCO_2$ is a danger sign if it presages exhaustion (see Fig. 3.39), and with acidosis is an indication for mechanical ventilatory assistance. But chronic hypercapnia is neither dangerous nor damaging and may accompany advanced stable lung disease.

The clinical signs of hypoxaemia and hypercapnia are insensitive and nonspecific, but Table 1.2 indicates some similarities and differences.

### Interpretation

Examples of ABG abnormalities are:
- ↓ $PaO_2$ with ↑ $PaCO_2$: hypoxaemia, e.g. exacerbation of COPD, in a patient who is becoming too exhausted to ventilate adequately;
- ↓ $PaO_2$ with ↓ $PaCO_2$: hypoxaemia in a patient who is breathless, e.g. pneumonia, fibrosing alveolitis, pulmonary oedema, pulmonary embolus;
- normal $PaO_2$ with ↓ $PaCO_2$: emotion causing hyperventilation, e.g. painful arterial puncture or hyperventilation syndrome.

Hypercapnia is likely to be longstanding if pH is >7.35 (BTS 2008).

Reduced minute volume raises $PaCO_2$ and lowers $SaO_2$, but the reverse is not true. Increased minute volume blows off $CO_2$, but $SaO_2$ does not rise above normal because Hb cannot be supersaturated. However, MV with a high $FiO_2$ can raise $PaO_2$ above normal when the extra oxygen dissolves in the plasma.

### Other Indices of Oxygenation

Gas exchange is best documented in relation to the inspired oxygen, described as the $PaO_2$:$FiO_2$ ratio. Less easy to measure, but useful in identifying the cause of hypoxaemia, is the difference between alveolar and arterial oxygen, known as the alveolar–arterial gradient, the 'A–a gradient', or $PAO_2$–$PaO_2$. A raised gradient indicates greater difficulty in getting oxygen across the alveolar–capillary membrane, as occurs in diffusion impairment. Hypoventilation or reduced $FiO_2$ does not affect the $PAO_2$–$PaO_2$.

### Acid–Base Balance

> **Normal pH in the human body**: 7.35–7.45

The degree of acidity or alkalinity is measured by pH, which shows the hydrogen ions in solution, but negatively, namely:
- low pH means more hydrogen ions and greater acidity
- high pH means fewer hydrogen ions and greater alkalinity

Neutral is 6.8, but body functions occur on the alkaline side of neutral. **Acidosis** occurs when arterial pH falls below 7.35. The term means increased acidity in the body, while **acidaemia** means increased acidity of blood plasma, but the former is normally used for both. Acidosis can lead to myocardial depression, arrhythmias and hypotension, while hypercapnic acidosis weakens the respiratory muscles and can increase inflammation (Bruno 2012). **Alkalosis** occurs at pH over 7.45.

The pH independently predicts intensive care unit (ICU) admission and 12-month mortality (Stokes et al. 2016a). It responds to metabolic and respiratory change but it cannot differentiate between them.

The following identify acid–base imbalances:
- **Respiratory acidosis** occurs when the drop in pH is caused by increased $PaCO_2$ and is due to hypoventilation, leading sometimes to ventilatory failure.
- **Respiratory alkalosis** occurs when a patient hyperventilates, which washes out $CO_2$. This always accompanies a raised minute volume and often accompanies breathlessness, though the rapid shallow breathing pattern of a breathless person is not necessarily efficient, nor synonymous with hyperventilation.
- **Metabolic acidosis** occurs when the body produces too much acid or the kidneys cannot remove enough

acid, leading to haemodynamic instability (Celotto et al. 2016). Metabolic acids include all the body acids except dissolved $CO_2$. They are not respirable and have to be neutralized, metabolized or excreted by the kidney. Lactic acidosis is a form of metabolic acidosis caused by the build-up of lactic acid if oxygen supply is inadequate.

- **Metabolic alkalosis** raises pH out of proportion to changes in $PaCO_2$, a common occurrence in critically ill patients due to fluid volume loss, diuretics or low potassium (Oh 2010).

Patients can have mixed acid–base disorders, e.g. a patient with acute hypercapnic COPD may have $CO_2$-induced respiratory acidosis, but comorbidities such as diabetes or the side effects of diuretics can induce a metabolic alkalosis, with the knock-on effects of a depressed respiratory drive and increased airway resistance (Terzano et al. 2012).

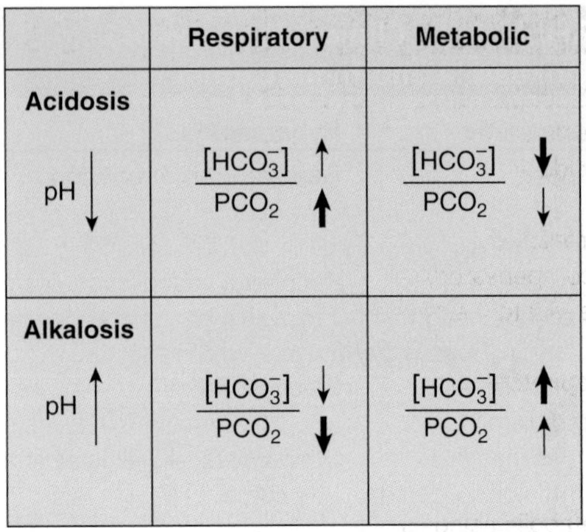

## Buffers

A buffer is a weak acid or base that mitigates an upset pH by mopping up or squeezing out hydrogen ions like a chemical sponge. **Bicarbonate** ($HCO_3^-$) is a buffer whose value provides an estimate of the metabolic component of acid–base balance, although it is affected by both metabolic and respiratory components. Values for $HCO_3^-$ are:

- normal: 22–26 mmol/L
- metabolic acidosis: <22 mmol/L
- metabolic alkalosis: >26 mmol/L.

**Standard bicarbonate** (SBE) is the bicarbonate concentration under standard conditions, being adjusted as if $PaCO_2$ were 5.3 kPa, i.e. it is similar to bicarbonate in a person with normal acid–base status.

**Base excess** (BE) is a calculated value from SBE, being positive with metabolic alkalosis and negative with metabolic acidosis. It represents the quantity of acid required to restore pH to normal if $PCO_2$ were adjusted to normal. Like $HCO_3^-$, it measures metabolic acid–base balance, but takes buffering by red blood cells into account and provides a more complete analysis of metabolic buffering than $HCO_3^-$. BE is calculated from pH, $PaCO_2$ and haematocrit. Values are:

- normal: minus 2 to plus 2 mmol/L
- metabolic acidosis: < minus 3 mmol/L
- metabolic alkalosis: > plus 3 mmol/L

Along with clinical assessment, ABG analysis helps identify the main causes of acidosis or alkalosis, although

**FIGURE 1.14** Four examples of acid–base imbalance showing the process of compensation. *Thick arrows* in each box indicate which way a value has gone in order to create the acidosis or alkalosis. *Thin arrows* indicate which way the other value is going in order to compensate.

one may dominate and the other partially compensate (Fig. 1.14). The prime mover is the one on which to focus and it is a mistake to treat a compensation.

> **KEY POINT**
>
> If the primary acid–base disturbance is metabolic, pH and bicarbonate/BE change in the same direction, while if the primary problem is respiratory, pH and $PaCO_2$ change in opposite directions (see Fig. 1.14).

## Regulation

Acid–base balance is disturbed if removal of $CO_2$ from the lungs is abnormal (respiratory acidosis or alkalosis) or production of acid from the tissues or elimination elsewhere is abnormal (metabolic acidosis or alkalosis). Any deviation of pH from normal is fiercely resisted, at whatever cost, by three homeostatic mechanisms:

1. The buffer system neutralizes acids or bases by giving up or absorbing hydrogen ions, all within seconds. The following equation represents the dissociation of carbonic acid in solution, acting as a sink for hydrogen ions:

$$H_2O + CO_2 \leftrightarrow H_2CO_3 \leftrightarrow H^+ + HCO_3^-$$

| TABLE 1.3   Interpretation of arterial blood gas trends | | | |
|---|---|---|---|
| **Status** | **Causes** | **Effects** | **Recognition** |
| Acute respiratory acidosis | Hypoventilation, e.g. exhaustion, weakness | $PaCO_2$ ↑, pH ↓, $HCO_3^-$ N (no renal compensation yet) | Shallow breathing, drowsiness, severe acute respiratory disease |
| Chronic (compensated) respiratory acidosis | Chronic hypoventilation | $PaCO_2$ ↑, pH N, $HCO_3^-$ ↑ (retention of $HCO_3^-$ to restore pH, i.e. full compensation) | Severe chronic respiratory disease, e.g. COPD |
| Respiratory alkalosis | Acute hyperventilation, e.g. anxiety, pain, acute cardiorespiratory disease, fever, CNS injury | $PaCO_2$ ↓, $HCO_3^-$ ↓ , pH ↑ (partial compensation) | Breathlessness |
| Metabolic acidosis | Shock, lactic acidosis, diabetic acidosis, severe diarrhoea or dehydration, kidney failure | $HCO_3^-$ ↓, pH ↓, $PaCO_2$ ↓, BE < −2 (partial compensation) | Hyperventilation (respiratory compensation to blow off $PCO_2$) |
| Metabolic alkalosis | Sepsis, heart failure, diuretics, severe vomiting, ↓ albumin | $HCO_3^-$ ↑, pH ↑, $PaCO_2$ ↑, BE > +2 (partial compensation) | Delirium |

*BE*, Base excess; *CNS*, central nervous system; *COPD*, chronic obstructive pulmonary disease; *N*, normal.

An increase in $PaCO_2$ shifts the equilibrium to the right, increasing $H^+$ and causing respiratory acidosis. A decrease in $PaCO_2$ shifts it to the left.
2. If buffering is not adequate, the lungs then present an avenue for regulating $CO_2$. Hyperventilation or hypoventilation can stabilize acid–base balance in 1–15 min.
3. If this is still not adequate, the kidneys take over, but they need 3–5 days to do so (Ayers & Warrington 2008).

These mechanisms work to dispose of the acids that are continually produced by the body's metabolic processes, caused mostly by the hydration of $CO_2$ to create carbonic acid.

### Interpretation

Step 1. Look at the pH:
  • ↓ pH means acidosis
  • ↑ pH means alkalosis
Step 2. Look at the $PaCO_2$: does it account for an abnormal pH? If breathing is the prime mover:
  • ↑ $PaCO_2$ means respiratory acidosis
  • ↓ $PaCO_2$ means respiratory alkalosis
Step 3. Look at the $HCO_3^-$ or BE: does it account for an abnormal pH? If breathing is not the prime mover:
  • ↓ $HCO_3^-$ or BE means metabolic acidosis
  • ↑ $HCO_3^-$ or BE means metabolic alkalosis

To help decide if a change in pH is respiratory or metabolic (if this is not obvious clinically), any change outside the following is likely to be metabolic in origin (Williams 1998):
  • For every increase in $PaCO_2$ of 2.6 kPa (20 mmHg) above normal, pH falls by 0.1.
  • For every decrease in $PaCO_2$ of 1.3 kPa (10 mmHg) below normal, pH rises by 0.1.
When pH is restored to normal, full compensation has occurred. The stages can be identified as follows:
  • Abnormal pH + change in $PaCO_2$ or $HCO_3^-$/BE = noncompensation, i.e. an acute process.
  • Abnormal pH + change in $PaCO_2$ and $HCO_3^-$/BE = partial compensation.
  • Normal pH + change in $PaCO_2$ and $HCO_3^-$/BE = full compensation.
Table 1.3 clarifies the causes, effects and recognition of ABG imbalances. Examples are in Appendix A.

Table 1.4 shows how two respiratory disorders can affect ABG readings. $PaCO_2$ values reflect breathlessness in acute asthma and hypoventilation in COPD. $HCO_3^-$ and pH values reflect an acute noncompensated condition in acute asthma, and full compensation in COPD.

## THE OXYGEN CASCADE

The *raison d'etre* of the cardiorespiratory system is to get oxygen to the tissues by means of oxygen cascading from the outside to the subcellular environment. Even when ventilation, diffusion and perfusion are in order, oxygen still has to reach and get into the tissues.

Oxygen **transport** is the passage of oxygen to the tissues via the arteries and capillaries. The arterial circulation also acts as a cushion to soften the pulsations generated by the heart so that capillary blood flow is stable. The term 'oxygen transport' is often used synonymously with, and is virtually the same as, oxygen **delivery**, which is the oxygen presented to the tissues. Oxygen **consumption** or **uptake** by the tissues is usually equivalent to oxygen **demand**, determined by the metabolic

needs of the tissues and approximating 250 mL/min in a resting person. Oxygen delivery depends on cardiac output (CO), haemoglobin and $SaO_2$, supplying approximately 1000 mL/min, so that about 25% of the arterial oxygen content is used every minute (Law & Bukwirwa 1999).

Oxygen moves down a pressure or concentration gradient from a high level in air, through alveolar gas, arterial blood, capillaries and finally the cell, where energy is produced by the mitochondria (Fig. 1.15).

Oxygen availability to the tissues depends on:
- $SaO_2$, $PaO_2$ and Hb
- cardiac output
- distribution of CO and tissue perfusion
- oxygen extraction
- the oxygen dissociation curve

Tissue oxygenation reflects the balance between supply (oxygen delivery or $DO_2$) and demand (oxygen consumption or $\dot{V}O_2$). The cardiorespiratory system, as with most other systems, has plenty of reserve capacity, and $DO_2$ is normally four times greater than $\dot{V}O_2$, creating an oxygen extraction ratio ($\dot{V}O_2/DO_2$) of 25%.

$\dot{V}O_2$ varies with metabolic rate, individual tissue blood flows adjusting according to need (Wolff et al.

**TABLE 1.4   Examples of arterial blood gas values in two disorders[a]**

|  | Normal | Acute asthma | COPD |
|---|---|---|---|
| $PaO_2$ | 12.7 (95) | 9.3 (70) | 7.3 (55) |
| $PaCO_2$ | 5.3 (40) | 3.3 (25) | 8 (60) |
| pH | 7.4 | 7.5 | 7.4 |
| $HCO_3^-$ | 24 | 24 | 29 |

[a]Numbers in brackets indicate mmHg.
*COPD,* Chronic obstructive pulmonary disease.

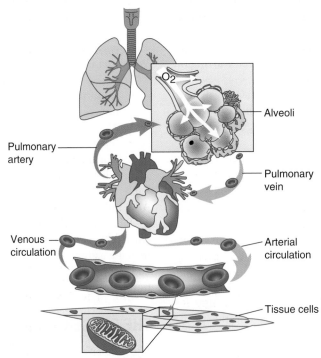

**FIGURE 1.15** Oxygen journey through cardiovascular system to mitochondria.

Labels: $O_2$ · Alveoli · Pulmonary artery · Pulmonary vein · Venous circulation · Arterial circulation · Tissue cells

2016). An increase is usually met without difficulty by increased $DO_2$ (mostly through increased CO, partly through increased minute ventilation) and increased oxygen extraction by the tissues. Once maximum oxygen extraction is reached, consumption no longer drives delivery but becomes dependent on it, leading to anaerobic metabolism and lactic acidosis.

Some organs are greedier than others, e.g.:
- The brain comprises 2.2% of body weight and receives 1.5% of CO.
- The myocardium comprises 0.5% body weight and receives 5% of CO.
- The kidneys comprise 0.5% body weight and receive 20% of CO.
- Skeletal muscle and skin comprise 50% body weight and receive 10% of CO (Epstein 1993).

Tolerance to hypoxia also varies:
- The brain suffers irreversible damage within 3 min.
- The kidneys and liver can tolerate 15–20 min of hypoxia.
- Skeletal muscle withstands 60–90 min and vascular smooth muscle 24–72 h.
- Hair and nails continue to grow for some days after death (Leach & Treacher 2002).

Septic patients may need 50%–60% extra oxygen delivered to their tissues, while patients with multiple trauma, septic shock or burns may require 100% extra (Epstein 1993). At the same time, critically ill patients may be affected by:
- impaired $DO_2$ because of cardiorespiratory dysfunction;
- cellular oxygen extraction hindered by toxins associated with sepsis, leading to mitochondrial dysfunction (Van Boxel et al. 2012);
- loss of autoregulation, leading to disordered regional distribution of blood flow, both between and within organs;
- hypoxic kidneys and a liver unable to detoxify by-products of the shocked state.

Some cells can produce energy for a short time without oxygen, using anaerobic metabolism, while sensitive organs such as the brain are dependent on aerobic metabolism. If tissues are not able to acquire, transport, extract and utilize sufficient oxygen, lactic acidosis occurs.

Compared to gas exchange in the lung, which is easily monitored in arterial blood, tissue oxygenation is usually estimated indirectly from the leftover oxygen in pulmonary artery blood, where it is at the end of its journey before being reoxygenated in the lungs (p. 471).

## VARIATIONS

### Effects of Obesity

Worldwide, obesity has more than doubled since 1980, driving cardiopulmonary morbidity and mortality (Chung 2016). It is second only to tobacco as the leading preventable cause of death (DeTurk & Cahalin 2011, p. 477).

Obesity loads the respiratory system, pushing up the diaphragm so that FRC approaches residual volume (Fig. 1.16), leading to closure of dependent airways and $\dot{V}_A/\dot{Q}$ mismatch (Salome et al. 2010). Breathing tends to be rapid, shallow and apical.

Obesity may also cause:
- a mixed obstructive/restrictive respiratory defect (Reynolds 2011) and limited ability to take a deep breath, thus hindering some forms of physiotherapy and affecting some lung function test results (Enright 2015);
- breathlessness, which increases in supine (Perino et al. 2016), ↑ WOB and ↑ $\dot{V}O_2$ (Murphy & Wong 2013);
- attenuated response to hypoxic and hypercapnic ventilatory drives, ↓ exercise capacity (Mesquita et al. 2015);
- tissue hypoxia, causing insulin resistance and systemic inflammation (Ban et al. 2016), the inflammation leading to airway inflammation, infection risk

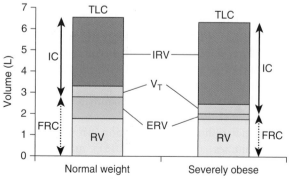

**FIGURE 1.16** Effect of obesity on lung volumes, showing how FRC can approach residual volume. Compare with Fig. 2.30A. *ERV,* Expiratory reserve volume; *FRC,* functional residual capacity; *IC,* inspiratory capacity; *IRV,* inspiratory reserve volume; *RV,* residual volume; *TLC,* total lung capacity.

(Almond 2013) and reduced muscle mass (King et al. 2013);

- further loss of muscle mass during the metabolic stress of illness, and lack of micronutrients (Abdelhamid et al. 2016);
- stress on the heart with exercise (Vella et al. 2012), sudden cardiac death (Adabag 2015), risk of heart failure (Alpert et al. 2016) and, in children, cardiovascular risk (Philip et al. 2015);
- urinary incontinence (Wang et al. 2017), osteoporosis (Zhang et al. 2016a) and some cancers (Blackadar 2016);
- barotrauma during MV (Pedoto 2012);
- obesity hypoventilation syndrome (Piper et al. 2016);
- bias in the health care system (O'Brien et al. 2012).

On the surgical wards, an obese patient should barely have emerged from anaesthesia before the physiotherapist becomes involved in pain control and positioning, closely followed by incentive spirometry and early mobilization, along with regional analgesia if possible (Bluth et al. 2016). Morbidly obese people show a 30% likelihood of atelectasis or pneumonia after abdominal surgery and a greater propensity for thrombosis and wound infections (Licker et al. 2007).

On the medical wards, obesity is associated with asthma (Ulrik 2016) and COPD (Katz et al. 2015). It can disrupt pharmacokinetics, e.g. steroids can augment obesity (Cooper 2011) while obesity itself causes reduced response to steroids and bronchodilators (Sismanopoulos 2013).

In the ICU, obesity prolongs length of stay (Goh et al. 2016) and increases the complications of immobilization, the latter being moderated by early rehabilitation (Genc et al. 2012). There is a greater need for MV (Tafelski et al. 2016) along with a requirement for elevated airway pressures (Kaese et al. 2016). Paradoxically, obesity is also associated with improved ICU survival, possibly by secretion of antiinflammatory adipokines (Yusuke et al. 2015).

Multidisciplinary rehabilitation is required for comorbidities (Capodaglio 2013), including pain management because of altered physiology and drug utilization (D'Arcy 2016). Physiotherapy is based on developing a long-term exercise habit, along with joint protection. Oxygenation may increase during exercise because of the effect of deep breathing on expansion of collapsed lung units (Sood 2009). Exercise training itself improves breathlessness as well as fitness (Bernhardt & Stickford 2016), with cycle ergometry and cycling being especially effective for testing and training (Bott 2016).

## Effects of Smoking

*Tobacco is the single most preventable cause of death in the world today … it kills up to half of those who use it.*

**World Health Organization 2008**

Smoking is the world's leading cause of preventable death (Siqueira 2017). It disproportionately affects the poorest members of societies and is rising rapidly in the Third World (Agrawal 2016) as multinational companies offload their stocks. Each smoker loses at least a decade of life (Jha et al. 2013). The 5000 toxic chemicals in tobacco smoke (Freire et al. 2016) include cyanide, carbon monoxide, arsenic and over 50 known carcinogens (BMA 2015). The litany of destruction is outlined in Table 1.5 and below.

Smoking shortens life by an average 11 min for each cigarette (Warren 2001). It increases the risk of postoperative complications, although it eases postoperative nausea and vomiting in patients who can escape the ward (Talbot & Palmer 2013). It worsens Crohns disease but improves ulcerative colitis (Siqueira 2017). The effects can even jump a generation, the grandchildren of smokers being more likely to develop asthma independent of the mother's smoking status (Magnus et al. 2015).

Smoking is neither virile nor sexy, tobacco being toxic to ovaries (Camlin et al. 2016) and testes (Yang et al. 2016b). Smoking during pregnancy increases the risks of stillbirths (Westreich 2017), infant deaths and harm that lasts into adulthood, e.g. impaired cognition, increased impulsivity, hyperactivity and risk of developing an addiction (Siqueira 2017). It increases the likelihood of lower birth weight (Duby 2015), gestational diabetes in daughters (Bao et al. 2016) and causes as much damage to the foetus as if it was smoking itself (Le Souëf 2000).

> **KEY POINT**
>
> *It is never too late to quit.*
>
> Schroeder 2013

Passive smoking can cause heart disease or lung cancer in people who have never smoked, 50% of childhood asthma and the majority of infant deaths (BMA 2015). The effect on infant mortality is ameliorated by cigarette

| TABLE 1.5 | Effects of smoking related to physiotherapy practice |
|---|---|
| Cardiorespiratory | Carnage to both respiratory and cardiovascular systems (Chapters 3 & 4)<br>Risk of pneumothorax 13-fold (Light 1993)<br>Risk of sleep apnoea, asthma exacerbations, tuberculosis (Jayes et al. 2016)<br>↓ Vitamin C, which would otherwise repair some of the lung damage (Banerjee et al. 2008)<br>↑ Dosage requirements for corticosteroids, theophylline (Sohn 2015) and opioids (Talbot & Palmer 2013)<br>Inflammatory damage and mucus production (Yang et al. 2016a), ↓ mucociliary clearance (Freire et al. 2016) |
| Musculoskeletal | Damage to diaphragm and quadriceps (Ramirez-Sarmiento 2004)<br>Lumbar disc herniation (Huang et al. 2016a)<br>Osteoarthritis (Amin et al. 2007)<br>Muscle weakness, osteoporosis, rheumatoid arthritis (Pignataro 2012)<br>Nonunion of fractures (Clement et al. 2016)<br>Ankylosing spondylitis (Ward et al. 2008) |
| Neurological | Some neurological diseases and neuropathic pain (Pignataro 2012)<br>Risk of ulnar neuropathy (Richardson 2009)<br>↑ Postoperative pain in males (Chiang et al. 2016) |
| Other | Cough, dyspnoea, reflux, dry throat, irritable upper airway, taste and smell disorders, bad breath, toothache, nasal congestion, snoring, nasal discharge (Şanlı et al. 2016)<br>↓ Immunity (Bauer et al. 2013)<br>↓ Hearing (Chang et al. 2016)<br>Rotten teeth (Vettore et al. 2016)<br>Depression (Berk et al. 2013), ↑ risk of drugs misuse (Reed 2017)<br>↓ Sleep (Mehari et al. 2014)<br>Wrinkles (Vierkötter et al. 2015)<br>Kidney injury, erectile dysfunction (Siqueira 2017)<br>Doubling of the risk of dementia (Pignataro 2012) |

taxes (Patrick et al. 2016). Children may also suffer ear and chest infections, dental caries, hearing loss and some learning disabilities (Duby 2015).

In adults, passive smoking impairs lung function, reduces mucociliary clearance (Freire et al. 2016) and exercise tolerance (Arjomandi et al. 2012), upsets the circadian rhythm (Sundar et al. 2015) and increases heart and lung disease (Talbot & Palmer 2013), cancers of the lung, larynx and pharynx (Rafiq et al. 2016) and stroke (Kwon et al. 2016). Third-hand smoke is a risk to children who ride in cars where others have smoked (Talbot & Palmer 2013).

Nicotine is more addictive than heroin and seven times as addictive as alcohol (Haas & Haas 2000), reaching the brain 7 secs after inhalation (Siqueira 2017). Exposure to e-cigarettes is more than twice as damaging to children as exposure to cigarettes (Kamboj et al. 2016), while vaping itself can cause nicotine addiction in adolescents (Liberman 2017).

*A custom loathsome to the eye, hateful to the nose, harmful to the brain and dangerous to the lungs.*
**King James I**

## Effects of Stress

All ill people suffer stress at times, often as a result of and sometimes as a predisposing factor to illness. The following effects of stress have been identified:

- ↑ RR, blood pressure (BP) and heart rate (HR) (Schwartz et al. 2011), ↑ myocardial oxygen consumption, myocardial ischaemia and arrhythmias (ICS 2014a);
- shift of breathing from the diaphragm to the chest (Schleifer et al. 2002);
- inflammation, with links to asthma, cardiovascular disease, some cancers and depression (Shields et al. 2016);
- exacerbation of respiratory infections (Stover 2016);
- neurocognitive deficit (Bharwani et al. 2016);

- immunosuppression (Fawcett et al. 2012), which in children can last into adult life (Slopen et al. 2013). Anxiety has now been claimed as perhaps the most important risk factor for cardiovascular disease (Allgulander 2016).

## Effects of Sleep

*Nurses and doctors frequently overestimate how much sleep patients are getting, and underestimate the importance of sleep.*

**Gelling 1999**

Sleep is necessary for the regulation of mood, memory (Kanda et al. 2016) and metabolism (Borbély et al. 2016). It brings cardiorespiratory changes:

- bronchoconstriction, which is only of consequence with asthma (Kamdar et al. 2012);
- ↓ respiratory drive, hypotonia of respiratory muscles, ↑ $PaCO_2$ and ↑ upper airway resistance (Sowho et al. 2014) especially during rapid eye movement (REM) sleep (Fig. 1.17);
- dips in $SaO_2$ to 90% or less (BTS 2008), which may drive $SaO_2$ down the steep part of the dissociation curve (see Fig. 1.12);
- ↓ lung volume due to the horizontal position, which along with ↓ muscle tone leads to $\dot{V}_A/\dot{Q}$ mismatch and a doubling of airway resistance (Xie 2012);
- ↓ metabolic rate, HR, and sympathetic tone, ↑ vagal activity (Garcia et al. 2013).

Most people accommodate all this quite happily, but those with little cardiorespiratory reserve can suffer nocturnal desaturation, sometimes dramatically

(p. 150–151 & 160) as well as nights disturbed by breathlessness or coughing.

A full 90-min cycle is needed to gain the benefits of REM sleep, which comprises a quarter of the sleep cycle and is associated with dreaming and perceptual learning. The brain is highly active during this restorative phase and consumes more oxygen than when awake at rest. It is the time when memories are consolidated (McDevitt et al. 2015) and is particularly important for critically ill patients to prevent memory distortion.

Sleep is regulated by melatonin from the pineal gland, which is released at about 2200, peaks by 0300 and is lowest around 0900. Sleep deprivation, poor sleep quality or obliteration of REM sleep contributes to cardiovascular disease, increased mortality (Rittayamai et al. 2016), stroke, multiple sclerosis (Palma 2013), dementia, impaired learning (Qiu et al. 2016a) and musculoskeletal pain (Li et al. 2017). Poor sleep quality is frequent in people after a cardiac event and may affect prognosis or impede cardiac rehabilitation (Le Grande et al. 2016). Rest, both physical and cognitive, may also be limited due to illness or the environment, and some cardiorespiratory diseases are subject to diurnal rhythms, e.g. COPD symptoms are worse in the morning, those of heart failure escalate during the day and are worst at night, thromboembolism occurs commonly between 1030 and 1230 h and cardiac arrest occurs most frequently between 0600 and 1200 (Smolensky et al. 2015).

## EFFECTS OF IMMOBILITY

*The pandemic of physical inactivity is associated with a range of chronic diseases and early deaths.*

**Ding et al. 2016**

Immobility predisposes to:

- ↓ muscle mass by up to 1%–5% per day, cardiovascular deconditioning and thromboembolism (Mah 2013);
- orthostatic intolerance, ↓ $\dot{V}O_2$max (Fig. 1.18) and cardiovascular instability during position change (Vollman 2013);
- ↓ survival and quality of life (BTS 2013);
- constipation (Giorgio et al. 2015), depression (Hamer et al. 2013), incontinence (Jerez-Roig et al. 2016) and osteoporosis (Armstrong et al. 2016);

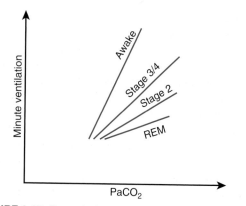

**FIGURE 1.17** Control of ventilation during sleep, showing reduced respiratory drive at deeper sleep stages. *REM*, Rapid eye movement. (From Douglas et al. 1982.)

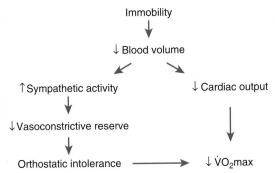

FIGURE 1.18 The effect of immobility on maximum oxygen consumption ($\dot{V}O_2$max).

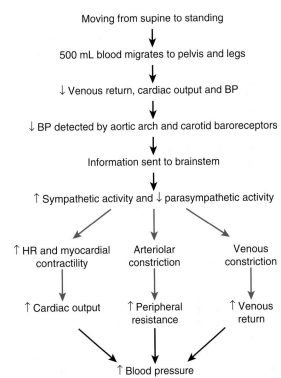

FIGURE 1.19 Typical circulatory response to postural change. *BP*, Blood pressure; *HR*, heart rate.

- for critically ill patients: pneumonia, delayed weaning, pressure sores (Vollman 2013), myopathy and delirium (Pawlik 2012), muscle inflammation (Kang & Ji 2013) and joint contractures (Brower 2010).

Contractures begin immediately, especially for joints held in extension (Trudel et al. 1999), although this is unlikely to be significant for a patient who is immobile for just a few days.

Loss of gravitational stimulus to the cardiovascular system causes a negative fluid balance within 24 h, impairing vasoconstrictive ability and augmenting deconditioning. Deterioration occurs more rapidly in the cardiorespiratory system than the musculoskeletal system, and deterioration is quicker than recovery (Dean & Ross 1992).

Inactive people are said to be contributing to a mortality burden as large as tobacco smoking (Wen & Wu 2012), with 60% of the world's population not being physically active enough for health (Vrdoljak 2014).

## Turning, Sitting and Standing Up

Regular position change as a preventive measure reduces haemodynamic instability on movement (Vollman 2013). Moving from supine to standing increases minute volume (Bahadur et al. 2008) and redistributes blood from the thorax to the lower body, followed by compensatory vasoconstriction in most patients to restore BP (Fig. 1.19).

Orthostatic intolerance occurs with inadequate haemodynamic compensation, e.g. with hypovolaemia or autonomic dysfunction, after prolonged bed rest or if the patient is elderly or dehydrated. Slow deep breathing improves orthostatic tolerance (Lucas 2013).

## Effects of Exercise

*Physical activity can increase life expectancy by 1.3–3.5 years.*

*Serón 2015*

During exercise, tidal volume initially rises then RR increases rapidly while tidal volume stabilizes (Tsukada et al. 2016). Exercise increases oxygen delivery, consumption and extraction by several mechanisms:

- The cardiovascular response can increase CO fivefold, accomplished by a near doubling of stroke volume and an increase in HR to about 220 minus the person's age (MacIntyre 2000).
- The respiratory response is represented by increased diffusion, more uniform lung perfusion, recruitment of dormant capillaries and, except with asthma, bronchodilation (Dominelli & Sheel 2012).
- Intense exercise can increase $\dot{V}O_2$ 20-fold (Owens 2013).
- Cerebral oxygenation rises during mild exercise and drops during hard exercise (Peltonen 2012).

- Acid–base balance is usually maintained by increased ventilation, but metabolic acidosis may develop if buffering mechanisms are unable to cope with the extra $CO_2$ and lactic acid.
- $PaO_2$ remains steady throughout.

Exercise also enhances mucous transport (p. 205), helps prevent low back pain (Steffens et al. 2016), reduces the risk of postoperative delirium (Abelha et al. 2013) and a single session helps stabilize posture (Fukusaki et al. 2016). Gait is worsened by smoking (Verlinden et al. 2016).

Regular exercise brings the following benefits:

- ↓ mortality (Khan et al. 2017), cardiovascular disease, diabetes and obesity, ↑ mental health and quality of life (Chaddha et al. 2017), protection against immune dysfunction, some cancers, musculoskeletal disorders, dementia (Di Raimondo et al. 2016) and some of the damage caused by smoking (Nesi et al. 2016);
- ↓ inflammation related to COPD (Davidson 2012), sepsis (Araújo et al. 2012), heart failure (Vlist & Janssen 2010) and knee osteoarthritis (Gomes et al. 2014);
- ↑ oxygen delivery and extraction (Hellsten & Nyberg 2015);
- healthier semen in men (Vaamonde et al. 2012);
- ↑ bone mineral density to a greater degree than the drug alendronate (Macias et al. 2012);
- ↓ falls (Yoo et al. 2013) and depression (Stanton et al. 2015), ↑ sleep, ↓ stress (Williams 2016);
- the vascular changes shown in Figs 1.20 and 4.2.

A physically active life is reported to add 8–10 years of freedom from chronic illness (Di Raimondo et al. 2016), the recommended level being at least 150 min a week of moderate intensity aerobic activity or 75 min of vigorous activity (Wise 2017a), but there is no lower threshold for benefits to be seen (Wilson et al. 2016).

For people with cardiopulmonary disease, regular exercise may be inhibited by dyspnoea or lack of social support, in which case motivation is available via online forums video blogs, self-monitoring devices and phone apps (Chaddha et al. 2017).

The evidence base for prescribing exercise for 26 different diseases is described by Pedersen and Saltin (2015).

> *Exercise is 'a miracle drug'.*
>
> ***Wen & Wu 2012***

## CASE STUDY: MS LL

*A 62-year-old patient from Cape Town is admitted with an exacerbation of COPD. Answer the questions below.*

### Relevant medical history

- Heart failure
- Hypertension
- Increased dyspnoea for 2 weeks

### Subjective

- Cannot stop coughing
- Occasionally bring up phlegm

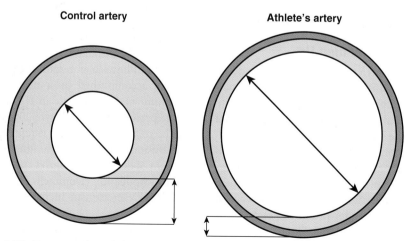

**FIGURE 1.20** Cross section of the artery of a healthy nonathlete (left) and an endurance athlete (right) which conveys performance and health benefits. (From Green et al. 2012.)

- Cannot sleep
- Daren't lie down
- Exhausted

### Objective

- Apyrexial
- Oxygen via nasal cannulae at 2 L/min
- Rapid shallow breathing with prolonged expiration
- Fluid chart and clinical assessment indicate dehydration
- No oxygen prescription or monitoring charts
- Speaking sets off paroxysms of wheezy coughing, usually nonproductive
- Clutches between legs when coughs
- Sits in chair day and night
- Can mobilize slowly
- Blood gases on air: $PaO_2$ 10.2 kPa (76.7 mmHg), $PaCO_2$ 6.4 kPa (48.1 mmHg), pH 7.4, $HCO_3^-$ 28 mmol/L

### Questions

1. Analysis?
2. Problems?
3. Goals?
4. Plan?

---

**CLINICAL REASONING**

*Comment on the logic of the following conclusion to a research study.*

*'Our data suggest that the use of postural drainage and chest percussion in patients without sputum production is not indicated …'*

*Chest* (1980), 78, 559–564

---

### Response to Case Study

1. Analysis
   - Breathing pattern suggests ↑ WOB.
   - Blood gases indicate hypoxaemia, hypercapnia and compensated respiratory acidosis.
   - Oxygen therapy is uncontrolled.
   - Coughing is largely ineffective and contributes to fatigue.
   - Coughing, stress incontinence, immobility and fluid restriction are likely to be interrelated.
2. Problems
   - Inaccurate and unmonitored oxygen
   - Dyspnoea

- Uncontrolled cough
- Fatigue
- Anxiety
- Sputum retention
- Stress incontinence
- ↓ Mobility

3. Goals
   - Short term: optimize oxygen, control cough, clear chest, balance rest and exercise.
   - Long term: educate patient and liaise with family for home management.

4. Plan
   - Liaise with the team about the need for a Venturi mask, oxygen prescription and monitoring (Chapter 5).
   - Positioning for comfort, breathlessness and sputum clearance.
   - Identify cause of poor sleep e.g. dyspnoea/cough/noise/anxiety, then remedy as possible with the team.
   - Educate on cough suppression for use when cough is uncontrolled and nonproductive.
   - Educate on mucociliary clearance, including fluid intake. Patient chose manual techniques at first, then autogenic drainage.
   - Educate on effective cough for when secretions are accessible.
   - Explain connection between coughing and stress incontinence, teach preliminary pelvic floor exercises and refer to continence service.
   - Show breathlessness management strategies.
   - Mobilize to toilet.
   - Provide written daily programme for self chest management and mobility.
   - Liaise with ward staff re. getting dressed and mobilizing.
   - Rehabilitate to independence, including family.

---

**RESPONSE TO CLINICAL REASONING**

It is not indicated to do an unnecessary treatment.

---

### RECOMMENDED READING

Berryman, N., 2017. Relationships between lower body strength and the energy cost of treadmill walking in a cohort of healthy older adults. Eur. J. Appl. Physiol. 117 (1), 53–59.

Bonhomme, V., Hans, P., 2001. Mechanisms of unconsciousness during general anaesthesia. Curr. Anaesth. Crit. Care 12 (2), 109–113.

Bruno, P.C., 2017. Effects of caffeine on neuromuscular fatigue and performance during high-intensity cycling exercise in moderate hypoxia. Eur. J. Appl. Physiol. 117 (1), 27–38.

Busha, B.F., Banis, G., 2017. A stochastic and integrative model of breathing. Resp. Physiol. Neurobiol. 237, 51–56.

Cavanaugh, M.T., Döweling, A., Young, J.D., 2017. An acute session of roller massage prolongs voluntary torque development and diminishes evoked pain. Eur. J. Appl. Physiol. 117 (1), 109–117.

DeTroyer, A., Wilson, T.A., 2016. The action of the diaphragm on the rib cage. J. Appl. Physiol. 121 (2), 391–400.

Dominelli, P.B., Sheel, A.W., 2012. Experimental approaches to the study of the mechanics of breathing during exercise. Respir. Physiol. Neurobiol. 180, 2–3.

Dunham-Snary, K.J., Wu, D., Sykes, E.A., et al., 2016. Hypoxic pulmonary vasoconstriction: from molecular mechanisms to medicine. Chest 151 (1), 181–192.

Fähling, M., Persson, P.B., 2012. Oxygen sensing, uptake, delivery, consumption and related disorders. Acta. Physiol. (Oxf.) 205 (2), 191–193.

Feiner, J.R., Weiskopf, R.B., 2017. Evaluating pulmonary function: an assessment of PaO2/FIO2. Crit. Care Med. 45 (1), e40–e48.

Frantz, T.L., Gaski, G.E., Terry, C., et al., 2016. The effect of pH versus base deficit on organ failure in trauma patients. J. Surg. Res. 200 (1), 260–265.

Fronius, M., Clauss, W.G., Althaus, M., 2012. Why do we have to move fluid to be able to breathe? Front. Physiol. 3, 146.

Gittemeier, E.M., 2017. Effects of aging and exercise training on the dynamics of vasoconstriction in skeletal muscle resistance vessels. Eur. J. Appl. Physiol. 117 (1), 397–407.

Gopal, K., Ussher, J.R., 2017. Sugar-sweetened beverages and vascular function. Am. J. Physiol. Heart Circ. Physiol. 312 (2), H285–H288.

Henderson, M.A., Runchie, C., 2017. Gas, tubes and flow. Anaesth. Int. Care Med. 18 (4), 180–184.

Jenkins, L.A., Mauger, A.R., Hopker, J.G., 2017. Age differences in physiological responses to self-paced and incremental $\dot{V}O_2$max testing. Eur. J. Appl. Physiol. 117 (1), 159–170.

Kang, M.Y., Katz, I., Sapoval, B., 2015. A new approach to the dynamics of oxygen capture by the human lung. Respir. Physiol. Neurobiol. 205, 109–119.

López-Barneo, J., 2016. Oxygen-sensing by arterial chemoreceptors: mechanisms and medical translation. Mol. Aspects Med. 47–48, 90–108.

Lumb, A.B., 2017. Nunn's Applied Respiratory Physiology, 8th ed. Elsevier, Oxford.

Magder, S., 2016. Volume and its relationship to cardiac output and venous return. Crit. Care 20, 271.

Matsuo, K., Palmer, J.B., 2010. Coordination of mastication, swallowing and breathing. Jpn. Dent. Sci. Rev. 45 (1), 31–40.

Miles-Chan, J.L., 2017. Standing economy: does the heterogeneity in the energy cost of posture maintenance reside in differential patterns of spontaneous weight-shifting? Eur. J. Appl. Physiol. 117 (1), 795–807.

Mutolo, D., 2017. Brainstem mechanisms underlying the cough reflex and its regulation. Resp. Physiol. Neurobiol. 243, 60–76.

Nakajima, K., Oda, E., Kanda, E., 2016. The association of serum sodium and chloride levels with blood pressure and estimated glomerular filtration rate. Blood Press. 25 (1), 51–57.

Rae, D.E., Chin, T., Dikgomo, K., 2017. One night of partial sleep deprivation impairs recovery from a single exercise training session. Eur. J. Appl. Physiol. 117 (1), 699–712.

Roman, M.A., Rossiter, H.B., Casaburi, R., 2016. Exercise, ageing and the lung. Eur. Respir. J. 48 (5), 1471–1486.

Ruprecht, A.A., De Marco, C., Pozzi, P., et al., 2016. Outdoor second-hand cigarette smoke significantly affects air quality. Eur. Respir. J. 48 (3), 918–920.

Teboul, J.L., Scheeren, T., 2017. Understanding the Haldane effect. Intensive Care Med. 43 (1), 91–93.

Verbanck, S., Van Muylem, A., Schuermans, D., et al., 2016. Transfer factor, lung volumes, resistance and ventilation distribution in healthy adults. Eur. Respir. J. 47 (1), 166–176.

Wagner, P.D., 2015. The physiological basis of pulmonary gas exchange: implications for clinical interpretation of arterial blood gases. Eur. Respir. J. 45 (1), 227–243.

Wains, S., 2017. Impact of arousal threshold and respiratory effort on the duration of breathing events across sleep stage and time of night. Resp. Physiol. Neurobiol. 237, 35–41.

Weibel, E.R., 2013. It takes more than cells to make a good lung. Am. J. Respir. Crit. Care Med. 187 (4), 342–346.

Wiles, J.D., Goldring, N., Coleman, D., 2017. Home-based isometric exercise training induced reductions resting blood pressure. Eur. J. Appl. Physiol. 117 (1), 83–93.

Zampieri, F.G., Kellum, J.A., Park, M., et al., 2014. Relationship between acid-base status and inflammation in the critically ill. Crit. Care 18, R154.

# 2

# Assessment

## LEARNING OBJECTIVES

*On completion of this chapter the reader should be able to:*
- interpret medical notes and nursing charts;
- analyse a patient's subjective report in order to develop, with the patient, problem-based goals and plans;
- develop the skills of observation, palpation and auscultation;
- analyse radiology findings;
- interpret respiratory function tests;
- use clinical reasoning to identify cardiorespiratory problems.

## INTRODUCTION

*It is more important to know what sort of a patient has a disease than what sort of disease a patient has.*
                                      ***William Osler***

Accurate assessment is the linchpin of physiotherapy and forms the basis of clinical reasoning. A problem-based assessment leads to thinking such as:
- This patient cannot cough up her sputum by herself. Why?
- Because it is thick. Why?
- Because she is dehydrated. Why?
- Because she feels too ill to drink.

Illogical assessment leads to reasoning such as: 'This is chronic bronchitis therefore I will turn the patient side-to-side and shake her chest'.

A thoughtful assessment encourages both efficiency and effectiveness. Efficiency saves time by avoiding unnecessary treatment. Effectiveness is assisted by incorporating the domains of the International Classification of Functioning, Disability and Health (ICF), which includes environmental and social factors and provides a standardized language on rehabilitation and what matters to the patient, i.e.:
- body function and structure
- activity limitation
- participation (Stucki 2016)

The last two concepts relate in particular to the multidisciplinary team within which the physiotherapist works. Patient participation is embedded in shared decision making, particularly for patients who have difficulty communicating due to dyspnoea or intubation.

Relevant parts of the patient assessment should be repeated after treatment to assess outcome. Specific assessment and outcomes for different conditions are in the pertinent chapters.

# BACKGROUND INFORMATION

*Not everything that counts can be measured. Not everything that can be measured counts.*

**Albert Einstein**

## Handover

It is the physiotherapist's job to clarify the indications for physiotherapy to other staff, and to explain which changes in a patient's condition should be reported. No patient is too ill or too well for physiotherapy.

The ward report or handover also provides the opportunity to ask three oft-neglected questions:
1. Is the patient drinking?
2. Is he eating?
3. Is he sleeping?

Apart from a daily report from the nurse in charge, any other opportunity to communicate should be taken, such as ward rounds and meetings. For physiotherapists working in the community, much communication will be on the phone, but visits to other teams usually benefit all concerned.

If physiotherapy notes are kept separate from the medical notes, verbal communication can be reinforced by writing physiotherapy information in the medical notes, e.g. a résumé of physiotherapy treatment or request for a minitracheostomy.

## Notes

Relevant details from the medical notes include:
- applicable medical history, e.g. other disorders needing physiotherapy, and conditions requiring precautions in relation to certain treatments, e.g. light-headedness, bleeding disorder, history of falls or swallowing difficulty;
- relevant investigations, medical treatment and response;
- social history and home environment;
- recent cardiopulmonary resuscitation (requiring X-ray inspection for aspiration or fracture);
- possibility of bony metastases;
- longstanding steroid therapy, leading to a risk of osteoporosis;
- history of radiotherapy over the chest.

The last four findings are a warning to avoid percussion or vibrations over the ribs until sufficient information is available to ensure that there is no risk of rib fracture.

## Charts

The charts record:
- the vital signs of temperature, blood pressure (BP), heart rate (HR), respiratory rate and arterial oxygen saturation ($SpO_2$);
- prescription and monitoring for oxygen and drugs;
- fluid balance.

**Respiratory rate** (RR) is normally 10–16 breaths/min. It increases with exercise, anxiety and sometimes heart or lung disease.

**Core temperature** is one of the most tightly guarded of physiological parameters and is usually maintained at 37°C, but may vary by up to 1°C in health. For acute patients, the chart should be checked at every visit because fever is the main harbinger of infection.

Fever may be accompanied by increased RR and HR because excess heat raises oxygen consumption and metabolic rate. Clinical examination helps distinguish respiratory from other infection. Pyrexia can also have a noninfectious origin, e.g. atelectasis, dehydration, thromboembolism, blood transfusion or drug reaction (Cunha 2013).

Fever is an adaptive response to infection, some microorganisms being adversely affected and some defence mechanisms performing better at higher body temperatures (Richardson et al. 2015), but it may have adverse effects with noninfectious conditions (Walter et al. 2016).

> **KEY POINT**
>
> A pyrexial patient may be referred for physiotherapy with a 'chest infection'. Sputum retention can accompany a chest infection but does not itself cause pyrexia. The treatment for a bacterial chest infection is antibiotics while the treatment for sputum retention is physiotherapy. The physiotherapist works on the problem rather than the diagnosis.

**Blood pressure** indicates the force that the blood exerts on the walls of the vessels. Normal at rest is 120/80. A systolic BP <90 mmHg in adults indicates hypotension. These patients should be mobilized only with close observation for light-headedness, and with a chair close behind. A systolic pressure >140 or a diastolic pressure >90 indicates hypertension. The relevance of BP to exercise training, heart surgery and manual hyperinflation is discussed in the relevant chapters.

Normal **heart rate** at rest is 60–100 beats/min (bpm). More than 100 bpm indicates tachycardia, which increases myocardial oxygen demand and may indicate sympathetic activity, hypoxaemia, hypotension, hypoglycaemia, dehydration, anxiety, pain or fever. Less than 60 bpm indicates bradycardia, which may reflect profound hypoxaemia, arrhythmias, heart block or vagal stimulation due to suctioning. Moderate bradycardia is normal during sleep and in the physically fit. Both tachycardia and bradycardia can impair cardiac output. Voluntary regulation of HR is achievable by yogi masters, or by others with the help of biofeedback (Jones et al. 2015a).

**Oximetry** gives instant feedback on $SpO_2$ and is accurate even in hypoxic or shock states (Overbeck 2016). The different absorption of light by saturated and unsaturated haemoglobin (Hb) is detected by a pulse oximeter, which displays the percentage of Hb saturated with oxygen. The sensor is attached close to a pulsating arteriolar bed on the ear, finger or toe. Average values for normal adults breathing air is 97.1% at 18 years old and 95.4% at 70 years old, the lower limits of normal being 96%–94%, respectively (Pretto et al. 2013). It is interpreted in relation to the fraction of inspired oxygen ($FiO_2$).

The relationship between $SpO_2$ and arterial blood gases is shown in Fig. 1.12 and Table 1.1. Oximetry becomes less accurate if Hb desaturates below 83% (NGC 2001) or if there is too much motion or ambient light, or too little signal (cold peripheries, anaemia, vasoconstriction, peripheral arterial disease, hypotension, hypovolaemia, hypothermia or finger clubbing). With nail polish, the probe can be turned sideways so that the light does not pass through the nail. The delay between application and an accurate reading may be 30 s for a finger probe, and most probes have a light to indicate maximum pulsation. Gentle rubbing may be needed to encourage vasodilation.

**Arterial blood gases** may be required in the following situations:

- unreliable oximetry readings
- critically ill patients
- if there is an unexplained drop in $SpO_2$
- clinical signs of hypercapnia (p. 40)
- breathless patients at risk of metabolic conditions such as diabetic ketoacidosis or renal failure

In smokers, a fall in $SpO_2$ during a 20-s breath-hold at end-exhalation may identify lung damage before symptoms become apparent (Inoue 2009).

### TABLE 2.1  Examples of criteria for calling the outreach team

| Vital sign | Patient at risk |
|---|---|
| Airway | Threatened airway, excessive secretions or stridor |
| Breathing | RR <8 or >25 breaths/min |
| Circulation | HR <50 or >150 beats/min |
| | Systolic BP <90 mmHg, >200 mmHg, or drop of >40 mmHg |
| | BP below patient's normal values |
| Consciousness | Sustained fall in Glasgow coma scale of >2 in past hour |
| Oxygen | $SpO_2$ <90% on >.50 $FiO_2$ |
| Urine output | <30 mL/h for >2 h (unless normal for the patient) |
| General | Clinically causing concern |
| | Not responding to treatment |

*BP*, Blood pressure; *FiO_2*, fraction of inspired oxygen; *HR*, heart rate; *RR*, respiratory rate.

The vital signs may be correlated by a 'track-and-trigger' Modified Early Warning Score (MEWS) system (Table 2.1) or an electronic automated system (Schmidt et al. 2015) to identify patients at risk. Vital sign streaming with Google Glass holds promise (Liebert et al. 2016).

Prescribed **drugs** and **oxygen** are documented on the prescription chart and their effects documented on the observation chart, e.g. peak flow or $SpO_2$.

The **fluid** chart documents input and output. It should show a positive daily balance of about 500–1000 mL due to insensible loss from the skin and respiratory tract. There are many reasons for a wide variation in fluid balance, including ambient temperature and major fluid shifts after surgery.

Fluid overload may cause hyponatraemia and systemic or pulmonary oedema. Dehydration is accompanied by reduced urine output and can be caused by diuretics, laxatives, lack of thirst in old age, dementia, inability of a patient to reach or manage their drink, or conscious fluid restriction due to anxiety about reaching the toilet. A urine colour chart can be used to assess patients at home or in residential care (Malisova et al. 2016), but is only reliable for early morning specimens and so long as the colour has not been affected by medication (Heneghan et al. 2012). Table 2.2 shows the fluid balance of a healthy adult.

| TABLE 2.2   Sources of normal fluid gain and loss over 24 h in a 70 kg male | | | |
|---|---|---|---|
| **INTAKE AND CATABOLIC PROCESSING** | | **OUTPUT** | |
| Water via fluids (mL) | 1500 | Urine (mL) | 1500 |
| Water via food (mL) | 500 | Evaporation from skin and lungs (mL) | 800 |
| Water via metabolism (mL) | 400 | Faeces (mL) | 100 |
| Total (mL) | 2400 | Total (mL) | 2400 |

Dehydration is common in older patients (McCrow et al. 2016) and predisposes to:

- sputum retention
- pressure sores
- constipation
- confusion, short-term memory loss and impaired cognition (Rush 2013)
- kidney dysfunction
- headache
- delayed BP response to position change (Yadav et al. 2016)
- muscle cramps
- fatigue
- impaired motor control (Holdsworth 2012)
- ↑ HR and orthostatic intolerance after exercise (Charkoudian et al. 2016)

Fluid loss from the vascular to the interstitial space is caused by altered hydrostatic or oncotic pressures, or increased capillary membrane permeability, leading to effective hypovolaemia.

## Biochemistry

Normal values are in Appendix A.

### Urea and electrolytes

Below are the urea and electrolyte results that are most relevant to physiotherapy.

**Sodium** is the commonest electrolyte in the blood and is regulated by the kidneys. Low levels (hyponatraemia) are due to fluid retention or inappropriate antidiuretic hormone secretion, while high levels (hypernatraemia) indicate dehydration.

**Potassium** is the principal intracellular electrolyte. High or low values can weaken muscles, including the diaphragm. Low levels (hypokalaemia) predispose to cardiac arrhythmias, and can be caused by loss from diarrhoea or vomiting, inappropriate steroids (Blann 2006, p. 62) or too-rapid correction of respiratory acidosis (Hammond et al. 2013). High levels (hyperkalaemia) suggest acidosis or kidney failure and are the commonest electrolyte emergency, requiring insulin and glucose to force potassium back into the cells.

**Urea** is formed from protein breakdown and is excreted by the kidneys. High levels may be caused by impaired kidney perfusion from heart failure or shock. **Creatinine** is formed from muscle breakdown and is also renally excreted. Levels rise with kidney failure and drop with malnutrition. Both urea and creatinine rise with dehydration.

### Albumin

This antioxidant is the main protein in plasma and the interstitium, providing 15% of the buffering capacity and 80% of the osmotic pressure of blood (Vincent 2001). Reduced levels, due to hypermetabolism, malnutrition, blood loss, liver or kidney problems, burns, ascites, chronic inflammation or critical illness, cause metabolic alkalosis and reduce osmotic pull from the vascular space so that fluid escapes, causing systemic and pulmonary oedema.

### Microbiology

Microorganisms are identified by culturing specimens, e.g. blood, sputum or pleural fluid, on various media that promote their growth. Most bacteria grow in 24–48 h, but the tubercle bacillus may require 6 weeks. Sensitivity tests identify which antibiotics can then tackle the bacteria.

### Haematology

A full blood count analyses the components of blood to assess blood cells and coagulation.

**Red blood cells** (erythrocytes) are the most abundant cell in blood and contain no nucleus so they can penetrate the smallest capillaries. Relevant abnormalities are the following:

- Reduced haemoglobin indicates anaemia, which causes fatigue and is poorly tolerated in people with lung or heart disease. Mobilizing a patient with low Hb requires close attention to a patient's colour and the same precautions as for hypotension. A high concentration of Hb, known as polycythaemia, is the body's adaptation to chronic hypoxaemia due to disease or living at high altitude.

- Haematocrit (packed cell volume) is the proportion of total blood volume that is composed of red cells. Red blood cell count provides the same information.
- Erythrocyte sedimentation rate is raised following myocardial infarction or if there is inflammation, tuberculosis (TB), cancer or anaemia.

**White blood cells** (leucocytes) are part of the immune system, working to ingest unwelcome microorganisms by phagocytosis. A raised white cell count (WCC) indicates infection or other condition such as cancer, rheumatoid arthritis or the postoperative state. Neutrophils are the most common white cells and their number is raised with bacterial infection or inflammation. They become overactive in sepsis and start to destroy healthy tissue as well as pathogens. Cytotoxic drugs reduce WCC (leukopenia) e.g. with cancer or following transplantation, indicating that the patient is immunocompromised and extra infection control precautions are required.

**Clotting studies** (see the Glossary) which indicate that a patient might bleed easily include low platelet count (thrombocytopaenia), prolonged prothrombin time or raised international normalized ratio. Patients on heparin are at risk.

### Cytology and histology

Cytology is the study of fluids, e.g. in sputum or blood, to identify abnormal or cancerous cells. Histology does the same with tissues such as biopsied lung tissue.

### Arterial blood gases

Arterial blood is usually taken from the radial artery by a doctor, as opposed to other blood tests in which blood is taken from a vein by the phlebotomist. Patients should be undisturbed and stay in the same position for 20 min beforehand. Interpretation is on p. 17.

## SUBJECTIVE ASSESSMENT

*Osler supposedly said, 'Listen to the patient. He is telling you the diagnosis', to which I would*

*add, 'And she just might be telling you the best management too'*

**Pitkin 1998**

The subjective assessment is what matters to the patient. Problems such as breathlessness are more closely related to quality of life than physiological measurements, and subjective wellbeing is associated with longevity (Xu & Roberts 2010). When possible, patients should be assessed in a well-lit area that is quiet, private, warm and well ventilated. Respect for privacy includes awareness of those within hearing.

> **KEY POINT**
>
> *If a patient's curtain is drawn, it is equivalent to their front door and you need to knock.*
> Beaven 2012

The patient requires an explanation because the public perception of physiotherapy is often limited to football and backache.

The inequality of the relationship is minimized by:
- positioning ourselves at eye level if possible;
- addressing adults by their surname (Wilkins et al. 2010, p. 12) unless they ask otherwise;
- asking permission before assessment.

Permission not only encourages patients' self-respect, it is a legal necessity in most countries. It is also good practice to ask before moving a patient's personal items or opening their locker. In relation to addressing patients, for elders it can be seen as disrespectful rather than friendly to address them by their first name unprompted.

Patients are then asked to define their problems and how these influence their life. Empathy is then facilitated by using the patient's words and phrases rather than our own. Acknowledging a patient's experience and respecting their opinion are also potent motivating factors.

### Patient History

*'I know what my body is telling me'.*

**Morgan 2012**

The history from the notes is supplemented with questions about how the patient's condition is affecting their lifestyle, from which goals can be developed.

Unreliability of recall may be caused by anxiety, according to Barsky (2002), who also suggests that patients should be asked to describe the most recent events first. If the patient is unable to give a history, relatives can be questioned, but there is often disparity between relatives' and patients' perception of their quality of life (Carr 2001).

## Cardiorespiratory Symptoms

How long have symptoms been troublesome? What is their frequency and duration? Are they getting better or worse? What are aggravating and relieving factors?

### Breathlessness

> *Dyspnoea can be as powerfully aversive as pain … Documentation of dyspnoea is the first step to improved symptom management.*
> **Stevens et al. 2016**

Shortness of breath (SOB) is the most common symptom in advanced cardiopulmonary disease (Booth et al. 2008) but it can also be metabolic, neurogenic or neuromuscular in origin. Respiratory causes usually relate to excess WOB, which is abnormal if inappropriate to the level of physical activity. Significant SOB is indicated by the inability to complete a full sentence. Visual analogue scales (Fig. 2.1) and numeric rating scales have been validated (Johnson et al. 2010), or a key question at each visit can be a comparative measurement, e.g.:

- 'How much can you do at your best/worst?'
- 'What are you unable to do now because of your breathing?'

If SOB increases in supine it is called **orthopnoea**. In lung disease, this is caused by pressure on the diaphragm from the abdominal viscera. In heart failure, a poorly functioning left ventricle is unable to tolerate the increased volume of blood returning to the heart in supine. **Paroxysmal nocturnal dyspnoea** is caused by orthopnoeic patients sliding off their pillows during sleep, leading them to seek relief by sitting up over the edge of the bed.

Distinguishing SOB due to lung or heart disorder is achieved by clinical reasoning using peak flow readings, auscultation, imaging, exercise testing and history.

The quality of SOB can only be judged by the patient, typical descriptors being identified by Scano et al. (2005), and, specifically for heart failure, by Parshall (2012). Patients may deny SOB if it has developed

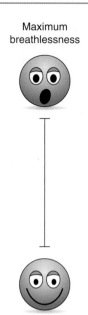

Maximum breathlessness

No breathlessness

**FIGURE 2.1** Visual analogue scale for shortness of breath.

gradually, but they often complain of its functional effects such as difficulty in getting upstairs, which underlines the relevance of the ICF approach. Detailed measurement of SOB is on p. 251. Table 2.3 indicates possible causes in relation to onset.

### Cough

Coughing is abnormal if it is persistent, painful or productive of sputum. It may be underestimated by smokers and people who swallow their sputum. Acute cough is normally benign, self-limiting and associated with upper respiratory tract infection, in which the virus hijacks the cough to propagate itself (Atkinson et al. 2016). Chronic cough is one that lasts more than 8 weeks and may be associated with gastro-oesophageal reflux disease (GORD), asthma, hyperventilation syndrome (Benoist 2015), smoking, lung disease, pleural effusion, heart failure, post-nasal drip, habit, Tourette syndrome, some drugs, and occupational or environmental factors (Song et al. 2016a).

> **KEY POINT**
>
> A cough should be reported if is chronic and of unknown cause, or if it is accompanied by unexplained haemoptysis.

**TABLE 2.3  Approximate time to the onset of dyspnoea**

| Immediate | Hours | Days or weeks | Months or years |
|---|---|---|---|
| Pneumothorax | Asthma | Pleural effusion | Chronic obstructive pulmonary disease |
| Pulmonary embolus | Pulmonary oedema | Lung cancer | Lung fibrosis |
| Foreign body aspiration | Chest infection | | Heart failure |
| | Myocardial infarct | | Neuromuscular disorder |

**TABLE 2.4  Characteristics of cough**

| Type of cough | Possible causes |
|---|---|
| Dry | Chronic asthma, ILD, pollutants, hyperventilation syndrome, airway irritation, ACE inhibitor drugs, viral infection |
| Productive | COPD, bronchiectasis, CF, PCD, acute asthma, chest infection |
| With position change | Asthma, bronchiectasis, CF, PCD, pulmonary oedema |
| With eating or drinking | Aspiration of stomach contents, e.g. with neurological disease or in elderly people |
| With exertion | Asthma, COPD, ILD |
| Inadequate | Weakness, pain, poor understanding |
| Paroxysmal | Asthma, aspiration, upper airway obstruction, croup, whooping cough |

*ACE*, Angiotensin-converting enzyme; *CF*, cystic fibrosis; *COPD*, chronic obstructive pulmonary disease; *ILD*, interstitial lung disease; *PCD*, primary ciliary dyskinesia.

Serious conditions presenting as an isolated cough include cancer, TB and foreign body aspiration. A chronic cough is only considered idiopathic after assessment at a specialist cough clinic (Morice 2006).

Suggested questions relating to a cough are:

• What started it (e.g. infection)?
• What triggers it (e.g. smoking)?
• Is there sputum?
• Does the cough occur at night (GORD and/or asthma)?
• Does it cause pain (see 'pleuritic pain', p. 36)?

Clinical reasoning can then be used, with the help of Table 2.4, to identify possible causes.

A cough caused by asthma or GORD should disappear once the condition is controlled. A quarter of patients taking angiotensin-converting enzyme inhibitor drugs develop a dry cough, which usually dissolves in 2–3 months (Li et al. 2012). Other nonproductive

and habit coughs, such as those following viral infection, usually disappear over time, but a dry cough can perpetuate itself by irritating the airways, in which case it can be controlled by the measures on p. 218.

The cough reflex may be oversensitized by upper respiratory tract infection, mouth-breathing, GORD or irritants such as aerosols and cigarette smoke (Morice 2013).

Listening to the cough will help identify weakness or pick up sounds that may be missed on auscultation but stimulated by a cough. It is best to ask patients to show how they would cough to clear phlegm rather than to ask them to 'show me a cough'. Cough questionnaires include the Leicester Cough Questionnaire (Ward 2016) and Cough-specific Quality of Life Questionnaire (Spinou & Birring 2014). Severity can be measured with a visual analogue scale (Morice et al. 2007).

## Secretions

Can the patient clear their secretions independently? If not, do they need advice or physical assistance? For acute patients, are secretions interfering with gas exchange? For people with a chronic condition, are secretions impairing their lifestyle or contributing to a vicious cycle that perpetuates hypersecretory disease (p. 88)? Has sputum changed in quality or quantity?

## Wheeze

Airways narrowed by bronchospasm increase the WOB and may cause wheezing. The feeling should be explained to patients as tightness of the chest on breathing out, not just noisy, laboured or rattly breathing. If aggravated by exertion or allergic reaction, asthma is a likely cause. Airways which are narrowed by factors other than bronchospasm may also cause a wheeze, but less consistently. Objectively, wheeze is confirmed by auscultation.

## Other Symptoms

**Pain** and SOB activate common areas in the brain (Kohberg et al. 2016). Chest pain may be musculoskeletal, cardiac, alimentary or respiratory in origin. Many patients associate chest pain with heart attacks, and anxiety may modify their perception and description of it. Lung parenchyma contains no pain fibres, but chest pains relevant to the physiotherapist are the following:

1. Pleuritic pain, which denotes the nature of the pain rather than the pathology. The pleura is replete with nerve endings, and pleuritic pain is sharp, stabbing and worse on deep breathing, coughing, hiccupping, talking and being moved. Causes include pleurisy, lobar pneumonia, pneumothorax, fractured ribs or pulmonary embolism.
2. Angina pectoris, a crushing chest pain due to myocardial ischaemia, which should be reported.
3. Musculoskeletal pain, e.g. costovertebral tenderness, which may be due to hyperinflation, when the muscles are obliged to work inefficiently, or chronic coughing, which may cause muscle strain. Musculoskeletal pain around the neck or shoulders may interfere with the accessory muscles of respiration.
4. Raw central chest pain, worse on coughing, caused by tracheitis and associated with upper respiratory tract infection or excessive coughing.
5. Bronchiectasis pain, which is a deep ache localized to areas of inflammation.

Postoperative pain is discussed on p. 297.

**Fatigue** is a common and often wretched symptom, closely associated with SOB and depression (Radbruch 2008). Patients may prefer to say that they are tired rather than admit to depression, which carries a stigma. The word 'fatigue' is not found in all languages, in which case the word 'weakness' can be used for the physical dimension and 'tiredness' for the cognitive dimension. Cognitive fatigue complicates activities such as reading, driving and other activities of daily living. The sensation fits all domains of the ICF and is characteristic of many chronic conditions which may overlap, including chronic obstructive pulmonary disease (COPD), heart failure, cancer and neurological disease. Causes include inflammation, anaemia, infection, stress, dehydration, cachexia or sedatives (Radbruch 2008). Fatigue is severe if it cannot be relieved by rest or sleep.

Fatigue and weakness feel similar but may require opposite management strategies, e.g. exercise for weakness and rest for acute fatigue. However, many patients have both and require energy conservation, pacing and graded exercise. If a patient is not able to describe the sensation, it is noteworthy that carers may overestimate and staff may underestimate fatigue (Radbruch 2008). Visual analogue scales fail to assess the impact of fatigue on daily functioning, and valid measurements are in Appendix A or described by Butt et al. (2013). Fatigue serves a protective function (Boullosa & Nakamura, 2013) and can lead to exhaustion, which, if accompanied by ventilatory failure, may indicate the need for noninvasive ventilation.

**Sleep** may be impaired by anxiety, SOB, a noisy environment, loss of day/night rhythm, pain or depression. **Appetite** may be impaired by depression, feeling ill, hospital food or the side effects of drugs.

**Dizziness** may be associated with postural hypotension, hyperventilation syndrome or a lesion of the 8th cranial nerve or brain stem. A history of **falls** requires investigation of the risks on p. 412. **Fainting** (syncope) or near-fainting may be caused by hyperventilation syndrome, prolonged coughing or cardiovascular disorder.

---

**KEY POINT**

If a patient spends their day flopped in front of their screen, is this because of preference, exercise limitation or depression?

---

How does the patient feel about their disease? This question provides the opportunity for patients to describe their feelings but does not pressurize them. **Anxiety** affects the neural processing of respiratory sensations, which may underlie the increased perception of respiratory sensations in anxious individuals (Leupoldt et al. 2012), particularly if symptoms are unpredictable. Anxiety may also reinforce frustration, embarrassment or restricted social function or loss of control. People in some cultures may express emotions in terms of bodily sensations.

It is useful to adopt the practice of asking patients what they think is the cause of their symptoms, because their perceptions are often surprisingly accurate.

## Activities of Daily Living

*Many patients express a desire for quality of life equal to or greater than their desire for quantity of life.*

*O'Neil et al. 2013*

Is it difficult to bathe, dress or shop? How much daily exercise does the patient take? Limitation of activity is not an accurate indicator of cardiorespiratory disease because patients gradually reduce their activities of daily living as they experience slowly increasing breathlessness or fatigue, thus perpetuating a vicious cycle. But questions can be asked such as 'what have you stopped doing because of your breathing?' Reduced mobility may lead to constipation, which is exacerbated by dehydration, and to urinary incontinence, which is exacerbated by coughing.

How many stairs are there at work or home? Is the environment well-heated, smoky, dusty? Does the patient live alone, smoke, eat well? Is nutrition affected by SOB or dysphagia? What support is available? Problems with personal care, employment, finance and housing also loom large for people with cardiorespiratory disease. Measures of physical functioning are more related to quality of life than spirometry (Geijer et al. 2007).

Questionnaires are described in the relevant chapters.

## OBSERVATION

Any part of the body not being observed should be kept covered throughout, with awareness of the needs of different cultures (Wilson et al. 2012).

### Breathing Pattern

The breathing pattern should be observed while approaching the patient because it will change once they are aware of the physiotherapist's presence. Normal breathing is rhythmic, with active inspiration, passive expiration and an inspiratory to expiratory (I:E) ratio of about 1:2. There should be synchrony between chest and abdominal movement, but a relaxed person may show only abdominal movement. Individual variations achieve the same minute volume by different combinations of rate and depth or varied chest and abdominal movements.

**Laboured breathing** represents increased WOB, e.g.:
- forced exhalation with active contraction of the abdominal muscles to propel air out through narrowed airways;
- obvious accessory muscle contraction (Fig. 2.2);
- indrawing/recession/retraction of the soft tissues of the chest wall on inspiration (Fig. 2.3), caused by excess negative pressure in the chest which sucks in supraclavicular, suprasternal and intercostal spaces, thus destabilizing the chest wall and further increasing the WOB.

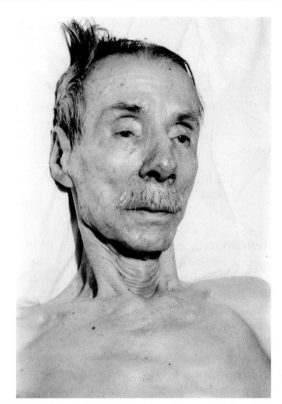

FIGURE 2.2 Soft tissues draped over the bones and prominent sternomastoid muscles, indicating malnutrition and muscle hypertrophy.

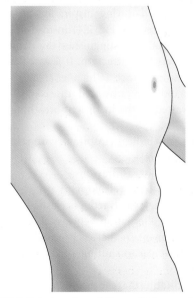

FIGURE 2.3 Indrawing of the soft tissues between the ribs due to extra work of breathing during inspiration.

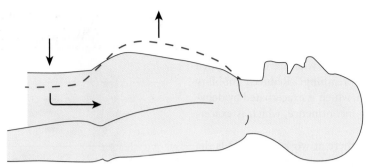

**FIGURE 2.4** Paradoxical inward movement of the abdomen on inspiration due to weakness or fatigue of the diaphragm.

**Disturbed speech** may represent increased WOB, e.g. prolonged inspiration (which increases the silences), short expiration (which reduces the time available for speech), faster RR, smaller tidal volumes or inability to speak in complete sentences (Tehrany et al. 2016).

**Paradoxical breathing** may be evident by the following:

- indrawing of soft tissues (as above);
- Hoover's sign, which occurs in a hyperinflated chest when the flattened diaphragm (see Fig. 2.6) pulls in the lower ribs on inspiration, becoming, in effect, an expiratory muscle;
- flail chest due to rib fractures (p. 534);
- abdominal paradox, in which a weak or fatigued diaphragm is sucked up into the chest by negative pressure generated during inspiration so that the abdomen is sucked in (Fig. 2.4) instead of swelling outwards. Palpation distinguishes this from active abdominal muscle contraction. It is associated with poor exercise tolerance (Chien et al. 2013) either because it indicates advanced disease or because energy is wasted on the inefficient breathing pattern itself.

The following may indicate inspiratory muscle fatigue, weakness and/or overload:

- abdominal paradox, as previous;
- ↑ RR, ↓ $PaCO_2$, ↑ pH (alkalosis);
- shallow breathing, which reduces elastic loading;
- less commonly, alternation between abdominal and rib cage movement so that each muscle group can rest in turn, similar to shifting a heavy bag between arms.

Exhaustion, indicating that the patient requires mechanical assistance, is evident by:

- ↓ RR, ↑ $PaCO_2$, ↓ pH (acidosis)

Periods of apnoea interspersed with waxing and waning of the rate and depth of breathing are called **Cheyne–Stokes** breathing when regular or **Biot's** breathing when irregular. These indicate neurological damage, but Cheyne–Stokes breathing is also associated with heart failure (Olson 2014) or nearing the end of life, or it may be normal in some elderly people.

**Irregular breathing** indicates tension or may occur during normal rapid eye movement sleep. **Sighs** above the normal rate of 0–3 in 15 min may indicate hyperventilation syndrome (Barker & Everard 2015).

## General Appearance

Is the patient obese, thus compromising diaphragmatic function, or cachectic, indicating poor nutrition and weakness? If the patient is unkempt, does this reflect difficulty with self care or a measure of how disease has affected self esteem? Is the patient restless or incoherent, possibly due to hypoxia?

Does the posture suggest fatigue, pain, altered consciousness or respiratory distress? Breathless people may brace their arms so that their shoulder girdle muscles can work unhindered as accessory muscles of respiration. For mobile patients, gait gives an indication of mood, balance, coordination or dyspnoea.

## Confusion

Clinical reasoning helps to identify which of the following could be the cause of confusion:

- hypoxia
- hypercapnia
- infection
- pain
- polypharmacy

- poor sleep
- fatigue
- constipation
- depressive illness
- sensory deficit
- disorientation, e.g. from 'relocation stress'
- dementia
- dehydration or electrolyte imbalance

A notorious case occurred in the UK in 2009 when a young man became confused from dehydration, was sedated, and subsequently died from the dehydration.

## Respiratory rate

Average RR is 12–16 breaths/min but there is a wide adult range of 10–20.

A rate below 8 breaths/min increases $PaCO_2$ and may lead to respiratory acidosis. Above 40 breaths/min (tachypnoea) blows off $PaCO_2$, sometimes leading to respiratory alkalosis, and increasing WOB because of the extra turbulence. Rapid breathing is inefficient and if combined with shallow breathing increases dead space so that breathless patients can also be acidotic. Table 2.5 outlines abnormalities.

## Chest shape

The chest and abdomen should be as visible for observation as the patient feels comfortable with. The chest should be mobile and normally inflated (Fig. 2.5). Obstructive lung disease may cause hyperinflation by increasing its anteroposterior diameter (Fig. 2.6).

| TABLE 2.5  Some causes of abnormal respiratory rate | |
| --- | --- |
| ↑ RR | ↓ RR |
| Lung or heart disease | Drug overdose |
| Inspiratory muscle fatigue or weakness | Exhaustion |
| Brain injury | Brain injury |
| Anaemia | Diabetic coma |
| Pain, nausea, anxiety or fever | |
| Pulmonary embolism or pneumothorax | |

RR, Respiratory rate.

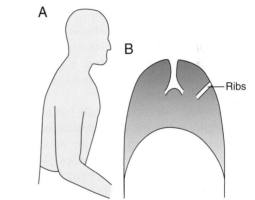

FIGURE 2.5 (A) Normal chest shape with (B) domed diaphragm and oblique ribs.

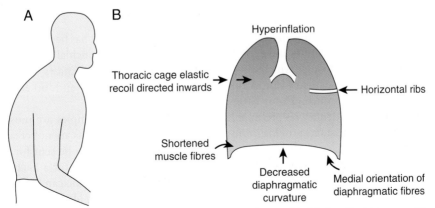

FIGURE 2.6 (A) Hyperinflated, barrel-shaped and rigid chest with (B) flat diaphragm and horizontal ribs.

Hyperinflation may assist in keeping obstructed airways open, but at the cost of increased WOB.

Other abnormalities of the chest wall may cause a restrictive defect and increase WOB (p. 113).

## Colour

*When the lips are blue the brain is too.*

*Clapham 2005*

**Pallor** is associated with anaemia, reduced cardiac output or hypovolaemic shock. A **plethoric** appearance is a florid colour indicating polycythaemia. Haemoglobin is red when saturated with oxygen, but desaturation turns it blue, leading to a dusky blue colour of the skin known as **cyanosis**, best appreciated under fluorescent lighting. Causes are circulatory disorder for peripheral cyanosis and respiratory disorder for central cyanosis.

Peripheral cyanosis shows at the fingers, toes and ear lobes, and indicates stagnant blood that has given up its oxygen and is not being replenished. Causes include peripheral arterial disease or a cold environment which causes peripheral vasoconstriction.

Central cyanosis shows peripherally but also at the lips and tongue, indicating a pulmonary or cardiac problem. It is a useful warning sign but an unreliable guide to hypoxaemia, being identified at $SpO_2$ levels that vary from 72% to 95% (Martin 1990). Its detection depends not just on Hb in the blood, but also on skin pigmentation and the patency of vessels. It can be exaggerated by polycythaemia, masked by anaemia, and missed in a patient with $SpO_2$ <85% Hb <11 g/dL (Oechslin 2015).

## Hands

The hands are a rich source of information. Poor cardiac output causes cold hands. $CO_2$ retention is indicated by warm hands due to peripheral vasodilation, and a coarse flapping tremor of the outstretched hands which disappears when the hands drop to the patient's side. A fine tremor may be a side effect of bronchodilator drugs, particularly in the elderly. For patients who are unable to give a smoking history, nicotine stains provide irrefutable evidence of the deadly habit.

Finger clubbing (Fig. 2.7) is a reduced angle between the nail and nail bed, possibly related to abnormal capillary growth pattern (Rutherford 2013). Causes are:
- pulmonary: 75%;
- cardiac: 10%;

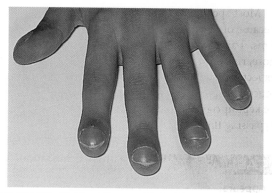

**FIGURE 2.7** Clubbed fingers. (From Lissauer et al. 2012).

- liver or gut: 10%;
- other, e.g. thyroid disease or laxative abuse: 5% (Jefferies & Turley 1999, p. 117).

Pulmonary causes include fibrosing alveolitis and suppurative disorders such as bronchiectasis, cystic fibrosis, empyema or abscess. Clubbing is of supreme disinterest to the physiotherapist because it is not affected by physiotherapy, but it should be reported if it appears unexpectedly in a smoker because it may be the first sign of lung cancer (White 2016).

## Oedema

Oedema is excess fluid in interstitial spaces. Peripheral oedema accumulates around the ankles or sacral area, depending on posture, and is usually caused by kidney, liver or cardiorespiratory disease such as COPD or heart failure.

## Sputum

Sputum is mucus that has been expectorated. It is always abnormal because bronchial secretions are swallowed in healthy people. Colour charts help identify purulence (Reychler et al. 2016) and other characteristics are shown in Table 2.6.

Green or yellow samples are most likely to contain bacteria, but if secretions are not creamy, white or clear, a sputum specimen may be sent for culture to identify the pathogen responsible for a likely chest infection so that an accurate antibiotic can be given. Eosinophils or neutrophils can also be identified, which indicate allergy or inflammation respectively, and occasionally some cancers may be identified (Yu et al. 2010).

Most specimens have low sensitivity and specificity because of contamination with upper respiratory organisms. This can be minimized by patients blowing their nose, rinsing their mouth and spitting out saliva before expectorating. For patients who require suction, a sterile mucous trap is incorporated into the circuit. This should be kept upright during suction to prevent the specimen bypassing the trap.

Table 2.7 helps distinguish sputum and pulmonary oedema.

If a specimen cannot be produced by chest clearance or suction, or if specimens are required from the lower respiratory tract, e.g. to identify inflammation, sputum induction using hypertonic saline can be used to facilitate the production of a specimen (Langridge et al. 2016) (see Appendix A).

**Haemoptysis** is expectoration of sputum containing blood, which can be an alarming experience for patients who see TV dramas in which coughing up blood presages instant death. Haemoptysis varies from slight streaking to frank bleeding. It is bright red if fresh, pink if mixed with sputum, or rusty brown if it is old blood. Causes are:

- bronchiectasis (intermittent, fresh);
- lung cancer (persistent);
- pulmonary tuberculosis (intermittent);
- lung abscess (copious);
- pneumococcal pneumonia (rusty red);
- pulmonary oedema (frothy, and pink or white);
- pulmonary embolus (bright red);
- blood clotting abnormality (fresh);
- trauma such as intubation, tracheostomy, lung contusion or frequent/rough tracheal suction (fresh).

**Haematemesis** occurs when blood is vomited, and it may be confused with haemoptysis. It is more likely to be mixed with food than with mucus, and is distinguished by acidity and a dark brown colour, which resembles coffee grounds. It may be associated with melaena (digested blood passed per rectum) or nausea.

### TABLE 2.6    Characteristics of sputum

| Appearance | Possible causes |
| --- | --- |
| Mucoid, i.e. clear, gooey, grey or white (like raw egg white) | Chronic obstructive pulmonary disease |
| Thick | Infection or dehydration |
| Purulent, yellow or green | Infection, allergy, or stasis of secretions e.g. neglected bronchiectasis |
| Stringy | Asthma or poor oral hygiene |
| Plugs | Asthma |
| Green or yellow | Presence of eosinophils |
| Thick, green, musty-smelling | Pseudomonas infection |
| Smelly | Abscess, aspiration, anaerobic infection, bronchiectasis |
| Frothy (mixed with air) and sometimes pink (blood squeezed into alveoli) | Pulmonary oedema |
| Containing blood | See below |

### TABLE 2.7    Comparative signs of excess bronchial secretions and pulmonary oedema secretions

| | Bronchial secretions | Pulmonary oedema |
| --- | --- | --- |
| History | Lung disease or chest infection | Heart disease (may be secondary to lung disease) |
| Temperature | May be raised | Normal |
| Fluid balance | Normal | Fluid retention usually |
| Crackles (heard at the mouth or by auscultation) | Patchy | Bilateral, late-inspiratory, dependent |
| Cough | Caused by secretions, productive | Caused by irritation of lung receptors, usually dry |
| Secretions | Mucoid or purulent | Frothy, white or pink |
| Clearance of secretions | Cough or suction | Diuretics |
| Radiology | Normal, or related to lung disease | Bilateral hilar flare, often enlarged heart, sometimes pleural effusion |
| Albumin | Normal | May be reduced |

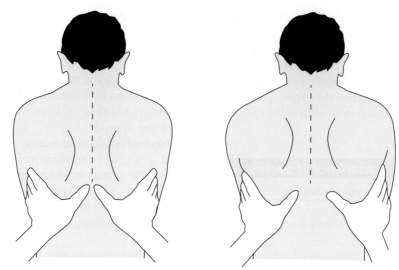

**FIGURE 2.8** Palpation for rib cage expansion. The fingers hold the sides of the chest and the thumbs rest lightly on each side of the spine. On inspiration, symmetrical separation of the thumb tips indicates equal chest expansion (From Wilkins et al. 2010).

Careful questioning is needed to identify whether expectorated blood has been swallowed and vomited, or if vomited blood has been aspirated and expectorated.

## PALPATION

### Abdomen

The abdomen enjoys a close relationship with the diaphragm. After obtaining permission it should be palpated at every assessment. A distended abdomen inhibits diaphragmatic movement, restricts lung volume and increases WOB. Causes of distension include pain and guarding spasm, obesity, flatulence, paralytic ileus, enlarged liver, ascites, acute pancreatitis and constipation.

### Chest Expansion

Chest movement reflects lung expansion. The patient sits over the edge of the bed if possible and their chest observed or palpated from behind as they take a deep breath (Fig. 2.8), unequal expansion suggesting loss of lung volume.

While palpating for expansion, other signs may be felt such as the crackling of sputum or, around the neck and upper chest, the popping of subcutaneous emphysema, which feels like Rice Krispies under the skin.

### Percussion Note

The percussion note (PN) is elicited by tapping the chest wall with a stiff curved finger from the dominant hand onto a finger from the other hand placed flat on the patient's chest (Fig. 2.9). To avoid dampening the sound, the dominant finger should recoil sharply, like a woodpecker striking a tree. All the movement is in the wrist.

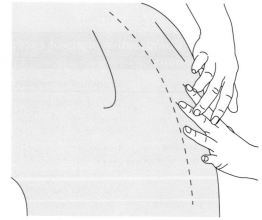

**FIGURE 2.9** Eliciting a percussion note. One finger is placed firmly along an intercostal space and struck by a finger of the opposite hand.

The PN evaluates the density of underlying tissue to a depth of 5–7 cm (Wilkins et al. 2010, p. 79). It is useful for confirming auscultation findings, and is especially helpful if patients are unable to take a deep breath or if breath sounds are obscured by a noisy environment or loud wheezy crackles. Each side of the chest should be percussed alternately for comparison, remembering that the upper lobe predominates anteriorly and the lower lobe posteriorly (Fig. 2.10).

The PN is **resonant** over normal lung tissue. **Hyper-resonance** indicates excess air, as with hyperinflation or a large pneumothorax. A **stony dull** note is unmistakable

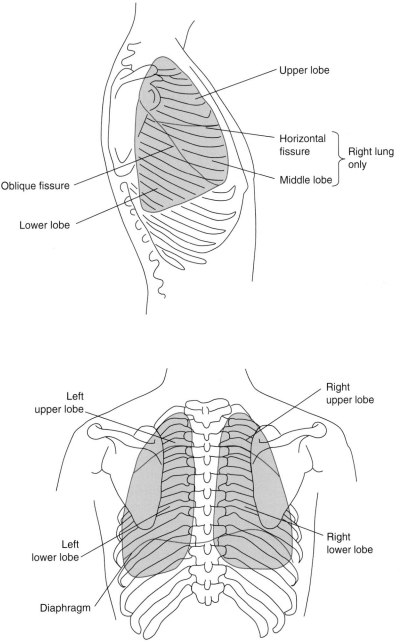

**FIGURE 2.10** Lateral and posterior views of the lobes and fissures of the lungs.

and heard over a pleural effusion larger than 500 mL. However, both these conditions are detected more clearly radiologically unless the patient is supine. Most useful to the physiotherapist is the **dull** note of atelectasis or consolidation, in which the air that should be in the lung is replaced by solid (albeit squashy) tissue.

## Hydration

The 1500 mL fluid intake that is normally required per day may not be achieved by people who are ill or in an unfamiliar environment. Patients at risk are:

- older people
- those who feel too sick to drink
- some who are not on intravenous fluids
- those who are constipated or pyrexial

A patient who has heart failure and does not have swollen ankles should be closely examined for dehydration.

Dehydration causes inelastic skin, but so does ageing; it causes a dry tongue and lips, but so do mouth-breathing and oxygen therapy. Clinical assessment for dehydration is imperfect but the following are suggestions:

1. The skin over the sternum preserves its elasticity with age, and when pinched gently, should bounce back. If it stays creased, it is called 'tenting' and indicates reduced skin turgor and dehydration.
2. The axilla has a dry, velvety feel in most dehydrated people (Eaton et al. 1994).

Dehydration is also suspected in a patient with dark urine, a white coating on the tongue, slow capillary refill (see below), postural hypotension with a racing pulse, or increased urea, creatinine, sodium and potassium levels. Weakness, malaise, headache, nausea, vomiting, cramps, weight loss, dry mouth, thirst, oliguria, tachycardia and low-grade fever are indicative of, but not specific to, dehydration.

## Trachea

**Tracheal deviation** is detected by gentle palpation in the suprasternal notch. In the absence of thyroid enlargement, deviation is due to a shift of the mediastinum away from a large pleural effusion or tension pneumothorax, or a shift towards upper lobe atelectasis or fibrosis, which can be confirmed radiologically (see Fig. 2.16). A hyperinflated chest causes a **tracheal tug**, which is descent of the trachea on inspiration, when it is pulled downwards by the low flat diaphragm.

## Capillary Refill Time

With good circulation, pressing briefly on the nail or pulp of a finger to obstruct the circulation is followed by rapid return of normal colour. If this capillary refill is >2 s, reduced cardiac output or hypovolaemia is suspected.

## Tactile Vocal Fremitus

A hand flat on the chest can feel the vibration of the voice, which is the palpatory equivalent of vocal resonance (p. 47).

# AUSCULTATION

Auscultation is used to verify observed and palpated findings before and after treatment. Prior to reaching for the stethoscope, it is worth listening for sounds at the mouth, which are just audible in a person with normal lungs. Noisy breathing indicates airflow turbulence due to obstructed upper airways. Crackles heard at the mouth should be cleared by coughing to prevent them masking other sounds during auscultation.

## Technique

The basic positions for placement of the stethoscope are in Fig. 2.11, but further positions may be necessary if required. Fig. 2.10 is a reminder to avoid listening optimistically for breath sounds over the kidney, inferior to the posterior surface markings of the lower lobes. The diaphragm of the stethoscope is used for the high frequencies of breath sounds. The bell is used for the low frequencies of heart sounds, or with small children. The ear pieces face forward into the ears and the diaphragm is pressed firmly onto the skin to reduce extraneous sounds including the rustle of chest hair. The patient is asked to breathe steadily in and out through the mouth. Each area of lung is compared on alternate sides, asymmetrical sounds usually indicating pathology.

The patient is best positioned sitting upright over the edge of the bed with arms forward to protract the scapulae and the physiotherapist standing behind. A compromise is with the patient in bed leaning forward from long sitting, but this position compresses the lung bases so that breath sounds over this important area may be indecipherable. In patients who cannot sit up, side-lying may be used, with allowance for sounds from the underneath lung usually being quieter. The diaphragm of the stethoscope should be cleaned between patients.

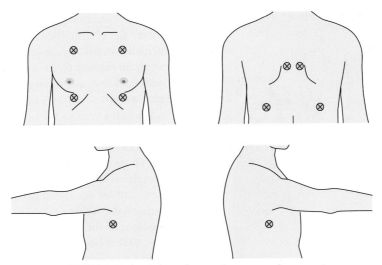

FIGURE 2.11 Locations for stethoscope placement.

## Breath Sounds

Breath sound intensity indicates regional ventilation or factors which affect transmission of the sound. Breath sounds are generated by turbulent airflow in the large airways but not beyond lobar or segmental bronchi because the total cross-sectional area is too wide to create turbulence (see Fig. 1.4). They are then transmitted through air, liquid and solid to the chest wall, each medium attenuating the sound to a different degree so that sounds at the surface are filtered versions of those in the large airways. The term 'breath sounds' is more accurate than 'air entry' because air may enter the lung but the transmission of sound can be affected by pathology.

Breath sounds may be normal, abnormal or diminished. **Normal** breath sounds are muffled because air in the alveoli is a poor conductor of sound. They are quieter in the base than the apex because the greater volume in the lung bases filters the sound further. Inspiration is louder than expiration because of turbulence created by airway bifurcations (Fig. 2.12).

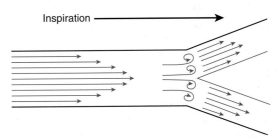

FIGURE 2.12 Turbulence at airway bifurcation creating noises on inspiration.

**Bronchial breathing** is an abnormal sound that is distinguished by a hollow blowing quality on expiration and a pause between inspiration and expiration. It indicates loss of functioning lung volume and is heard over the following:

- consolidation, which acts acoustically like a lump of meat in the lung, the solid medium transmitting sounds more clearly than air-filled lung (Fig. 2.13);
- a small area of collapse, when there is a patent airway to transmit the sound, but it then has to pass through collapsed lung tissue before reaching the surface;
- above a pleural effusion because the compressed lung increases sound transmission (Sapira 1995).

**Diminished** breath sounds are heard if:

- there is no air entry to generate the sound, e.g. a larger area of collapse than that causing bronchial breathing, i.e. there is an occluded airway;

### PRACTICE TIP

If the patient is unable to take a deep enough breath, the deep breathing following exertion can be utilized by listening immediately after the patient has talked, coughed, turned or been suctioned.

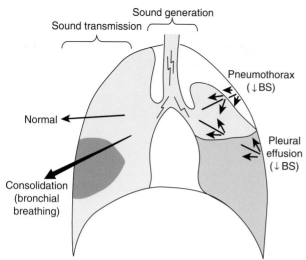

**FIGURE 2.13** Mechanism of the creation of different breath sounds. *BS*, breath sounds.

- there is air entry but transmission of the sound is blocked by an acoustic barrier such as a pneumothorax or pleural effusion (Fig. 2.13);
- there is air entry but excess air in the lung filters the sound, e.g. hyperinflation as in emphysema or acute asthma;
- the patient is obese, in a poor position or not breathing deeply.

Inaudible breath sounds over the chest of a person with acute asthma are a danger sign (p. 83).

## Added Sounds

Added sounds may be superimposed on breath sounds. They are sometimes more obvious and can mask breath sounds.

> ### PRACTICE TIP
>
> If added sounds are louder on one side, this may be due to increased added sounds on this side, or reduced breath sounds through which to hear the added sounds on the other side.

**Crackles** indicate secretions or parenchymal disorders such as pneumonia, fibrosis or pulmonary oedema. They are created when air is forced through airways which have been narrowed by inflammation, excess secretions or pulmonary oedema fluid that has migrated up from the alveoli (Bennett et al. 2015a). They are principally heard on inspiration, and their timing depends on the source. As a generalization:

- early and mid-inspiratory crackles arise in the large airways, are sometimes heard at the mouth and are often heard with COPD;
- early and midinspiratory crackles are characteristic of bronchiectasis or cystic fibrosis;
- late-inspiratory crackles originate in alveoli and peripheral airways as they open at the end of inspiration, and are associated with pneumonia, fibrosis or pulmonary oedema.

The weight of the lung itself causes a degree of airway closure so that late-inspiratory crackles may be heard in dependent regions, especially in elderly obese people who have been recumbent for some time. Late-inspiratory crackles are sometimes called crepitations, fine crackles, dry crackles or velcro crackles (Sellarés et al. 2016). Crackles are heard predominantly on inspiration, but both inspiratory and expiratory crackles are heard in bronchiectasis (coarse) and fibrosing alveolitis (fine). Absence of coarse crackles does not always indicate absence of secretions (Jones & Jones 2000).

**Wheezes** are generated by the vibration of narrowed airways as air rushes through. Expiratory wheeze, combined with prolonged expiration, is usually caused by bronchospasm. Wheeze on inspiration and expiration can be caused by inflammation, pulmonary oedema, bronchial secretions, tumours or foreign bodies. These are termed polyphonic wheezes. Less common is a monophonic (single note) wheeze, denoting upper airway obstruction from a foreign body or tumour. It is greater on inspiration and is also heard without a stethoscope.

**Stridor** is an inspiratory strangled sound that can also be heard without a stethoscope. It denotes laryngeal or tracheal narrowing to a diameter of just 5 mm (Thomas & Manara 1998) and is a warning that nasopharyngeal suction should be avoided and the patient's head kept elevated to minimize oedema. Treatment of stridor is by steroids, heliox or stenting.

A **pleural rub** occurs in pleurisy, when the roughened inflamed pleural surfaces rub on each other and produce a sound similar to boots crunching on snow. It is localized to the affected area, but may be heard best over the lower lobes because excursion of the pleura is greater basally.

Nonrespiratory sounds occur independently of the breathing cycle and may be transmitted from the abdomen, the patient's voice or the environment.

## Voice Sounds

The vibrations of speech can be felt by the hands (tactile vocal fremitus) or heard through the stethoscope (vocal resonance). The patient is asked to say '99', or engaged in conversation.

Voice sounds are normally an unintelligible mumble because vowels are filtered through air-filled lung. **Increased voice sounds** create a clearer sound, heard when it is transmitted through a denser medium, e.g. consolidation, or a small area of atelectasis with a patent airway. This is usually associated with bronchial breathing and is sometimes known as *bronchophony*. Voice sounds transmitted above the liquid/air interface at the top of a pleural effusion have a characteristic nasal bleating quality, a slightly different form of increased vocal resonance called *aegophony*.

**Reduced voice sounds** are heard when there is a pneumothorax, pleural effusion or large patch of atelectasis with a blocked airway. Voice sounds tend to follow the breath sounds, i.e. they increase with bronchial breathing and decrease with quiet breath sounds.

Another confirmatory test is to ask the patient to whisper '99'. Over normal lung tissue, whispered words are barely audible, but through a solid medium such as consolidation, individual syllables are recognizable. This is known as **whispering pectoriloquy.**

The digital stethoscope transforms sound data into electrical signals, which can be amplified, stored and replayed, making it useful in telemedicine (Lakhe et al. 2016).

## IMAGING

> **AP**: anteroposterior
> **PA**: posteroanterior
> **L**: left, **R**: right,
> **LL**: lower lobe, **UL**: upper lobe

The chest radiograph provides a unique insight into the lungs and chest wall, but it has limitations:

1. A two-dimensional representation of a three-dimensional object can obscure the relationship between structures.

2. Radiology findings tend to lag behind other measurements, e.g. they are a later indication of chest infection than pyrexia, and pneumonia may have resolved for days or even weeks while X-ray signs still linger.

3. A normal radiograph does not rule out disease because its contribution is structural only, e.g. the physical damage of emphysema is more apparent than the hypersecretion of chronic bronchitis because secretions do not normally show on X-ray.

If possible, a posteroanterior (**PA**) view is taken, in which the beam is directed from the back, the patient standing up and taking a deep breath with shoulders abducted so that the scapulae do not obscure the lungs. The posterior ribs are clearly visible but become more obscure anteriorly (Fig. 2.14). In the erect position it is easy to detect a pleural effusion because of its visible fluid line, or a medium-sized pneumothorax because gas passes upwards.

An anteroposterior (**AP**) film is used when it is unsafe for patients to go to the radiology department due to immobility or impaired immunity. Patients sit up ('erect portable') or lie down, and a portable machine sends the rays from front to back. The patient may not be able to raise their arms or take a deep breath, leaving the lung fields partly obscured by the scapulae and diaphragm. The heart appears larger and the anterior ribs are less clear than in a PA film. In supine, the fluid of a pleural effusion spreads throughout that side of the thorax, giving a haze-like appearance which differs from parenchymal densities in that vascular markings are visible through the density. Fig. 2.15 indicates the location of structures.

## Systematic Analysis

A methodical approach avoids the viewer becoming diverted by the first obvious abnormality. Previous films should be viewed for comparison. Allowance needs to be made for normal variations between individuals such as different shaped diaphragms. Chest films show bilateral symmetry for many structures, enabling opposite sides to be compared.

Abnormalities can be classified into whether they are:
- too white
- too black
- too big
- in the wrong place (Corne & Kumaran 2015)

Dense structures absorb rays and are opaque, while air has low density and appears black.

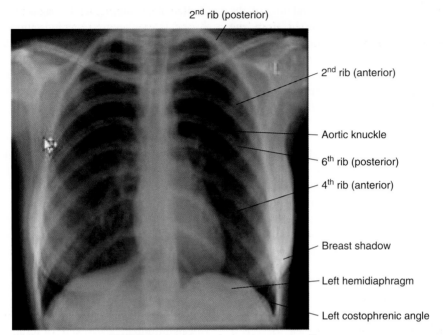

FIGURE 2.14 Normal posteroanterior film.

2nd rib (posterior)

2nd rib (anterior)

Aortic knuckle

6th rib (posterior)

4th rib (anterior)

Breast shadow

Left hemidiaphragm

Left costophrenic angle

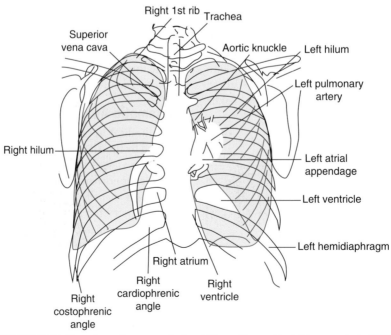

Right 1st rib   Trachea

Superior
vena cava

Aortic knuckle    Left hilum

Left pulmonary
artery

Right hilum

Left atrial
appendage

Left ventricle

Left hemidiaphragm

Right atrium

Right
cardiophrenic
angle

Right
ventricle

Right
costophrenic
angle

FIGURE 2.15 Drawing of a normal chest X-ray (From Hodgkinson et al. 1993).

## Preliminary checks

The patient's **name** and the **date** should be identified. Then the **projection** is checked to see whether it is a PA or AP film. The **exposure** is then noted: an overexposed film appears too black and low density lesions can be missed, while an underexposed film appears falsely white. Correct exposure allows vertebral bodies to be visible through the upper but not the lower heart shadow.

**Symmetry** is correct if the spinous processes, which appear as teardrop shapes down the spine, are midway between the medial ends of the clavicles. This check avoids misinterpretation about displacement of the heart, which is at the front of the chest so that if the patient rotates to either side, the heart shadow appears shifted towards that side.

## Trachea

The vertical dark column of air overlying the upper vertebrae represents the trachea, which is in the midline down to the clavicles, then displaced slightly to the right by the aortic arch, before branching into the main bronchi. Abnormal deviation occurs if it is pushed, for example by a tumour, or pulled, for example by atelectasis or fibrosis (Fig. 2.16).

## Heart

The heart is sandwiched between the lungs and is the main occupant of the mediastinum. Points to note are:

**Size**. The transverse diameter is normally less than half the diameter of the chest in a PA film. An enlarged heart could be due to heart failure (see Fig. 4.3), an AP film or poor inspiratory effort. A narrow heart is caused by hyperinflation, when the diaphragm pulls down the mediastinum (Fig. 2.17), or it may be normal in tall thin people.

**Shape**. In right ventricular hypertrophy, the heart appears enlarged and boot-shaped. A rounded heart might indicate pericardial effusion.

**Position**. The heart normally extends slightly left of midline. If displaced, it is pushed away from a large pleural effusion (Fig. 2.18) or tension pneumothorax

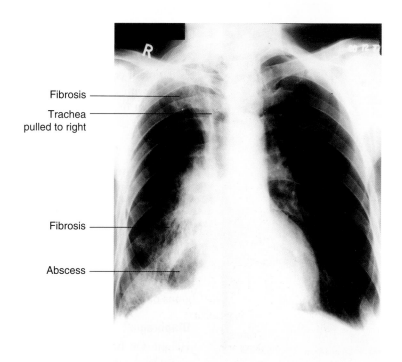

**FIGURE 2.16** Fibrosis in the right upper lobe pulling the trachea to the right. Fibrosis and an abscess are visible in the right mid- and lower zones. The patient has tuberculosis.

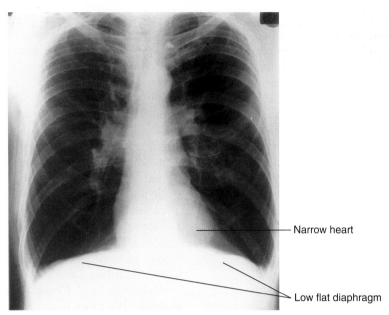

FIGURE 2.17 Hyperinflated chest as indicated by a low flat diaphragm and narrow heart, suggesting emphysema.

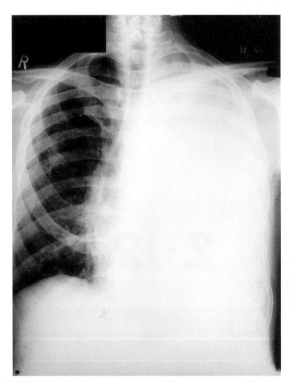

FIGURE 2.18 A large pleural effusion in the left chest is obliterating the left lung and pushing the mediastinum away from the effusion.

(see Fig. 21.29), and pulled towards a significant unilateral collapse (Fig. 2.19), resection (see Fig. 14.23a) or fibrosis (see Fig. 2.16).

**Borders**. These are obscured (silhouette sign) if there is a lesion abutting the heart, e.g. middle lobe consolidation or collapse. Apposition of the extra density of lung with a contiguous structure such as the diaphragm or heart obliterates the boundary between the two.

## Hila

Blood and lymph vessels make up the hilar shadows, the left being slightly higher because of the heart. Hila are abnormally pulled up if there is upper lobe (UL) fibrosis, atelectasis or lobectomy, and pulled down by lower lobe (LL) atelectasis. Ring shadows near the hilum are normal large airways seen in cross section. Bilateral enlargement of hilar shadows could be due to pulmonary hypertension. Unilateral enlargement raises suspicions of malignancy.

## Diaphragm

**Height**. On full inspiration, the diaphragm should be about level with the 6th ribs anteriorly, 8th laterally and 10th posteriorly. The right side is about 2 cm higher than the left because it is pushed up by the liver while

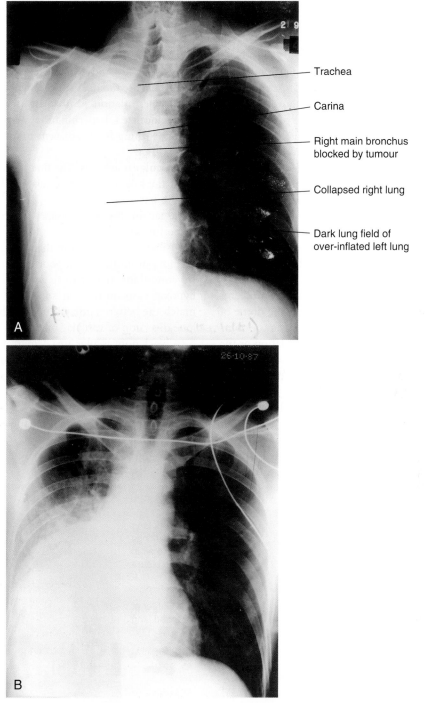

Trachea

Carina

Right main bronchus blocked by tumour

Collapsed right lung

Dark lung field of over-inflated left lung

**FIGURE 2.19** (A) Atelectasis of the right lung, showing the mediastinum pulled towards the opacity. The right main bronchus was blocked by a tumour. (B) Atelectasis of the right lower lobe, showing shift of the mediastinum towards the lost lung volume on the patient's right.

the left is pushed down by the heart. A low flat diaphragm suggests hyperinflation (Fig. 2.17). An elevated diaphragm could be:

- positional as in an AP film;
- physiological due to lack of a full inspiration;
- pathological due to pressure from below, e.g. abdominal distension, or a shrinking lung above, e.g. lung fibrosis (Fig. 2.20).

If one side of the diaphragm is raised, this could be due to lower lobe atelectasis or resection, a paralysed hemidiaphragm or, on the left, excess gas in the stomach.

**Shape**. The diaphragm should be dome-shaped and smooth. Hyperinflation flattens it, while fibrosis can pull it up upwards into two peaks (see Fig. 2.20). Loss of the smooth surface may be caused by lower lobe or pleural abnormality.

**Costophrenic angles**. These delineate the ribs and diaphragm, being of interest to the physiotherapist because they provide the first clue to problems lurking in the base of the lung behind the dome of the diaphragm. The normal acute angle may be obliterated by the patchy shadow of consolidation or the smooth meniscus of a pleural effusion, although 200–300 mL of fluid needs to accumulate in the pleura before blunting the costophrenic angle.

**Subphrenic area**. Air under the right hemidiaphragm is expected after abdominal surgery. If it persists for more than a week, or appears spontaneously, it may indicate a subphrenic abscess or perforated gut. An air bubble under the left hemidiaphragm, sometimes containing a fluid line, is usually in the stomach and therefore normal.

## Lung fields

Lungs that are too white usually indicate infiltrates. Lungs that are too dark suggest hyperinflation. Generalized hyperinflation is normally due to lung disease, while localized hyperinflation may be due to overexpanded lung tissue adjacent to lobar collapse. Other observations are below.

**Vascular markings**. The fine white lines fanning out from the hila are blood vessels and lymphatics, which should be:

- larger in the lower zones to reflect the greater perfusion;
- visible up to 2 cm from the lung margin;
- more prominent with poor inspiration.

In conditions that reduce ventilation to the bases, hypoxic vasoconstriction squeezes blood upwards to match the better-ventilated upper lobes, causing upper lobe diversion of vascular markings (see Fig. 4.3).

A black nonvascular area demarcated medially by the white line of the visceral pleura indicates a pneumothorax (Fig. 2.21). A small pneumothorax is easier to see on an expiratory film and a tiny pneumothorax may be seen in a lateral decubitus view (patient side-lying). Reversing black and white by changing from positive to negative may also be helpful.

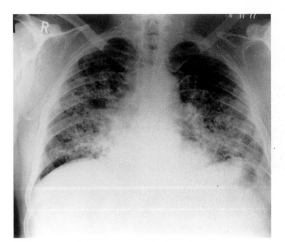

**FIGURE 2.20** Diaphragm pulled up by the contracting lung tissue of fibrosing alveolitis.

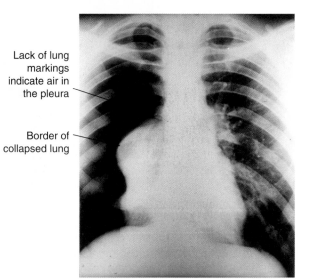

Lack of lung markings indicate air in the pleura

Border of collapsed lung

**FIGURE 2.21** Large right pneumothorax.

**Horizontal fissure**. This is a thin white line visible in 60% of normal films, from the right hilum to the 6th rib in the axilla. It is pulled upwards by UL collapse and downwards by LL collapse.

**Diffuse shadowing**. Examples are:
- ground glass appearance indicating alveolar pathology such as inflammation;
- reticular or a coarser honeycomb pattern, representing progressive damage, e.g. inflammation progressing to fibrosis in interstitial disease (see Fig. 2.20);
- 'batswing' pattern fanning out from the hila, suggesting pulmonary oedema (see Fig. 4.3);
- infiltrates as in diffuse pneumonia;
- the snowstorm appearance of acute respiratory distress syndrome (see Fig. 22.19).

**Unilateral whiteout**. Dense opacities can be caused by lung collapse (see Fig. 2.19) or pneumonectomy (see Fig. 14.4) both of which pull the mediastinum towards the lesion, or a large pleural effusion, which pushes the mediastinum away (see Fig. 2.18).

**Ring shadows**. These represent:
- bullae, which have hair-line borders, are air-filled and usually associated with emphysema;
- a cyst, with wall thickness >1 mm, often associated with bronchiectasis or cystic fibrosis;
- a thick-walled abscess, often containing a fluid level (Fig. 2.22).

**Air bronchogram**. Airways are visible if they are contrasted against an opacity such as pulmonary oedema or consolidation (Fig. 2.23). If an area of collapse has no air bronchogram, the airway is obstructed.

**Fluid line**. This is a horizontal line, sometimes with a meniscus at the edge, atop a dense opacity. It may indicate the level of pus in an abscess (see Fig. 2.22), fluid in a stomach bubble under the left hemidiaphragm or, if it spans the width of the lung, a pleural effusion (Fig. 2.24).

**Opacities with no shift of adjacent structures**. Consolidation is represented by a patchy opacity, often indicating pneumonia, frequently displaying air bronchograms and usually occupying a lobe or segment (see Figs 2.23 and 3.31). Opacities of about 3 cm diameter may be pulmonary masses, those of 5–10 mm are called pulmonary nodules and those of 1–2 mm are miliary nodules. Bronchial tumours are usually located proximally, while metastases may be scattered.

**Opacities with shift of adjacent structures**. Loss of lung volume causes shift of a moveable structure, e.g. the diaphragm (see Fig. 14.22), mediastinum (see Fig. 2.19), fissure or hilum, towards the area of lost volume. There may also be crowding of vascular markings, with compensatory hyperaeration of adjacent lung tissue which appears darker, and loss of a border if the collapse is on the same plane as a structure such as the heart or diaphragm. A large collapse may cause rib crowding.

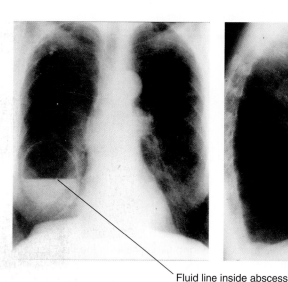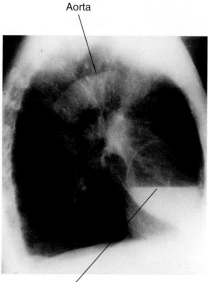

Aorta

Fluid line inside abscess

**FIGURE 2.22** Posteroanterior and lateral film showing a lung abscess in the middle lobe.

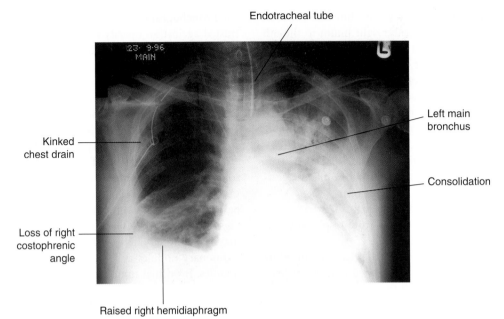

Endotracheal tube

Left main
bronchus

Consolidation

Kinked
chest drain

Loss of right
costophrenic
angle

Raised right hemidiaphragm

**FIGURE 2.23** Left lower lobe pneumonia showing air bronchograms. Loss of right costophrenic angle suggests there is also some infiltration of the right lower lobe, and raised right hemidiaphragm indicates right lower lobe lost volume. Patient is intubated, rotated to his left and has a kinked right apical chest drain.

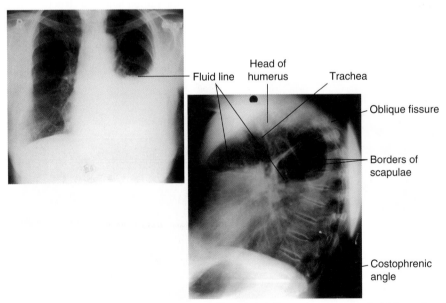

Fluid line

Head of
humerus

Trachea

Oblique fissure

Borders of
scapulae

Costophrenic
angle

**FIGURE 2.24** Posteroanterior (left) and lateral film (right) films showing the fluid line of a pleural effusion. The lateral picture shows fluid seeping up into the oblique fissure (which is invaginated pleura). Crossing this fissure can be seen the two borders of the scapulae and anterior to these is the black trachea. The head and shaft of the humerus can also be seen.

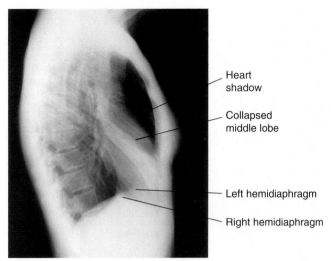

Heart shadow

Collapsed middle lobe

Left hemidiaphragm

Right hemidiaphragm

**FIGURE 2.25** Lateral film showing dense opacity of a collapsed wedge-shaped middle lobe against the less dense opacity of the lozenge-shaped heart. The upper border of the wedge is the horizontal fissure and the lower border the oblique fissure. The patient is facing towards the right of the picture.

The RUL collapses into a triangular opacity, with the horizontal fissure migrating upwards. LUL collapse shows loss of the left upper cardiac border and elevation of the left hilum. Middle lobe collapse shows silhouetting of the R heart border but is more obvious in a lateral film (Fig. 2.25).

A fuzzy and raised hemidiaphragm suggests LL collapse. The heart border remains clear because the lower lobes are posterior. LLL collapse may form a straight line, or 'sail' shape, either behind the heart, or overlapping and obliterating the heart border (see Fig. 3.13).

The following lobes may be collapsed or consolidated if these borders are obscured:
- LLL: L hemidiaphragm
- RLL: R hemidiaphragm
- LUL: aortic arch
- RUL: R upper mediastinum
- lingula: L heart border
- middle lobe: R heart border

## Bones

The bones are examined with care following cardio-pulmonary resuscitation or other trauma, or if the patient is suspected of having osteoporosis or malignant secondary deposits. A fresh rib fracture is seen as displacement of the border of the rib, which helps distinguish it from other overlapping structures. Old fractures are identified by callous formation. Bony secondaries may appear as densities. Cough fractures may show up in bones weakened by malignancy or osteoporosis.

If any positive-pressure treatment is planned for a patient who has fractured ribs, a radiologist should be asked to check the film because a pneumothorax may be hiding, for example, behind the cluster of rib shadows at the apex.

## Artefact

Extrathoracic tissues cause shadows that may project onto the lung fields, e.g. rolls of fat or breast shadows. Hardware may also be apparent, e.g. the radio-opaque tip of a nasogastric tube in the stomach or a tracheal tube above the carina. Other tubes and lines are discussed in Chapter 21.

## Lateral Film

A lateral film (Fig. 2.26) shows the lungs superimposed on each other. Different structures may be either more or less distinguishable than on the PA film. Lesions that were concealed behind the diaphragm or heart may now be apparent, e.g.:
1. Lower lobe collapse may appear as a white triangle in the costophrenic angle.

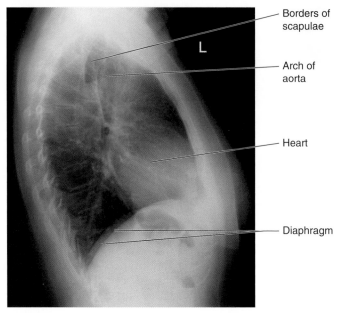

Borders of scapulae

Arch of aorta

Heart

Diaphragm

FIGURE 2.26 Lateral film of a normal lung (https://radiopaedia.org). (Copyright 2017 Dr Henry Knipe. Image courtesy Dr Henry Knipe and Radiopaedia.org. Used under licence.)

2. A pleural effusion of just 50 mL can now blunt the costophrenic angle.
3. If the oblique fissure is visible, any lesion behind it is in a lower lobe.

Fig. 2.27 illustrates the different structures visible on a lateral film.

## Other Tests

### Tomography

Computed tomography (CT) scans provide computed digital images from cross-sectional films, viewed as if from a supine patient's feet (Fig. 2.28). Manipulation of the data produces images in any plane, creating greater sensitivity to soft tissues than conventional X-rays and without interference from overlying structures, at the cost of a greater radiation dose.

For diagnosis, CT scans identify interstitial lung disease, lung cancer, pulmonary embolism, TB and the thick-walled dilated airways of advanced bronchiectasis, as well as determining the distribution of emphysema in anticipation of surgery. For physiotherapy, CT scans detect consolidation, atelectasis, abscesses, cavities, pleural effusion, pneumothorax and bullae (Saure et al. 2016).

Variations are:
• high-resolution CT scans, which achieve greater sensitivity for diffuse lung diseases by using thinner slices;
• spiral CT, which scans the whole chest with one breath-hold, reducing radiation exposure and motion artefact from breathing;
• contrast agents to highlight blood vessels, e.g. for detecting pulmonary embolism.

Ventilation–perfusion CT maps the distribution of ventilation and perfusion in the lung, and has the potential to identify airway obstruction (Mistry et al. 2010).

Electrical impedance tomography delivers information on regional ventilation and has been suggested as a guide to patient positioning (Lehmann et al. 2016).

### Magnetic resonance imaging

Magnetic resonance imaging is cross-sectional imaging free of ionizing radiation, which, amongst other things, can detect mucous plugging (Wielpütz et al. 2016).

### Fluoroscopy

Fluoroscopy projects moving images onto a monitor, e.g. to identify diaphragmatic paralysis. Videofluoroscopy is a modified barium swallow to identify dysphagia (Park & Lee 2012).

### Functional respiratory imaging

Functional imaging techniques offer the possibility of visualizing lobe volumes and airflow distribution in three dimensions (Hajian et al. 2016).

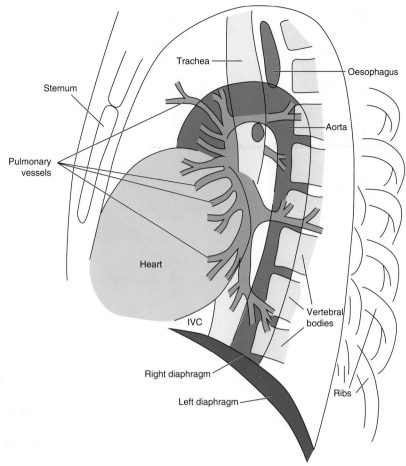

**FIGURE 2.27** Representation of lateral film in a patient facing to the left of the picture. *IVC,* inferior vena cava. (From Hodgkinson et al. 1993.)

# RESPIRATORY FUNCTION TESTS

**ERV**: expiratory reserve volume
**FEV₁**: forced expiratory volume in one second
**FRC**: functional residual capacity
**FVC**: forced vital capacity
**IRV**: inspiratory reserve volume
**L**: litre
**PCF**: peak cough flow
**PEFR**: peak expiratory flow rate (peak flow)
**RR**: respiratory rate
**RV**: residual volume
**TLC**: total lung capacity
**VC**: vital capacity
**V$_T$**: tidal volume
**V̇O$_2$**: oxygen consumption

Respiratory function tests quantify lung function in order to:

- define an abnormality, e.g. distinguish COPD from asthma;
- indicate the progress of disease or response to treatment;
- provide risk assessment, e.g. before surgery.

Tests are particularly useful for detecting an impending asthma attack or identifying ventilatory failure in progressive neurological disease. However, they bear little relation to quality of life (Fig. 2.29) and are rarely affected by physiotherapy.

Measurements vary with posture, ethnic origin, stature, smoking status (Mirabelli et al. 2016), sex and age (Verbanck et al. 2016), the last two variables relating

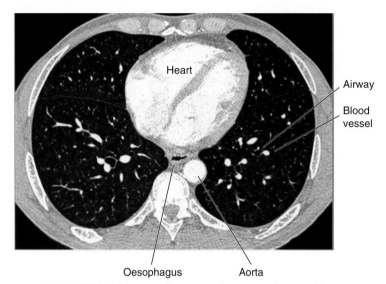

**FIGURE 2.28** Computed tomography scan of normal lung.

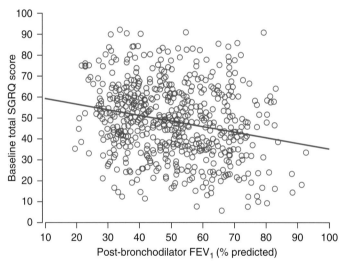

**FIGURE 2.29** Lack of correlation between forced expiratory volume in one second and quality of life, as measured by the St George's Respiratory Questionnaire (From Jones 2001).

to muscle strength and therefore most relevant to tests requiring effort. Some measurements depend on fitness and time of day or year.

## Working Definitions

If two or more subdivisions of lung volume are taken together, the sum is called a capacity.

All values are approximate.

**Peak expiratory flow rate** or **peak flow** (PF) is the highest flow that can be achieved during a forced expiration from a full inspiration. It is one of the parameters measured on the flow-volume loop (Fig. 2.33).

- Normal value: 300–600 L/min;
- Elderly males: 340 L/min (Sandhu et al. 2016);
- Severe airways obstruction: <100 L/min, or unrecordable.

**Vital capacity** (VC) is the volume of gas that can be exhaled after a full inspiration (Fig. 2.30) and represents the three volumes under volitional control: inspiratory

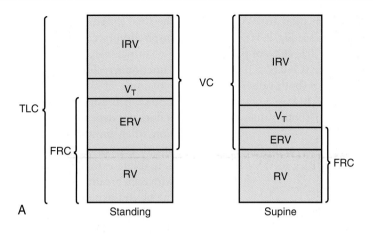

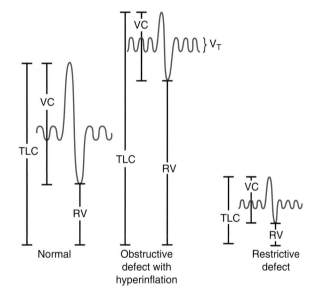

**FIGURE 2.30** (A) Volumes and capacities in standing and supine (From Levitzky 2013). (B) Lung volumes for different conditions. *RV,* Residual volume; *TLC,* total lung capacity; *VC,* vital capacity; $V_T$, tidal volume.

reserve volume (IRV), tidal volume ($V_T$) and expiratory reserve volume (ERV).

- Normal: 3–6 L, or approximately 80% of total lung capacity (TLC);
- For adequate cough: >1 L;
- Swimmers: above normal (Lazovic et al. 2016).

**Forced vital capacity** (FVC) is similar to VC but with forced exhalation (Fig. 2.31).

- Normal: equal to VC
- COPD: less than VC if the manoeuvre causes airway collapse

**Forced expiratory volume in one second** (FEV$_1$) is the volume of gas expelled in the first second by a forced exhalation from a full inhalation (see Fig. 2.31).

- Normal: 80% of VC, or 2–4 L;
- Severe airways obstruction: <30%–50% predicted.

**FEV$_1$/FVC** expresses FEV$_1$ in relation to FVC and is more accurate than FEV$_1$ alone (see Fig. 2.31).
- Normal: 0.7–0.8, i.e. FEV$_1$ = 70%–80% of FVC;
- Moderate airflow obstruction: 0.5–0.6;
- Severe airflow obstruction: 0.3 (both values reduced but with a greater dip in FEV$_1$);
- Restrictive disease: up to 1.0 (both values reduced but a greater dip in FVC).

**Total lung capacity** (TLC) is the sum of the four primary lung volumes (residual volume [RV], ERV, V$_T$, IRV), i.e.

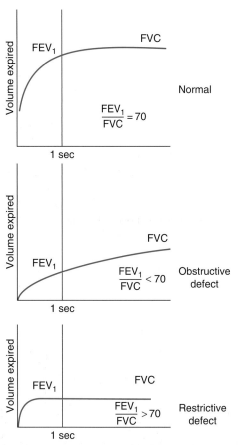

the total volume of gas in the lungs after maximum inspiration (see Fig. 2.30).
- Normal: 3–8 L

**Functional residual capacity** (FRC) is the volume of gas remaining at the end of a tidal exhalation (see Fig. 2.30A). It is a useful indicator of lung volume because it does not depend on effort, reflecting the resting position when inward and outward elastic recoil are balanced. The reasons for the normal large volume of FRC is to dilute extreme changes in alveolar oxygen tension with each breath, and to protect the alveoli from collapsing at end-expiration and then having to open again, causing atelectrauma. FRC is reduced with restrictive disorders and increased with lung hyperinflation.
- Normal in standing: about 40% of TLC, or approximately 2.4 L;
- Normal in supine: up to 2.2 L;
- COPD: up to 80% of TLC.

**Tidal volume** (V$_T$) is the volume of air inhaled and exhaled during one respiratory cycle (see Fig. 2.30). It mixes fresh gas with residual gas, as when the sea refreshes a tidal pool.
- Normal: 10% of VC, approx. 300–800 mL, average 7 mL/kg body weight;
- On exercise: up to 50% of VC.

**Inspiratory reserve volume** (IRV) is the extra volume of gas that can be inhaled voluntarily from end-inspiratory V$_T$ (see Fig. 2.30A). It is used during deep breathing exercises or with exertion. It is decreased in people with hyperinflated lungs because the breath starts from a higher FRC. IRV is determined by inspiratory muscle strength, effort and size of the starting point (FRC + V$_T$).
- Normal: 3.1 L

**Expiratory reserve volume** (ERV) is the extra volume of gas that can be exhaled forcefully from end-expiratory V$_T$ (see Fig. 2.30A). It is decreased with obesity, ascites or after upper abdominal surgery.
- Normal: 1.2 L

**Residual volume** (RV) is the volume of gas remaining in the lungs after maximum exhalation (see Fig. 2.30). It is inhaled with the first breath at birth and not exhaled until death because the outward recoil of the chest wall prevents the lungs emptying completely. RV prevents the lungs collapsing at low lung volumes, causing atelectrauma, and avoids the need for a mighty inspiratory effort for reinflation. It is measured by gas dilution or body plethysmography (see p. 62). It is reduced with restrictive disease and increased with age or gas

**FIGURE 2.31** Spirograms. **Normal**: most of the forced expiratory volume is expelled within 1 s, the decreasing slope of the curve being caused by progressive airway compression and lower elastic recoil during exhalation. **Obstructive**: prolonged exhalation. **Restrictive**: reduced forced vital capacity, all of which is expelled within a second due to augmented recoil.

trapping, the ratio of RV to TLC being an index of hyperinflation.

- Normal: 20%–30% of TLC, average 1.2 L

**Minute volume/ventilation** is the volume of gas breathed in or out per minute, i.e. $V_T \times RR$.

- Normal: 5–7 L/min;
- COPD: approx. 9 L/min;
- Acute respiratory failure: up to 10 L/min, but the patient may not be able to sustain the work of breathing required, leading to ventilatory failure;
- On brief maximum exercise: up to 150 L/min.

**Maximum voluntary ventilation** is the volume of air inhaled and exhaled with maximum effort over 12–15 s. It relates to endurance, energy expenditure and functional performance (Cavalheri et al. 2012).

- Normal: 50–200 L/min

## Airflow Obstruction

Measurements should be taken with the patient in loose clothing, not after a heavy meal or recent vigorous exercise, with an empty bladder, without smoking for at least an hour beforehand and with the head in neutral (Han et al. 2016a). The same position must be used for subsequent readings, preferably standing (Wallace et al. 2013) with a stable chair behind the patient because forced exhalation can cause dizziness.

If bronchodilators are to be tested, caffeine should be avoided in the previous 4 h (Welsh et al. 2010), and if the patient needs to take their inhaler during this time, it should be recorded. $FEV_1$ is normally higher in the morning (Lange 2009) except for people with asthma, and the same time of day should be used for comparative readings when possible. Accuracy is assisted by giving specific instructions and asking patients to keep dentures in place.

### Peak flow

The PF provides a quick and simple indication of airflow obstruction but varies with effort and expiratory muscle strength. Three tests are performed, with a rest in between, and the best test result recorded. A 'windmill' trainer helps children, elderly people and those with learning disabilities to master the technique (Clare & Teale 2001).

Suggested technique is to:

- explain the purpose of the test;
- check that the marker is at zero;
- demonstrate the technique with a separate device;

- ask the patient to take a deep breath, then, with a firm seal on the mouthpiece, blow 'short, sharp and as hard as possible'.

Dependence on motivation means that it is inaccurate for children under age four. It reflects only resistance in the large airways and is therefore invalid for people with COPD except to distinguish it from heart failure (Gough & Brewer 2012). PF is most usefully expressed as a percentage of the patient's previous best value, or if this is not available, as a percentage of that predicted for the patient's age and stature (as with spirometry, below). PF meters are available on prescription in the UK.

## Spirometry

Spirometry tells us how much and how fast air comes out of lungs. A spirometer tests volumes and is used for forced expiratory tests by measuring volume against time (see Fig. 2.31). As with any forced manoeuvre, it is difficult for breathless people, may bring on bronchospasm in susceptible patients and is affected by weak muscles. Contraindications are pneumothorax, haemoptysis of unknown origin, aneurysm, cardiovascular or cerebral instability, and recent surgery to the chest, abdomen or eyes (Ranu et al. 2011).

$FEV_1$ is more tiring than PF but more accurate because the first second is the most sensitive to airway resistance. After a standardized inspiration (Centanni 2003), patients are exhorted to 'blast the living daylights out of the machine, and keep blowing until your lungs are empty'. When exhalation is nearly complete, it is best to emphasize continuing as long as possible rather than as hard as possible because forceful blowing can reduce expiratory time due to airway collapse. The recording needs to continue until a plateau is reached, which can take up to 15 s in someone with severe COPD. The expiratory volume/time trace should be smooth and free from irregularities. Much uninhibited encouragement is required, repeated on subsequent measurements.

Three technically satisfactory readings are required for accuracy, with at least two within 100 mL or 5% of each other. $FEV_1$ is subject to day-to-day fluctuations and declines with smoking (Fig. 2.32) and age, normal lungs losing 25% to 30% of their $FEV_1$ over a lifetime (Washko 2012). It also declines with air pollution and some occupational exposures, e.g. in New York firefighters after 9/11 (Holguin 2012). Many researchers take account of the above, but the results are also

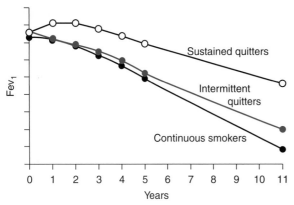

**FIGURE 2.32** Decline in forced expiratory volume in one second with age in smokers and in those who have quit smoking, which can be used as a motivating tool for people who are still smoking.

affected by pain (invalidating research involving pre- and postoperative comparisons), muscular effort and motivation.

**Vital capacity** is useful for measuring ventilatory reserve, indicating the ability to breathe deeply and cough. VC is sometimes reduced in obstructive disorders and always in restrictive disorders. It is also diminished with respiratory muscle weakness and is subject to day-to-day fluctuations. Measurement requires the patient to blow out from maximal inspiration and at a comfortable and sustained speed until no more can be exhaled. **FVC** is done with maximal and forceful exhalation. The **FEV$_1$/FVC** ratio is a standard diagnostic test for COPD (p. 76).

A **flow-volume loop** is produced when a patient performs maximum inspiration followed by maximum expiration (see Fig. 2.33). During inspiration, flow is dependent on effort throughout. During expiration, the highest flow occurs initially, where it is dependent on effort and represents large airway function. After a small proportion of VC has been exhaled, flow is independent of effort because increased driving pressure will not increase flow due to the small airways collapsing under the pressure of dynamic compression (p. 206). Flow then depends solely on elastic recoil and small airway resistance.

In obstructive disease, expiratory flow shows a concave appearance representing attenuation of expiration as floppy airways collapse or narrowed airways obstruct. Restrictive disease shows a limited ability to generate flow.

'Lung age' can be identified from spirometry but this is a frightening concept for patients, who should be reassured that having '120-year-old lungs' is simply a technical term, that lungs have a large reserve capacity and that the septuagenarian Pope lost a lung in childhood and was in fine fettle at the time of writing.

## Measurements independent of effort

Maximum mid-expiratory flow (MMEF, MEF$_{50}$), or the mid-forced expiratory flow (FEF$_{25-75}$ or FEF$_{50}$), is the mean forced expiratory flow during the middle half of FVC and is independent of effort. It is measured by the pneumotachograph, which detects pressure drop across a resistance placed in the airstream. When related to FVC (MMEF/FVC) it suggests early COPD (Mirsadraee et al. 2013).

## Lung Volumes

Lungs cannot be completely emptied voluntarily and always retain their RV, so lung volumes are measured indirectly by one of the following:

- Plethysmography: the patient sits inside a sealed box in which the air is compressed, the resulting change in pressure enabling RV, FRC and TLC to be calculated. For more accurate results, e.g. to predict complications prior to lung surgery, high-resolution CT is required (Takahashi et al. 2016).
- Gas dilution: air in the lungs is mixed with an inert gas such as helium, the dilution of which gives an indication of lung volume.
- Nitrogen washout: nitrogen makes up 80% of air, so lung volume can be calculated by having the patient breathe nitrogen-free gas and measuring the expired nitrogen.

TLC and RV can also be measured by using one of the above plus spirometry.

Miller et al. (2005) provide standardization for some lung function tests, and Table 2.8 compares results for obstructive and restrictive disease.

Tidal and spirometric volumes can also be measured by inductive or light plethysmography, which measures chest and abdominal wall movement (Laouani et al. 2016). Unlike spirometry, effort is not required, and the physiotherapist can identify the relative contributions of chest and abdominal movement. Light plethysmography can also measure volume recruitment in ventilated patients (Fig. 2.34).

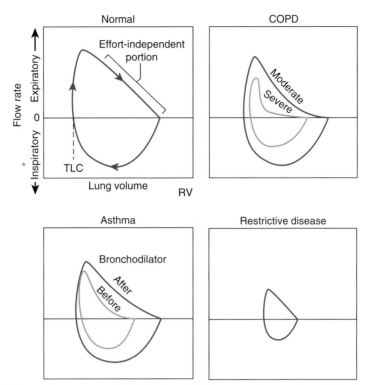

**FIGURE 2.33** Flow-volume loops. A dip in the effort-independent portion of the expiratory loop, above the line, indicates the obstructed airways of chronic obstructive pulmonary disease and asthma. A restrictive pattern is represented by a small loop and rapid expiration.

## Respiratory Muscle Function

These tests need to be done in the same position each time (Costa et al. 2015). More than one test is advised because individual tests of respiratory muscle strength tend to overdiagnose weakness (Steier et al. 2007).

1. **VC** is simple but relatively insensitive. Small pressures are required to inflate the lung, therefore reduced VC only occurs with severe muscle weakness. A fall of 25% or more in supine compared to upright may indicate diaphragmatic paralysis. Once it falls below 1 L, ventilatory support may be required (Ranu et al. 2011). Results are also influenced by effort, fitness and compliance of the lung and chest wall.

2. **Mouth pressures** comprise:
   - maximum inspiratory pressure (MIP), indicating diaphragmatic strength, measured from FRC and maintained for one second;
   - maximum expiratory pressure (MEP), indicating expiratory muscle and cough strength, measured from TLC.

**TABLE 2.8  Effect of obstructive and restrictive disease on volume and flow measurements**

|  | Obstructive | Restrictive |
|---|---|---|
| Tidal volume | Normal (N) | N or ↓ |
| VC | N or ↓ | ↓ |
| PF | ↓ | N or ↓ |
| FEV₁ | ↓ | N |
| FVC | N or ↓ | ↓ |
| FEV₁/FVC | ↓ | N or ↑ |
| RV | N or ↑ | N or ↓ |
| FRC | N or ↑ | ↓ |
| TLC | N or ↑ | ↓ |

$FEV_1$, Forced expiratory volume in one second; *FRC*, functional residual capacity; *FVC*, forced vital capacity; *PF*, peak flow; *RV*, residual volume; *TLC*, total lung capacity; *VC*, vital capacity.

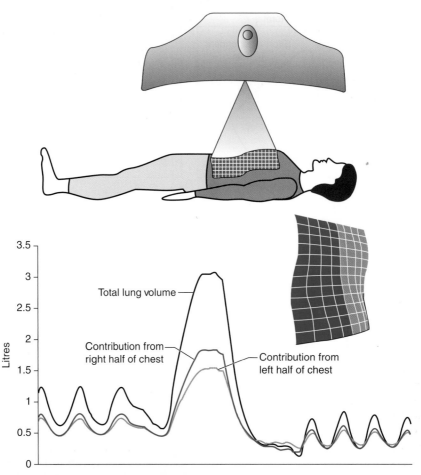

**FIGURE 2.34** Representation by light plethysmography of the chest and abdominal wall, with corresponding volume–time curve

Keeping a firm lip seal, the patient inhales or exhales sharply against a blocked mouthpiece with a small leak to prevent pressure being generated by the mouth muscles. The best of three efforts is recorded. Technique must be meticulous and the patient's position standardized because values vary with effort, initial lung volume and the learning effect of the test. Values are:

- Normal MIP: –100 cmH$_2$O;
- Inspiratory muscle weakness: MIP below (less negative than) –80 cmH$_2$O;
- Weaning failure: below –30 cmH$_2$O (Cairo 2012, p. 327);
- Neurological patients at risk of ventilatory failure: <60% predicted (Mangera et al. 2012) or below –20–30 cmH$_2$O (Cairo 2012, p. 52).

3. **Sniff nasal inspiratory pressure** is easier for some patients and does not require a mouth seal, consisting of a short sharp maximal inhalation through one or both nostrils (Benício et al. 2016). Values should be more negative than –70 cmH$_2$O for men and more negative than –60 cmH$_2$O for women.

4. **Peak cough flow** is the velocity of air expelled from the lungs during a cough, measured by a pneumotachometer or, less accurately, by an insufflator–exsufflator (Kulnik et al. 2015). The patient is asked to inspire to TLC and then cough into the device via a tightly-fitting face mask or mouthpiece. For intubated patients, the cuff is deflated and tube occluded. Normal is 720 L/min (Suárez et al. 2002). At least 270 L/min is required to prevent complications during chest infections, and 160 L/min for an

effective cough (Bianchi et al. 2012). Weak patients can precede the test with breath-stacking (p. 112). More invasive tests are transdiaphragmatic pressure and twitch diaphragmatic pressure. Nonvolitional tests include cervical magnetic stimulation of the phrenic nerves (Fitting 2012).

## Other Tests

### $O_2$ and $CO_2$

Blood **oxygen levels** are measured by $PaO_2$ or $SpO_2$, and **$CO_2$ levels** by $PaCO_2$ (p. 14), or less painfully by capnography or transcutaneous monitoring (p. 466–467).

**Pulmonary gas exchange** can be evaluated by the alveolar-arterial gradient (p. 17). The diffusion component of this reflects the integrity of the alveolar-capillary membrane and is monitored by diffusion capacity/gas transfer/transfer factor, or the total lung transfer capacity for carbon monoxide (TLCO). Normal values are 17–25 mL/min/mmHg. Reduced TLCO occurs with emphysema (Lee et al. 2016a), advanced age, heavy smoking, alveolar ventilation to perfusion ($\dot{V}_A/\dot{Q}$) mismatch (Nishimura 2011) or a thickened alveolar-capillary membrane, as occurs with fibrosis or pulmonary oedema. However, even if TLCO is <50% predicted, there is enough reserve for diffusion to be adequate for normal metabolic demands (Hughes 2007).

A measure of **gas exchange at tissue level** is given by the saturation of haemoglobin with oxygen in the pulmonary artery (p. 471).

### Maximum oxygen consumption ($\dot{V}O_2$max)

$\dot{V}O_2$max quantifies maximum exercise tolerance, reflecting the integration of the central nervous, cardiopulmonary and metabolic systems. By measuring expired air while workload is increased, it identifies the point at which oxygen demand exceeds supply, when the anaerobic threshold is reached and lactic acid produced. It is a lengthy and exhausting test that is used for research or to assess a patient's suitability for lung resection. For clinical purposes it can be estimated from the 6-min walk test (p. 251), but the correlation is less accurate for patients with COPD if peak exercise is limited by dyspnoea (Fregonezi et al. 2012). Normal $\dot{V}O_2$max is >25 mL/kg/min, or 25 times the resting level.

### Oxygen cost of breathing

This is assessed by determining the oxygen consumption at rest and the increased level of ventilation produced by hyperventilation, the added oxygen uptake being attributed to metabolism of the respiratory muscles. This is small at rest but can be 10% of total oxygen consumption on exercise and up to 15% in endurance athletes (Dominelli & Sheel 2012).

### Ventilation/perfusion distribution

$\dot{V}_A/\dot{Q}$ mismatch can be monitored at the bedside by electrical impedance tomography (Baumgardner & Hedenstierna 2016).

### Ultrasonography

Ultrasound waves act as visual stethoscopes and monitor aeration by reflecting off an air/tissue interface. They help identify the cause of dyspnoea (Shah et al. 2016) and can distinguish atelectasis, gas trapping (Lobo et al. 2014), pneumothorax, pneumonia, pulmonary oedema, pleural effusion (Irwin & Cook 2016), consolidation, diaphragm excursion (Le Neindre et al. 2016) and even readiness to wean (Soummer 2012). Ultrasound can also be used to reduce the need for repeated arterial puncture (Haynes & Mitchell 2010).

### Exhaled breath

An electronic nose provides distinctive smell-prints of volatile breath biomarkers for respiratory conditions such as COPD, asthma and lung cancer (Mazzatenta 2013), for lower respiratory tract infections in ventilated patients (Fowler et al. 2015) or to detect smokers (Maga et al. 2017).

### Exercise tests

Functional tests for patients with chronic disease are shown on p. 251. For patients hospitalized with acute disease, step tests are safe and can identify desaturation (José 2016).

## CASE STUDY: MS DT

*Ms DT has late stage COPD and is visited at home.*

### Relevant medical history

- Depression

### Social history

- Lives alone
- Help with shopping from son

## Drug history

- Multiple COPD drugs on repeat prescription including oral steroids
- Sleeping tablets
- Long-term oxygen therapy

## Subjective

- Stopped going to shops since panic attack
- Can just manage stairs
- Use oxygen when I need it

## Objective

- Unable to speak in complete sentences due to dyspnoea
- Breathing pattern rapid and apical
- Thin
- $SpO_2$ 90% at rest and 87% on exercise

## Question

What is your plan of action?

---

**CLINICAL REASONING**

*'… we compared … five subjects affected with chronic ventilatory failure due to Duchenne muscular dystrophy and treated with nasal intermittent positive pressure ventilation [with] an unventilated comparison group … who refused long-term mechanical ventilation …'*
Chest (1994), 105, 445–448

Is this a suitable comparison group?

---

## Response to Case Study

1. First visit
- Education on COPD to ensure that fears are addressed that might contribute to depression or panic attacks.
- Desensitization to breathlessness.
- Exploration with patient on when she feels that she 'needs' oxygen. Ms T says this is when she feels breathless or anxious. Explanation provided about (a) the lack of association between breathlessness and oxygen, and (b) the need for oxygen at night and when possible in the day: 'the more the merrier'.
- Provision of hand-held fan.
- Discuss how Ms T would like to address her depression, with suggested options being to talk to her son, talk to a counsellor and/or take antidepressants.

- Breathing re-education.
- Initiation of sitting exercises and paced walking, with personalized tick chart for home practice.
- Leaflets on COPD, sleep, panic attacks and breathlessness (Appendix B).
- Referral to community occupational therapist for management of panic attacks, insomnia and activities of daily living.
- Referral to community pharmacist for drug review and inhaler technique.
- Referral to dietician.
- Letter to general practitioner requesting bone density scan and referral to respiratory consultant.

2. Plan for next visit
- Address end-of-life wishes;
- Further breathless management strategies (Chapter 8);
- Paced walking in garden;
- Stairs and progression of exercise programme;
- Assessment for ambulatory oxygen;
- Discuss pulmonary rehabilitation.

---

**RESPONSE TO CLINICAL REASONING**

Patients unwilling to try assisted ventilation differ from those accepting the treatment and are therefore not a suitable comparison group.

---

# RECOMMENDED READING

AARC, 2013. Clinical practice guideline: blood gas analysis and hemoximetry. Respir. Care 58 (10), 1694–1703.

Albert, T.J., Swenson, E.R., 2016. Circumstances when arterial blood gas analysis can lead us astray. Respir. Care 61 (1), 119–121.

Amin, S.B., Slater, R., Mohammed, T.L., 2015. Pulmonary calcifications: a pictorial review and approach to formulating a differential diagnosis. Curr. Probl. Diagn. Radiol. 44 (3), 267–276.

Bohadana, A., Izbicki, G., Kraman, S.S., 2014. Fundamentals of lung auscultation. N. Engl. J. Med. 370 (8), 744–751.

Bordoni, B., Marelli, F., Morabito, B., et al., 2016. Manual evaluation of the diaphragm muscle. Int. J. Chron. Obstruct. Pulmon. Dis. 11, 1949–1956.

Boros, P.W., 2012. Reversibility of airway obstruction vs bronchodilation. COPD 9 (3), 213–215.

Bruusgaard, D., Tschudi-Madsen, H., Ihlebæk, C., et al., 2012. Symptom load and functional status. BMC Public Health 12, 1085.

Cheuvront, S.N., 2013. Physiologic basis for understanding quantitative dehydration assessment. Am. J. Clin. Nutr. 97 (3), 455–462.

Desborough, M.J., Keeling, D.M., 2013. How to interpret a prolonged prothrombin time or activated partial thromboplastin time. Br. J. Hosp. Med. 74 (1), C10–C12.

Elder, A., Japp, A., Verghese, A., 2016. How valuable is physical examination of the cardiovascular system? BMJ 354, i3309.

Foo, J.Y., Chua, K.P., Tan, X.J., 2013. Clinical applications and issues of oxygen saturation level measurements obtained from peripheral sites. J. Med. Eng. Technol. 37 (6), 388–395.

Fortis, S., Corazalla, E.O., Qi, W., et al., 2015. The difference between slow and forced vital capacity increases with increasing body mass index. Respir. Care 60 (1), 113–118.

Frerichs, I., 2017. Chest electrical impedance tomography examination, data analysis, terminology, clinical use and recommendations. Thorax 72 (1), 83–93.

Hansell, D.M., Bankier, A.A., MacMohon, H., et al., 2008. Fleischner society: glossary of terms for thoracic imaging. Radiology 246, 697–722.

Hansen, K.B., Westin, J., Andersson, L.M., et al., 2016. Flocked nasal swab versus nasopharyngeal aspirate in adult emergency room patients. Infect. Dis. (Lond.) 48 (3), 246–250.

Heavens, K.R., Charkoudian, N., O'Brien, C., et al., 2016. Noninvasive assessment of extracellular and intracellular dehydration in healthy humans using the resistance-reactance–score graph method. Am. J. Clin. Nutr. 103, 724–729.

Hughes, J.M.B., 2007. Assessing gas exchange. Chron. Respir. Dis. 4, 205–214.

Jain, S.N., 2011. A pictorial essay: radiology of lines and tubes in the intensive care unit. Indian J. Radiol. Imaging 21 (3), 182–190.

Janssen, R., Wang, W., Moço, A., et al., 2016. Video-based respiration monitoring with automatic region of interest detection. Physiol. Meas. 37 (1), 100–114.

Mohrmann, M.E., Shepherd, L., 2012. Ready to listen: why welcome matters. J. Pain Sympt. Manag 43 (3), 646–650.

Muñoz, C.X., 2013. Assessment of hydration biomarkers including salivary osmolality during passive and active dehydration. Eur. J. Clin. Nutr. 67, 1257–1263.

Nakada, T.A., Masunaga, N., Nakao, S., et al., 2016. Development of a prehospital vital signs chart sharing system. Am. J. Emerg. Med. 34 (1), 88–92.

Pasterkamp, H., Brand, P.L., Everard, M., et al., 2016. Towards the standardisation of lung sound nomenclature. Eur. Respir. J. 47 (3), 724–732. doi:10.1183/13993003.01132-2015.

Pryor, T., Page, K., Patsamanis, H., 2014. Investigating support needs for people living with heart disease. J. Clin. Nurs. 23 (1-2), 166–172.

Rush, E.C., 2013. Water: neglected, unappreciated and under researched. Eur. J. Clin. Nutr. 67 (5), 492–495.

Sarkar, M., Madabhavi, I., Niranjan, N., et al., 2015. Auscultation of the respiratory system. Ann. Thoracic Med 10 (3), 158–168.

See, K.C., Ong, V., Wong, S.H., et al., 2016. Lung ultrasound training: curriculum implementation and learning trajectory among respiratory therapists. Int. Care Med. 42 (1), 63–71.

Singh, V., Meena, P., Sharma, B.B., 2012. Asthma-like peak flow variability in various lung diseases. Lung India 29 (1), 15–18.

Weiszhar, Z., Horvath, I., 2013. Induced sputum analysis. Breathe 9, 300–306.

# 3

# Respiratory Disorders

## LEARNING OBJECTIVES

*On completion of this chapter the reader should be able to:*
- recognize the pathological processes underlining obstructive and restrictive disorders, infections, lung cancer, the cardiorespiratory manifestations of systemic disease and respiratory failure;
- identify the general management of these conditions;
- use clinical reasoning to ascertain strategies for the physiotherapy management of each disorder.

## OUTLINE

## INTRODUCTION

*Clinical medicine places too much emphasis on labelling disorders and too little emphasis on the integrative mechanisms which bridge these disorders.*
**Killian 1998**

Lung diseases are often slowly progressive and are usually incurable except for infections. Physiotherapy, however, can have a gratifying impact on a patient's quality of life (QoL). Lung disorders are usually divided into obstructive and restrictive disease, both of which share an association with heart disease (Eriksson 2013), and disorders that fit neither or both categories.

Obstructive disease involves the narrowing of airways, which increases airflow resistance and the work of breathing (WOB). Causes are:

- reversible factors, e.g. inflammation, bronchospasm or mucous plugging;
- irreversible factors, e.g. fibrotic airway walls, or floppy airways due to loss of the elastic recoil which normally supports them;
- localized lesions, e.g. upper airway tumour or foreign body.

Restrictive disorders reduce lung volume and compliance, increasing elastic resistance and WOB by means of:
- shrinkage of lung tissue, e.g. fibrosis;
- compression from inside the chest wall, e.g. pleural effusion or pneumothorax;
- compression by the chest wall, e.g. skeletal disorders;
- reduced ability to expand the lung, e.g. neurological disorders.

Lung disease is notoriously underreported, over 40% more people living with COPD than reported, twice as many with idiopathic pulmonary fibrosis and four times as many with bronchiectasis (BLF 2016). The lung's vulnerability to the environment leads to tobacco or pollution causing damage both prenatally (Morales et al. 2015) and postnatally (Grigg 2016).

Medical management is discussed in Chapter 5, and physiotherapy management is discussed in Chapters 6–9. When specific to a disease, management is discussed in this chapter.

# CHRONIC OBSTRUCTIVE PULMONARY DISEASE

*The insidious onset, lacking the jolt of a first heart attack, may take away its ability to provide a sharp motivational shock.*

**Jarvis 1995**

COPD is a group of disease subtypes characterized by airflow obstruction that is progressive and largely irreversible. It is associated with an abnormal inflammatory response to nasty substances such as cigarette smoke and includes significant systemic effects, leading to disability from pulmonary and extrapulmonary factors (Singer 2013).

The clinical diagnosis of chronic bronchitis and the pathological diagnosis of emphysema usually occur together as COPD, with some patients having a preponderance for one or other disease entity.

A COPD–asthma overlap syndrome (Fig. 3.1) occurs in patients who demonstrate the fixed airways obstruction that defines COPD plus symptoms more typical of asthma. This dual diagnosis brings a higher burden of disability than each condition on its own (Barnes 2016).

COPD is suspected in smokers or ex-smokers aged over 35 who develop chronic productive cough, winter chest infections and shortness of breath (SOB). Accelerated decline in $FEV_1$ occurs in half of patients (Jones 2016), and spirometry is used to stratify severity:

- Grade 1 or mild: $FEV_1 \geq 80\%$ predicted, plus smoker's cough and little or no SOB.
- Grade 2 or moderate: $FEV_1 \leq 80\%$ predicted, plus SOB on moderate exertion.
- Grade 3 or severe: $FEV_1 \leq 50\%$ predicted, plus hyperinflation, peripheral oedema and SOB at rest.
- Grade 4 or very severe: $FEV_1 < 30\%$ predicted, plus end-stage symptoms (GOLD 2016).

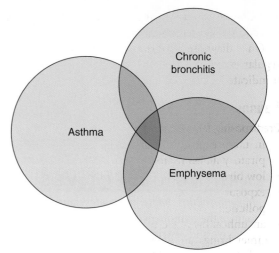

**FIGURE 3.1** Overlap of the commonest obstructive lung diseases.

Spirometry, however, shows wide variability (Tashkin 2013) and is an unreliable marker of exercise limitation, health status or breathlessness (Jones et al. 2012a), which are of most concern to patients (Barrecheguren 2016). The relevant ICF domains are severity of symptoms and functional impairment, which are also poorly related to physiological measurements (Vercoulen 2012). Physical inactivity is the strongest independent predictor of mortality (DePew et al. 2013). Physiotherapy is aimed mainly at the management of breathlessness and physical activity, both directed at the individual's functional needs.

COPD is laden with gloomy statistics:

- It kills as many people as lung cancer (Neerkin 2006), is the third leading cause of death worldwide (Zanforlin et al. 2016), affects roughly 10% of the global population and its prevalence continues to rise (Mulhall 2016).
- Disadvantaged people are 14 times more likely to have COPD than rich people (DoH 2010a).
- Half of elderly smokers have the disease (Lindberg et al. 2012).

Both overdiagnosis and underdiagnosis are common, the former leading to unnecessary medication and the latter known as 'the silence of COPD' (Spyratos et al. 2016), partly attributed to discrimination against smokers (Winstanley et al. 2007) and patients' tendency to misattribute their symptoms to ageing (Pinnock 2012). Diagnosis can be refined with sputum or saliva biomarker tests, and self-monitoring with smartphone-based spirometry could assist in the early detection of exacerbations (Dixon et al. 2016).

Once diagnosed, mortality can only be reduced by regular exercise (Garvey 2016), smoking cessation and, if indicated, home oxygen (Lahousse et al 2016).

## Causes

Predisposing factors are:

- in utero exposure to smoking, and childhood respiratory illness (Soto-Martinez 2010);
- low birth weight and malnutrition (Duijts 2012);
- exposure to tobacco, biomass fuel or occupational pollution (Vestbo & Lange 2016);
- an 'unhealthy/Western-style' diet (Zheng et al. 2016).

Summer brings air pollution and sometimes a heavy heat that increases morbidity (Hansel et al. 2016), while patients are also extra sensitive to cold, with winter doubling the exacerbation rate (Jenkins et al. 2012). People with COPD, such as those with rheumatoid arthritis, are barometers for impending weather change.

## Pathophysiology, Clinical Features and Comorbidities

*'You're frightened about things, you get yourself worked up, then your breathing is worse'*

***Toms & Harrison 2002***

The natural history of COPD spans 20–50 years, bringing little or no symptoms until there is loss of up to 50% of lung function (Hodgkin et al. 2009) because airflow obstruction begins in the small airways (Martin 2013) where there is a wide total cross section and little resistance to airflow.

Inhaled irritants stimulate epithelial cells (in chronic bronchitis) and alveolar macrophages (in emphysema) to release inflammatory mediators that damage airways and alveoli. Inflammatory products disseminate around the body, where, along with other effects of the disease and its treatment, they predispose to comorbidities linked to inflammation such as bronchiectasis (Svenningsen 2017), inflammatory bowel disease (Triantafyllakis et al. 2016) and a two–five times higher risk of major cardiovascular diseases (Triest et al. 2016). Triest et al. (2016) also found that only 21% of patients who had had a myocardial infarction were previously known with this diagnosis, which has implications for pulmonary rehabilitation (PR). Other organs are affected by hypoxia due to impaired gas exchange (Gulbas et al. 2013). Physical inactivity and smoking are more strongly associated with comorbidities than the airflow obstruction (Remoortel et al. 2014).

### Chronic bronchitis

Chronic bronchitis is characterized by excess mucus secretion due to a rampant increase in the size and number of goblet cells. This contributes to airflow obstruction (Craig 2017), risk of exacerbations, a 50% risk of bronchiectasis (Svenningsen 2017) and a **productive cough**, first in the morning and then throughout the day, often dismissed by the patient as a smokers' cough but increasing the risk of urinary incontinence (Burge et al. 2017). Chronic bronchitis may be present without airflow obstruction at first (Kim & Criner 2013), but repeated irritation of the airways leads to inflammation, fibrotic changes and sometimes bronchospasm (Fig. 3.2). Patients experience bronchospasm as **chest tightness** or a **wheeze**.

### Emphysema

Emphysema is a disease of alveoli and the smallest airways, with secondary effects on the larger airways. Repeated injury from cigarette smoke causes proteolytic degradation of the alveolar walls and destruction of elastic fibres. In the alveoli, erosion of alveolar septa leads to enlargement of airspaces (Fig. 3.2), sometimes breaking down into bullae (Fig. 3.3), which are air-filled spaces with thin walls of attenuated emphysematous lung tissue. In the distal airways, bronchioles are destabilized by loss of the elastic recoil, which normally splints them open. These floppy airways then collapse, trapping gas distally.

**Hyperinflation** (see Fig. 2.17) occurs when $FEV_1$ has declined to roughly half normal (Enright & Crapo 2000); it is caused by gas trapping and the following:

- Loss of elastic fibres reduces inward lung elastic recoil, which loses the fight to balance outward chest wall recoil, leading to static hyperinflation.
- Active inspiratory muscle contraction to hold open the floppy airways, even during exhalation, leading to dynamic hyperinflation.

Hyperinflation worsens with exercise because the rapid respiratory rate makes it difficult for the lungs to empty (Cooper et al. 2014), creating one of the mechanisms of **dyspnoea**. Hyperinflation impairs the function of the now-shortened inspiratory muscles, which are already struggling with inflammation and sometimes malnutrition (Itoh et al. 2013).

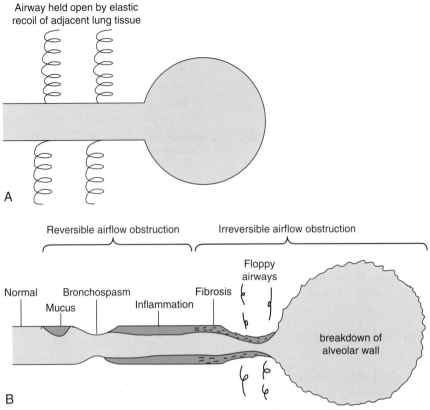

**FIGURE 3.2** Airway and alveolus in (A) normal lungs, (B) COPD lungs.

The flattened diaphragm inactivates the bucket handle action of the ribs and works paradoxically by pulling in the lower ribs on inspiration (**Hoover's sign,** p. 38), thus becoming expiratory in action (Courtney 2009). Dynamic hyperinflation may prevent full expiration before the next inspiration starts, trapping more gas and leading to positive pressure in the chest known as intrinsic PEEP (Fig. 3.4). This stabilises on a higher, less compliant, portion of the pressure volume curve (see Fig. 1.6), leading to the inspiratory muscles having to overcome an inspiratory threshold load of up to 6–9 cmH$_2$O, and sometimes working at near total lung capacity (Lahaije et al. 2012).

Work of breathing is also increased by active exhalation if air needs to be forced out through obstructed airways, contributing to fatigue of the abdominal muscles on exercise (Hopkinson et al. 2010). Thoracic **pain** is reported in 21%–77% of patients, but under-treatment is common (Janssen et al. 2016).

Inefficient **abdominal paradox** (p. 38) may be evident and some patients can only inhale by lifting up their entire rigid rib cage, contributing to fatigue and leading to **hypertrophied accessory muscles**.

**Breathlessness** is the most disabling symptom and a marker of disease severity (Han et al. 2015). It is caused by airway narrowing, hyperinflation, muscle dysfunction and hypermetabolism, exacerbated on exercise by lactic acid production which increases ventilatory drive (Jolley & Moxham 2009). **Exercise intolerance** is particularly troublesome during activities of daily living (ADLs) when the accessory muscles of respiration may have to switch from assisting breathing to supporting upper limb activity. Other causes of exercise intolerance are deconditioning (Vogiatzis et al. 2013) and reduced venous return due to positive intrathoracic pressure created by dynamic hyperinflation (Tzani et al. 2011). Physical inactivity appears to be a better predictor of mortality than clinical status (Lahaije et al. 2012).

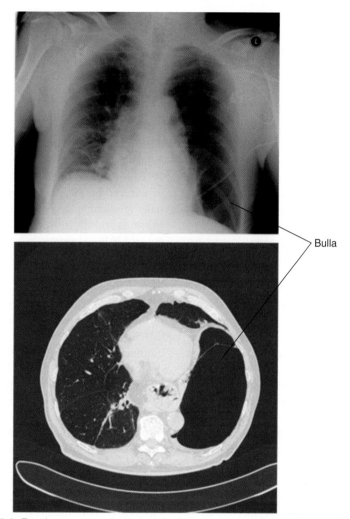

Bulla

**FIGURE 3.3** Emphysematous bulla in left *(L)* lower zone. (From Noppen et al. 2006.)

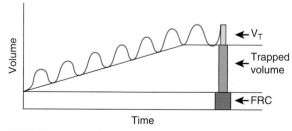

**FIGURE 3.4** Gas trapping, leading to increased resting lung volume, $V_T$ being unchanged but FRC stabilizing at a higher volume. *FRC,* Functional residual capacity; *$V_T$,* tidal volume (From Cairo 2012).

**KEY POINT**

Breathlessness affects the patient mostly as exercise intolerance.

### Alpha₁-antitrypsin deficiency

Emphysema that develops in the third to fifth decade of life may be due to a congenital lack of $\alpha_1$-antitrypsin (AAT), a plasma protein that protects the alveoli from digesting themselves (p. 4). The disease takes on average 6 years to be diagnosed, especially as 50% of cases mimic asthma by showing reversibility to bronchodilators (Barker 2010), but it occurs in 1% of people who have COPD (Soriano 2017). Suspicions are raised if a non-smoker develops COPD symptoms or a smoker develops symptoms earlier than expected, especially if there is a family history of emphysema and/or liver disease. Diagnosis is by low serum AAT levels, protease inhibitor analysis or an electronic nose (Hattesohl et al. 2011).

Treatment is by normal COPD management, especially smoking cessation, plus augmentation therapy with infusions of purified AAT (Balbi et al. 2016), sometimes lung transplantation or, in the future, gene therapy. Relatives planning parenthood are offered genetic counselling because of a 25% incidence in the children of two carriers. Breathlessness has the greatest impact on quality of life and is the focus of physiotherapy.

### Chronic bronchitis and emphysema

Whether either of these entities predominates, COPD inexorably progresses. Chronic hypoxia leads to compensatory proliferation of red cells (**polycythaemia**). This increases the oxygen-carrying capacity of blood at first and improves survival (Kollert et al. 2013), but once packed cell volume reaches 55%, the thickened blood impedes oxygen delivery, burdens the heart, causes pulmonary hypertension and may lead to headaches.

The tenuous alveolar–capillary membrane means that alveolar damage brings capillary damage. This combines with widespread hypoxic pulmonary vasoconstriction (p. 13) to augment pulmonary hypertension, increasing the load against which the right ventricle must pump, leading to hypertrophy and dilation of its ventricle, a condition known as cor pulmonale. When the myocardium can no longer cope, right-sided heart failure develops, which is present in 20% of patients (Zeng & Jiang 2012). Systemic blood pressure (BP) rises in order to overcome the increased right atrial pressure, which strains the left ventricle and eventually leads to left-sided heart failure, impairing cerebral oxygenation and cognition (Oliveira et al. 2016). Lung damage continues (Fig. 3.5), but a third of patients die from cardiovascular causes (Rothnie 2016a).

### Further comorbidities and clinical features

COPD brings an extra risk of **cardiovascular disease, diabetes, osteoporosis, sleep apnoea,** and **sarcopaenia,** comorbidities for which specific treatments are available and associated with better COPD outcomes (Brown & Martinez et al. 2016). **Fatigue** is a problem in 90% of patients (Lewko et al. 2009). This is worsened in up to a third of patients who have **anaemia**, caused by systemic inflammation and some drugs, which further compromises the patient by increasing SOB, decreasing exercise tolerance and possibly creating an independent predictor of death (Budnevsky et al. 2016).

As many as 50% of patients suffer from **anxiety** and **depression** (Robertson 2010), which both worsen QoL, reduce exercise capacity, increase SOB (Martinez et al. 2016) and worsen prognosis (GOLD 2016). Both can also be reduced by PR (Tselebis et al. 2016) and are potentially modifiable targets to reduce COPD-related readmissions and the 'revolving door syndrome' (Yohannes & Leroi 2016). However, in only half of patients are these recognized and treated (Pommer et al. 2012). **Frustration** is common, and COPD has been described as one of the most isolating of the chronic diseases (Toms & Harrison 2002). **Panic attacks** are 10 times greater than in the general population (Livermore et al. 2010).

Objectively, there is a rich tapestry of signs such as a plethoric **appearance**, **oedema** and a breathing pattern of **forced expiration**, **pursed lips breathing**, **prolonged expiration** with an inspiratory:expiratory (I:E) ratio up to 1:4, and **soft tissue recession** (p. 37). Patients may lean forward on their elbows to force the diaphragm into a more efficient dome shape and stabilise the shoulder girdle for optimum accessory muscle action. **Clinically**, emphysema shows hyperresonance to percussion and diminished breath sounds, and chronic bronchitis shows inspiratory crackles and expiratory wheezes (Jacome & Marques 2015).

A third of patients suffer from **malnutrition**, caused by excess energy demand, reduced energy supply and inflammation. More common in emphysema, it cannibalises the respiratory muscles for their protein and predisposes to cachexia, decreased exercise capacity, increased risk of exacerbations and higher mortality (Hsieh et al. 2016). **Obesity** can coexist with malnutrition and has been found in 53% of patients (Katz et al. 2016a). Combined obesity and sarcopaenia increases the systemic inflammatory burden (Joppa et al. 2016).

**Muscle atrophy** (Box 3.1) ranges from 20% to 40% (Silva et al. 2016) but is potentially reversible by PR (Jones et al. 2015b). It is a predictor of mortality, affecting respiratory and limb muscles, especially the quadriceps (Ausín et al. 2017). Upper limb muscles are often preserved because of their accessory role in breathing

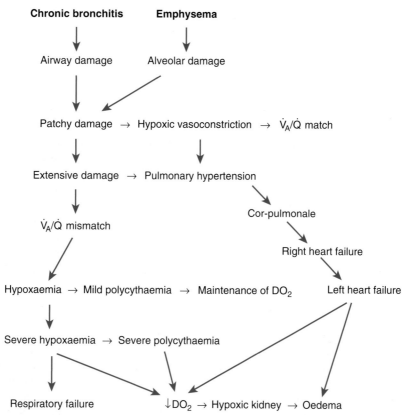

**FIGURE 3.5** Progression of COPD to respiratory failure and heart failure. $DO_2$, Oxygen delivery to the tissues; $\dot{V}_A/\dot{Q}$, ventilation/perfusion.

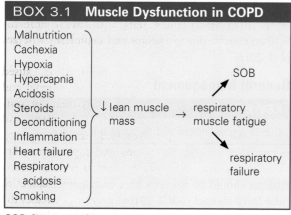

### BOX 3.1 Muscle Dysfunction in COPD

*SOB*, Shortness of breath.

normal activities. The strength of the diaphragm may be preserved by working against obstructed airways, but its action is impaired by operating at a mechanical disadvantage in expanding a hyperinflated chest, leading to functional muscle weakness (Lahaije et al. 2012). This can lead to exercise limitation, risk of exacerbations and ventilatory failure (Barreiro & Gea 2016).

Respiratory acidosis exacerbates muscle loss through oxidative stress and inflammation (Hsieh et al. 2016). Greater abdominal muscle activation during breathing impairs ability to recover balance (Smith et al. 2016a), which, along with muscle dysfunction, some drugs and cognitive impairment, increases the risk of **falls** (Roig et al. 2011) which occur four times more than in the healthy elderly population (Harrison et al. 2015a).

**Hypoxaemia** is greatest at night. Studies have reported that 27%–70% of patients who are not hypoxaemic when awake experience substantial desaturation at night, partly due to hypotonia of the accessory muscles (Owens 2013). Patients with severe disease may desaturate by

(Donaldson et al. 2012). Exercise tolerance is often limited by lower limb weakness more than SOB (Vlist & Janssen 2010), indicating the importance of quadriceps exercises for any patient unable to perform their

20% during non-REM sleep and 40% during REM sleep, which is greater than with maximal exercise (Ezzie 2011). The resulting **pulmonary hypertension** may affect exercise tolerance independent of lung function (Cuttica et al. 2011) and can be predicted by hypoxaemia on exercise without severe resting hypoxaemia (Nakahara et al. 2016). Cerebral hypoxia secondary to hypoxaemia contributes to **cognitive impairment,** which is thought to progress to **dementia** in over half of patients within 3–5 years (Dag et al. 2016).

Hypoxaemia leads to **chronic renal failure** in a third of patients, which contributes to **oedema** and further **cardiovascular disease** (Bruno & Valenti 2012).

Hypoventilation at night, and sometimes in the day, causes **hypercapnia** in some patients, when the 'wisdom of the body' decides to protect the inspiratory muscles as the disease progresses rather than strive for untenable normocapnia at all costs (Poon et al. 2015). **Sleep disturbance** occurs in 78% of patients (Price et al. 2013), exacerbated by SOB, coughing, steroids (Greenberg et al. 2009) and nocturnal oxygen desaturation, which itself predisposes to nocturnal cardiac dysrhythmias (Toraldo et al. 2012). **Restless legs syndrome** may occur at night (Budhiraja et al. 2015); infrared physiotherapy claims to modulate the symptoms (Guffey et al. 2016).

Cardiovascular complications are exacerbated by inflammation and smoking, which also contribute to a twofold to fourfold increase in **lung cancer** risk (Gonzalez et al. 2016). **Osteoporosis** is found in nearly half of patients (Silva 2011), favouring those who are inactive or taking steroids. This worsens with an exacerbation (Kiyokawa et al. 2012) and should not await fracture for diagnosis. COPD is a risk factor for hip fracture (Huang et al. 2016b), and vertebral fractures have been found in 48% of patients never exposed to steroids, 57% of those on inhaled steroids and 63% of those on oral steroids (Ionescu 2005).

Uncoordinated breathing combines with swallowing dysfunction (Cvejic 2011) to cause **gastro-oesophageal reflux disease** in 37% of patients (Shimizu et al. 2012), predisposing to exacerbations (GOLD 2016). Chronic **laryngitis** has been found in 70% of patients (Gilifanov et al. 2016).

## Tests

Screening is by **questionnaire** (Lyngsø 2013) and diagnosis by **spirometry**, the latter being done after a bronchodilator so that COPD is not misdiagnosed because of the normal reduction of $FEV_1$ with ageing (Dyer 2012). Confirmation is by $FEV_1$/FVC of <70%, along with relevant symptoms and/or a history of exposure to risk factors. Low **diffusing capacity** distinguishes emphysema from chronic bronchitis and is more descriptive of deconditioning than gas exchange (Weinreich et al. 2015).

**Radiology** is unhelpful at first, except to exclude other smoking-related diseases such as cancer. Upper lobe diversion (p. 139) may then become apparent. Emphysema shows the signs of hyperinflation (see Fig. 2.17) and sometimes bullae.

**Oximetry** may indicate whether **blood gases** are required, either arterial, or venous combined with oxygen saturation (McKeever et al. 2016). **Blood tests** include a full blood count to identify anaemia or polycythaemia. **ECG** and **echocardiography** are advised (de Miguel Díez 2013).

**Sputum induction** (Appendix A, Chapter 2) usually shows a high neutrophil count (Gupta 2013), but if eosinophils are present, the patient is likely to respond to steroids (Calverley 2017). Neutrophilic inflammation is not controlled by steroids, which can actually prolong the survival of neutrophils (Barnes 2003).

Exercise tests are on p. 251. For people with comorbid heart failure, cardiopulmonary exercise tests help distinguish pulmonary and circulatory dysfunction (Patel 2016). Heart failure along with COPD increases SOB on exercise due to a heightened neural drive (Arbex et al. 2016).

## General Management

**KEY POINT**

COPD is preventable and treatable but not curable.

Patients should be issued with a management plan by their third contact (NICE 2010a).

Smoking cessation is the most effective intervention to stop disease progression (Ito et al. 2015). Otherwise, treatment is like running a bath without the plug.

Multidisciplinary education has been found to pay for itself nearly five times over (Gallefoss & Bakke 2002), partly by reducing admissions (Siddique 2012). This is best incorporated into a PR programme, either in a group setting or at home, followed by telephone backup (Vitacca et al. 2016). Anxiety and depression need to be addressed because they limit participation in education (Schüz et al. 2015) and increase the fear associated with exercise (Nici 2000). Helpfully, exercise itself can reduce anxiety and depression (Hopkins et al. 2012).

Accurately-prescribed oxygen therapy for patients with chronic hypoxaemia improves cognitive function, QoL, exercise capability and survival (Katsenos 2011). Assessment should include 24-h oximetry because diurnal desaturations impair cognition (Rizzi 2016).

The dietician may advise on nutrients to improve exercise tolerance (GOLD 2016), including those with antioxidant and antiinflammatory properties (Chambaneau et al. 2016), and vitamin D to help prevent osteoporosis (Persson et al. 2012). For hospitalized patients, oral nutritional supplements speed discharge (Snider et al. 2015).

Referral to specialist services for comorbidities is required, especially for cardiovascular conditions. Palliative care is associated with the end of life, but is suitable for COPD before this stage because palliation emphasises patient's goals, function and QoL (Reticker et al. 2012).

## Drug Management

*Participants reported great concerns over their use of multiple drugs. 'And slowly, you have to take more and more'*

**Boeckxstaens 2012**

Airflow obstruction cannot be appreciably reversed by medication (Smolensky et al. 2015) and no drug has been found to modify long-term decline in lung function, but bronchodilators and/or steroids may help reduce symptoms (GOLD 2016). Assessment is usually based on spirometry (Fig. 3.6) but exercise tests can be included (Sava et al. 2012). Over half of patients choose to discontinue their long-active bronchodilators (Arfè et al. 2016), and choosing a device to suit the patient is as important as the drug (Melani & Paleari 2016). For hospitalized patients, inhalers allow earlier discharge than nebulisers (NICE 2010a) and are indicated unless nebulisers are objectively more effective (Smyth et al. 2001).

Combining drugs with different mechanisms and durations may improve their effect, sometimes with less side effects (GOLD 2016). Triple combination therapy has shown improved QoL and reduced exacerbations (Lee et al. 2016b), e.g. once-daily vilanterol trifenate, umeclidinium and fluticasone (Malerba et al. 2016).

Precautions on drugs for airflow obstruction are the following:

- The cardiac safety of LABAs and LAMAs (Fig. 3.6) is uncertain in patients with substantial cardiovascular disease or polypharmacy (Lahousse et al. 2016).
- Short-acting $\beta_2$-agonists are for symptom relief, but overuse is common and associated with increased disease severity (Fan et al. 2016). Long-acting bronchodilators are for maintenance and may be used in combination (Oba et al. 2016). An ultra

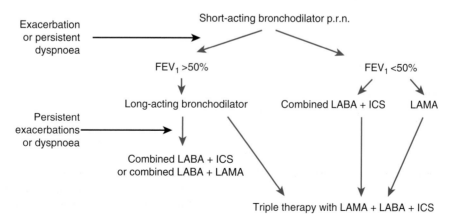

**FIGURE 3.6** Inhaled drugs for COPD. *ICS,* Inhaled corticosteroid; *LABA,* long-acting $\beta_2$-agonist bronchodilator; *LAMA,* long-acting muscarinic antagonist (anticholinergic) bronchodilator; *p.r.n,* as required, i.e. according to symptoms. (Adapted from NICE 2010a.)

long-acting β₂-agonist called indacaterol can reduce SOB and improve right-sided heart performance (Santus et al. 2015).

- Swift et al. (2012) advise against using systemic steroids in the long term, and Alifano (2010) warn that inhaled steroids given for advanced disease increase the incidence of pneumonia by 64%.

Other drugs are below:

- Diuretics are widely used for peripheral oedema but may worsen hypercapnia, disturb acid base balance and upset electrolytes (Terzano et al. 2012).
- β-Blockers may reduce exacerbations (Bhatt et al. 2016).
- Patients with bacterial exacerbations generally benefit from antibiotics. Prophylactic antibiotics are usually frowned on, but macrolide antibiotics have been suggested for prevention (Djamin et al. 2016).
- Exercise capacity may be increased by udenafil (Park & Lim 2012).
- Breathlessness may be relieved by accurately up-titrating opioids (Rocker & Cook 2013).

Neither antitussives to control cough nor mucolytics to loosen mucus are advisable routinely (GOLD 2016).

## Surgical Management

Surgery is occasionally indicated for symptom control in emphysema, e.g. laser ablation of giant bullae, bronchoscopic lung volume reduction (Jarad 2016) or the insertion of coils to restore some elasticity (Wise 2016). Lung transplantation is occasionally indicated for severe diffuse disease, which can increase exercise tolerance, improve QoL and prolong life (Lahzami 2009), but comorbidity and organ shortage limit this option. Anaesthesia is best administered regionally when possible.

## Physiotherapy

*Exercise training is the most powerful intervention that is currently available to provide symptomatic relief in COPD.*

**Ribeiro et al. 2013**

Physiotherapy begins with information to reduce anxiety, continues with assistance to reduce WOB and, sometimes, clear secretions. Then PR is the cornerstone of treatment, followed by a lifelong daily programme of small sustained increases in physical activity.

> ### PRACTICE TIP
>
> Preliminary advice to patients: 'COPD does two different things: it lowers your oxygen and makes you breathless. These need different treatments. Lack of oxygen is a chemical problem and requires oxygen therapy, which nourishes your brain and takes the strain off your heart. Breathlessness is a mechanical problem and requires physiotherapy…'

## Stable Disease

Research has identified the following:

- Pulmonary rehabilitation improves QoL and exercise capacity, including immediately after exacerbation (Man et al. 2016).
- A multidisciplinary community programme reduces respiratory admissions, more so in patients who have completed PR (Chung et al. 2016a).
- If secretions are subjectively troublesome, the active cycle of breathing (ACBT) is often helpful, but for patients with floppy airways, when forced exhalation may cause them to collapse, the huff can be modified or the patient may choose autogenic drainage (AD) or a positive pressure device (Svenningsen et al. 2016).
- For chronic ventilatory failure, noninvasive ventilation (NIV) at home may improve gas exchange, QoL (Bhatt 2013) and exercise tolerance (Alifano 2010).
- Benefits have been found with rib cage muscle stretch (Barros de Sá 2017), diaphragmatic release, osteopathic techniques (Rocha et al. 2015, Zanotti et al. 2012) and some spinal manipulative techniques (Wearing et al. 2016).

## Exacerbation

*When it comes to breathing, fear is the worst enemy.*

**Kvangarsnes et al. 2013**

Worsening symptoms for at least 48 h indicate an exacerbation, a distressing event that accelerates disease progression (Merinopoulou et al. 2016), triggered by infection or sometimes pollution (GOLD 2016). There is increased risk of cardiovascular incidents, particularly myocardial infarction, and markers of myocardial injury and heart failure may be elevated (Hatipoglu 2016).

Symptoms include lethargy, increased sputum volume and purulence, loss of appetite, poor sleep, SOB, fear (Kvangarsnes et al. 2013) and weakened quadriceps and respiratory muscles (Barreiro & Gea 2016). Rapid shallow breathing increases intrinsic PEEP so that up to half of inspiratory muscle effort may be required to overcome it (Peigang & Marini 2002), while the gap between energy intake and energy expenditure widens (Sanders et al. 2016). Between 24 and 50% of hospitalized patients get panic attacks (Dowson et al. 2010), and two or more exacerbations nearly double the incidence of posttraumatic stress symptoms (Teixeira et al. 2015), which is a reminder of the importance of education from the start.

Patients should have sufficient medication at home to begin self-management by:

- starting antibiotics if their sputum becomes purulent;
- increasing fluid intake;
- adjusting bronchodilators to control symptoms;
- starting oral steroids if increased SOB interferes with ADL (NICE 2010a).

Supervision is advised because steroids or diuretics may disturb acid–base balance (Bruno & Valenti 2012). Steroid-induced muscle weakness is significant during an exacerbation (Liao et al. 2016a), but oral steroids may be avoided by doubling the dose of a LABA and inhaled steroid, which are claimed to eliminate cardiovascular events (Bourbeau et al. 2016).

COPD accounts for 10% of medical admissions (BTS 2014) but a multidisciplinary 'Hospital-at-Home' service may reduce this, as well as decreasing readmissions and mortality (Jeppesen et al. 2012). Table 3.1 assists in the decision about home or hospital.

For patients admitted to hospital, a multidisciplinary clinical pathway can reduce length of stay and complication rates (Ban et al. 2012). Oxygen therapy is usually by venturi mask, but if $FiO_2$ and $SpO_2$ are closely monitored, high-flow nasal cannulae can be used, which bring the added benefit of reducing WOB and lowering $PaCO_2$, though less so than NIV (Bräunlich et al. 2016). CPAP may be beneficial for type 1 respiratory failure if oxygen therapy is inadequate (Luiz et al. 2016).

Type 2 respiratory failure occurs in a quarter of patients (DoH 2010a), for which NIV is required if there is respiratory acidosis despite maximum medical treatment. NIV reduces hospital stay and the need for intubation (Amri et al. 2016), and a generous $FiO_2$ does not appear to upset the respiratory drive in hypercapnic patients (Savi et al. 2013). If invasive ventilation is required (p. 519), subsequent extubation straight to

### TABLE 3.1   Factors to consider when deciding where to treat a patient

| Factor | Treat at home | Treat in hospital |
|---|---|---|
| Able to cope at home | Yes | No |
| Breathlessness | Mild | Severe |
| General condition | Good | Poor/deteriorating |
| Level of activity | Good | Poor/confined to bed |
| Cyanosis | No | Yes |
| Worsening peripheral oedema | No | Yes |
| Level of consciousness | Normal | Impaired |
| Already receiving home oxygen | No | Yes |
| Social support | Good | Living alone |
| Acute confusion | No | Yes |
| Rapid onset | No | Yes |
| Significant comorbidity (particularly cardiac disease and diabetes) | No | Yes |
| $SpO_2$ <90% | No | Yes |

From NICE 2012a.

NIV may reduce morbidity and mortality (Ornico et al. 2013), and ongoing NIV at home may be required for patients with continued hypercapnia (Altintas 2016).

Attention to depressive symptoms should be included because these are associated with frequent exacerbations and SOB (Tse et al. 2016), and can send patients into a downward spiral (Gysels & Higginson 2009).

Patients admitted to hospital must be cared for by a respiratory team, have access to an early discharge scheme with community support and be reviewed within 2 weeks of discharge (DoH 2011a). Early supported discharge and a 'Hospital at Home' service shows a trend towards lower mortality (Echevarria et al. 2016), but without follow-up support, two-thirds of patients show functional decline (Medina et al. 2016).

Physiotherapy involves sputum clearance with minimum effort from the patient. ACBT/AD may need to be modified (p. 208) and manual techniques may be preferred by those with significant breathlessness or fatigue, as long as there is no osteoporosis, and percussion is rhythmic, steady and intermittent rather than continuous (Hill et al. 2010).

Little-and-often quadriceps exercises should be started immediately, using an exercise diary for encouragement, followed by an early exercise programme, which more than compensates for the immobility of hospitalization (Martín-Salvador et al. 2016) and motivates patients to exercise after discharge (Tang et al. 2013). Troosters et al. (2010) found that a programme of 70% 1RM, using three sets of eight repetitions and Borg scores for dyspnoea and fatigue, improved walking distance at discharge and was well tolerated by patients even with severe exacerbations. Some patients prefer electrostimulation, although benefits are not maintained after cessation (Maddocks et al. 2016a). TENS over acupuncture points has shown promise in improving exercise capacity (Öncü & Zincir 2017).

Written self-management action plans can reduce the duration of exacerbations and are cost-effective (Dritsaki et al. 2016). A trip to the physiotherapy gym before discharge enables patients to feel and understand the degree of SOB on exertion that is required to build up and maintain exercise tolerance, e.g. 'breathless but not speechless'. Premature discharge increases readmission and mortality (Reid et al. 2012), while discharge bundles reduce readmissions (Ospina 2017).

After an exacerbation, functional impairment worsens over the following month (Torres-Sánchez et al. 2017), and physical inactivity is the strongest predictor of dying in the following year (Esteban et al. 2016). Ongoing exercise training has been found to reduce mortality and hospitalization, as well as improve QoL and exercise capacity (Emtner & Wadell 2016).

### End Stage Disease

*It is essential that advance care planning and end of life discussions are initiated in advance of a life threatening situation.*

**Lodewijckx et al. 2012**

There is a striking difference between the management of people with end-stage COPD and those dying from cancer. COPD patients may experience more anxiety, depression and dyspnoea but are prescribed less palliative medication and have less access to comprehensive care, despite the UK guidelines stipulating that they and their carers should be offered specialist palliative care (GOLD 2016).

Physiotherapists can be instrumental in ensuring recognition of the patient's needs. This should include

opportunities for discussion of prognosis and preferences for end-of-life care (Carlucci et al. 2016) and support for patients who prefer to die at home, which brings less risk of cognitive disturbance and depression (Escarrabill 2009). Teamwork includes acute, community, respiratory and palliative care services (Crawford et al. 2013).

Prioritizing palliation of symptoms does not preclude hospital admission or mechanical ventilation (Pinnock 2012). One of these milestones, or the initiation of home oxygen, may provide the opportunity to initiate a discussion on the patient's future wishes. Patients usually die at night, which is thought to be due to the effect of nocturnal hypoxaemia on the cardiovascular system (Owens 2013).

### Outcomes

What matters to most patients are physical function, SOB, cough, anxiety and fatigue, for which self-reported outcomes are available (Ekström et al. 2016). A plethora of other functional outcome measures are described by Liu et al. (2016a), who also recommend the 6-min walk test, 4-m gait speed and endurance treadmill test for function and exercise tolerance. Other outcome measures are described by GOLD 2016, Marques et al. 2016, Slok et al. 2016, Sundh et al. 2016, or, for an ICF approach, by Oliveira et al. 2013a.

## ASTHMA

*Facilities for breathing retraining need to be available as part of the overall management of asthmatic patients.*

**Thomas et al. 2001**

Asthma is defined as 'recurrent and (somewhat) reversible airflow obstruction due to airway inflammation, bronchospasm and mucus hypersecretion' (Rubin 2015a). It is caused by undue responsiveness to stimuli that are normally innocuous, a mechanism known as hyperreactivity. The condition is increasing in prevalence and severity, partly due to Westernized diets (Lynch 2016) and sedentary lifestyles (Groth et al. 2016). Mortality is low, but most asthma deaths in the UK are preventable (Levy & Winter 2015). People die if they, their relatives or doctors do not see asthma as a potentially fatal disease, nor grasp the importance of prevention, nor recognise deterioration.

| TABLE 3.2 | Distinguishing features of asthma and COPD | |
|---|---|---|
| | **Asthma** | **COPD** |
| Smoking history | Not necessarily | Usually |
| May start in childhood | Yes | No |
| Onset | Variable | Slow |
| Symptoms under age 35 | Often | Rarely |
| Atopy | Most patients | No |
| $FEV_1$ | Variable | Reduced |
| TLCO | Normal | Reduced with emphysema |
| Timing of symptoms | Episodic, diurnal, seasonal | Minor fluctuations only |
| Provocation of symptoms | Often weak stimulus, e.g. inhaled irritant | Often strong stimulus, e.g. infection |
| Cough | Usually dry | Usually productive |
| Nocturnal cough | Patient wakes coughing | Wakes, then coughs |
| Diurnal variability | Common | Uncommon |
| Breathlessness | Variable | Persistent and progressive |
| Induced sputum | More eosinophils | More neutrophils |
| Prognosis | Normal, except for refractory asthma | Progressive deterioration |

*Atopy,* Allergic hypersensitivity; *TLCO,* total lung transfer capacity for carbon monoxide (a measure of diffusion).

Asthma predisposes to an individual to COPD, both conditions being characterized by chronic inflammation and remodelling of the airways and vasculature (Olivieri 2014). The two may be difficult to distinguish in later life, leading to underdiagnosis by as much as 50% (Gillman & Douglass 2012) or unnecessary medication. Differences are in Table 3.2.

## Causes

Genetic, environmental and inflammatory causes have been identified, with allergy involved in most patients (Dennis et al. 2012a). Perinatal risks include maternal malnutrition or obesity, maternal smoking, prenatal stress (Khashan 2012), in utero or early life exposure to air pollution (Liu et al. 2016a), in vitro fertilization (Källén 2013), early antibiotics, possibly because these devour friendly gut flora that would normally help educate the immune system, Caesarean delivery due to lack of exposure to maternal microbes and separation from the mother in the first weeks of life (Azad & Kozyrskyj 2012).

Later contributors include:
- in childhood, food allergy (Wang & Liu 2012), stress (Rosenkranz et al. 2016), obesity (Black et al. 2012a) and fast food (Ellwood 2013);
- anxiety, with which asthma has a bidirectional relationship (Lee et al. 2016c);
- hyperventilation syndrome (HVS), which could be cause or effect, or which may be misdiagnosed as asthma (Meuret & Ritz 2010), studies finding that a third of people treated for asthma have HVS (Grammatopoulou et al. 2014);
- vocal cord dysfunction due to reflux (Hamdan et al. 2016), which may simply be mimicking asthma (Matrka 2014) or may relate to HVS; one distinction being that an expiratory wheeze often indicates asthma while an inspiratory wheeze is more likely due to vocal cord dysfunction;
- house dust mite, for which test kits are available (Winn et al. 2016);
- mould (Kespohl et al. 2016), poverty and stress (Koinis-Mitchell 2014).

The original cause of asthma may or may not be the same as the stimuli which typically trigger an asthma attack:
- diesel exhaust, which penetrates deep into the lung (Carlsten et al. 2016);
- allergic reaction to warm-blooded pets, pollen, some foods (Lee et al. 2013a) or cleaning sprays (Bédard et al. 2014);
- active, passive or prenatal smoking (BTS/SIGN 2016);
- change in temperature or thunderstorms, which sweep up pollutants (D'Amato et al. 2013);
- chest infection, exercise without warm-up, certain drugs such as aspirin, nonsteroidal antiinflammatory drugs and some β-blockers (Mathew et al. 2012).

Comorbidities include diabetes, depression and cardio-vascular disease (Cazzola et al. 2013).

## Pathophysiology

Three phases of response take place (Fig. 3.7):
1. The *sensitization* stage occurs in atopic people: exposure to allergens stimulates mast cells to release bronchoconstrictor mediators such as histamine and leukotrienes. Over time, removal from the allergen does not prevent the development of asthma.
2. The *hyperreactive* stage occurs with or without an allergic component: continued exposure to allergens, or response to other stimuli, leads to release of inflammatory cytokines such as eosinophils, and sometimes secretion of excess mucus. Once asthma is established, inflammation is present even in the chronic state (Barbers et al. 2012).
3. *Bronchospasm* occurs in response to various stimuli acting on hyperreactive airways.

Airflow obstruction is caused by inflamed airways and, in the acute phase, by bronchospasm. The narrow distal airways may also be obstructed by mucus, which is tethered to the goblet cells and thicker than the secretions of COPD or bronchiectasis because of inflammatory neutrophils (Loughlin et al. 2010), leading to mucous plugging being a feature of fatal asthma (Rogers 2004). The airways of some people who have died of acute asthma may be so clogged with mucus on postmortem that the lungs do not collapse when the chest cavity is opened (Wanner et al. 1996). Persistent inflammation leads to remodelling, fibrosis and some irreversibility.

Gastro-oesophageal reflux disease has been found in 50% of patients, either because prolonged coughing and wheezing increase abdominal pressure (Hamdan et al. 2016) or because oesophageal acid stimulated by steroid medication tips into the airways (Lazenby 2002).

A modest silver lining is that if the patient develops Alzheimer's disease, this might ameliorate their asthma because of progressive cholinergic failure (Ohrui et al. 2002).

## Classification and Clinical Features

Classic symptoms are wheeze, chest tightness, dyspnoea and cough, particularly at night or in the early morning. Impaired QoL correlates more with psychosocial factors than lung function (Thomas & Bruton 2014). Allergic asthma, known as extrinsic, usually develops in early life. Intrinsic asthma tends to develop in adulthood, and is more fulminant and less responsive to drug treatment. Variations are described as follows:

**Chronic** asthma, if well controlled, should cause no more trouble than an intermittent dry cough or occasional morning wheeze. Peak flow (PF) varies by <25%.

**Severe chronic** asthma is characterized by frequent exacerbations and symptoms that significantly affect QoL. PF varies by >25%, and patients tend to have a poor response to steroids, which paradoxically leads to higher doses being administered (Barnes 2011).

**Refractory** asthma is severe and unstable, occurring in less than 5% of patients (Bakal 2013). There is a chaotic PF day and night, persistent symptoms despite multiple drugs, significant mortality (Dennis et al. 2010) and complications from oral steroid use (Sweeney et al. 2016). Patients need individual arrangements for direct hospitalization if an attack occurs. The alternative term 'brittle asthma' is sometimes preferred by patients because it validates their experience of the disease. Another term 'Ferrari asthma' is not beloved by patients because it reminds them that they can go from 0 to intensive care in minutes.

**Acute** asthma is as 'like being in the sea when you can't swim' (Casteldine 1993) and reflects failure of preventive management or exposure to a specific stimulus. WOB is increased by bronchospasm of large airways and oedema of small airways. Recognition is by:

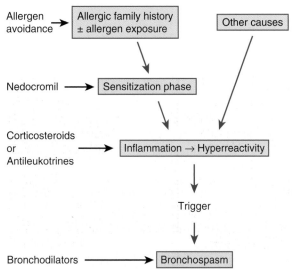

**FIGURE 3.7** Development of asthma, with drug treatment on the left.

- increasing SOB, wheeze and/or cough;
- difficulty in speaking, eating or sleeping;
- reliever inhaler being less effective.

There is sometimes chest pain, which may cause diagnostic confusion and patient anxiety. Arterial blood gases are required if $SpO_2$ falls below 92% (BTS 2012a). Nebulized treatment should be driven by oxygen, but if this is not available, an air compressor can be used with supplementary oxygen via nasal cannula.

**Severe acute** asthma can present deceptively. Patients tend to have a reduced sensitivity to SOB (Kuniyoshi et al. 2012) and, if drowsiness develops, they may appear less distressed. Salbutamol must be accompanied by high-concentration oxygen because of potential interaction of the drug in the presence of severe hypoxaemia (Lipworth 2001). Hypercapnia indicates exhaustion and the need for mechanical assistance. Medical help should be sought immediately if the patient shows a reduced response to bronchodilator or the signs in Table 3.3.

If there are no breath sounds or wheeze on auscultation, the chest is too hyperinflated to transmit sound, which is an ominous sign known as a 'silent chest'. Dehydration, due to SOB preventing fluid intake and causing loss of fluid from the respiratory tract, contributes to the mucous plugging (Fig. 3.8) that is usually found in fatal asthma (Kuyper 2003).

**Status asthmaticus** describes an asthma attack prolonged over 24 h and refractory to medication.

**Asphyxic** asthma, also known as catastrophic asthma or near-fatal asthma, occurs when status asthmaticus progresses to respiratory failure with $PaCO_2$ > 6.66 kPa (50 mmHg) and sometimes altered consciousness, requiring mechanical ventilation (D'Amato et al. 2016). If the patient stops breathing before intubation, one person can administer assisted ventilation and, if the chest is dangerously hyperinflated, another can kneel astride the patient and squeeze the chest, either at end-expiration, or, according to Fisher et al. (1989) at end-inspiration. Using this method, paramedics have managed to avoid out-of-hospital fatalities in patients who were asystolic on their arrival.

**Exercise-induced** asthma is caused by mouth breathing cold dry air, leading to evaporation of airway surface liquid and bronchospasm (Parsons 2014). It occurs during or after exertion, with recovery about 30 min later. Preventive measures include training to improve physical fitness, warm-up and cool-down, a scarf over the mouth on cold days, antileukotrines (Kansra 2013) or a bronchodilator or nedocromil before exercise (BTS/SIGN 2016).

**Nocturnal** asthma, identified by a morning dip in PF >20% compared to the previous evening, may be triggered by allergens in bedding, reflux in the supine position or an exaggeration of the normal circadian

| TABLE 3.3 | Some features of acute asthma | |
|---|---|---|
| | **Severe** | **Life-threatening** |
| $SpO_2$ | ↓ | <92% |
| $PaO_2$ | ↓ | <8 kPa (60 mmHg) |
| RR | >25 | ↓ |
| $PaCO_2$ | ↓ | >6 kPa (45 mmHg) |
| HR | >110 | ↓ |
| BP | ↑ | ↓, or arrhythmia |
| Peak flow | <50% predicted, or <200 L/min | <33% or unrecordable |
| Speech | Inability to complete sentence in one breath | Impossible |
| Auscultation | Wheeze | Silent chest |
| Colour | | Any change |
| Consciousness | | Any change |

*BP*, Blood pressure; *HR*, heart rate; *RR*, respiratory rate. Adapted from NICE 2013a.

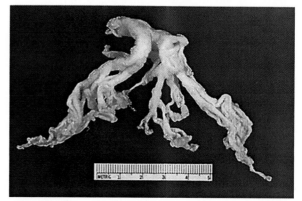

**FIGURE 3.8** Mucous cast of bronchial tree coughed up by an asthmatic patient during a severe exacerbation.

rhythm, which sees most asthma deaths at night (Smolensky et al. 2015).

**Occupational** asthma is usually diagnosed by a fall in $FEV_1$ of >20% over the working day or week, but may not become apparent for weeks or years. This is more likely in adult-onset asthma (BTS/SIGN 2016).

**'Difficult'** asthma presents with symptoms that do not match up or respond to medication. This is sometimes because the symptoms mimic asthma (Aguilar et al. 2014), which explains the high proportion of misdiagnosis and treatment failure, common misdiagnoses being HVS and vocal cord dysfunction (Löwhagen 2015). Patients should be under the care of a multidisciplinary 'difficult asthma service' (BTS/SIGN 2016).

## Tests

Misdiagnosis occurs in a third of adults (Wise 2017b), sometimes circuitously if a patient is given a bronchodilator inaccurately because they feel breathless, then labelled as asthmatic because they have a bronchodilator. Accurate diagnosis is in three stages (BTS/SIGN 2016):

1. Suspicions are raised by a history of acute attacks with wheeze, chest tightness, SOB and cough, including at night.
2. $FEV_1/FVC$ <0.7 indicates a likelihood of asthma.
3. A >400-mL improvement in $FEV_1$ after a $\beta_2$-agonist or steroid trial strongly suggests asthma.

Other tests use exhaled breath (Michils et al. 2016) or induced sputum (Wagener et al. 2015). Green or yellow sputum suggests the presence of eosinophils, which respond to steroids. Imaging is only used to identify complications or mimics of asthma (Richards et al. 2016).

## General Management

Goals of treatment include insignificant symptoms day or night, no limitation on physical activities, no asthma attacks, no need for rescue medication and minimal side effects from medication (BTS/SIGN 2016). This should be achievable with all but refractory asthma so long as education is at the heart of treatment, particularly as patients tend to tolerate unnecessary symptoms (Al Busaidi 2009). Less than a quarter of people who die have evidence of a personal asthma action plan (Levy & Winter 2015).

Examples of prevention and education are:

- a written personal asthma action plan for all patients, with details of their own triggers and current treatment, information on how to prevent relapse and when and how to seek help, to be reviewed and updated at each annual review (RCP 2016);
- education that smoking reduces the efficacy of steroids as well as creating the normal damage (Bakakos et al. 2016);
- immunotherapy (desensitization), e.g. against house dust mite (Devillier et al. 2016);
- advice on the management of panic attacks, which can halve panic symptoms, reduce medication and maintain asthma stability (Lehrer et al. 2008);
- information that air conditioners may be helpful (Boyle et al. 2012) but not room humidifiers, which tend to nurture house dust mite.

Self-monitoring (Fig. 3.9) and self-management (NICE 2013) improve adherence to medication, reduce the need for oral steroids (Clark et al. 2012) and help patients anticipate exacerbations (Honkoop et al. 2013). People with severe chronic asthma may benefit from nocturnal continuous positive airway pressure (D'Amato et al. 2014) or bronchoscopic thermoplasty to reduce smooth muscle mass in the airway walls (Zein et al. 2016a).

## Medical Management

Underuse, overuse and inappropriate use of medication are common. Patients are fond of their reliever bronchodilators, and anxious people tend to use them unnecessarily (Bakal 2013), but they do not prevent inflammatory damage to the airways. Levy and Winter (2015) and asthma deaths have been linked to a 'scarcely believable overprescription of reliever inhalers'. Use of more than one bronchodilator inhaler per month indicates a need for urgent review. Except with acute or refractory asthma, they should be used 'as required' only. Routine and unnecessary use of $\beta_2$-agonists may:

- reduce their effectiveness and increase airway hyperreactivity (Bakal 2013);
- encourage patients to rely on them when they should be seeking assistance;
- worsen prognosis (Athanazio 2012) and increase mortality (Dennis et al. 2012).

The paradox is that $\beta_2$-agonists are often beneficial, even life-saving, but may be detrimental if not used accurately.

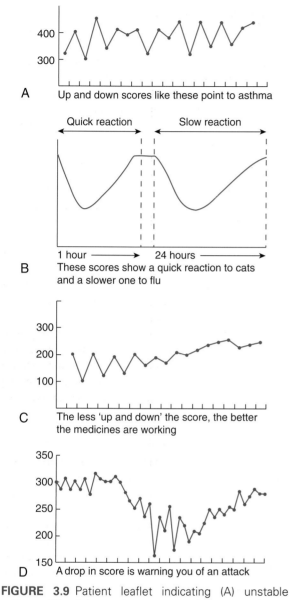

A    Up and down scores like these point to asthma

B    These scores show a quick reaction to cats and a slower one to flu

C    The less 'up and down' the score, the better the medicines are working

D    A drop in score is warning you of an attack

**FIGURE 3.9** Patient leaflet indicating (A) unstable asthma, (B) quick reaction to cats and slow reaction to influenza, (C) chronic asthma responding to medication, (D) acute asthma responding to medication.

## Drugs for chronic asthma

The principles of prevention should be considered at three levels (Warner & Warner 2000): the primary treatment (before sensitization), followed if required by secondary treatment (after sensitization but before disease development), then followed if necessary by tertiary treatment (of the disease itself). When possible, inhaled drugs should be by inhaler rather than nebuliser (Clark et al. 2010), and always after training and assessment in inhaler technique (BTS/SIGN 2016).

This principle has been developed into a stepwise approach (Appendix A). People with mild disease can often be maintained at step one with just a bronchodilator as required (after education on 'as required'), but newly diagnosed patients begin with a regular inhaled steroid to discourage them from the habit of grabbing their bronchodilator to relieve nonspecific symptoms. If patients on step 1 need their 'rescue' bronchodilator more than three times a week, they should be under the care of a specialist (asthma nurse, respiratory physiotherapist, respiratory physician or GP specializing in asthma) (BTS 2012a). Stepping up or down can be instigated by patients online (Hashimoto 2011).

Steroids begin at step 2, but control is often poor on these drugs if the patient does not receive regular medication reviews (Roche et al. 2016). Steroids are discussed on p. 167.

Drugs specific to asthma include omalizumab to dampen allergy and modulate immunity (Cusack et al. 2016). Antileukotrienes such as montelukast mobilise inflammatory products to the circulation, allowing 75% of patients on low-dose steroids to switch to these drugs, which come with few side-effects (Ciółkowski et al. 2016). Nedocromil is no longer under patent and therefore of no interest to the pharmaceutical industry (Montuschi 2011). It inhibits the release of inflammatory mediators and is one of the safest asthma drugs (Kewalramani et al. 2008), being derived from plant extract and with few side effects (Barnes 2006). It is inconvenient because of the need for q.d.s. dosing, and may take several weeks to show an effect. It brings the added bonus of reducing obesity (Wang & Shi 2012), which may itself reduce asthma symptoms (BTS/SIGN 2014).

Other options are biological drugs, nebulized heparin (Mathew et al. 2012), coffee (O'Keefe et al. 2013), agents that act on taste receptors in the airways (Weaver 2013) and hookworms (Biggelaar et al. 2004).

## Drugs for acute asthma

One puff of short-acting bronchodilator should be taken every 30–60 s, up to a maximum 10 puffs, preferably by inhaler with spacer. Outside hospital, if this does not alleviate symptoms, an ambulance should be called.

If this takes longer than 15 min to arrive, the inhaler can be used again, as above. Patients on the 'Symbicort SMART' or 'Fostair MART' regimens will have their own procedure to follow.

People with severe acute asthma may require bronchodilators delivered intravenously (BTS/SIGN 2016), subcutaneously (Sahadevan 2016) or by continuous nebulization (Dennis et al. 2012a). Hypoxaemia is a major contributor to asthma deaths (Rubin & Pohanka 2012) and $SpO_2$ should be kept above 94% (BTS/SIGN 2016). Steroids, antileukotrines, magnesium sulphate or glucagon (Cavallaria et al. 2017) may be used, but antibiotics are not recommended. Sedatives can be dangerous in a severe attack, when patients may already be drowsy.

---

**CLINICAL REASONING TIP**

O'Byrne et al. (2013) describe an article displaying benefits aplenty from steroids for asthma, but not the detriments. The disclosures showed all the authors to be either employees of pharmaceutical companies or recipients of their generosity.

---

## Physiotherapy

Physiotherapy is most helpful for people with severe chronic asthma (Bakal 2013). Benefits include improved QoL and exercise tolerance, plus reduced symptoms and medication use (Bruurs et al. 2013). Details are as follows.

### Breathing retraining

*Breathing retraining should now be a standard part of the range of treatments.*
**Thomas & Bruton 2014**

Specific techniques have shown the following benefits with chronic asthma:

- abdominal breathing: ↑ QoL (Prem et al. 2013);
- relaxation and reducing minute volume: ↑ QoL and PF, ↓ need for medication (Slader et al. 2006);
- 10 min of diaphragmatic breathing, pursed lips breathing and yoga pranayama techniques: ↑ ADL ability, ↓ use of rescue inhaler (Karam et al. 2017);
- relaxation, reducing minute volume, abdominal breathing and nasal breathing: ↑ QoL and ↓ anxiety (Holloway & West 2007);

- reducing minute volume plus capnography: ↑ QoL, ↓ symptoms, PF variability and bronchodilator use (Ritz et al. 2014);
- pursed-lips breathing in a relaxed posture, manual reinforcement of exhalation, abdominal breathing and posture correction: ↑ QoL, ↓ panic, agoraphobia and need for bronchodilators (Laurino et al. 2012).

The emphasis is on gentle improvements in the efficiency of breathing, usually in the form of rhythmic breathing and/or abdominal breathing, but not deep breathing, which can exacerbate bronchospasm (Pyrgos et al. 2012). Nose breathing should be encouraged throughout. These techniques are particularly useful for people with refractory asthma (Bakal 2013).

Two techniques were developed when drugs were less effective but can still assist patients who feel out of control of their breathing:

- Innocenti (1974) describes how patients can gain control by learning to change back and forth between abdominal and upper chest breathing, and to alter, breath by breath, the rate and depth of breathing.
- Weissleder (1976) taught patients to first feel the quality of their breathing, then inhale through the nose, slowly to eliminate any wheeze, increasing abdominal, lateral costal and upper chest expansion, then exhale in reverse order. Muscle tension is controlled throughout.

The 'Buteyko' technique is based on reducing minute volume by slowing the respiratory rate, using breath-counting to build up $CO_2$, and rocking and walking as a distraction from the resulting air hunger. At night, patients may be asked to lie on their left side and/or tape their mouth closed with micropore, to help maintain nose breathing. The rationale is that hyperventilation causes bronchospasm, which is true but simplistic because there are many causes of bronchospasm. However, the technique can improve asthma control (Prem et al. 2013) and it may be that the patients who benefit also coincidentally have hyperventilation syndrome (HVS), because the treatment of HVS is to reduce minute volume. The physiotherapist's role is to give any patient diagnosed with asthma the Nijmegen questionnaire to identify HVS (p. 391), and if it is positive, either treat them for HVS or refer them to a respiratory colleague or Buteyko practitioner.

Other techniques are inspiratory muscle training (Göhl et al. 2016), acupuncture (Thorax 2003), TENS on acupuncture points (Chan et al. 2012) and yoga

(Sodhi et al. 2014). A dry cough can stir up bronchospasm and patients may need advice on cough control.

## Exercise

Asthma and exercise have a topsy-turvy relationship. Exercise can trigger an acute episode, but regular aerobic exercise with appropriate precautions has shown the following benefits:

- ↓ severity of asthma (Dugger 2013), ↑ exercise tolerance, confidence and independence (Emtner et al. 1996);
- ↓ asthma symptoms and QoL (Eijkemans et al. 2012);
- ↓ bronchospasm and morbidity in children (Philpott et al. 2010).

Explaining that SOB is not harmful benefits patients who dislike exercise because they associate breathlessness with an asthma attack, leading to reduced fitness (Bahmer 2017). Outdoor exercise is best taken in the least polluted areas and times of day. Asthma is the most common chronic medical condition in Olympic athletes, which may relate to inhaled pollutants (Kippelen et al. 2012). Face masks protect against some pollutants but the filter must be changed regularly.

### Physical assistance for acute asthma

*'Most conversations in A & E are directed over and about me, and rarely involve me in any meaningful way'*

***Carter 1995***

Some patients do not want to be touched during an attack but most do not want to be left alone. Some do not want to talk but all want to be consulted. Noise and crowding should be minimal. Medication takes precedence over physical input.

Early attention to hydration and warm humidification may be required. Relaxed and rhythmic chest percussion, without upsetting the breathing pattern, may promote relaxation by input to receptors in the chest wall, with the occasional bonus of clearing secretions.

Some of the following advice may be beneficial for some patients.

- Sit upright, or lean slightly forward resting your arms on a table, or sit astride a chair backwards with your arms resting on the chair's back.
- Keep warm.

- Sit near fresh but not cold air, or use a fan.
- Take sips of warm water (some prefer cold), though this should not be attempted in the throes of a bad attack.
- Breathe through the nose unless breathlessness makes this impossible.
- Dizziness and tingling hands or feet mean that breathing is faster than it needs to be, which does not do harm but is a reminder of the innocuous cause of the symptoms.
- Practice previously learned techniques of relaxation, abdominal breathing and control over breathing. These should be started at the first intimation of an acute episode as they will not be possible later.
- Cuddle a warm hot water bottle or vibrating pillow.
- High-frequency oscillation may help clear stubborn thick secretions (Bose 2013).

In hospital, patients may need intravenous hydration, and acidosis indicates the need for mechanical assistance. Continuous positive airway pressure at 3–8 cmH$_2$O relieves inspiratory muscles from their exhausting work of holding open the obstructed airways (Phipps & Garrard 2003), but noninvasive or invasive mechanical ventilation may be needed if ventilatory failure supervenes (Stefan et al. 2016). If positive pressure assistance is required, the X-ray should be checked beforehand in case of a pneumothorax. Within 24 h of discharge, information should be sent to the patient's GP, who must follow the patient up within 2 days (BTS/SIGN 2016).

Children's asthma is on p. 367.

## Outcomes

Validated outcome measures include the Asthma Control test, Mini-Asthma Quality of Life Questionnaire (Karam et al. 2016) and Asthma Control Questionnaire (Schuler et al. 2016).

## BRONCHIECTASIS

Bronchiectasis is a chronic obstructive lung disease characterized by permanent distortion and dilation of the airway walls. The incidence of this 'orphan disease' is rising (ElMaraachli et al. 2016) but is underestimated in prevalence, incidence and morbidity (Goeminne 2010), probably because of a low level of clinical suspicion, or symptoms being ascribed to smoking (Smith et al. 2010). It disproportionately impacts countries where children are not vaccinated against whooping cough and measles (Chang & Marsh 2012).

## Causes

Bronchiectasis represents the final common pathway of a number of infectious, genetic, autoimmune and allergic disorders predisposing to persistent lung infection. The cause is unknown in 50% of cases (Metersky 2012), but associated factors are in Box 3.2.

A common process of inflammation or autoimmunity links the condition to inflammatory bowel disease, rheumatoid arthritis (Koch et al. 2016a) and, in up to

---

**BOX 3.2   Conditions Linked to Bronchiectasis**

- Congenital: cystic fibrosis or primary ciliary dyskinesia
- Infective: bacterial, viral or fungal, including ABA and TB
- Inflammatory: rheumatoid disease, inflammatory bowel disease, SLE or GORD
- Predisposition: immune deficiency, severe childhood respiratory infection
- Aspiration: foreign body or corrosive substance e.g. gastric acid

*ABA,* Allergic bronchopulmonary aspergillosis; *GORD,* gastro-oesophageal reflux disease; *SLE,* systemic lupus erythematosus; *TB,* (lung) tuberculosis.

---

half of patients, COPD (Suhling et al. 2016). If no cause is found, patients should be tested for α1-antitrypsin deficiency (Stoller & Aboussouan 2012).

## Pathophysiology

Inflammatory damage to the bronchial walls stimulates excess thick mucus secretion (Tambascio et al. 2013) which may be focal or diffuse, the latter often accompanied by sinusitis or other comorbidity (Ramakrishnan et al. 2013). The warm moist environment of the lung combines with the mucus to set up a vicious cycle of infection, inflammation and further obstruction (Fig. 3.10), compounded by oxidative stress (Olveira et al. 2013). Thick mucus crushes the tender cilia and causes additional damage. An overexuberant immune response to the colonizing microbes releases toxic inflammatory chemicals, particularly neutrophils, further contributing to the vicious cycle. Persistent inflammation leads to fibrosis and sometimes sets off bronchospasm. Abscesses may develop in florid disease. The airways are chronically colonized in 60% of patients (Goeminne 2010).

'Traction' or 'dry' bronchiectasis is not actually bronchiectasis but an offshoot of pulmonary fibrosis (see Fig. 3.23) in which lung tissue is pulled apart by scarring (Piciucchi et al. 2016). It favours the upper lobes, which are more stretched by gravity, but does not produce excess mucus and chest clearance is not indicated.

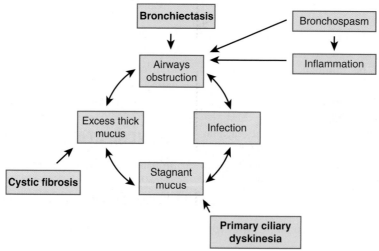

**FIGURE 3.10** Vicious cycle of the diseases of impaired mucociliary clearance.

## Clinical Features

Voluminous quantities of sputum are produced but are inefficiently cleared because of corrugated airways and damaged cilia. Secretions cause coarse wheezes, crackles and squeaks on auscultation.

Respiratory and musculoskeletal factors contribute to exercise intolerance (Hill et al. 2012). Muscle dysfunction is caused by inflammation, hypoxia, inactivity, malnutrition and some drugs (Ozalp et al. 2012). Dyspnoea on exertion is experienced by an average 75% of patients, chest pain by 50%, snoring by 44% and finger clubbing by 3% (Athanazio 2012). SOB is felt more keenly by those with hypoxia-driven cognitive dysfunction (Gülhan et al. 2015). Fatigue can be disabling, caused by persistent cough, recurrent infection and SOB (Hester et al. 2012). Other features are loss of appetite, depression, anxiety, embarrassment, reduced confidence and altered relationships (Tomkinson & Bruton 2009). Stress incontinence is a frequent result of excess coughing. Chest pain may reflect pneumonitis adjacent to the sensitive pleural surface and tends to lessen once the patient has an effective chest clearance regimen.

Exacerbations occur on average several times a year and are identified by four or more of the following: change in sputum, ↑ SOB, ↑ cough, fever >38° C, ↑ wheeze, ↓ exercise tolerance, fatigue, let hargy and radiographic signs (Goeminne 2010). Acute infection may erode the airway lining and cause haemoptysis, leaving the airways more vulnerable to infection. For children with the disease, exacerbations can be identified by specific clinical features and systemic markers (Kapur et al. 2012).

## Tests

Spirometry may indicate airflow obstruction but does not aid in clinical decision making (Guan et al. 2016). If the disease progresses, a restrictive pattern may develop (Athanazio 2012).

High-resolution CT scan is the gold standard for diagnosis and its sensitivity is thought to be the reason for a 10-fold increase in the rate of diagnosis (King & Daviskas 2010) and possibly the reason for some patients emerging distressed from being told their scan results by someone who does not know that they have minimal symptoms. Parallel tramlines on the scan indicate thickened airway walls, and ring shadows represent dilated airways seen in cross-section (Fig. 3.11). Neglected disease shows 'glove finger shadows' that are dilated bronchi full of solidified secretions, and sometimes ring shadows with fluid levels (Fig. 3.12). A bronchogram outlines the dilated airways (Fig. 3.13) but is rarely necessary.

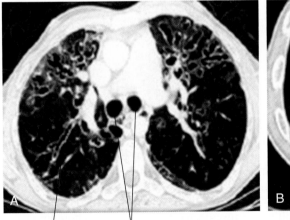
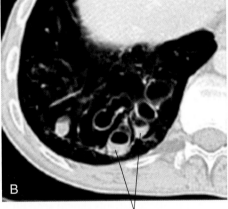

Tramlines        R and L main bronchi            Dilated airways containing mucus

**FIGURE 3.11** Bronchiectasis scans showing thickened airway walls: (A) as tramlines and (B) in cross section. (From Ibrahim et al. 2016.)

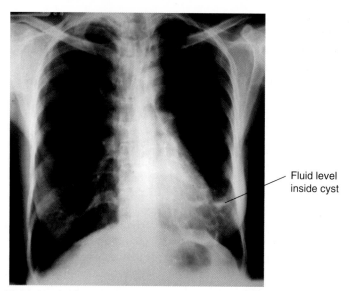

**FIGURE 3.12** Fluid levels in cysts behind the left breast shadow, indicating neglected bronchiectasis.

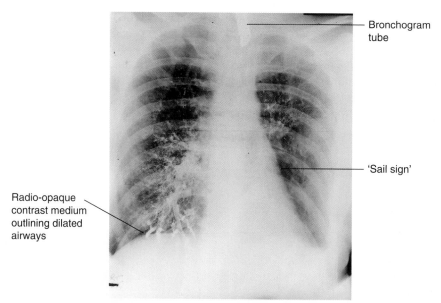

**FIGURE 3.13** Bronchogram illustrating the dilated airways of bronchiectasis in the right lower lobe. The straight left heart border ('sail sign') indicates previous left lower lobectomy.

During an exacerbation, microbiology identifies the offending organisms. Stable patients should send off an annual sputum sample (BTS 2012a). Murray (2009) found a 5% incidence of bacterial colonization in mucoid sputum, 43.5% in mucopurulent sputum and 86.4% in purulent sputum. Patients should also be investigated for allergic bronchopulmonary aspergillosis, immune deficiencies (BTS 2012a), cardiovascular disease and osteoporosis (Gale et al. 2012). Table 3.4 clarifies the difference with COPD.

**TABLE 3.4  Distinguishing features of bronchiectasis and COPD**

|  | Bronchiectasis | COPD |
|---|---|---|
| Age | Varied | Older |
| Smoking history | Not necessarily | Usually |
| Auscultation | Noisy, may be localized | Diffuse crackles if chronic bronchitis |
| Sputum | Excessive, often thick and green | Moderate if chronic bronchitis |
| Haemoptysis | Sometimes | No |
| Finger clubbing | Sometimes | No |
| Imaging | Specific | Variable |

## Medical Treatment

Patients should be issued with a management plan (NICE 2010a) and are best referred to a specialist centre, where education and systematic management are provided (French et al. 2007).

**Antibiotics** are used as needed, alternating one or more antibiotics. For patients who deteriorate every winter, regular antibiotics can be taken in the cold months. Patients need a store of antibiotics specific to their usual organisms, to be taken at the first sign of colour change in their sputum. The macrolide erythromycin has antibiotic and antiinflammatory effects, and may reduce exacerbations (Burr et al. 2016). An exacerbation may require intravenous antibiotics, preferably managed at home. A blitz of oral, intravenous and nebulized antibiotics is sometimes able to eradicate the dreaded pseudomonas infection (White et al. 2012a).

Antibiotics do not control the persistent inflammation which may be progressively damaging the airways, but inhaled **steroids** reduce inflammatory markers and sputum volume (Athanazio 2012), although they should not be used routinely (Judson et al. 2014). **Mucolytics** have antiinflammatory, antioxidant and mucoregulatory properties (Kim & Kim 2012a). Inflammation is exacerbated by lack of vitamin D, from which the majority of patients suffer (Chalmers et al. 2013). Hyperosmolar agents such as **hypertonic saline** or **mannitol** may assist mucociliary clearance (Hart et al. 2014). Bronchodilators are unhelpful unless hyperreactive airways are present (Athanazio 2012).

If symptoms such as pain are intractable, surgical resection of nonperfused lung is occasionally indicated for localized disease. Transplantation may be possible for some patients in late stage disease (Rademacher et al. 2016).

## Physiotherapy

Bronchiectasis reduces mucociliary clearance to an average 15% of normal (Houtmeyers et al. 1999). Untreated, patients will compensate with excessive coughing, which is antisocial, tiring and weakens the pelvic floor. Mucus retention is associated with exacerbations and mortality (Herrero et al. 2016). Daily chest clearance enhances lung function (Lee et al. 2013b) and dampens down the vicious cycle of secretions and inflammation (Volsko 2013).

Treatment begins with cough control (p. 218), patients being discouraged from coughing until they are ready to expectorate. A daily chest clearance programme must be sufficient to clear the airways enough to eliminate coughing between sessions. Hydration, an exercise programme and ACBT/AD may be adequate. Some patients find home-based humidification helpful (Rea et al. 2010) and regular inhaled 7% hypertonic saline can improve QoL (Kellett & Robert 2011). Other airway clearance techniques may be required (Chapter 7), and some patients prefer to choose a device:

1. The Flutter speeds sputum removal and may reduce airflow resistance (Figueiredo et al. 2012) but for some patients it is less effective than ACBT (Eaton et al. 2007).
2. The Acapella increases sputum clearance, exercise capacity and QoL (Murray & Pentland 2009) and some patients have found this more convenient than ACBT (Patterson et al. 2005).
3. Some patients find benefit with percussors (Paneroni et al. 2011) or oscillators (Nicolini et al. 2013).

Pelvic floor exercises may be required, but stress incontinence usually needs referral to the continence service. Pulmonary rehabilitation should be offered to those whose SOB affects their activities of daily living (BTS 2012a), but patients must skip sessions when they have an infection in order to minimize cross-infection. All patients must gel their hands, and equipment should be wiped down between sessions.

Outcome can be assessed by questionnaires on cough, QoL and function (Spinou et al. 2016) or the Seattle Obstructive Lung Disease Questionnaire (Bulcun et al. 2015). CT scans can identify mucus clearance and MRI the resulting ventilation improvements (Svenningsen

2017). Reduced stress incontinence and fatigue are often what matter most to patients.

---

**MINI CLINICAL REASONING**

*Article title: Airway clearance in bronchiectasis: a randomized crossover trial of active cycle of breathing techniques (incorporating postural drainage and vibration) versus test of incremental respiratory endurance*
           *Chron Respir Dis* (2004) 1, 127

We need read no further: a technique aimed at clearing secretions is going to be more effective in clearing secretions than a technique that is not aimed at clearing secretions.

---

# CYSTIC FIBROSIS

Cystic fibrosis (CF) is no longer a disease of childhood. The majority of patients are now adults (Wielpütz et al. 2016) and median survival is 50 years (Castellani 2017).

Although CF exists in every ethnic group, among European-derived populations it is the commonest life-shortening genetic disease, affecting approximately 90,000 humans worldwide (Kerem 2016), plus orangutans (Stringer et al. 2016). The gene is carried by 1 in 25 Caucasians and expressed when inherited from both parents. Two carriers have a 25% chance of each of their children having CF, and a 50% chance that each child will be a carrier.

Despite progress in organ transplantation, improved survival is mainly due to advances in conventional treatment, with patients fitting their lives around chest clearance, inhaled drugs and cleaning their equipment. One patient responded when asked about her job: 'I'm a full-time cystic'.

## Pathophysiology

CF is a chronic progressive disorder of the exocrine glands, manifesting mainly as an obstructive airways disease. In most cells the gene encoding CF is dormant, but in epithelial cells it is switched on, impairing ion and water transport across epithelial surfaces and obstructing various body lumens. In the gut, pancreatic insufficiency leads to malabsorption and fat intolerance. In the male reproductive system, blockage causes infertility in most patients (Hotaling 2014), but sexual function is not affected and fatherhood is possible artificially.

In the lungs, dehydrated and acidic airway surface liquid impairs antimicrobial function and thickens mucus (Haq et al. 2016) so that it acts more like pus than mucus (Rubin 2015b). Mucociliary clearance may come to a standstill (Sturm 2012), but the cough mechanism, now much needed, is compromised by the mucins in mucus getting glued to the epithelium (Knowles & Boucher 2002). A neutrophil-dominated inflammatory response releases DNA, whose strands bind together and thicken secretions further.

Airway abnormalities are present at birth (VanDevanter et al. 2016) and bronchiectasis develops before school age, leading to inflammation disseminating systemically (Sly 2016). Intractable infection becomes established by adolescence (Dickson et al. 2016), even when the child is clinically well, leading to progressive damage and regular exacerbations (VandenBranden 2012).

*Staphylococcus aureus* is the commonest pathogen in infants and young children. Adults infected by the methicillin-resistant *Staphylococcus aureus* (MRSA) have double the rate of airflow obstruction (Vanderhelst et al. 2012). *Pseudomonas aeruginosa* may impair respiratory muscle function (Magnet 2017) and hides from antibiotics in biofilm macrocolonies (Solé & Girón 2016). A minority of patients carry the feared onion rot organism *Burkholderia cepacia*, which brings a risk of pneumothorax (Mohan 2004), increases mortality (Kitt et al. 2016) and requires segregation of patients, at great personal cost for those who have previously socialized freely. Even sibling separation is tolerated by some families. The bacteria has been found in nebulisers and hospital sink drains (Ida et al. 2016), so respiratory equipment and treatment locations are segregated.

## Comorbidities

**Gut problems** occur early in life and can severely impair QoL. Patients may suffer obstruction or inflammatory bowel syndrome. Frequent coughing may cause gastro-oesophageal reflux disease (GORD) (Demeyer et al. 2016), which should be treated with CF-specific medication rather than conventional drugs (Pauwels 2012).

**Sleep problems** relate mostly to breathing difficulties (Silva et al. 2016).

**Malnutrition** compromises respiratory defence. It may be caused by liver disease, pancreatic insufficiency or inflammation, sometimes contributing to **respiratory muscle fatigue**. The respiratory muscles themselves show normal or increased strength because of their work in breathing through obstructed airways (Dassios 2015) but other muscles may succumb to **peripheral neuropathy** (Chakrabarty 2013).

Longer survival has given rise to new problems:

- **Osteoporosis** occurs in a quarter of adults due to malabsorption, delayed puberty, steroid therapy and, for some, immunosuppressive drugs after transplantation (Quon 2012). Fracture rates are nine times higher than in age-matched controls (Stahl et al. 2017).
- **Pain** interferes with airway clearance and occurs in 77% of adults and 42% of children, including back, abdomen, chest, limbs and, due to chronic sinusitis or uncontrolled coughing, headaches (Lee et al. 2016d). Inflammatory joint damage can be identified by ultrasound or MRI (Fitch et al. 2016).
- Pancreatic damage and steroid use predispose to **diabetes** (Fig. 3.14) in up to 40% of adults (Bilodeau et al. 2016).
- **Cardiac dysfunction**, caused by systemic inflammation, diabetes, or pulmonary hypertension from prolonged hypoxaemia (Almajed & Lands 2012), contributes to impaired exercise tolerance (Van Iterson et al. 2016).
- **Liver disease** may cause portal hypertension and coagulopathy, leading to it becoming the third leading cause of death (Stonebraker et al. 2016). If complicated by ascites, sputum clearance is best done as upright as convenient for the patient.

- Bronchial artery hypertrophy may lead to **pulmonary haemorrhage.**
- **Pneumothorax** may occur in the later stages. High percentage oxygen assists reabsorption of the gas (ACPCF 2011). A chest drain may be required but the lung takes longer than average to reexpand (MacDuff et al. 2010). Chest clearance should continue, but without unnecessary coughing.

## Clinical Features

*'It doesn't do too much for one's confidence to know that one has probably got halitosis, so I tend to talk to people sideways on'*

*Hall 1984*

The antisocial nature of CF relates to delayed puberty, flatus, unrelenting weariness, nasal discharge and incessant coughing. The fact that patients usually look well leads to misunderstandings about invisible symptoms such as fatigue, and up to a third of patients have anxiety or depression (Quittner et al. 2016).

Objectively, wheezes and widespread crackles are heard on auscultation. Hyperinflation increases the inspiratory work of breathing and is associated with reduced exercise capacity, but the extra volume assists the airways to stay open and reduces expiratory resistance (Sovtic et al. 2013).

Exacerbation, indicated by weight loss or worsening respiratory symptoms, increases morbidity and mortality

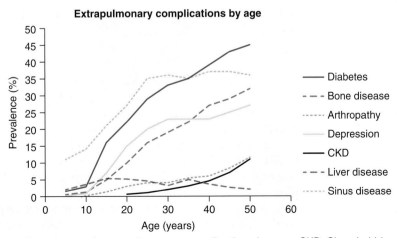

**FIGURE 3.14** Prevalence of extrapulmonary complications by age. *CKD,* Chronic kidney disease. (From Quon 2012.)

(Heltshe & Goss 2016). If the cause is respiratory, secretions are thicker than normal and the patient may become less rather than more productive.

In the later stages, $PaO_2$ falls and eventually $PaCO_2$ rises. The inexorable deterioration is anticipated by patients, who each respond in their individual way. They often form strong attachments to each other, which provides comradeship but can be devastating when one dies. Palliative specialists need to be part of the team throughout, and most patients want to discuss end-of-life care (Chen et al. 2017).

## Tests

Screening is possible at three stages:

1. Carrier screening has been found to be cost-effective (Norman 2012).
2. Prenatal diagnosis is available for pregnancies known to be at risk because of family history.
3. Universal screening of newborns is recommended (Wielpütz et al. 2016).

After birth, CF is suspected if an infant fails to thrive or has repeated chest infections. The skin tastes salty, and confirmation is by a test for abnormally salty sweat at 6 weeks old. By puberty, lung function tests begin to show an obstructive pattern (Vermeulen et al. 2014).

Structural changes show up first on CT scan (Fig. 3.15), then on X-ray (Fig. 3.16). Mucous plugging can be demonstrated by CT, MRI (Wielpütz et al. 2016) or tomosynthesis (Kim 2010).

Exercise tests have been found more sensitive than spirometry to detect structural changes in the lungs (Hatziagorou et al. 2016).

## General Management

The aim is to reduce infections and prevent organ damage. Both children and adults must be under the care of a multidisciplinary CF team (Doull & Evans 2012). Passage from paediatric to adult care requires a

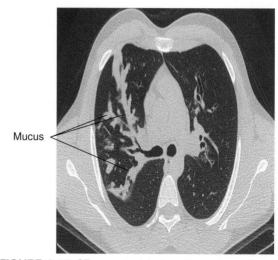

**FIGURE 3.15** CT scan just below the carina, showing mucous plugging. (From Sheikh et al. 2015.)

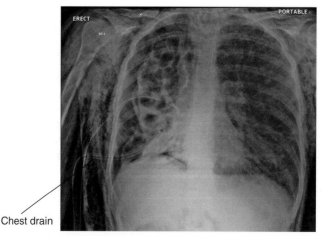

**FIGURE 3.16** Cystic fibrosis lungs with extensive subcutaneous emphysema and, on the right, a pneumothorax. (From Lord et al. 2016a.)

flexible age of transfer, prior visits to the adult centre and good communication between all parties.

Patients require frequent needle sticks for assessment and treatment, and should be advised to request topical anaesthesia.

## Education

When a baby with CF is born, education begins as soon as the parents have accommodated sufficiently to the diagnosis. General points are:

- CF children should, within any limitations, take part in normal physical activities.
- They should share with healthy siblings the disciplines and standards of the family.
- CF children are not infectious.
- No-one should smoke in the home, and infection control measures are required (Miroballi et al. 2012).

Professional support reduces family isolation and improves attention for siblings, while cascade carrier testing offers relatives the opportunity to know their status (Duguépéroux et al. 2016). At adolescence, seven out of eight patients do not follow treatment recommendations (Ernst et al. 2010), and self-help groups may be useful. Daily chest clearance is the greatest chore, and time-related factors are the main reason for low adherence (Flores et al. 2013).

## Oxygen therapy

Acute oxygen may be required to achieve a target $SpO_2$ of 94%–98%, or 88%–92% for those at risk of hypercapnia. For chronic disease, home oxygen is required if stable $PaO_2$ drops below 7.3 kPa (55 mmHg) when breathing air, or <8 kPa (60 mmHg) in the presence of peripheral oedema, polycythaemia or pulmonary hypertension.

## Nutrition

Nutritional status is strongly associated with pulmonary function and survival, and management includes exclusive breast feeding in infancy, energy intake adapted to achieve normal weight and height, pancreatic enzyme and fat soluble vitamin treatment, enteral tube feeding if required, glucose tolerance testing from 10 years old and bone mineral density checks from age 8–10 years (Turck et al. 2016). Extra attention is required for low-birth-weight babies (Darrah et al. 2016).

## Medication

The underlying cause of the disease can treated by ivacaftor, which facilitates chloride transport, and lumacaftor, which increases trafficking of mature protein to the cell surface, both of which combine as Orkambi (Schneider 2017).

An unremitting onslaught against bacteria is provided by high-dose antibiotics. These may be pumped into the body by home nebulisers or specialized inhalers (Moore et al. 2016). Inhaled microparticles may be able to penetrate the thick mucus (Craparo et al. 2017) but the intravenous route is generally used, either electively every 3 months or symptomatically (Breen 2012), usually by central line and a small reservoir called a portacath implanted under the skin of the lateral chest wall. This may be managed at home, which avoids hospital infections, or the patient is admitted to a specialist centre, which provides mutual support and family respite.

Mucolytic agents may loosen secretions so that they are easier to clear, e.g. mannitol, N-acetylcysteine, bicarbonate (Stigliani et al. 2016) or dornase alfa. Dornase alfa can overliquify secretions so that chest clearance is 'like eating soup with a fork', according to one patient. Specialist assessment is required.

Bronchodilators should not be used unless there is evidence of benefit (Barry & Flume 2017).

## Assisted ventilation

NIV improves survival in critically ill patients, but invasive mechanical ventilation brings high mortality (Sheikh et al. 2011). NIV may also be used nocturnally for chronic ventilatory failure, as a bridge to transplantation, as palliation, or to help clear secretions in an exhausted patient (Rodriguez et al. 2017). Patients should be given the opportunity to discuss their preferences before the need arises.

## Surgery

A patient with a pneumothorax has a 50%–90% chance of recurrence, and pleurodesis is often required. This does not contraindicate subsequent transplantation (Flume 2009).

Evaluation for transplant of heart, lungs and/or liver occurs when pulmonary hypertension supervenes. Success can transform a chair-ridden invalid into an active person within weeks. Most of the pulmonary problems of CF are eliminated because donor lungs do not have the genetic abnormality, but bone loss is accelerated in the first year (Rosenblatt 2009).

Problems of transplantation are formidable, including the stress of waiting for donor organs, life-long immunosuppressive drugs for the successful transplant, and devastated families if the wait is too long or the transplanted organs rejected. Ambulatory extracorporeal membrane oxygenation allows some patients to participate in physiotherapy and eat normally during their wait (Hayes et al. 2012). Palliative specialists should be on the team (Bourke et al. 2016) so that patients can choose the balance of symptom relief and/or vigorous gastrostomy feeding, mechanical ventilation and other heroics.

### Future therapies

Gene transfer therapy allows genetic material to be transferred by inhalation of a normal gene on a virus or other vector. Stem cell therapies would target stem and progenitor cells in the lungs. Gargling with egg yolk immunoglobulins has been suggested as prophylaxis against pseudomonas infection (Thomsen et al. 2016).

### Physiotherapy

Long-term trials of chest clearance are limited, possibly because it might be considered unethical to deprive a control group of a treatment that makes physiological sense. However, studies suggest that physiotherapy brings short-term benefit (Warnock & Gates 2015) and clinical reasoning suggests that this might be prolonged.

Once CF has been diagnosed, chest clearance usually starts immediately in order to minimize chronic infection (Rand et al. 2013). Adherence rates are well below 50% in the early years (Schechter 2007) and gruelling regimens produce no immediate improvement in well-being, with sputum quantity the only reinforcement. Goal setting, daily tick charts and a reward system can improve outcomes (Ernst et al. 2010).

If convenient for the patient and family, chest clearance should be coordinated with nebuliser treatments, i.e. before antibiotics so that absorption of the drug is not hampered by mucus, and after bronchodilators or nebulized saline. Details of sputum clearance techniques are in Chapter 7, with evidence specific to CF as follows:

- Inhaled **hypertonic saline** can improve mucociliary clearance (Fig. 3.17), speed the resolution of exacerbation symptoms (Dentice et al. 2016) and work in a similar way to mannitol, but it is time consuming and the side effects include the salty taste, bronchospasm and cough. It is used before or during airway clearance and is usually preceded by a bronchodilator, then nebulized in concentrations of 3%–10%, in volumes of 3–10 mL (Rand et al. 2013), depending on tolerance of the saltiness. Delivery under positive pressure may be beneficial (O'Connell et al. 2011). Hypertonic saline also eases sinusitis symptoms.
- **Exercise** has the advantage that most patients will do it, so long as they choose the type of exercise, e.g. Internet-based programmes (Cox et al. 2015) and it is started early, e.g. bouncing on a gym ball. Regular exercise reduces airflow obstruction and

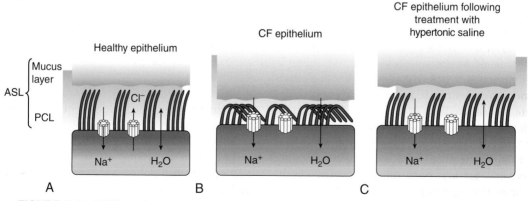

**FIGURE 3.17** (A) Normal mucus hydration, (B) CF thick mucus, (C) restoration of hydration with hypertonic saline. *ASL,* Airway surface liquid; *CF,* cystic fibrosis; *PCL,* periciliary layer.

hospital admissions (Cox et al. 2016), increases bone health (Tejero et al. 2016), enhances airway clearance and increases survival (Williams 2010). The 6-min walk test, although tedious for these busy patients, identifies those who might desaturate (Chetta 2001). Assessment and outcomes can be performed remotely, to save another trip to the clinic, using the 3-min step test (Cox 2013). Patients with advanced disease may be suited to muscle electrostimulation (Vivodtzev et al. 2013).

- **Autogenic drainage** (AD) is the most popular treatment (Herrero et al. 2016) and if combined with hypertonic saline, reduces treatment time (Van Ginderdeuren et al. 2011).
- The **active cycle of breathing** (ACBT) helps clear secretions from peripheral airways (Hristara & Tsanakas 2007). For both AD and ACBT, the huff may need modification to avoid small airway closure (Kilpatrick et al. 2001).
- **Positive expiratory pressure** (PEP) can be used from age 4. It clears secretions by stabilizing floppy airways and can reduce exacerbations (McIlwaine et al. 2013). **Oscillating PEP** has also been found to improve QoL (Lee et al 2015).
- Young children respond well to **blowing bubbles** and **bubble PEP.**
- **High-frequency chest compression** has shown benefit in the short term (Fainardi et al. 2011).
- If **postural drainage** is the chosen treatment, drainage time is about 15 min in younger children, and more in adolescents and adults, depending on patient preference, quantity of secretions and the effectiveness of other measures. **Manual techniques** are included if they produce more sputum or the patient finds them effective. This can be a burden for the family, but may reduce airflow obstruction when added to ACBT (Williams et al. 2001). The patient's history should be checked for GORD, and the head-down tip avoided if it brings on symptoms, although in young children this has not been shown to exacerbate the reflux.

The priority of patient choice is underlined by studies finding little difference in outcome between techniques (MAS 2009, Flume 2012). Chest clearance is usually done once or twice daily, or, during an exacerbation, up to four times a day, depending on the quantity of secretions. Each treatment session is continued until sputum is no longer expectorated or a rest is needed.

Musculoskeletal input helps ease stiffness in thoracic joints (Havermans et al. 2013). In supine, for example, patients can breathe out and depress their shoulder girdles, then on breathing in raise their arms above their head, holding the stretch for a few seconds. Some gain benefit from a rolled up towel placed vertically under their thoracic spine. If this is done on waking or before sleeping it barely interferes with the patient's lifestyle. Hands-on input for noninflammatory pain includes mobilizations to the rib cage and thoracic spine, advice based on the Alexander technique (Sandsund et al. 2011) and postural interventions (Massery 2005). Claims have been made that this can partially correct thoracic kyphosis and slow the decline in $FEV_1$ (ACPCF 2011). Precautions include a check for osteoporosis.

Early independence should be encouraged, with young children actively participating, and 10-year-old children able to do their own treatment during sleepovers. Older children are advised against cough suppression for social reasons, and reminded that clearing their chest before socializing reduces the need to cough.

Patients of any age may have difficulty expectorating, sometimes because they don't like the taste. Children can be congratulated for coughing up anything, even saliva, with extra praise and stickers if they manage to produce 'froggies'. Swallowing large amounts of sputum can lead to vomiting up precious nutrition.

The 'optimum' programme is not always the most effective in the teenage years. Management is best negotiated, people with CF being particularly worth listening to because they are medically streetwise and understand much about their treatment. Motivation in hospitalized patients is enhanced by simple measures such as offering a choice of treatment times and techniques. Patients can also be invited to video their session, which helps them remember details of technique and can be updated when required.

Patients will not always volunteer that they have stress incontinence, so they should be asked in private whether they wet themselves on coughing, with reassurance that this is common in people with CF and a continence service is available. Urinary incontinence affects 11% of men and 68% of women over 11 years of age, leading to a quarter of patients refraining from coughing out their sputum (Reichman et al. 2016). Patients may balk at the phrase 'incontinence', which they often interpret as floods of urine rather than the more acceptable leaking.

Once the optimum regimen has been negotiated, patients require a review every 3 months.

### Precautions

Patients should not be asked to cough unnecessarily because of the resulting stress incontinence, fatigue and collapse of central airways with impaired sputum clearance (Zapletal 1983).

Haemoptysis occurs in 10% of patients, caused by hypertrophied bronchial arteries from chronic airway inflammation (Fitzgerald 2012). Blood streaking of sputum is common and should be disregarded, but if >50 mL is coughed up over 24 h, chest clearance, including exercise training, should be halted and the medical team notified. Frank haemoptysis usually indicates late-stage disease and the patient will need hospital admission and sometimes bronchial artery embolization. Modified physiotherapy can continue once the patient is stabilized.

Measures to prevent cross infection include scrupulous hand washing, covering of sputum pots and single-patient use of all devices.

Patients with an $FEV_1$ <50% predicted are likely to show desaturation on exercise, which may be avoided by interval training (p. 256), a lower workload or supplemental oxygen. Fluids and sometimes extra salt are needed in hot weather because of the salty sweat.

In advanced disease, physiotherapists should be alert to the breathlessness and pleuritic pain of a pneumothorax. If NIV is used, high pressures should be avoided because of this risk (Haworth et al. 2000).

Anaemia may cause dyspnoea and reduced ability to exercise. Coagulopathy may contraindicate manual techniques. Oesophageal varices or haematemesis contraindicates all physiotherapy except abdominal breathing.

### Outcomes

Both lung function and exercise capacity are used to evaluate treatment, as well as being predictors of prognosis (Doeleman et al. 2016). Outcome measures include the Cystic Fibrosis Questionnaire (Solé et al. 2016), quality of life questionnaires (Bradley et al. 2013, Havermans et al. 2013, Vermeulen et al. 2014) and single-breath washout tests for airway clearance (Abbas 2013). Exercise tests are described by Radtke et al. (2016) and Vallier et al. (2016). The incremental shuttle walk

test is a better reflection of exercise tolerance in CF than the 6-min walk test (Saglam et al. 2016).

## PRIMARY CILIARY DYSKINESIA

Primary ciliary dyskinesia (PCD) is a recessively inherited group of disorders in which disorganized motility of cilia leads to uncoordinated mucociliary action similar to an escalator malfunctioning in rush hour, leaving the lungs vulnerable to airflow obstruction by the vicious cycle on page 88. There is virtually no mucociliary clearance and the patient compensates by coughing. Half the patients have dextrocardia (Fig. 3.18) and their middle lobe on the left, indicating Kartagener syndrome, a combination of bronchiectasis, sinusitis, situs inversus (mirror image of internal organs), and infertility (due to dyskinetic cilia in fallopian tubes or on sperm tails) (Fretzayas & Moustaki 2016).

Children may also have glue ear, a perpetually runny nose, chronic sinusitis and frequent chest infections. Early diagnosis helps prevent progression to bronchiectasis, but the condition is rare and often missed. Suspicions are raised in people with bronchiectasis who have a history of otitis media and family members with a similar history, including male subfertility. Patients should be referred to a specialist centre, where clinical tests are available (Behan et al. 2016).

Medical treatment is by microbiological surveillance, selective antibiotics, vaccinations and avoidance of smoking. Exacerbation is followed by around 25% of children failing to recover baseline lung function within 3 months, which is similar to CF (Sunther et al. 2012)

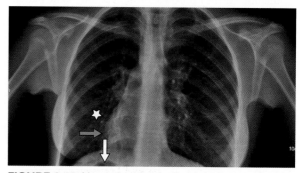

**FIGURE 3.18** X-ray showing in the right lower zone the bronchiectatic changes of PCD *(white star)*, dextrocardia *(purple arrow)* and right-sided gastric bubble *(white arrow)*. (From Raoufi et al. 2016.)

and is a reminder of the importance of accurate antibiotics and meticulous chest clearance. Gene editing offers hope for the future (Lai et al. 2016).

Physiotherapy is by daily chest clearance (Chapter 7). Exercise can improve lung function (Gokdemir et al. 2013) and cause better bronchodilation than a $\beta_2$-agonist (Daniels & Noone 2015). Questionnaires are available as outcome measures for children and adolescents (Dell et al. 2016).

## INHALED FOREIGN BODY

Inhaling an unwanted object usually occurs in children, or in adults who are elderly, have neurological disease or are intoxicated. If the object becomes stuck, it may trap air or induce inflammation, causing atelectasis (Fig. 3.19) or pneumonia respectively (Salih et al. 2016). It may also lead to bronchiectasis (Pellissier et al. 2016), and accounts for 40% of unintentional deaths in infants (Lluna et al. 2017).

There is usually a history of paroxysmal coughing, followed by a relatively asymptomatic interval. In some cases, clinical signs may then arise, such as reduced breath sounds, stridor, persistent cough, haemoptysis, nonresolving consolidation or a localized wheeze, sometimes leading to a misdiagnosis of asthma (Metin et al. 2016). Foreign bodies lodge preferentially in the right main stem bronchus because of its larger diameter and more vertical orientation than the left.

Small objects can be retained for months or, in the case of one patient who inhaled a pen cap, 41 years (Pellissier et al. 2016). Many foreign bodies are made of vegetable matter and do not show on X-ray. Most are capricious, and in young children difficult to diagnose.

Physiotherapy is contraindicated because of the risk of shifting the object to a more dangerous location. The foreign body is usually removed by bronchoscopy, following which there can be inflammatory secretions or a localized collapse that may require physiotherapy.

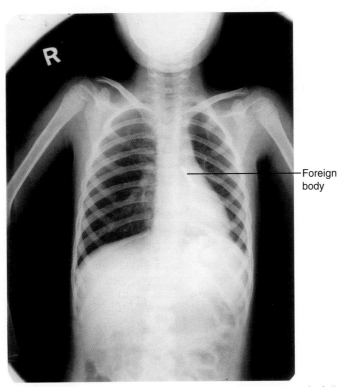

**FIGURE 3.19** Left lower lobe collapse, with mediastinum shifted to the left, following aspiration of a foreign body by a child.

# INTERSTITIAL LUNG DISEASE

Diseases that affect the parenchyma rather than the airways are covered by the umbrella term interstitial lung disease (ILD), indicating inflammation and fibrosis. These shrink the lung, categorizing it as a restrictive disease. Causes include immune disturbance and exposure to toxic agents such as coal dust, cigarette smoke (Fig. 3.20), asbestos or stomach acid.

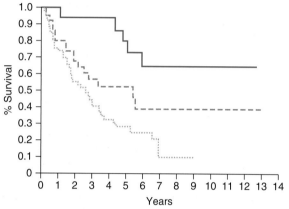

**FIGURE 3.20** Kaplan-Meier survival curves of patients with pulmonary fibrosis by smoking status. Current smokers *(—)*, never smokers *(- -)* and previous smokers *(...)* with 5-year survival: 75.5%, 53.8% and 28.3%, respectively. (From Greene et al. 2002.)

## Pathophysiology and Comorbidities

Macrophages engulf the inhaled particles, but inflammatory mediators are also released. The resulting alveolitis either resolves or progresses to an aberrant repair mechanism and the remodelling of parenchyma into fibrosis (Fig. 3.21). The differentiation of normal lung fibroblasts into myofibroblasts occurs by means of a 'Yin-Yang' factor (Lin et al. 2011), which is not as serene as it sounds and allows invasion of the damaged basement membrane in a similar way to metastatic cancer (Li et al. 2011). This may explain why the disease brings increased risk of lung cancer (Puglisi et al. 2016). As with all alveolar disorders, the capillaries are also affected, and pulmonary hypertension may develop, indicating the importance of cool-down after exercise to avoid a rapid fall in cardiac output and risk of syncope (Markovitz 2010). Other comorbidities are bronchiectasis (Plantier et al. 2016), rheumatoid arthritis (Nurmi et al. 2016), COPD, obstructive sleep apnoea, cardiovascular disease and gastro-oesophageal reflux (Agrawal et al. 2016), the antacids for which may increase the risk of infection (Kreuter et al. 2016).

The main effects are:

- lung stiffness, which increases the WOB;
- hypoxaemia due to disorganized lung architecture and ↓ diffusion (Craig 2017)
- ↓ surface area of the alveolar–capillary membrane, which impairs gas exchange;

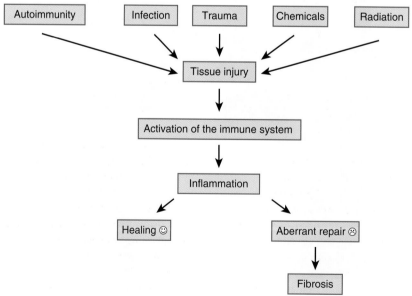

**FIGURE 3.21** Pathogenesis of injury progressing to healing and fibrosis.

- respiratory and limb muscle dysfunction (Panagiotou et al. 2016).

Worsening SOB and new opacities on high resolution CT (HRCT) scan suggest exacerbation, possibly caused by aspiration or drug toxicity. Prognosis is poor (Puglisi et al. 2016).

## Classification

Some of the 200 disorders (Spagnolo et al. 2012) are described below.

**Fibrosing alveolitis** is the commonest and most devastating form of ILD. Causes include drugs such as amiodarone (Nasri et al. 2016) or anticoagulants (Tomari et al. 2016) and occupational pollutants such as cement, metal or wood dust. Its incidence is rising, and progression of the disease is relentlessly aggressive, with a median survival of 3–5 years, but sometimes with rapid decline and death over months (Agrawal et al. 2016). If there is no obvious cause, it is called cryptogenic or idiopathic pulmonary fibrosis (IPF) and is probably the result of complex interactions between genetic and environmental factors, its incidence increasing with age (Jo et al. 2016). If there is a known inhaled cause, such as occurs with occupational exposure, it may be called extrinsic allergic alveolitis or hypersensitivity pneumonitis (Feary & Szram 2016). The term fibrosing alveolitis can incorporate the end result of other disorders such as those described in the following section, which may or may not be classified separately.

**Bird fancier's lung** and **farmer's lung** lead to fever and malaise 4–8 h after exposure to the organic dust. Lung fibrosis may develop if birds or farming cannot be avoided.

The **pneumoconioses** are slowly developing inhalation diseases. The body reacts to each inhaled particle by creating an inflammatory wall of cells around it. Miners' lung and silicosis are forms of this occupational exposure.

**Asbestosis** is characterized by a delay of up to 50 years between inhaling asbestos dust and developing the disease (Wright et al. 2002). Radiologically there is a 'shaggy heart' appearance and sometimes pleural involvement indicating mesothelioma (p. 120) or non-malignant pleural fibrosis (Dale et al. 2013).

**Rheumatoid disease** is a systemic condition best known for inflamed joints, but in 10%–15% of patients it also manifests as 'rheumatoid lung', which incorporates pleural, vascular, airway and fibrotic components, sometimes exacerbated by arthritis drugs (Diamanti et al. 2011).

ILD may combine with pulmonary hypertension to complicate systemic connective tissue diseases such as scleroderma, polymyositis, Sjögren syndrome and the following (Mathai 2016):

**Systemic lupus erythematosus** (SLE) involves chronic inflammation of skin, nervous system, kidneys, blood vessels, joints and lungs, the latter causing pleurisy, pleural effusion and fibrosis. Complications include pneumonia due to treatment by immunosuppressive agents and, for some, a 50-fold increased risk of myocardial infarction (Goodman 2012).

**Systemic sclerosis** affects the skin and internal organs. It is characterized by a disrupted microvasculature and immune system, deposition of collagen and sometimes a pulmonary vascular disorder (Hassoun 2012). If pulmonary hypertension develops, exercise training may improve QoL and possibly prolong survival (Grünig et al. 2012). The term **scleroderma** indicates that the skin is the most obvious organ involved.

**Sarcoidosis** is a chronic multisystem granulomatous disorder commonly presenting at ages 20–40, some patients being symptom-free but with radiological lymphadenopathy and often pulmonary infiltrates. Lung disease is the most common manifestation, but skin, eyes and joints may be affected. Infiltration of the myocardium can affect the heart (Holland 2010), and exercise may be impaired by peripheral muscle dysfunction. Causes are unknown but it is sometimes triggered by stress (Trombini 2012), and World Trade Center dust has been identified in fire fighters who developed the disease after 9/11 (De Boer & Wilsher 2010). Sarcoidosis stabilises or clears in the majority of patients, but others suffer irreversible fibrosis, requiring steroids, sometimes immunosuppressive drugs and occasionally transplantation (Soto-Gomez et al. 2016). Fatigue, psychological health and physical function can improve with a physical training programme (Marcellis et al. 2015).

A double whammy has been identified in which the deranged remodelling of ILD is combined with the tobacco-induced oxidative damage of COPD. Lung volumes are commonly within normal limits due to the opposing effects of fibrosis and hyperinflation, but the combination leads to premature lung ageing and sometimes lung cancer (Chilosi et al. 2012), the chemotherapy for which may worsen lung injury (Ozawa et al. 2016).

## Clinical Features

> **PRACTICE TIP**
>
> The rapid shallow breathing pattern that is adopted by most patients is probably the most efficient, so long as it is synchronous.

The lungs have a large reserve capacity and the following only emerge after considerable damage:

- progressive and unrelenting SOB, leading to anxiety, depression, insomnia, fatigue, social withdrawal and fear of disease progression (Russell et al. 2016);
- a tightly constrained breathing pattern, manifesting as shallow breathing to ease the elastic load and rapid breathing to maintain minute ventilation;
- incessant coughing due to lung distortion (Russell et al. 2016);
- on auscultation, fine end-inspiratory 'velcro' crackles, caused by peripheral airways popping open (Sellarés et al. 2016), unchanged by deep breathing, coughing or position change;
- 'ground glass' radiological signs, representing the inflammatory exudate of alveolitis, progressing to reticular patterning (Fig. 3.22) and honeycombing, representing fibrosis as alveoli are pulled apart to form cystic spaces (Fig. 3.23);
- ↓ $PaO_2$ due to $\dot{V}_A/\dot{Q}$ mismatch;
- ↓ $PaCO_2$ due to rapid breathing;
- ↑ $PAO_2$–$PaO_2$ due to a thickened alveolar–capillary membrane;

- further hypoxaemia on exercise, not predicted by resting $SpO_2$, and nocturnal hypoxaemia severe enough to affect cognition (Bors et al. 2015), QoL and physical functioning (Clark et al. 2010);

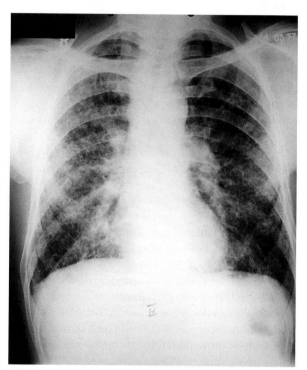

**FIGURE 3.22** Interstitial lung disease showing heart borders blurred by reticular patterning in lung fields.

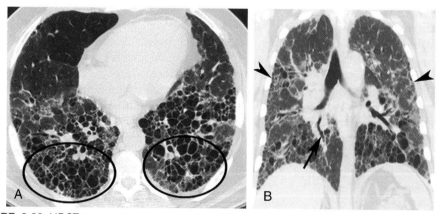

**FIGURE 3.23** HRCT scans through mid-lungs (A) and bases (B) show peripheral and basal-predominant reticulation (arrowheads), traction bronchiectasis (arrow) and honeycombing (circles). (From Ahuja et al. 2016.)

- exercise limitation, due to SOB in 65% of patients and leg fatigue in 35% of patients (Dale et al. 2013);
- finger clubbing in 20% of patients (Behr 2013);
- poor sleep, which severely affects QoL (Milioli et al. 2016).

## Tests

Suspicions are first raised by rapid shallow breathing following exercise. Respiratory function tests then show impaired gas transfer, and high resolution HRCT scan is usually diagnostic, negating the need for a risky lung biopsy (Martin et al. 2016a). Assessment should include the needs of the family (Boland et al. 2016).

## General Management

Patients should be referred to a specialist multidisciplinary centre, where regular assessment, pulmonary rehabilitation and gastro-oesophageal reflux therapy lead to improved survival (Kulkarni et al. 2016). Education includes information that smoking worsens outcome. An explanation of how scarring causes SOB by irritating nerve endings helps reduce the fear of SOB because patients understand that their SOB is the result of damage, not its cause.

New drugs pirfenidone and nintedanib have antifibrotic properties (Jo et al. 2016), and morphine or sildenafil may ease SOB (Ryerson et al. 2012). Cotrimoxazole, macrolides and high-dose steroids may be indicated if there is rapid progression to respiratory failure (Oda et al. 2016a), despite the consequence of steroid-induced muscle weakness (Hanada 2016). Two rather alarming drugs, thalidomide and carbon monoxide, have also been suggested (Rafii et al. 2013).

Oxygen may be required to achieve a target $SpO_2$ of 94%–98%, or 88%–92% for those at risk of hypercapnia. When delivered by high-flow nasal cannula, it can reduce the respiratory rate (Kim 2016). For chronic disease, home oxygen is required if stable $PaO_2$ drops below 7.3 kPa (55 mmHg) when breathing air, or <8 kPa (60 mmHg) if there is peripheral oedema, polycythaemia or pulmonary hypertension. This often requires high $FiO_2$, and a high-flow nasal cannula, which can be run off two concentrators at home. The outcome may be a reversal of pulmonary hypertension, increased exercise tolerance and improved QoL (Criner 2013). Ambulatory oxygen therapy is often required to keep $SpO_2$ >88%, assessed by a single 6-min walk test, and has shown improve-ments in exercise capacity and SOB on exercise (Ora et al. 2013).

Lung transplantation offers hope for some patients (Puglisi et al. 2016), but for most, an end-of-life pathway is required, which has traditionally been less accessible than to those with lung cancer (Ahmadi et al. 2016). Mechanical ventilation is unwise (Güngör et al. 2013).

## Physiotherapy

*Exercise training is one of the few treatments to induce positive changes in symptoms.*

**Dowman et al. 2013**

The patient's main problems are the distress of SOB and the limitation that this imposes on his or her life. Patients who are breathing asynchronously may benefit from instruction in stabilizing their breathing pattern, but this should not slow down their necessarily fast respiratory rate. Deep breathing is likely to increase SOB, but if a patient finds that this brings relief by stretching their rib cage, they may also have hyperventilation syndrome, which is not uncommon with this condition.

Pulmonary rehabilitation can enhance exercise tolerance, dyspnoea and QoL (Puglisi et al. 2016) and should be started as early as possible, to include practical advice for patient and family (Russell et al. 2016). Benefits from aerobic exercise training appear to be mediated by peripheral oxygen extraction rather than improved oxygen delivery (Keyser et al. 2016). Patients may prefer interval training, and rotation of exercises helps prevent fatigue of individual muscles (Elia et al. 2013). Limitations to exercise are impaired gas exchange, pulmonary hypertension and muscle dysfunction (Holland 2010). Oxygen desaturation, which may be more severe than the degree of SOB suggests (Miki et al. 2013), must be avoided, and ambulatory oxygen may increase walking distance even if patients do not require home oxygen (Hicks 2007). $SpO_2$ may also drop after exercise as they 'repay' their oxygen debt.

Patients may respond to other measures (Chapter 8), including judicious use of NIV (Bräunlich 2013), but with close monitoring because patients are at risk of barotrauma (Fig. 3.24).

Outcome measures include the MRC scale (p. 351), which correlates with physiological and functional parameters (Manali 2010) and, if not distressing for the patient, a 6-min walk test (Porteous et al. 2016), especially when combined with oximetry to measure the

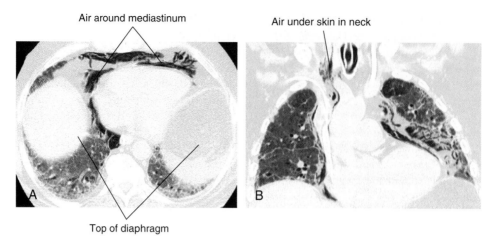

**FIGURE 3.24** Axial (A) and coronal (B) HRCT images showing pneumomediastinum and gas tracking up into the neck. (From Kusmirek et al. 2016.)

'desaturation distance ratio' (Pimenta et al. 2010). Questionnaires include the IPF-specific Health-Related Quality of Life, Chronic Respiratory Disease and IPF-specific St. George's Respiratory (Olson et al. 2016).

## PLEURAL DISORDERS

The pleural space normally contains <1 mL fluid, forming a film 10 μm thick (Davies et al. 2010a) but it is the conduit for 24 L of fluid a day, secreted by the parietal layer and resorbed by the visceral layer (Peek 2000), suggesting that its main function relates to fluid balance and the mechanics of breathing (p. 7).

### Pleurisy

Pleurisy is inflammation of the pleural membranes and is sometimes associated with lobar pneumonia. It causes a pleural friction rub on auscultation (p. 46) and a savage localized pain because the parietal pleura is richly innervated. Lung expansion is restricted because of shallow breathing due to pain. If a pleural effusion develops, the pain dissolves as the raw pleural membranes are separated by fluid.

### Pleural Effusion

Pleural effusion occurs when the pleural fluid filtration rate overwhelms the lymphatic removal rate. Excess fluid in the pleural cavity can be seen on X-ray (Figs 3.25, 2.18, 2.24).

Breathlessness is caused by the effort of breathing against the wall of fluid, and disturbed respiratory muscle mechanics as the diaphragm is displaced downwards (Thomas et al. 2015). Objective signs include lack of breath sounds locally, a stony dull percussion note, reduced fremitus over the affected area and bronchial breathing just above the fluid level. Some patients have a dry cough. Ultrasound or a CT scan confirms the diagnosis.

**Transudates** are clear straw-coloured fluids caused by increased hydrostatic pressure or decreased oncotic pressure. They are characteristic of simple effusions caused by liver, kidney or, most commonly, heart failure (Puchalski et al. 2013). **Exudates** are cloudy effusions that develop by fluid passing through damaged capillary beds and into the pleura. They are associated with pulmonary embolism, pneumonia or malignancy. Malignant pleural effusions may be secondary to a primary cancer or may relate to mesothelioma (p. 120) and are often recurrent, requiring pleurodesis or an indwelling pleural catheter. **Haemothorax** is blood in the pleura resulting from trauma or malignancy.

Medical treatment is directed at the cause when possible. Symptoms can be alleviated by needle aspiration or thoracentesis, which must be done slowly in order to avoid rebound pulmonary oedema (Ault et al. 2015). If the effusion does not resolve, one-way valves or drainage tubes can be used. Surgery may be needed for a thickened restrictive pleura (p. 313). For relentless malignant

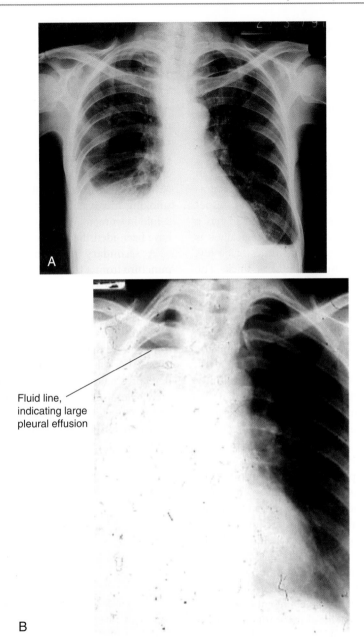

Fluid line, indicating large pleural effusion

**FIGURE 3.25** (A) The patient's right costophrenic angle shows the dense opacity of a pleural effusion, with a smooth horizontal border and meniscus laterally. The left shows a small effusion obliterating the costophrenic angle. (B) Large pleural effusion demonstrated by a dense opacity and fluid line on the right, with the heart pushed to the left.

effusions, pleuroperitoneal shunts or tunnelled pleural catheters can be used for palliation.

Positioning may improve comfort and gas exchange, guided by oximetry because a moderate unilateral effusion may benefit from side-lying with the affected side uppermost so that both ventilation and perfusion are greater in the lower lung and therefore better matched, whereas a large effusion may respond best with the patient lying on the affected side to minimize compression of the unaffected lung. Side-lying on the affected side may bring the added benefit of inhibiting a dry cough. Clinical reasoning suggests that physiotherapy beyond positioning cannot expand lungs under pressure from fluid, but Valenza-Demet et al. (2014) found that deep breathing exercises, incentive spirometry and mobilization improved radiological findings and shortened hospital stay.

## Empyema

Pus in the pleural cavity is known as empyema. It can complicate pneumonia, bronchiectasis, chronic aspiration, abscess or chest surgery (Alpert et al. 2014), especially oesophageal surgery (see Fig. 14.10), and has a 20% mortality (Davies et al. 2010a). Radiologically it is similar to a pleural effusion but sometimes has a less clear horizontal line because the fluid is thick. The patient may be asymptomatic or toxic, depending on the organism and volume of pus. Treatment is by local and systemic antibiotics, with sometimes needle aspiration, lavage, prolonged tube drainage into a bag or an underwater seal drain with strong suction, or surgery (p. 313).

Pus may break down the pleura, and the possibility of a fistula between pleura and lung means that the patient should not lie with the affected side uppermost in case infected fluid drains into the lung.

## Pneumothorax

If either the visceral or parietal pleura is ruptured, air rushes into the pleural space, causing a pneumothorax and disrupting the negative pressure that normally keeps the lungs expanded. Causes include lung disease, overdistension of alveoli, trauma, including some medical procedures, and occasionally the production of gas-forming organisms through infection. The lung shrivels towards the hilum until pressure is equalized or the collapsing lung seals the hole. Presentation varies from chest discomfort to life-threatening cardiorespiratory collapse. Loss of volume >15% requires chest drainage (p. 314).

Clinical features are dyspnoea, pain, diminished breath sounds over the affected area and sometimes a hyperresonant percussion note. Radiological signs are in Fig. 3.26, but half cannot be seen on X-ray. For a large pneumothorax, the lung collapses towards the hilum, sometimes with the mediastinum shifted away from the affected side, especially if the pneumothorax is under tension (see following section). A difficult-to-see pneu-

mothorax may be picked up by CT scan or oblique X-ray (Matsumoto et al. 2016).

### Types of pneumothorax

The apex of the upright lung is subject to greater mechanical stress than the base because the weight of the lung pulls down on it. A **spontaneous pneumothorax** usually occurs in this region, especially in tall thin young men (Pribadi et al. 2016) who are thought to grow faster than their pleura is able to keep up with (Chang et al. 2015). Although called 'spontaneous', smoking increases the likelihood 22-fold in men and 8-fold in women (Wakai 2011). Recurrence rates of 54% have been identified (Olesen et al. 2016).

A **secondary pneumothorax** may be caused by puncture from a fractured rib, inaccurate insertion of a cannula, high-volume mechanical ventilation, rupture of an emphysematous bulla or drug abuse with prolonged Valsalva breath-holds. It is termed an open pneumothorax if there is communication with the environment. A pneumothorax secondary to diseased lungs causes more severe symptoms and takes longer to heal. Rare precipitating factors are coughing fits, sneezing, breath-holding, loud music, playing a wind instrument and thunderstorms (Haga et al. 2013).

A **tension pneumothorax** is an emergency that occurs if a tear in the visceral pleura acts as a valve so

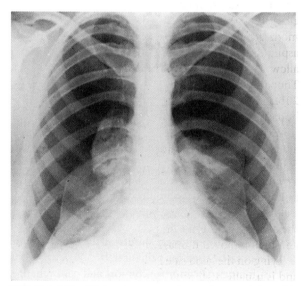

**FIGURE 3.26** Bilateral pneumothorax in a patient with emphysema.

that air enters the pleural space but cannot escape, usually in mechanically ventilated patients. Progressive positive pressure impedes cardiac output, and urgent action is required (p. 510).

## MINI CLINICAL REASONING
### (response below)

A 20-year-old male smoker presented with shortness of breath. Radiology identified a pneumothorax filling 80% of the hemithorax.
- 16 days later the pneumothorax had shrunk to 62%.
- 12 days after that the pneumothorax filled 33% of the hemithorax. He was advised on incentive spirometry 2–4 times a day for 5–10 min, with gradually increasing volumes.
- 12 days later the pneumothorax had resolved.

*The conclusion was that incentive spirometry had contributed to recovery.*

Pribadi et al. 2016

Is that your conclusion?

## Treatment

Medical management is aimed at expelling the unwanted air, facilitating pleural healing and preventing recurrence. If small and symptomless, a pneumothorax can be left to resolve itself and the patient is usually discharged, with advice to return if dyspnoea worsens. A moderate first pneumothorax can be managed by needle aspiration. If drainage is required, portable systems that allow air to escape but not reenter include a digital Thopaz drain, which monitors air leaks (Tunnicliffe 2014), and the Heimlich valve, which can be used at home (Gogakos et al. 2016).

A chest drain (p. 314) is required if simpler methods are inadequate or the patient is on a ventilator. Suction is occasionally necessary, at low-pressure to avoid 'air-stealing', perpetuation of the air leak or 'reexpansion pulmonary oedema' (Haga et al. 2016a). Once the air leak has sealed, i.e. when there is no more bubbling in the drainage bottle, the drain is clamped for some hours and then removed if imaging shows no recurrence.

Lying on the good side is often the most comfortable and is usually best for $\dot{V}_A/\dot{Q}$ matching, but lying on the affected side can speed reabsorption of air (Zidulka et al. 1982). There is no evidence to link exertion with

recurrence (MacDuff et al. 2010), and exercise can be as vigorous as the patient is willing if the cause is traumatic, e.g. after stabbing, in order to encourage lung expansion (Senekal 1994). However, exercise should be moderate after pleural surgery in case the pleura comes unstuck again.

In the unlikely event that the patient is admitted but has no chest drain, high concentrations of inspired oxygen should be given unless contraindicated. This speeds resolution by increasing the reabsorption of air fourfold, the inert nitrogen being displaced by absorbable oxygen.

Surgery by pleurodesis (p. 313) is required if these measures fail, if the condition is recurrent or bilateral, or if the patient's occupation involves rapid changes in atmospheric pressure such as scuba diving or flying.

Precautions for an undrained pneumothorax include avoidance of positive pressure techniques (CPAP, IPPB, NIV and manual hyperinflation). Patients should also be advised to avoid paroxysms of coughing and some intense yoga breathing techniques.

Once the pneumothorax has resolved, discharge advice is to avoid flying in the short term and scuba diving for life, but physical exertion can resume so long as there are no symptoms (Eccles 2013).

## RESPONSE TO MINI CLINICAL REASONING

It is possible that incentive spirometry contributed to recovery, but no causal link is proved, and the timing correlates with normal healing time.

## NEUROMUSCULAR DISORDERS

Neurological conditions that cause generalized weakness usually also cause respiratory muscle weakness. Weak inspiratory muscles cause a restrictive disorder by limiting lung expansion. Weak expiratory muscles impair the cough, leading to 90% of respiratory failure episodes (Auger et al. 2017). Compensatory respiratory plasticity may prolong breathing capacity (Fig. 3.27).

The cardiorespiratory needs of paediatric and critically ill patients with neurological conditions are in Chapters 16 and 22.

## Clinical Features and Monitoring

Any of the three physiotherapy problems may be present:

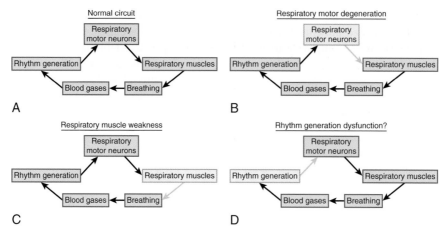

**FIGURE 3.27** (A) Normal respiratory control system: brainstem rhythm neurons modulate respiratory motor neurons, which activate respiratory muscles to generate breathing and regulate blood gases. (B) Respiratory motor neurons *(shaded)* degenerate, leading to ventilatory failure. (C) Respiratory muscles *(shaded)* become weak and atrophy from decreased activation. (D) Rhythm-generating neurons may also become dysfunctional, contributing to central sleep apnoea. (From Nichols et al. 2013.)

1. Increased WOB occurs if inspiratory muscles are weak.
2. Loss of lung volume results from limited expansion and sometimes spasticity. Lack of alveolar stretch inhibits production of surfactant.
3. Sputum retention is likely if there is impaired cough. Fatigue is ever present. Sleep disorders are common, due to further weakening of respiratory muscles at night and reduced chemoreceptor sensitivity, leading to sleep fragmentation, nocturnal hypoxaemia and excessive daytime somnolence (Fermin et al. 2016). Chronic pain affects 20%–40% of patients (Borsook 2012).

Monitoring is required for progressive conditions. Respiratory muscle weakness may go undetected if limb weakness reduces activity, and ventilatory failure can arrive unexpectedly. Peak cough flow (PCF) assesses cough and may predict aspiration risk (Silverman et al. 2016), whereas capnography and MIP (p. 64) provide warning of ventilatory failure (Kim et al. 2011). FVC below 50% of normal requires assessment for NIV (Carratù et al. 2009). Disease-specific values of pulmonary function can be used to assess the onset of ventilatory insufficiency in patients with amyotrophic lateral sclerosis, muscular dystrophy (Cho et al. 2016a) and Parkinson disease (Owolabi et al. 2016). A suggested pathway for investigating and managing patients is in Fig. 3.28.

The onset of hiccups, whose reflex arc is modulated by the central midbrain (Chang & Lu 2012) is a warning of potential brain stem dysfunction. Bulbar dysfunction is associated with dysphagia, dysarthria, weak mastication, facial weakness, nasal speech and/or a protruding tongue. Patients may need a face mask for spirometry (Wohlgemuth et al. 2003).

Dysphagia is suspected by the signs in Table 3.5 and a low PCF. It may develop insidiously, but usually parallels or shortly follows the development of speech problems. Patients require speech–language therapy (SLT), and sometimes drugs such as botulinum (Lee et al. 2009).

Dysphagia may lead to dehydration, which limits secretion clearance, and weight loss, which limits mobility. Other problems are malnutrition and aspiration, and scales are available to assess for the risk of aspiration pneumonia (Lee et al. 2016e). If assistance with eating is not adequate, feeding can be by PEG (p. 165), or, so long as it does not cause feelings of choking, nasogastric tube. Monitoring dysphagia is by:
- water swallow test combined with oximetry (Brodsky et al. 2016);
- videofluoroscopy to identify delayed swallowing, performed by a radiologist and SLT, sometimes with voluntary cough spirometry testing (Plowman et al. 2016); the physiotherapist stands by with suction equipment.

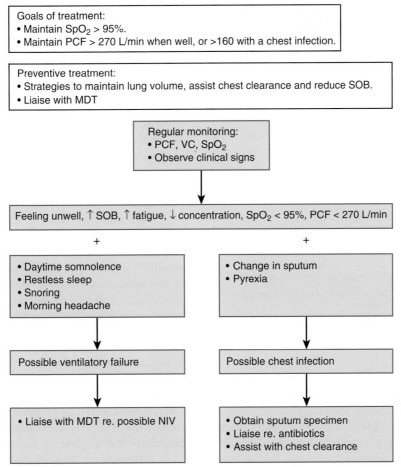

**FIGURE 3.28** Pathway for monitoring and managing patients with neurological disorders and potential ventilatory failure. *ADL,* Activities of daily living; *MDT,* multidisciplinary team including neuro-physiotherapist; *NIV,* noninvasive ventilation; *PCF,* peak cough flow; *SOB,* shortness of breath; *VC,* vital capacity. (From BTS/ACPRC 2009, Tzeng 2000, Mangera et al. 2012.)

Dysphagia rehabilitation is described by Malandraki et al. (2016).

## Classification

A weak cough is the main respiratory problem in **motor neurone disease** (MND), or its most common form **amyotrophic lateral sclerosis** (ALS). Patients with bulbar onset ALS usually have dysarthria and dysphagia, with communication problems having a greater impact on the patient than loss of physical function (Mora et al. 2012). Cortical atrophy predisposes to behaviour change and dementia (Finger 2016), and patients with nocturnal hypoxia require oxygen at night to protect the brain (Park et al. 2014). Dyspnoea may respond to some of the methods in Chapter 8 and can be relieved medically with opioids or, if exacerbated by anxiety, benzodiazepines (NICE 2016a). Excess salivation can be reduced by an anticholinergic such as atropine or hyoscine. Sleep disordered breathing carries over into daytime sleepiness, headaches and short-term memory problems, but once NIV is required, this improves sleep quality as well as easing respiratory symptoms and prolonging life (Nichols et al. 2013). Diaphragm pacing suits some patients (Sanli et al. 2016). Neurons controlling eye

TABLE 3.5   Identification of a swallowing problem

| Obvious indicators of dysphagia | Surreptitious indicators of dysphagia |
|---|---|
| • Difficulty with food or liquid in the mouth<br>• Drooling<br>• Difficulty swallowing<br>• Coughing or choking before, during or after swallowing<br>• Globus sensation ('lump in throat')<br>• Hoarse voice<br>• Feeling of obstruction<br>• Regurgitation of undigested food<br>• Nasal regurgitation<br>• Unintentional weight loss | • Change in breathing pattern<br>• Wet voice quality<br>• Tongue fasciculation<br>• Dry mouth<br>• Heartburn<br>• Change in eating e.g. eating slowly or avoiding social occasions<br>• Frequent throat clearing<br>• Recurrent chest infections or unexplained temperature spikes<br>• Lack of elevation of larynx on swallowing |

Adapted from NICE 2006.

movements and the bladder are generally spared up to the time of death (Nichols et al. 2013). Death occurs 3–5 years after diagnosis, usually from respiratory failure; it may happen suddenly but is usually peaceful (Baxter et al. 2013). Predicting longevity is assisted by the Amyotrophic Lateral Sclerosis Functional Rating Scale (Kaufmann et al. 2005).

**Parkinson disease** affects the brain and both sympathetic and parasympathetic nervous systems (Borghammer et al. 2016). It is the second most common neurodegenerative disorder after Alzheimer's disease. Exercise has a neuroprotective effect in reducing the risk of developing the disease or slowing its progression, and can improve cognition without excessive fatigue (Salgado et al. 2013), but autonomic disturbance blunts metabolic and cardiovascular responses to exercise tests (Kanegusuku et al. 2016). Group singing is an enjoyable way of improving respiratory muscle control (Stegemöller et al. 2016), and the ICF model is the most relevant for patient outcomes (Van Uem et al. 2016).

Expiratory muscles are disproportionately weak in people with **multiple sclerosis** (Klefbeck 2003), along with bulbar dysfunction and abnormalities of breathing control. Inspiratory muscle training, breath-stacking

(p. 112) and assisted cough can improve respiratory outcome and possibly increase survival (Macpherson & Bassile et al. 2016). Exercise has disease-modifying potential, but potential fatigue requires close adherence to the domains of the ICF, sometimes medication (Oral & Ayse 2013) and always energy conservation (Blikman 2013).

**Stroke** with hemiparesis may increase $CO_2$ sensitivity and decrease voluntary ventilation on the weak side (Lanini 2003). One-sided abdominal paradox on sniffing indicates unilateral diaphragmatic paralysis. Up to half of patients have dysphagia (Han et al. 2016b), and if they develop aspiration pneumonia, 20% die (Wilson 2012). Aspiration or reduced respiratory drive may cause hypoxaemia, especially at night (Roffe et al. 2003), and supplemental oxygen should be given if $SpO_2$ drops below 95% (Prasad et al. 2011). Increased tone in any of the core muscles can increase WOB. Lung function may improve with manually resisted inspiratory muscle exercise and pursed lips breathing, but it is unclear whether this helps the patient subjectively (Seo et al. 2013). The average 50% loss in lung function can be partly restored by game-based respiratory muscle training, which is probably more fun than inspiratory muscle exercise but still focuses on spirometry (Joo et al. 2015).

**Myasthenia gravis** is an autoimmune disease characterized by weakness of voluntary skeletal muscles, particularly the inspiratory muscles (Fregonezi et al. 2015), with recovery after rest. Medical treatment is by acetylcholine esterase inhibitors, immunosuppressive drugs and thymectomy for some (Melzer et al. 2016). Intermittent myasthenic crises may cause upper airway obstruction, sleep apnoea or respiratory failure. Respiratory muscle training may reduce symptoms in mild or moderate disease (Rassler et al. 2011).

**Muscular dystrophy** is a group of inherited disorders that involve progressive muscle weakness, particularly the expiratory muscles (Fregonezi et al. 2015). Respiratory problems are the main cause of morbidity and mortality, most patients not realizing the extent of their respiratory muscle weakness until complications arise (ATS 2004). Facilitation of respiration techniques can improve $SpO_2$ (Nitz & Burke 2002), and survival has been extended by giving patients a pulse oximeter, and, when $SpO_2$ drops below 95%, using a regimen of breath-stacking, NIV and in–exsufflation (AARC 2013).

**Postpolio syndrome** may occur 30–40 years after the acute illness, when metabolic demand on residual motor units triggers secondary neuronal death in 70% of patients, leading to chronic pain, extreme fatigue and progressive respiratory distress. Benefits have been found from judicious submaximal exercise, hydrotherapy, joint protection, TENS, acupuncture, rest periods during the day and NIV if required (Orsini et al. 2016).

**Diaphragmatic paralysis** may be caused by MND, infection, trauma or malignancy. Nocturnal hypoxaemia sometimes occurs because of $\dot{V}_A/\dot{Q}$ mismatch in supine. Bilateral paralysis effectively removes a portion of the chest wall, obliging patients to exhale by contracting the abdominal muscles in order to push up the diaphragm, with passive inspiration possible in the upright position. Signs of bilateral paralysis or severe weakness are the following:

- orthopnoea unexplained by heart or lung disease;
- accessory muscle activity unexplained by lung disease;
- abdominal paradox during inspiration, especially in supine when the diaphragm is unable to counteract pressure from the abdominal contents;
- postural fall in vital capacity (VC) of >50% in supine compared to upright;
- symptoms of nocturnal hypoventilation, e.g. daytime somnolence and hypercapnia (p. 16);
- nonspecific symptoms such as breathlessness or recurrent chest infections.

NIV may be required, especially at night (MacBruce et al. 2016).

## General Management

> **KEY POINT**
>
> Impaired communication can be the most difficult aspect for the patient and family.

Pulmonary complications are a major cause of morbidity and mortality (AARC 2013). Oxygen, if needed, is best prescribed after $CO_2$ levels have been measured because some patients have an inadequate hypercapnic drive (Chiou et al. 2016), and target saturation may need to be 88%–92% (O'Driscoll et al. 2008). Postpolio patients are particularly at risk because their respiratory centres may have been damaged by the original viral infection. For patients who have trouble sleeping, melatonin has been found to improve sleep quality (Zhang et al. 2016b). The multidisciplinary team includes occupational therapy, SLT and support groups.

## Management of Chronic Aspiration

Chronic aspiration is common in neurological disease if there is dysphagia or a poor gag reflex. A certain amount can be tolerated if mucociliary clearance is normal, but if symptoms are present, liaison with SLT, nursing staff and carers is required. Silent aspiration occurs without coughing but may cause any of the signs in Table 3.5.

Radiological signs of infiltrates can be regional or disseminated (Fig. 3.29), which may progress to fibrosis

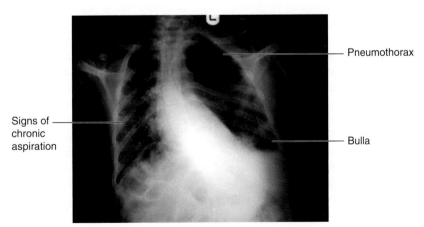

**FIGURE 3.29** Nodular shadows in the right lung, indicating chronic aspiration. The patient also has barotrauma on the left after prolonged mechanical ventilation, and scoliosis as result of cerebral palsy.

(Lee et al. 2010). Preventive measures are in Appendix A, and SLT may include isometric neck exercises to encourage laryngeal elevation (Logemann 1986) or neurostimulation (Michou & Hamdy 2013). The management of acute aspiration is on p. 115.

## Respiratory Physiotherapy

Some of the evidence-based techniques that have been found effective for specific disorders (discussed previously and p. 109–111) may be beneficial for other neurological conditions.

Any of the three physiotherapy problems may be helped by the techniques in Chapters 6–8, with specific approaches in relation to neurological disease as follows:

1. To assist sputum clearance, **manual** or **mechanical support** aids coughing for patients with PCF <270 L/min (AARC 2013). A mechanical insufflator–exsufflator simulates a cough by applying positive and then negative pressure to the airway (p. 217). For some patients with bulbar involvement, the insufflation can feel as if they are choking, or laryngeal adduction may occur, which can be managed by individually customized settings (Andersen et al. 2017). The machine is not suited to patients without significant weakness because their muscles automatically resist. Self-manual assistance is possible by patients manoeuvring their wheelchair against the edge of a suitable table to produce a thoracic and/or abdominal thrust timed to the opening of the glottis (Bianchi et al. 2014). If cough augmentation is ineffective, tracheostomy may best suit the patient, to avoid the distress of repeated suction (Toussaint et al. 2016a).

2. **Breath-stacking** or **lung recruitment** enables the patient to reach a mean peak cough flow >160 L/min (Toussaint et al. 2016b). It can also slow lung function decline in muscular dystrophy (Katz et al. 2016b) and helps reverse and helps prevent atelectasis in ALS (Bourke & Steer 2016). The patient takes a succession of deep breaths and stacks them behind the closed glottis. Assistance may be needed by an in–exsufflator, e.g. at +30 to −30 cmH$_2$O (Meric et al. 2017) a manual resuscitation bag and mask/mouthpiece, IPPB (Chen et al 2016f) or glossopharyngeal breathing (Bach et al. 2007). Caution is required with damaged lungs because of possible barotrauma (Westermann 2013). Incentive spirometry and regular position change also help maintain lung volume. If abdominal muscles show hypertonicity,

inspiration may be facilitated by inhibitory postures.

3. Carefully balanced **exercise training**, with adequate rest, is usually beneficial, and over time can reduce fatigue (Hedermann et al. 2016). A bedside exercise programme may enhance swallowing function (Kang et al. 2012a). Respiratory muscle training can increase respiratory muscle strength, but with little effect on exercise tolerance or function (Ferreira et al. 2016).

4. To reduce WOB, a balance of **rest and exercise** is advised, avoiding the overuse of compensatory muscles and sometimes using interval training (Aboussouan 2009). Fatigue does not necessarily correlate with disease severity and is partially reversible, e.g. by attention to hydration, nutrition and physical fitness, but it is made worse by excess physical activity or distress (Lou et al. 2010). Upright positioning may be more comfortable than other positions, and abdominal breathing enables some patients to use their muscles more efficiently. A useful side effect of in–exsufflation may be the reduction of dyspnoea (Jones et al. 2012b).

5. **Noninvasive ventilation** may need to be considered before an acute episode precipitates action. Patients should be told that if deterioration is progressive, weaning may be impossible. However, NIV can improve swallowing (Garguilo et al. 2016), reduce dyspnoea, enhance QoL and prolong survival (Jones et al. 2012b). When used overnight it can improve sleep and prevent orthopnoea. In the daytime, some patients may prefer to use a mouthpiece for ease of talking, eating and coughing (Nardi et al. 2016). The success of NIV can lead to loss of focus on the expiratory muscles, which may need expiratory muscle training.

6. **Glossopharyngeal breathing** is a technique that can be used to coax air into the lungs if FVC is <1 L. Patients use their lips, soft palate and tongue to collect 30–200 mL mouthfuls of air into their mouth and throat, then after 6–30 mouthfuls, gulp it all into their lungs, using their tongue and pharynx, then hold it there by a closed glottis and open their mouth to collect the next bolus of air, building up to a single breath of up to 3 L (Homnick 2007). Using a mirror, and in as upright a position as possible, training requires much concentration, with short daily sessions to avoid fatigue. The following benefits have been demonstrated (Filart et al. 2003, Maltais 2011, Johansson et al. 2012):

- several hours of ventilator-free time;
- a safety margin in case of ventilator backup failure;
- normalized speech, ability to cough, talk on the phone or call for help;
- easier defaecation;
- improved respiratory function.

Some patients can use the technique continuously, including at mealtimes when they briefly park the food at the side of their mouth.

An overview of respiratory physiotherapy for neurological patients is discussed by Jones et al. (2012b). For assessment and outcomes, a neurological ICF Core set has been validated (Bos et al. 2013).

## SKELETAL DISORDERS

As with neurological disorders, some skeletal conditions restrict lung expansion even though the lungs themselves are usually normal.

### Kyphosis, Scoliosis and Kyphoscoliosis

Degenerative changes in the spine contribute to a normal trend of kyphosis with increasing age, especially in those with osteoporosis. Prolonged computer use may also contribute (Decker et al. 2016). A thoracic kyphosis angle >40 degrees, or 'dowager's hump', occurs in about 30% of the older population, sometimes contributing to restrictive ventilatory dysfunction, pain, dyspnoea, decreased exercise tolerance and, as both cause and effect, vertebral fractures (Ailon et al. 2015). Surgery is occasionally required.

For people with adolescent idiopathic scoliosis, a scoliosis-specific exercise program can improve lung function and chest expansion (Moramarco et al. 2016).

Kyphoscoliosis increases WOB because of reduced chest wall compliance and a diaphragm forced to work inefficiently, occasionally requiring NIV if ventilatory failure occurs (Nicolini et al. 2016), which brings the added benefit of improving exercise capacity (Salturk et al. 2015). Exercise training can reduce dyspnoea and improve quality of life (Cejudo 2013).

### Ankylosing Spondylitis

This is a systemic inflammatory disease that restricts breathing because of a rigid thoracic cage and kyphotic spine. X-ray signs include apparent hyperinflation because the chest wall becomes fixed in an inspiratory position. Inflammation links it to cardiovascular disease in 2%–10% of patients (Ozkan 2016), and lung involvement occurs in up to 30% of patients, including pleural thickening, upper lobe fibrosis and sometimes apical bullae (Maghraoui & Dehhaoui 2012). Physiotherapy comprises attention to posture, thoracic mobility, exercise training (O'Dwyer et al. 2016) and inspiratory muscle training (Drăgoi et al. 2016).

### Pigeon Chest and Funnel Chest

Chest deformities include pigeon chest (pectus carinatum), which protrudes the sternum, and funnel chest (pectus excavatum), which depresses the sternum. These rarely restrict lung function but may reduce exercise tolerance by limiting the heart's ability to increase stroke volume (Koumbourlis 2015). If surgery is required, intensive rehabilitation is required (Bal-Bocheńska 2016).

## CHEST INFECTIONS

Infection from viruses, bacteria or fungi can occur anywhere from the nose to the lung parenchyma. Chest infections are a common cause of exacerbation of lung disease and are the commonest acute problem dealt with in primary care (NICE 2008). They include anything from acute bronchitis, a common and usually self-limiting viral infection of the upper airways, to life-threatening pneumonia. Chest infections in COPD, CF and bronchiectasis demonstrate bacterial persistence (Pragman et al. 2016) and purulent sputum is usually an indication for antibiotics, whereas purulent sputum during a mild infection of the upper airways in other patients does not itself indicate a need for antibiotics (Egger et al. 2016).

People at risk are those who are very old, very young, immunocompromised, stressed (Dhabhar 2009) or exposed to air pollution, which is the ninth leading risk factor for cardiopulmonary mortality (Kurt et al. 2016). Physiotherapy is required if patients are unable to clear secretions or need assistance with rehabilitation.

### Respiratory Tract Infection

Upper respiratory tract infection covers pharyngitis, laryngitis, sinusitis, otitis media, the common cold and influenza. Occasionally physiotherapy advice is required. The **common cold** is an infection of the nose, throat, sinuses and upper airways, caused by 200 different viruses, of which rhinoviruses are the commonest.

Susceptibility is increased with an inactive lifestyle (Nieman et al. 2010). Antibiotics are unhelpful and simply promote antibiotic resistance (Zanasi et al. 2016). Patients are contagious 2 to 3 days before symptoms emerge and remain contagious until symptoms have cleared.

The **influenza** virus can jump the species barrier and tends to occur in pandemics, including the 1918 episode that killed more people than the First World War (Aligne 2016). Flu slows mucociliary clearance and increases susceptibility to secondary bacterial infections (Pittet et al. 2010). Warm airways have an antiviral effect and the patient's subjective need to keep warm should be encouraged (Bender 2000). A cough or sneeze propels droplets up to a metre, which is a reminder to take precautions when a patient coughs or is suctioned (Thompson et al. 2013). Influenza leads all other illnesses in hospital bed-days and flu vaccination, if required, needs to be repeated annually because of virus mutation (Manning 2017).

## Pneumonia

### Mini case study: Ms TP

*A 24-year-old patient has been admitted with pneumonia.*

  *Background*
- Unemployed, mobile, independent
- Heroin user

  *Subjective*
- Well

  *Objective*
- Patient in nightie, tucked up in bed
- Apyrexial
- Fluid balance normal
- $SpO_2$ normal
- Auscultation – bronchial breathing left lower lobe, no crackles
- Respiratory rate normal
- Breathing pattern normal

  *Questions*
1. Identify the consolidation in Fig. 3.30
2. Analysis?
3. Problems?
4. Goals?
5. Plan?

Response on p. 117.

Pneumonia is inflammation of the alveoli caused by bacteria, fungi, chemical agents or viruses. These breach lung defences, inflame lung parenchyma and the smallest bronchioles, then fill and consolidate alveoli with fibrous exudate. Risk factors are stroke, poor nutrition, smoking, alcoholism, winter and the extremes of age. The incidence is growing as the population ages (Ebihara et al. 2016), as more critically ill patients survive, as transplantation increases and antibiotic resistance grows. A quarter of hospitalized patients with pneumonia develop a major cardiac complication (Corrales et al. 2013).

Clinical features include fever, SOB and tachycardia. If localized, the affected area is painful and may

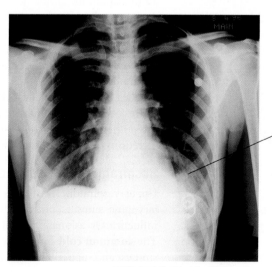

**FIGURE 3.30** Ms TP.

demonstrate a dull percussion note, pleural rub, decreased expansion and bronchial breath sounds or fine crackles on auscultation. Imaging often lags behind clinical presentation but tends to show a patchy opacity (Fig. 3.31), which may not resolve for some weeks. Radiological signs are reduced in dehydrated patients (Goudarzi 2000) but MRI or HRCT are helpful (Syrjala 2017).

A dry cough may later become productive of purulent or rust-coloured sputum as the consolidation resolves, but most of the exudate is removed by phagocytosis via the blood stream. Sensitized nerve endings may leave a dry irritating cough for some time.

The structure of the lung is preserved and resolution is usually complete, but there is a legacy of increased risk of cardiovascular disease (Soto-Gomez 2013).

Medical treatment is by oral or intravenous fluids, antimicrobial drugs, oxygen if indicated, CPAP if hypoxaemia persists, and NIV if ventilatory failure supervenes (Nicolini et al. 2016). Antibacterial drugs should not be given for viral pneumonia because it increases the risk of multidrug-resistant infections (Crotty et al. 2015). Physiotherapy is by positioning for $\dot{V}_A/\dot{Q}$ matching, sometimes assistance with chest clearance, and early mobility, which shortens hospital stay (Mundy et al. 2003). Rehabilitation helps reduce

subsequent complications such as cognitive impairment (Davydow et al. 2013), falls and delirium (Mody et al. 2012). Individualized programmes with pacing are advised because fatigue may continue for some months (NICE 2014a). Neuromuscular osteopathic techniques to relax the diaphragm and increase rib cage mobility have led to interesting reductions in hospital stay and the need for antibiotics (Noll et al. 2010).

Pneumonia is known as 'community acquired' unless it develops in hospital. Subdivisions are below.

### Bronchopneumonia

Bronchopneumonia is patchy and diffuse, often favouring the lower lobes and sometimes producing fine crackles on auscultation. It is most common in immobile or elderly people, over half of whom demonstrate dysphagia (Cabre 2010). Complications include dehydration and confusion.

### Lobar pneumonia

If pneumonia is confined to a lobe, localized pleuritic pain is a distinguishing feature, limiting tidal volume and mobility.

### Aspiration pneumonia

> **Regurgitation**: reflux of gastric contents into the oesophagus or oropharynx
> **Aspiration**: inhalation of foreign material into the airways beyond the vocal cords
> **Microaspiration**: repeated small episodes of aspiration that do not cause acute symptoms

Subclinical microaspiration is ubiquitous in healthy people (Dickson et al. 2016), but dysfunction of swallowing and coughing leads to pathological aspiration, causing cough, SOB, tachycardia, wheeze and diffuse crackles. The complication of aspiration pneumonia can develop within hours. Inflammatory mediators cause bronchospasm and a vicious pneumonitis that corrodes the alveolar–capillary membrane, depletes surfactant and may cause chemical pulmonary oedema, haemorrhage and necrosis.

Radiological signs of consolidation are rapidly apparent, then increase over 1–2 days, then either begin to resolve or show evidence of deterioration, e.g. acute respiratory distress syndrome or abscess. The location of

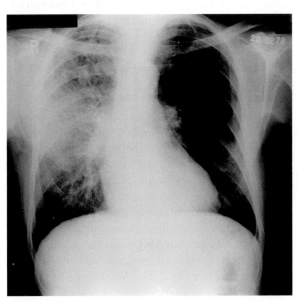

**FIGURE 3.31** Consolidation of right upper lobe.

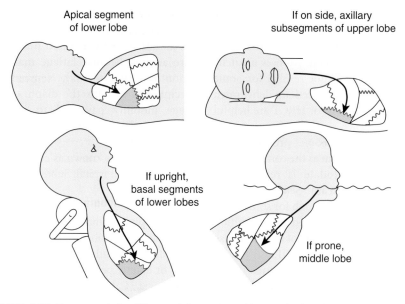

Apical segment
of lower lobe

If on side, axillary
subsegments of upper lobe

If upright,
basal segments
of lower lobes

If prone,
middle lobe

**FIGURE 3.32** Pneumonia in different lobes caused by aspiration in varying positions.

infiltrates helps identify the affected lobe (Fig. 3.32) and therefore the postural drainage position to use, if appropriate. The right lung is more likely to be affected, and supine patients typically show changes in the posterior segments of the upper lobes and superior segments of the lower lobes.

Risk factors are:

- suctioning of airway secretions (Manabe et al. 2015)
- intubation (Honold et al. 2015)
- presence of a nasogastric tube or tracheal tube (Raghavendran et al. 2012)
- impaired mobility
- poor dental hygiene
- old age, due to depression of the cough reflex (Yamanda et al. 2008)
- altered consciousness, e.g. sedation, brain injury, alcohol intoxication, seizure, sleep
- pregnancy or obesity, due to increased abdominal pressure
- gastro-oesophageal reflux (Lee et al. 2010)
- obstructive sleep apnoea (Chiner et al. 2016)
- unexpected loss of consciousness (LOC)

If the cause is unexpected LOC, the patient and X-ray are checked for trauma, then immediate physiotherapy is required in the form of postural drainage head-down and left lateral (Miles & Cook 2017), percussion, vibrations, shaking and cough or suction. If the patient

aspirated in supine, positioning the patient prone may assist postural drainage, improve oxygenation and help prevent progression to pneumonitis (Easby et al. 2003). If the patient is able, other techniques to clear secretions can be used. If aspiration occurred during intubation, manual hyperinflation is normally required. Once consolidation has set in, as indicated by bronchial breathing, and if there are no crackles on auscultation, airway clearance techniques are ineffective, but positioning may assist $\dot{V}_A/\dot{Q}$ matching. Mortality can reach 25% in hospitalized patients (Chowdhury et al. 2016).

### *Pneumocystis jiroveci* pneumonia

The fungus 'pneumocystis' normally lives innocuously in human lungs, but in people whose defence mechanisms are weakened, they can become agents for opportunist infection. The fungal organisms damage the alveolar lining, causing hypoxaemia, SOB, chills, sweats, pleuritic pain and a dry cough. Auscultation may be normal or demonstrate fine scattered crackles. Imaging is normal at first if immune deficiency delays the appearance of an inflammatory response, but later signs are disseminated reticular or granular opacities and air bronchograms (see Fig. 2.23). Weakening of the structure of the lung predisposes to pneumothorax and other barotrauma, suspected if there is sudden deterioration (Saleem et al. 2016). High-dose antibiotics and steroids are needed (Shaddock 2016), and physiotherapy may be required for acute SOB (Chapter 8).

### *Legionella pneumonia*

Legionnaires' disease is a severe bacterial pneumonia that often leaves survivors with permanent lung fibrosis (Caterino 2013). When hospital-acquired, it is three times as fatal as the community-acquired variant (Jespersen et al. 2010). It is not spread between humans but occurs in local outbreaks, especially near contaminated water systems, e.g. inadequately cleaned nebulisers (Mastro et al. 1991) or CPAP equipment (Stolk et al. 2016).

### BOOP or COP

Bronchiolitis obliterans organizing pneumonia (BOOP) or cryptogenic organizing pneumonia (COP) is characterized by granulation tissue filling the distal bronchioles and alveoli. It sometimes represents an indolent inflammatory extension of a primary process, e.g. bronchiolitis obliterans, cancer therapy, rheumatoid arthritis (Okada et al. 2016), transplantation (Costa et al. 2016) or toxicity from medication (Camus 2004). It responds to steroids or immunomodulatory macrolides.

### Hospital-acquired pneumonia

Pneumonia that develops more than 48 h after admission to hospital is known as hospital-acquired or nosocomial pneumonia. It involves different pathogens to community-acquired pneumonia and brings higher mortality (Bargellini 2013), being increasingly attributed to antibiotic-resistant bacteria (Micek et al. 2016). In the intensive care unit (ICU), ventilator-associated pneumonia is the commonest infection (Meyer et al. 2010) and the main cause of death (Khan et al. 2009b). Crossinfection between patients is the likely offender, usually carried by staff, or infection from the patient's own colonized sites such as invasive equipment or dental plaque (Wagner et al. 2016). Nosocomial MRSA pneumonia is by definition difficult to manage, with airway secretions being a major site for infection (Laguna et al. 2009).

### Response to mini case study

1. **Consolidation**
   - Area of consolidation is seen behind the left pierced nipple.
2. **Analysis**
   - There are no accessible secretions, no atelectasis, no desaturation.

- Bronchial breathing may linger but is not causing problems.
- It is not necessary to 'treat the X-ray'.

3. **Problems**
   - No physiotherapy problems are seen at present.
4. **Goals**
   - Self-rehabilitation
5. **Plan**
   - Advise patient to get dressed and mobilize.
   - Liaise with team re assistance for drug habit.

## Pulmonary Tuberculosis (TB)

TB is increasing in the UK (Nnadi et al. 2016). It is the world's most lethal infection, with nearly 10 million new cases a year (Evans et al. 2013). One-third of the world's population is infected by the TB bacillus (Fol et al. 2015), which resides discreetly in immunocompetent hosts but may become active if defence mechanisms are impaired by poor living conditions, drug dependency or HIV infection (Ahmed et al. 2016).

The lung is the commonest site of infection. Coughing disseminates infected aerosol, which can remain suspended in the air for some hours. Symptoms are fever, night sweats, cough, chest wall pain, weight loss, haemoptysis and SOB.

The tubercle bacillus is slow growing and tough, responding only to 6 months' treatment with a combination of powerful antibacterial drugs. The patient is no longer infectious after 2 weeks' treatment, so long as sputum is clear of the bacillus. 'Multidrug-resistant' TB requires second-line drugs for up to 2 years, bringing significant side effects and success rates of 65%–75%. 'Extensively drug-resistant' TB is still looking for effective drugs (Nam et al. 2016).

Miliary TB presents atypically with disseminated small nodular opacities on X-ray and is often not detected until autopsy (Savic et al. 2016).

The physiotherapist's role is usually confined to eliciting sputum specimens in a negative pressure room and devising ways to encourage exercise in an isolation cubicle. A high-efficiency particulate air-filtering mask must be used throughout.

## Aspergillosis

The *Aspergillus* fungus lives in the soil, is ubiquitous, and inhalation is common. Allergic bronchopulmonary aspergillosis (ABA) represents a spectrum of diseases resulting from an impaired or excessive immune response to inhaling the fungus. It may coexist with

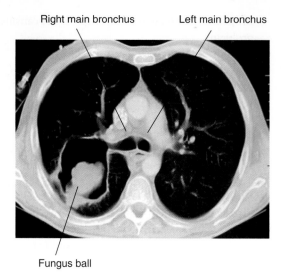

Right main bronchus    Left main bronchus

Fungus ball

**FIGURE 3.33** *Aspergillus.*

asthma, which traps the spores in its viscid mucus (Shah 2016), TB, bronchiectasis, cystic fibrosis, sarcoidosis, cancer, diabetes, malnutrition, alcoholism, steroid medication, lung transplantation (Geltner 2016), severe COPD or critical illness (Delsuc et al. 2015).

If *Aspergillus* spores germinate in the lung, they form a tangled mass called a fungus ball or aspergilloma, which resides in a cavity that it makes in the lung (Fig. 3.33). Early presentation is often silent, but patients may suffer malaise, weight loss, SOB, fever, haemoptysis and production of sputum containing brown plugs of the fungus. Both airways and lung tissue can be damaged, and diagnosis is by bronchoscopy, lavage or CT scan. Treatment is by antifungal agents, sometimes reduction of immunosuppressive therapy and occasionally surgical excision of the cavity along with its lobe (Denning et al. 2016). Prevention by inhaled medication shows promise for immunocompromised patients (Xia et al. 2015).

## Abscess

A lung abscess develops when infection leads to necrosis, producing a pus-containing cavity in the lung parenchyma. The commonest predisposing factors area swallowing impairment along with disorders of consciousness, e.g. alcoholic stupor or neurological problem, leading to aspiration of gastric contents. Other risks are aspiration of a foreign body, dental infections, bronchiectasis, lung cancer, frequent vomiting or immunocompromise.

Patients present with a spiking fever, night sweats, cough, putrid sputum, haemoptysis, pleuritic chest pain and fatigue. The X-ray shows an opaque lesion until communication with the airways is established, when natural drainage of the debris leaves a thick-walled ring shadow with a fluid line (see Fig. 2.22). Surgical drainage is unwise because it might unleash the infection, but prolonged antibiotics are required, and occasionally chest tube drainage, which may lead to empyema or bronchopleural fistula.

Postural drainage has been recommended (Kuhajda et al. 2016), combined with antibiotics (Zhou et al. 2016a), but it is only effective if the abscess is open to the airways, and only safe if the posture is accurate (Appendix E) and thorough, to avoid dissemination of infection. Both straight and lateral X-rays are required, and liaison with the radiologist helps to confirm the exact location of the abscess, common sites being:

- apical segment of the lower lobe of the right and sometimes left lung;
- posterior segment of the right upper lobe;
- middle lobe in case of vomiting and aspiration in prone, especially with intoxication (Kuhajda et al. 2016).

If there is doubt, treatment is best left to the antibiotics.

## LUNG CANCER

*Ageing has been described as the greatest of all carcinogens.*

**Gems 2011a**

Lung cancer kills more people and causes more distress than any other cancer (Polanski et al. 2016), usually because of late detection, with 5-year survival at around 16% (Khan et al. 2016). The risk is increased 5- to 10-fold in smokers and by 20% in passive smokers (Schwartz & Cote 2016). Most tumours arise in the large bronchi, whose bifurcation is the first to be hit by tobacco smoke (Fig. 3.34). This also makes them amenable to diagnostic endobronchial ultrasound and bronchoscopy. Comorbidities include TB, in whose scars the tumour may develop (Tamura 2016), and, for nearly half the patients, cardiovascular disease because of similar risk factors (Al-Kindi & Oliveira 2016)

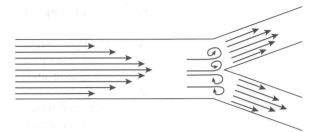

**FIGURE 3.34** Turbulent airflow at branching of airway.

including smoking, liberal consumption of processed meat (Miles et al. 2016) and lack of fruit and vegetables (Vieira et al. 2016).

Potential screening tests are sputum cytology, biomarkers and CT scan (Midthun 2016). An 'electronic nose' can pick up the disease in exhaled breath (Santini et al. 2016), as can dogs (Ferraris 2016). Early signs are unexplained cough or finger clubbing, recurrent pneumonia, and sometimes hypertrophic pulmonary osteoarthropathy, which causes pain and swelling of the wrists or ankles and may require bisphosphonates for pain control (Kilaru et al. 2012). A mass may hide behind the mediastinum on X-ray, or a tumour in a main bronchus may not be obvious until the lung collapses (Figs 3.35 and 2.19A).

## Clinical Features

The most distressing symptom is **shortness of breath** (SOB), caused by respiratory muscle weakness, radiotherapy or the tumour itself. It occurs in about 90% of patients and is less responsive to medication than is pain (Johnson et al. 2015). A persistent nonproductive **cough** occurs in 40%–70% of patients at initial presentation, caused by obstruction, pleural effusion, pneumonitis or comorbid COPD (Yorke et al. 2012).

Cancer **fatigue** can be unlike even the most profound fatigue of an otherwise well person. This is not always understood by health staff, who tend to think that pain is a more disruptive symptom (Radbruch 2008). Fatigue is the symptom that most affects quality of life (QoL), upsetting concentration (Borneman 2013) and sometimes continuing for months or years after treatment (Aynehchi et al. 2013). It is not proportional to recent activity and is often not relieved by rest, so pacing needs to be incorporated into all physiotherapy interventions. In the final stage of life, fatigue has been described as a protective mechanism (Radbruch 2008). Causes are

anaemia, inflammation, deconditioning, sleep disturbance, pain, chemotherapy, radiotherapy, depression or cachexia. Muscle wasting is the most important clinical feature of cancer cachexia and the principal cause of impaired physical function and respiratory complications (Bossola et al. 2016).

**Depression** is common, reduces adherence to treatment and increases mortality (Walker et al. 2013). Screening is required in advanced disease (Choi & Ryu 2016). It tends to be undertreated because of an assumption, according to Weinberger et al. (2012), that it is normal for cancer patients to be depressed. Normal does not mean OK.

Other clinical features are **hoarseness** if the recurrent laryngeal nerve is involved, **stridor**, a monophonic **wheeze**, and sometimes **haemoptysis**. **Chest pain** may be diffuse or aching, and neuropathic pain requires strong analgesia such as oxycodone/naloxone and pregabalin (De Santis et al. 2016). **Pleural effusion** is a poor prognostic sign (Porcel 2016).

## Classification

Lung cancers are subject to a high load of mutations and are regularly reclassified, but the following are generally recognized:

**Non-small cell lung cancers** make up 85% of cases (Garcia et al. 2016), comprising:

- adenocarcinoma, which are the most common in patients who never smoked (Rivera & Wakelee 2016);
- squamous cell carcinoma, which are usually located in large bronchi;
- large cell neuroendocrine carcinoma, which has the worst prognosis (Derks et al. 2016).

**Small cell lung cancers** mostly arise in the larger airways.

**Giant cell cancers** are, confusingly, a rare type of non-small cell cancer, with high mortality (Fujii et al. 2016a).

**Bronchoalveolar carcinoma** or **alveolar cell carcinoma** is a form of adenocarcinoma that develops in peripheral lung tissue, manifesting as local or diffuse infiltrates on X-ray and sometimes producing voluminous quantities of watery secretions. Chest clearance and some drugs may be beneficial (Rémi et al. 2016).

**Kaposi sarcoma** (KS) affects the skin, gut, connective tissue and lungs of immunocompromised people and is a frequent AIDS-defining cancer (Sigel et al. 2016). Pulmonary KS affects the parenchyma, lymph nodes or

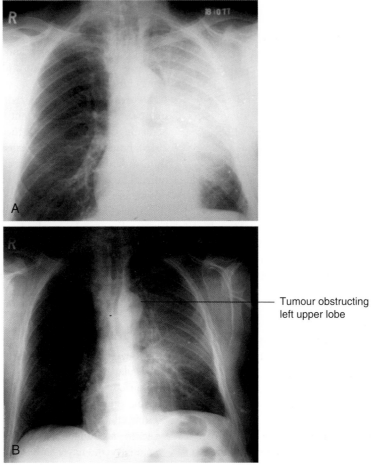

Tumour obstructing
left upper lobe

**FIGURE 3.35** (A) Dense opacity of left upper and mid zones partially obliterates a suspiciously shaped 'aorta'. (B) Darkened film shows 'aorta' to be a tumour squeezing the left main bronchus, reducing aeration of the left upper lobe. Loss of volume is reflected in a raised left hemidiaphragm.

pleura, manifesting as progressive SOB, cough and hypoxaemia.

**Mesothelioma** arises in the mesothelial cells of the peritoneum, pericardium or, most commonly, the pleura, where it is associated with malignant pleural effusion, finger clubbing and chest pain 'like being encased in concrete'. It is caused by asbestos exposure and will increase by 5%–10% per year in Europe over the next 25 years because of its decades-long latency period (Thompson et al. 2014). It is usually fatal, but pleurectomy-decortication or extrapleural pneumonectomy may extend life (Batirel et al. 2016).

Lung **metastases** are a poor prognostic sign but most have reached this stage by the time of diagnosis (Losanno 2016). Examples requiring particular attention are below:
1. Pancoast syndrome is an invasion of the chest wall, lymphatics and sympathetic chain, leading to loss of sympathetic tone and, if the upper rib is involved, shoulder pain.
2. Superior vena cava obstruction is an emergency that causes oedema, difficulty breathing, headache, nose bleeds, haemoptysis, stridor and faintness on bending down. It requires radiotherapy, steroids, stenting (Duvnjak 2012) and raising the head of the bed.

## General Management

The aim is to inflict the greatest damage to the cancer with the least damage to the patient. Chemotherapy may lead to 'chemo-brain', a form of cognitive decline that is often missed (Argyriou 2011), or 'chemo-lung', a form of lung fibrosis that can be aggravated by high concentration oxygen therapy (Allan et al. 2012). Radiotherapy may cause rib fracture (Abe et al. 2016).

Upper airway obstruction can be palliated by laser, stenting (which may cause a dry cough) or bronchoplasty. Immunotherapy may enable the immune system to recognise and destroy the cancer cells that conventional therapy misses (Steven et al. 2016). Targeted delivery of drugs without harming normal tissue may become available using stem cells (Yan et al. 2016) or nebulized liposome bubbles (Rudokas et al. 2016).

Surgical resection is minimally invasive when possible, leading to better shoulder range of motion and improved function than open surgery (Granger 2016), described on p. 309. The term 'resectable' indicates that the tumour can be completely excised, whereas 'operable' indicates that surgery brings an acceptably low risk of death or morbidity. Nonresectable tumours may respond to microwave ablation (Wei et al. 2016). A third of patients have bone metastases that can cause fractures and spinal cord compression, but surgery may be undertaken if life expectancy is long enough for patients to benefit from the resulting pain relief and improved mobility (Weiss 2011).

Most patients also have COPD (Granger 2016), which requires treatment, and long-term survivors need ongoing care because of a heavy burden of continuing symptoms (Yang et al. 2013), including fatigue, which may be a surrogate for depression (Goo et al. 2016). Undertreatment of lung cancer in elderly people is common (Peake 2003).

## Physiotherapy

*The cornerstone of physiotherapy management in lung cancer should be prescription and delivery of exercise.*

***Granger 2016***

Physiotherapists may be involved at any stage including sputum induction, prehabilitation before surgery, postoperative management, relaxation, acupuncture (Bauml et al. 2016), energy conservation, exercise and terminal care.

Dyspnoea management strategies decrease patient distress and anxiety, increase confidence and reduce costs (Man et al. 2016), for example, a single session of abdominal breathing, pacing and relaxation can reduce SOB, anxiety and depression (Johnson et al. 2015). Exercise is relevant at any stage:

- It appears to reduce the risk of developing lung cancer (Brenner et al. 2016).
- In established cancer, higher physical activity levels are associated with less symptoms, including depression, although it is unknown if fewer symptoms leads to more activity or if being active desensitises patients to their symptoms (Granger 2016).
- Exercise is recommended prior to medical treatment (Loughney et al. 2016).
- Before and after lung resection, the outcomes of exercise are described in Chapter 13.
- During palliative chemotherapy, patients find that prudent exercise enhances their activities of daily living (Henke et al. 2014).
- For survivors, physically activity patients live on average 4 years longer than those who are not active (Sloan et al. 2016).

## Complications

Before exercise prescription, the notes should be checked for anaemia. Pacing and falls prevention should be included, and interval exercise suits many patients.

Metastatic spinal cord compression develops in 28% of patients. Bladder symptoms or new lower limb weakness must be reported, and a scoring system helps identify the optimum management (Lei et al. 2016).

Occasionally a patient may cough up tumour tissue, so if a specimen has the appearance of a blood clot, it should be sent to cytology (Ochi et al. 2012).

Lung cancer is associated with a higher incidence of venous thromboembolism than other cancers (Walker et al. 2016).

## Outcomes

Outcome measures include the Lung Cancer Standard Set (Mak et al. 2016), dyspnoea scales (Ahmedzai et al. 2012, p.100), functional scales (Dean 2013), exercise tests (Henke et al. 2014) and the 'QLQ-C30 questionnaire' (Polanski et al. 2016).

## CARDIORESPIRATORY MANIFESTATIONS OF SYSTEMIC DISEASE

The cardiorespiratory system is influenced by most systemic disturbances. For example, oxygen delivery is impaired by anaemia, breathing is disrupted by acid–base imbalance and emotion, and the alveolar–capillary membrane is rendered leaky by sepsis. The following conditions are those with the most impact on cardiorespiratory function.

### HIV and AIDS

People with the chronic disease human immunodeficiency virus (HIV) require combination antiretroviral drugs to prevent the development of acquired immune deficiency syndrome (AIDS). The majority of patients live with the adverse effects of treatment and the consequences of immunodeficiency, e.g. TB, pneumonia, lung cancer, which is two to three times more prevalent in HIV-positive people (Collini 2016), emphysema, which is more than twice as common and lung fibrosis (Drummond et al 2017).

The physiotherapist's role is to assess for mobility and respiratory problems. Exercise can ease pain, fatigue and depression (O'Brien et al. 2016), but prolonged intense exercise can further suppress the immune system (Fig. 3.36).

### Sleep Apnoea

*'I literally fell asleep into my plate'*

*Sims 2003*

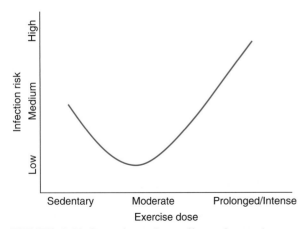

**FIGURE 3.36** Dose-dependent effect of exercise on risk and severity of respiratory tract infections. (Adapted from Nieman et al. 1989.)

Approximately 7% of road accidents have been attributed to sleep apnoea (Garbarino et al. 2015), with fatality rates similar to alcohol-related crashes (Goel et al. 2009). Sleep deprivation related to sleep apnoea has contributed to oil tanker spills, nuclear meltdowns and the Challenger space shuttle explosion (Howard 2005).

Sleep-disordered breathing is present in 5%–15% of the population (Punjabi 2013), or, according to Fox et al. (2016), 83% of those attending cardiac rehabilitation. Sleep apnoea occurs when breathing stops for more than 10 s. Desaturation stimulates the respiratory centres, and the subsequent arousal may be accompanied by spectacular snoring. The patient is affected by daytime sleepiness, poor concentration, morning headaches due to $CO_2$ retention, postural instability (Degache et al. 2016), memory loss and a disgruntled spouse. Hypoxaemia predisposes to cognitive, autonomic, sensorimotor (Park et al. 2016a), vascular and neural dysfunction (Deniz et al. 2016). Sympathetic activation during arousal causes spikes in blood pressure, leading over time to cardiovascular disease and increased mortality.

The risk of sleep apnoea is increased by smoking, excess alcohol (which suppresses pharyngeal muscle action) and being male (progesterone being a respiratory stimulant). Comorbidities include COPD, cardiovascular disease (Hang et al. 2016), stroke (Ifergane et al. 2016) and spinal cord injury (Chiodo et al. 2016). It can worsen in hospital because of sedative drugs, the supine position and sleep deprivation. It also worsens with age, when it is often not identified or treated (McMillan 2016). Diagnosis is made from symptoms, history and a sleep study.

Patients may misinterpret sleepiness as fatigue, and it is estimated that 90% of sufferers are not diagnosed (Mulchrone et al. 2016). Devasahayam (2012) found sleep disorders to be the commonest misdiagnosis for people referred to a chronic fatigue clinic. Physiotherapists may be the first to suspect the condition.

**Obstructive sleep apnoea** (OSA) is due to nocturnal upper airway obstruction. Comorbidities include obesity (because a thick neck can choke patients in their own fat when muscle tone wanes at night), impaired exercise capacity (Beitler et al. 2014), cardiovascular disease, erectile dysfunction (Taken et al. 2016) and Alzheimer's disease, the latter probably related to sleep-related deficiency in cerebral blood flow (Emamian et al. 2016). Childhood OSA may relate to enlarged adenoids and tonsils, and presents with hyperactivity and nocturnal enuresis rather than sleepiness (Tsubomatsu et al. 2016).

Screening is by the Epworth Sleepiness Scale (Sander et al. 2016) or the STOP-Bang Questionnaire (Chung et al. 2016b). Management is by weight loss and smoking cessation if required, exercise, avoidance of evening alcohol, stimulation of the genioglossus muscle, playing the didgeridoo (Chwiesko 2013), acupuncture (Lv et al. 2016) and avoiding sleeping supine (e.g. wearing a back-to-front bra with tennis balls in each cup). If lifestyle advice is not adequate, nightly CPAP is the gold standard (Kuźniar 2016). Pneumatically splinting open the upper airway (Fig. 3.37) is not always comfortable or elegant, but humidification helps those with nasopharyngeal symptoms (Soudorn et al. 2016). CPAP also reduces the risk of cardiovascular disease (Pépin et al. 2016), fatigue, sleep-related road accidents (Fig. 3.38) and OSA-associated urge incontinence (Ipekci et al. 2016), but may increase breathlessness in obese people (Xiao et al. 2016). Alternatives are high-flow nasal cannulae (Nishimura 2015), contraptions to hold open the upper airway (Gjerde et al. 2016), surgery such as uvulopalatopharyngoplasty (which is as complicated as it sounds) and either a minitracheostomy or a full tracheostomy (Camacho et al. 2016). Physiotherapy includes exercise training (Andrade 2016) and expiratory muscle training (Kuo 2017).

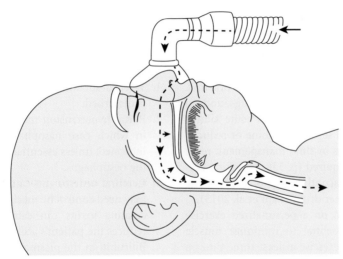

**FIGURE 3.37** Upper airway splinted open by CPAP.

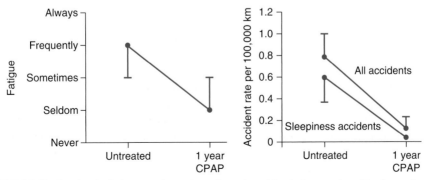

**FIGURE 3.38** Reduction in fatigue and number of road accidents in people with sleep-disordered breathing after a year of CPAP. (From Cassel 1996.)

**Central sleep apnoea** may overlap with OSA but involves no respiratory effort. It is associated with neurological disorders, heart failure or abnormal control of breathing (Malhotra & Owens 2010) including hyperventilation syndrome (Pevernagie 2012) and may require nocturnal NIV or $CO_2$ breathing (Mulchrone et al. 2016). **Restrictive sleep apnoea** can occur with scoliosis, ankylosing spondylitis or diaphragmatic paralysis.

Regular exercise for people with sleep disorders can reduce fatigue (Hargens et al. 2013), daytime sleepiness (Alves et al. 2013) and, in patients with coronary artery disease, the severity of apnoea (Mendelson et al. 2016).

## Kidney Disease

Kidney disease and its treatment may affect the cardiorespiratory system by causing:

• metabolic acidosis;
• fluid overload, leading to pulmonary oedema and sometimes pleural effusion;
• breathlessness due to pulmonary oedema or to compensate for metabolic acidosis;
• muscle wasting due to steroid treatment or uraemia.

Kidneys regulate the excretion of most drugs, and an adverse reaction to drugs is one cause of acute kidney injury, indicated by raised serum creatinine or reduced urine output. Treatment is by fluid management, renal replacement therapy if required (p. 538), smoking cessation (Siqueira 2017), discontinuation of nephrotoxic drugs and wary use of other drugs (Lapi et al. 2013).

Physiotherapy is based on a personalized exercise programme, which is essential to minimize muscle wasting. Thirty minutes' exercise at least three times a week improves physical functioning, BP, heart rate and QoL (Phan et al. 2016a), and may also help decrease osteoporosis, which is a risk factor with kidney disease (Marinho 2016). This is safe and effective for patients with chronic disease, including those in kidney failure and requiring dialysis (Dziubek et al. 2016), so long as BP is monitored. Hypertension and kidney disease augment each other in a vicious cycle (Ohno et al. 2016), and postexercise hypotension may occur in predialysis patients following aerobic exercise (Headley et al. 2017). Exercise also appears to offer some protection against cola-induced kidney damage (Cao et al. 2016a).

Exercise may be affected by problems related to kidney disease such as anaemia, fatigue, cardiomyopathy, respiratory dysfunction, muscle degradation and pulmonary oedema or pleural effusion caused by fluid overload. However, by taking suitable precautions such as avoiding fatigue, an exercise programme can improve muscle strength (Neto et al. 2016a).

## Liver Disease

The liver is the most metabolically active tissue by weight in the body, being served by two blood supplies and boasting over 500 functions. Most drug metabolism occurs in the liver, which complicates medical management when it malfunctions. The liver is sensitive to alcohol, malnutrition and the effect of more than 1000 drugs, including paracetamol (Kim & Hattori 2010)). If the cause of liver dysfunction is unknown, patients should be tested for $\alpha_1$-antitrypsin deficiency (p. 73).

Complications relevant to physiotherapy are muscle wasting (Dasarathy 2016) and dyspnoea, which can be caused by hepatomegaly, ascites, pulmonary vascular complications or cardiovascular disease (Francque et al. 2016).

Precautions relevant to physiotherapy are the following:

1. Tracheal suction is performed with caution if clotting is disturbed.
2. Portal hypertension may cause oesophageal varices, in which case nasopharyngeal suction is contraindicated, unless essential, in case the catheter enters the oesophagus.
3. Cerebral oedema can cause hyperventilation, which may need control by mechanical ventilation, and circulating toxins can cause encephalopathy, which reduces the patient's ability to cooperate.
4. Bilirubin in the plasma of jaundiced patients limits the accuracy of oximetry.
5. Following hepatic resection, blood glucose may be destabilized (Maeda 2010), which has implications for mobilizing patients.

Prehabilitation before liver resection has demonstrated improvements in exercise tolerance and QoL (Dunne et al. 2016).

## Sickle Cell Disease (SCD)

*The pain of sickle cell crisis is one of the most intense in medicine.*

**Nagel 2001**

SCD is a genetic disorder occurring mostly in black populations and characterized by red blood cells crystallizing into a rigid sickle shape, rendering them unable to squeeze through small vessels. The result is vasoocclusion, haemolytic anaemia, anaemic hypoxia and organ damage, including the risk of avascular necrosis, priapism and stroke, the latter requiring specific guidelines (Lawrence 2016). Death occurs at an average age of 45 (Adeniyi & Saminu 2011), or, for the majority not diagnosed by early screening, in childhood. An unexpected advantage is that SCD protects against malaria (Chakravorty 2015).

Sickling crises can be precipitated by nocturnal hypoxaemia (Owens 2013), pain, fatigue (Panepinto et al. 2014), dehydration, infection, extreme temperature change, smoking or sudden exercise. Some patients experience pain continuously (Bakshi & Morris 2016) and the ischaemic and neuropathic pain of a sickling crisis is notoriously undermanaged, particularly by staff who suspect that black people misuse narcotics (Ballas 2016). This has been found with other conditions, Hispanics being twice as likely as whites to receive no analgesia after trauma, and black patients 66% less likely to receive analgesia after leg fracture (Brockopp et al. 2003). People with sickle cell disease must be under the care of a specialist unit where morphine is provided in doses sufficient to compensate for the drug clearing 3–10 times faster than in the general population (Darbari et al. 2012). Patients should carry a note from their consultant specifying the analgesia required.

When vasoocclusion occurs in the pulmonary vasculature, an acute chest syndrome of pain, cough, production of characteristic golden sputum (Contou et al. 2015), breathlessness and hypoxaemia occurs, the latter being the leading cause of death (Nansseu et al. 2015). Pain causes diaphragmatic splinting and atelectasis, for which incentive spirometry has been found helpful (Adeniyi & Saminu 2011). CT scan or bedside ultrasound help locate lung opacities (Razazi et al. 2016). Chronic cardiorespiratory complications include pulmonary hypertension, venous thromboembolism, sleep-disordered breathing and wheezing (Mehari & Klings 2016).

Patients benefit from advice on joint protection and pacing. Regular physical activity helps control endothelial dysfunction (Chirico et al. 2012) but impaired parasympathetic function affects heart rate recovery (Alvarado et al. 2015). Exercise capacity is impaired by episodes of acute chest syndrome and peripheral microvascular occlusion, but inspiratory muscle training can bring some improvement in exercise tolerance, QoL,

SOB, fatigue and pain (Camcıoğlu et al. 2016). Precautions include:

- avoidance of overexertion, which can be fatal (Asplund 2016);
- checks for thromboembolism because of hypercoagulability;
- avoidance of ice treatment in case of rhabdomyolysis.

## Gastro-oesophageal Reflux disease (GORD)

GORD is the passage of gastric contents into the oesophagus. This occurs in >70% of people, usually during sleep (Dickson et al. 2016), but if frequent enough to damage the oesophageal mucosa or cause symptoms, it becomes a disease. Aspiration of this material can cause, trigger or exacerbate COPD, cystic fibrosis, sleep apnoea, asthma and interstitial lung disease (Bois et al. 2016). This association may relate to altered intrathoracic pressures or a shared vagal innervation by the oesophagus and bronchial tree.

Risk factors are heart failure (Arzt et al. 2016), the extremes of age, intellectual disability (May & Kennedy 2010), smoking, alcohol, chronic aspiration, obesity, frequent coughing, running (Herregods et al. 2016) and pregnancy through IVF (Turan et al. 2016a).

Stomach acid outside the mucus protection of its own environment causes heartburn, airway hyperreactivity, tooth erosion, morning hoarseness and a bitter taste in the mouth after recumbency or large meals. Aspiration into the lungs may cause pulmonary infiltrates on X-ray and a recurrent cough. Symptomatic children feed poorly and vomit, and in cystic fibrosis vomiting may be the only sign.

Management is by upright positioning when possible (Jung 2012), left side-lying in preference to right side-lying (Loots 2013), raising the head of the bed at night and modification of predisposing factors including drug review. Patients should avoid late or large meals, extreme exercise, smoking and if possible aminophylline, which relaxes the lower oesophageal sphincter. An antireflux diet excludes caffeine, fizzy drinks, alcohol, citrus fruit, chocolate and high fat products. Proton pump inhibitor drugs (PPIs) decrease gastric acid secretion but do not inhibit reflux because this is related to lower oesophageal sphincter relaxation. PPIs also increase the risk of pneumonia (Ojoo et al. 2013), fractures (Ozdil et al. 2013) and delirium (Otremba et al. 2016).

Physiotherapy, other than education, should be avoided after meals. The head-down postural drainage position is a risk, but the effect of different positions varies, with slumped sitting sometimes the worst because of increased abdominal pressure.

GORD increases the risk of oesophageal cancer via a transition phase called Barrett's oesophagus, in which metaplastic epithelium replaces the stratified squamous epithelium that normally lines the distal oesophagus (Song et al. 2016b).

## Diabetes Mellitus

An epidemic of type 2 diabetes is emerging due to the 1 billion overweight people worldwide, bringing also comorbid cardiovascular disease, which is the main cause of mortality (Pladevall et al. 2016). Predisposing factors for diabetes include cystic fibrosis, diet- and sugar-sweetened drinks, pollution (Nisell 2013), excess consumption of red meat (Ekmekcioglu et al. 2016) and transplantation (Wallia et al. 2016). Complications are hypotension, musculoskeletal problems (Baker et al. 2012), fracture risk (Choi et al. 2016a), cerebrovascular, kidney and eye disease (Weng et al. 2016), and for those with poor glycaemic control, impaired muscle quality (Yoon et al. 2016). Type 1 diabetes can occur from birth and brings added complications such as autonomic neuropathy (McCarty & Silverman 2016). Metformin is the most widely used drug, but it has been linked to pulmonary tumours (Deng et al. 2016).

With stable diabetes, regular exercise improves glycaemic control and reduces the risk of cardiovascular disease and early death (Hamasaki 2016). Precautions during exercise are to maintain hydration, look after the feet and when necessary increase insulin or carbohydrates to avoid hypoglycaemic events. Patients who have poor awareness of hypoglycaemia may benefit from setting a higher preexercise blood glucose goal (Lopez et al. 2011). Warning signs of hypoglycaemia include light-headedness, rapid breathing, weakness and fatigue. Patients need to bring a glucose tablet to exercise sessions and know their own glycaemic target (Cahn et al. 2016). Cardiac response to exercise is attenuated (Sydó et al. 2016) and exercise capacity may be further impaired by orthostatic intolerance or autonomic neuropathy. The metabolic cost of walking is higher than average (Petrovic et al. 2016) and many patients are already weak, so motivation is extra important, e.g. using rebound exercise (Maharaj et al. 2016).

For acute patients on the medical wards, fluid and acid–base disturbance may be present. On the surgical wards, blood glucose needs to be stabilized preoperatively, and infection is a risk (Kok et al. 2016).

## Inflammatory Bowel Disease

Systemic dissemination of inflammation may occur from ulcerative colitis or Crohn disease, predisposing to bronchiectasis, interstitial lung disease, BOOP and asthma (Zgraggen 2013). Respiratory symptoms may appear years after the bowel disease (Mahadeva et al. 2000) and the physiotherapist may be the first to make the connection.

## Drug-Induced Cardiorespiratory Disease

Adverse reactions to prescription drugs are a significant preventable cause of hospitalization, one study finding that 18.4% of hospital deaths were thought to be related to medication (Pardo et al. 2016). Cardiorespiratory examples are aspirin causing asthma, amiodarone causing lung fibrosis and cardiovascular drugs causing fatal bradycardias (Givens 2012). In the ICU, neuromuscular blocking agents and steroids increase the risk of secondary infection and ICU-acquired weakness (Annane 2016).

Reactions to illicit drug use depend on the substance, contaminants and route of administration. **Heroin** is a CNS depressant that is mainly smoked, leading to a high incidence of COPD and asthma, both usually undertreated (Lewis-Burke et al. 2016). Other effects related to physiotherapy include neuropathy (Coraci et al. 2016) and fatal chest rigidity (Burns et al. 2016), but the main cause of opioid-related deaths is respiratory depression (Hill et al. 2016). Acupuncture may help allay withdrawal symptoms (Wu et al. 2016a).

**Cocaine** is a CNS stimulant that can lead to arterial thrombosis, limb loss (Ali et al. 2017), stroke, myocardial infarction or multisystem failure (Zimmerman 2012). Exercise may protect against relapse in the early stages of abstinence (Beiter et al. 2016). **Crack cocaine** predisposes to cognitive decline (Sanvicente et al. 2016) and can cause 'crack lung', which brings fever, haemoptysis, dyspnoea, pulmonary oedema, alveolar damage, necrosis of the nasal septum and barotrauma (Mégarbane et al. 2013).

**Cannabis** can also cause barotrauma (Golwala 2012). Sustained use may impair cognitive and motor function (Ganzer et al. 2016) and predispose to cardiorespiratory disease (Kreuter et al. 2016). Early and heavy use may shorten life (Manrique et al. 2016). Inhaled cannabis brings complications related to the accompanying tobacco, delivering two–three times the carcinogens because of the inhalation pattern (Melvin & Markham 2015), and *Aspergillus* spores, which would be risky for immunocompromised people. Prenatal cannabis exposure can lead to neurodevelopmental deficit (Alpár et al. 2016). More optimistically, nonpsychoactive preparations have been used to reduce nausea, pain (Ablin et al. 2016), bronchospasm, osteoporosis (Kogan 2007), spasticity in multiple sclerosis (Corey-Bloom 2012), paediatric seizures (Isaacs & Kilham 2015) and some effects of spinal cord injury (Arevalo et al. 2016). Cannabinoids may even have some anticancer properties (Pyszniak et al. 2016).

Ecstasy can cause impaired cognitive processing (Betzler et al. 2017) and barotrauma.

Exercise training has been shown to reduce drug misuse in some individuals and decrease comorbid risk factors (Smith & Lynch 2012).

## RESPIRATORY FAILURE

The term **respiratory failure** (RF) is reserved for inadequate gas exchange as reflected in arterial blood gases, even though the process of respiration includes more than gas exchange in the lung. It can occur in acute or chronic disease, or in postoperative patients, one in five of whom die within 30 days of developing RF (Marseu 2016). **Respiratory insufficiency** is a vague term that suggests adequate gas exchange but at some cost, and may presage respiratory failure.

Type I (hypoxaemic) RF is failed oxygenation, represented by $PaO_2$ <8 kPa (60 mmHg). It is due to failure of the gas-exchanging function of the respiratory system and can be acute (e.g. pneumonia) or chronic (e.g. severe COPD).

Type II (hypoxaemic and hypercapnic) RF is failed ventilation, represented by $PaCO_2$ >6.7 kPa (50 mmHg) as well as hypoxaemia (Fig. 3.39). Raised $CO_2$ is caused by failure of the respiratory pump, e.g. impaired central respiratory drive or muscle weakness. It can be acute (e.g. severe acute asthma) or chronic (e.g. late-stage fibrosing alveolitis). Type II RF is also known as ventilatory failure and is accompanied by a fall in pH until renal compensation takes effect. Options for monitoring $CO_2$ are intermittent arterial or capillary blood gases, and continuous end-tidal $CO_2$ or transcutaneous $CO_2$ measurements. Ventilatory support may be required (BTS/ICS 2016).

In the later stages of COPD, patients who develop chronic ventilatory failure have been called 'physiologically wise' because they are thought to protect their diaphragm from fatigue by hypoventilating, leading to hypercapnia (Bégin 2000), albeit unwittingly. They pay the price by more rapid disease progression. Patients with type I RF keep their $PaCO_2$ under control but at the cost of dyspnoea. The relevance to physiotherapists is that the latter group in particular responds to breathless management techniques.

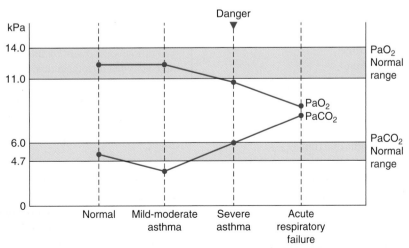

**FIGURE 3.39** Progressive changes in arterial blood gases during acute severe asthma.

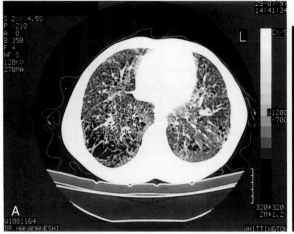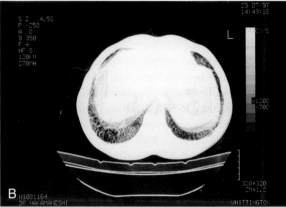

**FIGURE 3.40** CT scan of Mr MB (A) at chest level showing damaged lungs, (B) at diaphragm level.

## CASE STUDY: MR MB[a]

*This 25-year-old man from Nottingham has primary emphysema due to $\alpha_1$-antitrypsin deficiency.*

### Background

- Recurrent childhood infections
- Unemployed, lives alone, 'finished with girlfriend because I'm too busy with hospital appointments'. Nonsmoker.

### Subjective

- Grey sputum, cleared independently
- Shortness of breath worse since admission last April
- Watch TV much of the time
- Hoping for lung transplant

### Objective

- Hyperinflation
- Breathing pattern normal
- ↑ respiratory rate on slight exertion
- Stooped posture
- Scattered crackles on auscultation

### Questions

1. CT Scan: evidence of emphysema (Fig. 3.40)?
2. Analysis?
3. Problems?
4. Plan?

### CLINICAL REASONING

*The following study used lung inflation techniques to treat people with asthma. Has the correct problem been identified?*

*'Lung inflation techniques such as incentive spirometry, voluntary deep breathing, intermittent positive pressure breathing and continuous positive airways pressure, are used to increase lung volumes during acute attacks and to reduce atelectasis, but published studies have failed to document their usefulness in the treatment of asthma'.*

*Eur Resp J* (1993) 3, 353–5

### Response to Case Study

1. Scan
- Black areas in the lung fields indicate breakdown of alveoli into large airspaces.
- 'Double border' of the diaphragm is due to MB being unable to hold his breath for the scan.

[a]*CT*, Computed tomography; *SH*, social history.

2. Analysis
- Little ventilatory reserve
- Previous fitness not regained since hospital admission
- Inactive lifestyle
- Poor posture contributing to inefficient breathing

3. Problems
- Shortness of breath
- ↓ Exercise tolerance

4. Plan
- Educate on the relevance of exercise tolerance to eligibility for lung transplant
- Educate on breathless management
- Educate on posture correction
- Assess exercise tolerance
- Negotiate daily exercise programme
- Check that chest clearance techniques are not wasting energy, modify if necessary
- Follow up within a week to ensure motivation
- Adjust programme until optimum self-management
- Review 3-monthly

---

## RESPONSE TO CLINICAL REASONING

Is the patient's problem:
- Loss of lung volume? No, acute asthma causes hyperinflation and 'lung inflation techniques' would be counterproductive.
- Excess work of breathing? Yes, but the methods described would increase the work of breathing.
- Sputum retention? Maybe, but these methods are not designed for sputum clearance.

This is the type of article that is interpreted as 'physiotherapy' being ineffective for people with asthma.

---

# RECOMMENDED READING

Al-Dorzi, H.M., 2013. Life-threatening infections in medically immunocompromised patients. Crit. Care Clin. 29 (4), 807–826.

Beghi, G.M., Morselli-Labate, A.M., 2016. Does homeopathic medicine have a preventive effect on respiratory tract infections? Multidiscipl. Respir. Med. 11, 12.

Berdishevsky, H., 2016. Physiotherapy scoliosis-specific exercises – a comprehensive review of seven major schools. Scoliosis Spinal Disord. 11, 20.

Crinion, S.J., Ryan, S., McNicholas, W.T., 2017. Obstructive sleep apnoea as a cause of nocturnal nondipping blood pressure: recent evidence regarding clinical importance and underlying mechanisms. Eur. Respir. J. 49 (1), 1601818.

Dagan, N., 2017. External validation and comparison of three prediction tools for risk of osteoporotic fractures using data from population based electronic health records. Br. Med. J. 356, i6755.

Danoff, S.K., 2017. Toward understanding patient experience in idiopathic pulmonary fibrosis. Eur. Respir. J. 49 (1), 1602202.

Denipah, N., Dominguez, C.M., Kraai, E.P., et al., 2017. Acute management of paradoxical vocal fold motion (vocal cord dysfunction). Ann. Emerg. Med. 69 (1), 18–23.

Derdak, S., 2017. Prevention of COPD readmissions. Respir. Care 62 (1), 133–134.

Effing, T.W., Vercoulen, J.H., Bourbeau, J., et al., 2016. Definition of a COPD self-management intervention. Eur. Respir. J. 48 (1), 46–54.

Elborn, J.S., 2016. Cystic fibrosis. Lancet 388 (10059), 2519–2531.

El Maghraoui, A., Dehhaoui, M., 2012. Prevalence and characteristics of lung involvement on high resolution CT in patients with ankylosing spondylitis. Pulm. Med. 965956.

ERS, 2017. European Respiratory Society guidelines for the diagnosis of primary ciliary dyskinesia. Eur. Respir. J. 49 (1), 1601090.

Ford, B., 2017. CFTR structure: lassoing cystic fibrosis. Nat. Struct. Mol. Biol. 24 (1), 13–14. doi:10.1038/nsmb.3353.

Furukawa, T., Taniguchi, H., Ando, M., et al., 2017. The St. George's Respiratory Questionnaire as a prognostic factor in IPF. Respir. Res. 18, 18.

Gerber, L.H., 2014. Role of exercise in optimizing the functional status of patients with nonalcoholic fatty liver disease. Clin. Liver Dis. 18 (1), 113–127.

Ghannouchi, I., Speyer, R., Doma, K., et al., 2016. Swallowing function and chronic respiratory diseases: systematic review. Respir. Med. 117, 54–64.

Goyal, V., Grimwood, K., Marchant, J., et al., 2016. Pediatric bronchiectasis. Pediatr. Pulmonol. 51 (5), 450–469.

Guilleminault, L., 2017. Personalised medicine in asthma: from curative to preventive medicine. Eur. Respir. Rev. 26 (143), 160010.

Hoffman, L.R., Ramsey, B.W., 2013. Cystic fibrosis therapeutics. Chest 143 (1), 207–213.

Hu, S.T., Yu, C.C., Lee, P.S., 2014. Life experiences among obstructive sleep apnoea patients receiving CPAP. J. Clin. Nurs. 23 (1-2), 268–278.

Jones, R.L., Noble, P.B., Elliot, J.G., 2016. Airway remodelling in COPD: It's not asthma! Respirology 21 (8), 1347–1356.

Kalil, A.C., Metersky, M.L., Klompas, M., et al., 2016. Management of adults with hospital-acquired and ventilator-associated pneumonia: Clinical Practice Guidelines. Clin. Infect. Dis. 63 (5), e61–e111.

Kaneda, H., Nakano, T., Taniguchi, Y., et al., 2013. Three-step management of pneumothorax. Interact. Cardiovasc. Thorac. Surg. 16 (2), 186–192.

Karapanagiotis, S., 2017. Ventilatory limitation and dynamic hyperinflation during exercise testing in cystic fibrosis. Pediatr. Pulmonol. 52 (1), 29–33.

Kilcoyne, A., Lavelle, L.P., McCarthy, C.J., et al., 2016. Chest CT abnormalities and quality of life: relationship in adult cystic fibrosis. Ann. Transl. Med. 4 (5), 87.

Kline, J.N., Rose, R.M., 2014. Central nervous system influences in asthma. Adv. Exp. Med. Biol. 795, 309–319.

Ko, F.W., Cheung, N.K., Rainer, T.H., et al., 2017. Comprehensive care programme for patients with chronic obstructive pulmonary disease. Thorax 72, 122–128.

Kusmirek, J.E., Martin, M.D., Kanne, J.P., 2016. Imaging of idiopathic pulmonary fibrosis. Radiol. Clin. North Am. 54 (6), 997–1014.

Lahiri, T., 2016. Clinical Practice Guidelines from the Cystic Fibrosis Foundation for preschoolers with cystic fibrosis. Pediatrics 137 (4), e20151784.

López-Torres, I., 2016. Changes in cognitive status in COPD patients across clinical stages. COPD 13 (3), 327–332.

Lynch, J.P., Huynh, R.H., Fishbein, M.C., et al., 2016. Idiopathic pulmonary fibrosis: epidemiology, clinical features, prognosis, and management. Semin. Respir. Crit. Care Med. 37 (3), 331–357.

Megria, M., 2017. MRSA-induced pulmonary-renal syndrome. Respir. Med. Case Rep. 20, 42–44.

Meknes, D., 2012. Clinical effects of yoga on asthmatic patients. Ethiop. J. Health Sci. 20 (2), 107–112.

Meltzer, C., 2016. Visibility of structures of relevance for patients with cystic fibrosis in chest tomosynthesis. Radiat. Prot. Dosimetry 169 (1-4), 177–187.

Mizuguchi, S., Iwata, T., Izumi, N., et al., 2016. Arterial blood gases predict long-term prognosis in stage I non-small cell lung cancer patients. BMC Surg. 16 (1), 3.

Mnika, K., Pule, G.D., Dandara, C., 2016. An expert review of pharmacogenomics of sickle cell disease therapeutics: not yet ready for global precision medicine. OMICS 20 (10), 565–574.

Mochizuki, Y., Hayashi, K., Nakayama, Y., et al., 2016. ALS patients with ability to communicate after long-term mechanical ventilation have confined degeneration to the motor neuron system. J. Neurol. Sci. 363, 245–248.

Mogayzel, P., 2013. Cystic fibrosis pulmonary guidelines. Am. J. Respir. Crit. Care Med. 187 (7), 680–689.

Montgomery, S.T., Mall, M.A., Kicic, A., et al., 2017. Hypoxia and sterile inflammation in cystic fibrosis airways: mechanisms and potential therapies. Eur. Respir. J. 49 (1), 1600903.

Morisset, J., Dubé, B.P., Garvey, C., et al., 2016. The unmet educational needs of interstitial lung disease patients: setting the stage for tailored pulmonary rehabilitation. Ann. Am. Thorac. Soc. 13 (7), 1026–1033.

Murakami, M., 2013. Relationships between physical activity and pulmonary functions in Parkinson's disease. Hong Kong Physiother. J. 31 (1), 51.

NICE Guideline, 2013. Acute kidney injury [CG169].

NICE Guideline, 2013. Idiopathic pulmonary fibrosis [CG163].

NICE Guidance, 2017. Asthma management [GID-CGWAVE0743].

Nicholson, T.T., 2017. Relationship between pulmonary hyperinflation and dyspnoea severity during acute exacerbations of cystic fibrosis. Respirology 22 (1), 141–148.

Parati, G., Lombardi, C., Hedner, J., et al., 2013. Recommendations for the management of patients with obstructive sleep apnoea and hypertension. Eur. Respir. J. 41 (3), 523–538.

Patti, M.G., 2016. An evidence-based approach to the treatment of gastroesophageal reflux disease. JAMA Surg. 151 (1), 73–78.

Penafortes, J.T., Guimarães, F.S., Moço, V.J., et al., 2013. Relationship between body balance, lung function, nutritional status and functional capacity in adults with cystic fibrosis. Braz. J. Phys. Ther. 17 (5), 450–457.

Raghavan, D., Bartter, T., Joshi, M., 2016. How to reduce hospital readmissions in chronic obstructive pulmonary disease? Curr. Opin. Pulm. Med. 22 (2), 106–112.

Randerath, W., 2017. Definition, discrimination, diagnosis and treatment of central breathing disturbances during sleep. Eur. Respir. J. 49 (1), 1600959.

Reddy, A.P., Gupta, M.R., 2014. Management of asthma: the current US and European guidelines. Adv. Exp. Med. Biol. 795, 81–103.

Reich, J.M., 2014. Cough suppression disorders spectrum. Respir. Med. 108 (2), 413–415.

Remels, A.H.V., 2013. The mechanisms of cachexia underlying muscle dysfunction in COPD. J. Appl. Phys. 114 (9), 1253–1262.

Schoos, M., 2013. Echocardiographic predictors of exercise capacity and mortality in COPD. BMC Cardiovasc. Dis. 13, 84.

Seaburg, L.A., Sekiguchi, H., 2016. Two chronically ill patients presenting with hypoxemic respiratory failure. Chest 149 (4), e107–e110.

Shapiro, A.J., Zariwala, M.A., Ferkol, T., et al., 2016. Diagnosis, monitoring, and treatment of primary ciliary dyskinesia. Pediatr. Pulmonol. 51 (2), 115–132.

Shukla, S., Evans, J.R., Malik, R., et al., 2017. Development of a RNA-seq based prognostic signature in lung adenocarcinoma. J. Natl. Cancer Inst. 109 (1), djw200.

SIGN, 2016. British guideline on the management of asthma. Scottish Intercollegiate Guidelines Network [153].

Silver, P.C., Kollef, M.H., Clinkscale, D., et al., 2017. A respiratory therapist disease management program for subjects hospitalized with COPD. Respir. Care 62 (1), 1–9.

Simonds, A.K., 2016. Progress in respiratory management of bulbar complications of motor neuron disease/amyotrophic lateral sclerosis? Thorax 72 (3), 199–201.

Stolz, D., Leeming, D., Kristensen, J., et al., 2017. Systemic biomarkers of collagen and elastin turnover are associated with clinically relevant outcomes in COPD. Chest 151 (1), 47–59.

Terzi, N., 2007. Breathing-swallowing interaction in neuromuscular patients. Am. J. Respir. Crit. Care Med. 175, 269–276.

Turcios, N.L., 2012. Pulmonary complications of renal disorders. Paediatr. Respir. Rev. 13 (1), 44–49.

Vitacca, M., Vianello, A., 2013. Respiratory outcomes of patients with amyotrophic lateral sclerosis. Respir. Care 58 (9), 1433–1441.

Wallace, B., Vummidi, D., Khanna, D., 2016. Management of connective tissue diseases associated interstitial lung disease: a review of the published literature. Curr. Opin. Rheumatol. 28 (3), 236–245. doi:10.1097/BOR.0000000000000270.

Wan, E.S., DeMeo, D.L., Hersh, C.P., et al., 2012. Clinical predictors of frequent exacerbations in subjects with severe COPD. Respir. Med. 105 (4), 588–594.

Wand, S., Gong, W., Tian, Y., et al., 2016. FEVj/FEVg in primary care is a reliable and easy method for the diagnosis of COPD. Respir. Care 61 (3), 349–353.

Wedzicha, J.A., 2013. Mechanisms and impact of the frequent exacerbator phenotype in chronic obstructive pulmonary disease. BMC Med. 11, 181.

Wilkinson, E., 2016. Respiratory failure guidelines aim to reduce variation in care. Lancet Respir. Med. 4 (5), 352.

Wilt, T.J., 2013. Pharmacologic therapy for primary restless legs syndrome. JAMA Intern. Med. 173 (7), 496–505.

Younossi, Z.M., 2014. Obesity and liver disease. Clin. Liver Dis. 18 (1), xiii–xiv.

Zurek, M., Sladen, L., Johansson, E., et al., 2016. Assessing the relationship between lung density and function with oxygen-enhanced magnetic resonance imaging in a mouse model of emphysema. PLoS ONE 11 (3), e0151211.

# 4

# Cardiovascular Disorders

*Alison Draper, Jo Sharp*

## LEARNING OBJECTIVES

*On completion of this chapter the reader should be able to:*
- identify risk factors for the development of cardiovascular disorders;
- relate the pathological changes to the clinical features of hypertension, coronary heart disease and vascular disease;
- outline the medical management of cardiovascular disorders.

## OUTLINE

## INTRODUCTION

Neighbourly relations between heart and lungs are reflected in their integrated response to each other's disorders, especially when intravascular pressures are raised because they lie in series and are exposed to similar changes in intrathoracic pressure. Some heart and lung conditions also share aetiologies such as smoking and comorbidities such as diabetes and depression (O'Neil et al. 2013). Neurological and mechanical coupling between the two systems helps maintain homeostasis (Dick et al. 2014), but they can also affect each other negatively, e.g. myocardial damage can occur with exacerbations of chronic obstructive pulmonary disease (COPD) (Stone et al. 2013).

This chapter describes the pathophysiology and general management of commonly encountered cardiac and vascular disorders and facilitates clinical reasoning so that problems requiring physiotherapy can be identified. Physiotherapy is by education and exercise and is described in Chapters 10 and 11.

> **KEY POINT**
>
> 'Fast food and slow motion' are the main avoidable contributors to cardiovascular disease.

## HYPERTENSION

> **Systolic pressure**: pressure that the blood exerts on the blood vessels when the ventricles contract, normally 100–140 mmHg.
> **Diastolic pressure**: pressure exerted on the blood vessels when the ventricles relax, normally 60–90 mmHg.
> **Mean arterial blood pressure (MAP)**: cardiac output × peripheral vascular resistance, normally 80–100 mmHg.

**Stroke volume**: volume of blood ejected by the left or right ventricle in one contraction, normally about 70 mL.

**Cardiac output (CO)**: volume of blood pumped by the left ventricle per minute, i.e. stroke volume × heart rate (HR), normally 5 L/min.

**Peripheral vascular resistance (PVR)**: resistance to blood flow in the arteries.

**Systemic hypertension** is a chronic medical condition in which the pressure exerted by the blood on the arteries is elevated to a level that increases the risk of other cardiovascular diseases. Defined as 140/90 mmHg it is the leading cause of cardiovascular disease and death (van Kleef 2017). It is associated with impaired cognition (Piotrowicz et al. 2016) and can cause myocardial infarction (MI), stroke, kidney disease (Gassner 2016) and erectile dysfunction, the latter due to peripheral arterial disease (PAD) or antihypertensive drugs (Chrysant 2015). Over half of people over age 50 have hypertension, with those in higher income countries showing double the rate of those in lower income countries (Yang et al. 2016c).

**Pulmonary hypertension** occurs when the mean pulmonary artery pressure rises above 25 mmHg at rest. It may be idiopathic or caused by heart disease, obstructive or restrictive lung disease (Hoeper et al. 2017), or hypoxic pulmonary vasoconstriction (Craig 2017). The resulting increased workload exerted on the right heart leads to right ventricular hypertrophy and then failure. Symptoms such as dyspnoea, chest pain, fatigue and exercise intolerance (Bellofiore et al. 2017) are nonspecific and diagnosis is often missed, but electrocardiogram (ECG) and cardiac magnetic resonance imaging (MRI) are diagnostic. Medical treatment is with pulmonary vasodilator drugs (p. 460), pulmonary endarterectomy or heart/lung transplant. Exercise training can improve symptoms and function (Chia et al. 2016), including high-intensity interval training (Chia et al. 2017) but requires specific precautions (p. 323).

## Classification of Systemic Hypertension

Most common is **essential** or **primary** hypertension, which has no known cause. **Secondary** hypertension may result from vascular, endocrine or kidney problems (Loftus 2013). If the cause is corrected, blood pressure (BP) usually returns to normal.

Hypertension may also be classified according to its severity (Table 4.1). **Benign** hypertension is asymptomatic but not harmless because any sustained rise in BP carries the risks described above. **Resistant** hypertension is when BP is refractory to medication, occurring in 10%–15% of the hypertensive population (Acelajado et al. 2013). **Malignant** hypertension, also called a hypertensive emergency, occurs rapidly, with diastolic readings around 130 mmHg, causing damage to sensitive organs such as the kidneys (Amraoui et al. 2012) and requiring immediate medication.

## Physiology

The driving force behind blood flow to the tissues is arterial BP, regulated by peripheral vascular resistance (PVR) and cardiac output (CO). Fast-acting neural mechanisms respond to changes in posture and activity (Fig. 4.1A) and slow-acting hormonal mechanisms respond by adjusting fluid balance (Fig. 4.1B). Both mechanisms incorporate a negative feedback loop to maintain stability.

## Pathophysiology of Systemic Hypertension

Loss of elasticity in the large arteries and vasoconstriction of the smaller vessels drive up PVR and BP, with blood viscosity and inflammation playing a part (Schiffrin 2014). The kidneys respond by releasing renin and reducing sodium excretion. The resulting

**TABLE 4.1   Definitions and classification of blood pressure levels (mmHg)**

| Category | Systolic | Diastolic |
|---|---|---|
| Optimal | <120 | <80 |
| Normal | <130 | <85 |
| High-normal | 130–139 | 85–89 |
| Grade 1 hypertension | 140–159 | 90–99 |
| • Subgroup: borderline | 140–149 | 90–94 |
| Grade 2 hypertension | 160–179 | 100–109 |
| Grade 3 hypertension | >180 | >110 |
| Isolated systolic hypertension | >140 | <90 |
| • Subgroup: borderline | 140–149 | <90 |
| When a patient's systolic and diastolic pressures fall into different categories, the higher category applies. | | |

World Health Organization–International Society of Hypertension Guidelines for the Management of Hypertension (1999) *J Hypertension.* 17(2):151–183.

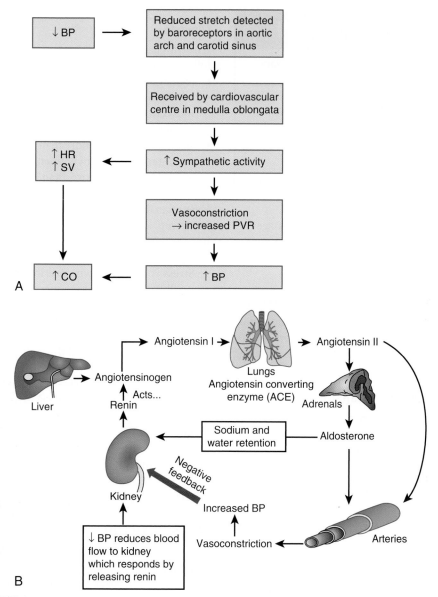

**FIGURE 4.1** (A) Neural mechanism that controls cardiac output and blood pressure *(BP)*. (B) Renal mechanism that regulates BP and circulating volume. Reduced blood volume releases aldosterone, which stimulates the kidneys to retain sodium, which promotes water absorption and expansion of the circulating volume. Aldosterone also causes vasoconstriction. Both these mechanisms increase BP, which is detected by the kidneys, leading to suppression of renin production as part of a negative feedback loop. *CO,* Cardiac output; *HR,* heart rate; *PVR,* peripheral vascular resistance; *SV,* stroke volume.

## TABLE 4.2   Predisposing factors for systemic hypertension

| Risk factors for essential hypertension | Causes of secondary hypertension |
|---|---|
| Genetic predisposition | Kidney disease |
| Obesity | Cushing syndrome |
| High salt or alcohol intake | Adrenal gland tumour |
| Psychogenic stress | Coarctation of the aorta |
| Low birth weight | Corticosteroid medication |
| Sedentary lifestyle | Oral contraceptive pill |

hypertension can thicken arterial walls, damage the kidneys further and contribute to cognitive dysfunction (Scuteri 2016), aided by genes and the environment (Table 4.2).

## Clinical Features of Systemic Hypertension

Some people may experience headaches, dizziness, nose bleeds or visual problems, but hypertension usually causes no symptoms and is usually detected during routine medical examination.

## Tests for Systemic Hypertension

A single high BP reading does not confirm the diagnosis. Systemic BP can be raised for many reasons, particularly in those who become anxious in a clinical environment ('white coat' hypertension). If BP is found to be 140/90 mmHg or higher, National Institute for Health and Care Excellence (NICE) (2011b) recommend two confirmatory tests:
- 24 h ambulatory BP monitoring, with at least two measurements per hour during the day, the average of at least 14 measurements being required;
- self-monitoring with two measurements at least 1 min apart, recorded morning and evening, in sitting, for at least 4 days; measurements on the first day are discarded and an average of the remaining values used.

## Treatment of Systemic Hypertension

### KEY POINT

Education forms the basis of treatment because of the need for lifestyle change, the frequent lack of symptoms, and patients' concerns about drug side effects.

## Lifestyle

Lifestyle changes have been shown to reduce BP and the following are recommended:
- regular aerobic exercise for 30 min on most days;
- weight loss for those with a body mass index >25 and waist circumference >102 cm in men and >88 cm in women;
- alcohol intake at no more than 3 units per day in men and 2 units per day in women;
- salt intake at no more than 6 g a day (Zoccali & Mallamaci 2016).

Vegetarian diets (Yokoyama et al. 2014) and garlic (Ried 2016) are associated with lower BP. Processed meat increases the risk of cardiovascular disease (Lacroix et al. 2017).

**Stress** is a well-known contributor to hypertension, especially in jobs where a person has little control (Kivimäki & Kawachi 2013). Relaxation, yoga (Apor 2016) or acupuncture may be beneficial (Gassner 2017).

Exercise is best provided through a multidisciplinary cardiac rehabilitation programme and is particularly helpful for resistant hypertension (Dimeo et al. 2012).

Head-down postural drainage is contraindicated.

## Drugs

Antihypertensive drugs should be considered alongside lifestyle changes if systolic pressure is persistently at or above 140–160 mmHg, or diastolic pressure at or above 90–100 mmHg (Table 4.3).

## HEART FAILURE

**End-diastolic volume**: volume of blood in the ventricle at the end of filling, just before it contracts, normally 120 mL.
**Ejection fraction**: stroke volume expressed as a percentage of end-diastolic volume, normally >55%.
**Systolic heart failure**: reduced or weakened pumping action of the heart, with ejection fraction <55%.
**Diastolic heart failure**: low compliance of myocardium, but with normal contraction and normal ejection fraction.
**Preload**: degree of stretch applied to the ventricle before contraction.
**Afterload**: load that the ventricle must overcome to eject blood.

**TABLE 4.3   Mechanism of action of the main classes of antihypertensive agents**

| Class | Example | Principal mechanisms of action |
| --- | --- | --- |
| β-Blockers | Atenolol, metoprolol | Reduction in cardiac output; reduction in α-adrenoceptor-mediated arteriolar tone; reduction in β-adrenoceptor-mediated renin release |
| Thiazide diuretics | Bendrofluazide, hydrochlorothiazide, indapamide (thiazide-related) | Promotion of salt and water excretion; direct arteriolar dilation |
| α-Blockers | Doxazosin, prazosin | Reduction in α-adrenoceptor–mediated arteriolar tone |
| ACE inhibitors | Captopril, enalapril, lisinopril perindopril | Blockade of effects of angiotensin on arteriolar tone, and aldosterone on salt and water retention |
| Angiotensin antagonists | Candesartan, irbesartan, losartan, valsartan | As for ACE inhibitors but selectively block the AT1 receptor subtype |
| Calcium channel blockers | Amlodipine, diltiazem, nifedipine, verapamil | Arteriolar dilation |
| Vasodilators | Hydralazine, minoxidil | Arteriolar dilation |
| Central acting | Clonidine, methyldopa, moxonidine | Central sympathetic blockade |

Brown et al. 2000.

If the heart cannot pump all the blood returned to it, it is said to have failed. It is either unable to meet the needs of the body, or can do so only with elevated atrial filling pressures.

**Acute** heart failure (HF) is sudden and severe and requires urgent medical treatment to restore CO. **Chronic** HF occurs gradually and is offset at first by compensatory mechanisms to maintain tissue perfusion, but eventually cardiac function declines and symptoms develop.

The incidence of chronic HF doubles with each decade of life (Strait 2013) and is present in 10% of individuals by age 70 (Currie et al. 2015). It is the leading cause of hospitalization in the elderly population (Ozierański 2015) and 50% of patients die within 5 years of diagnosis (Springer et al. 2013).

## Causes

HF may be instigated by cardiovascular disease (ESC 2016) or, in 30% of patients, by COPD. One or both ventricles are subject to excess workload due to one or more of the following:
- impaired contractility of the myocardium, e.g. acute coronary syndromes;
- increased afterload, e.g. hypertension or aortic valve stenosis;
- increased preload, e.g. mitral or aortic valve regurgitation.

Other risk factors are obesity, type II diabetes, atrial fibrillation (Aisu et al. 2017), kidney disease (ESC 2016),

social deprivation (Verma et al. 2017) and a surfeit of red meat (Wolk 2017).

## Classification
### Left ventricular failure

Left ventricular failure (LVF) is the most common form of HF, gradually pushing up pressure in the left atrium and pulmonary vascular system. The resulting pulmonary hypertension forces fluid into the alveoli, creating pulmonary oedema. The failing heart triggers compensatory mechanisms:
- Fast-acting neural systems increase sympathetic activity, raising HR and myocardial contractility (Fig. 4.1A).
- The slower response of the rennin–angiotensin mechanism (Fig. 4.1B) promotes the retention of sodium and water by the kidney, increasing preload and encouraging the myocardium to contract.

These raise the workload of the left ventricle further because angiotensin is an arterial vasoconstrictor and increases afterload. Other factors that increase the workload of the left heart are increased volume load, as in aortic valve regurgitation, or increased resistance to blood flow, as with systemic hypertension.

### Right ventricular failure

Right ventricular failure (RVF) occurs secondary to COPD (p. 74) or other causes of pulmonary hypertension such as interstitial lung disease or mitral valve disease. It is usually irreversible unless the ventricle is unloaded, e.g. by lung transplant for pulmonary hypertension.

Enlargement of the right ventricle that has resulted from lung disease is known as **cor pulmonale**, caused by hypoxic vasoconstriction and pulmonary hypertension.

### Congestive cardiac failure

Congestive cardiac failure (CCF) refers to combined LVF and RVF, with congestion in the pulmonary and systemic circulations.

## Pathophysiology

In LVF, the left ventricular myocardium hypertrophies in response to increased load. The greater size and number of myocytes raises myocardial oxygen demand and increases the diffusion distance for oxygen. Some muscle fibres become ischaemic, leading to patchy fibrosis, stiffness and reduced contractility. The workload may cause the ventricle to stretch and dilate (Fig. 4.2), leading to further force being required to maintain CO. Systolic failure is by reduced ejection fraction, and

diastolic failure is by reduced end-diastolic volume. Metabolic effects include loss of bone tissue, skeletal muscle and fat (Loncar et al. 2013).

Stiffness and reduced contractility raise end-diastolic pressure, which is transmitted back along the pulmonary veins to the pulmonary capillaries, from which fluid is forced into the interstitial spaces and, if severe, into the alveoli, causing pulmonary oedema. The increased pulmonary vascular pressure raises the afterload of the right ventricle, in the same way as chronic systemic hypertension raises the afterload of the left ventricle. Hypertrophy, patchy fibrosis, stiffness and reduced contractility of the right ventricular myocardium then ensue, as with the left ventricle, and congestive cardiac failure develops.

## Clinical Features

HF can progress over decades. The main symptom is **shortness of breath** (SOB) due to pulmonary oedema, first on exertion or bending down (Thibodeau 2017) and then at rest. This combines with **fatigue** and **muscle weakness** to cause **exercise limitation** (Brandão et al.

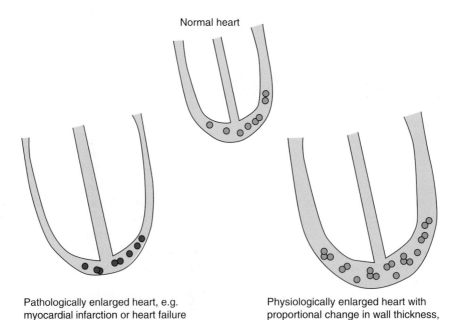

Normal heart

Pathologically enlarged heart, e.g. myocardial infarction or heart failure (myocyte death with fibrotic replacement)

Physiologically enlarged heart with proportional change in wall thickness, e.g. endurance exercise training

**FIGURE 4.2** Representation of normal heart, the pathologically enlarged heart of heart failure, and physiologically healthy exercise-induced cardiac growth. (Adapted from Wilson et al. 2015.)

2012), which is worsened by a 'complex dance' with anaemia, which itself increases mortality (Cleland 2016). These symptoms are often dismissed by the patient and medical staff as 'normal ageing' and it may fall to the physiotherapist to raise concerns so that a diagnosis can be made.

Cerebral oxygen deprivation leads to **cognitive impairment** in about half of patients (Currie et al. 2015), worsened by **insomnia** in 50%–60% of patients (Johansson et al. 2015), which itself is worsened by sleep apnoea, depression and a 49% incidence of incontinence (Hwang et al. 2013). Irritation of lung parenchyma causes a **cough**, and some patients manifest a complex **pain** pattern (Light et al. 2013). Functional limitations at different levels of severity are in Table 4.4.

Objective signs include **peripheral oedema** caused by venous congestion.

### Pulmonary oedema

Pulmonary oedema is extravascular water in the lungs caused by back pressure from a failing left heart. The main symptom is SOB, distinguished by **orthopnoea** and **paroxysmal nocturnal dyspnoea** (p. 34).

Interstitial pulmonary oedema barely affects lung function, but once the lymphatics become overloaded, fluid squeezes into alveoli, causing alveolar oedema, a widened $PAO_2$–$PaO_2$ gradient and hypoxaemia. If alveolar fluid moves into the airway, it mixes with air and may be coughed up as white **frothy secretions**, becoming pink if blood is also squeezed out.

Radiology shows an enlarged heart, with bilateral fleecy opacities spreading from the hila due to perivascular fluid, and sometimes diversion of vessels to the upper lobes to match perfusion to the better ventilated, less compressed, upper lung (Fig. 4.3). Fine crackles on auscultation may be heard over the lung bases, caused by the popping open of alveoli compressed by peribronchial oedema. Similar crackles can also be heard in immobile elderly people without HF when they take a deep breath and their closed alveoli pop open.

Noncardiogenic pulmonary oedema, distinguished by a normal-sized heart on X-ray, can be caused by fluid overload, systemic vasoconstriction, oncotic pressure changes (due to cirrhosis, malnutrition or nephrotic syndrome) or increased capillary permeability due to toxins or inflammatory damage.

### Tests

Diagnosis can be challenging and the condition is missed in up to 50% of patients (Hancock et al. 2013). A blood test identifies raised levels of a biomarker

| Class | Symptoms |
|---|---|
| I | No limitation of physical activity. Ordinary physical activity does not cause undue fatigue, palpitation, or dyspnoea. |
| II | Slight limitation of physical activity. Comfortable at rest, but ordinary physical activity results in fatigue, palpitation, or dyspnoea. |
| III | Marked limitation of physical activity. Comfortable at rest, but less than ordinary activity causes fatigue, palpitation, or dyspnoea. |
| IV | Unable to carry out any physical activity without discomfort. Symptoms of cardiac insufficiency at rest. If any physical activity is undertaken, discomfort is increased. |

**TABLE 4.4  Heart failure functional classification**

New York Heart Association.

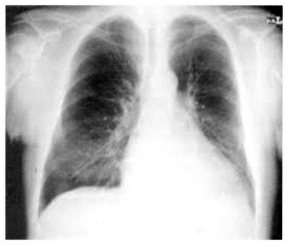

**FIGURE 4.3** X-ray showing the enlarged heart, hilar flare and upper lobe diversion of heart failure. (Courtesy Dr Claude Pierre-Jerome.)

secreted by the ventricles in response to excessive stretch, and an echocardiogram confirms the diagnosis by showing altered size, structure or function of the heart. Other tests include CO recovery after exercise (Myers et al. 2011). Cognitive screening is recommended (Alosco et al. 2013).

## Management

Patients with chronic disease should be under the care of a multidisciplinary HF team (Agvall et al. 2013). Education is best incorporated into a rehabilitation programme (Chapters 9 and 11) and helps clarify terminology and navigate patients through the maze of drug, salt and fluid management. Home management and remote monitoring suit some patients (Evangelista et al. 2015) and social support can reduce hospitalization, mortality, anxiety and depression (Årestedt et al. 2013).

---

**KEY POINT**

Drug management is based on a 'start low, go slow' principle.

---

Angiotensin-converting enzyme (ACE) inhibitors impede the conversion of angiotensin I to angiotensin II, and β-blockers reduce HR (Böhm & Reil 2013). Both drugs are uptitrated gradually over several weeks, balancing their beneficial effects on BP and HR with side effects such as cough, dizziness, hypotension or bradycardia.

Diuretics increase urine excretion and are considered if there is SOB or oedema. They are potent and non-selective, and overenthusiastic use can lead to dizziness on standing, and loss of calcium and potassium (Wile 2016). Distressing side effects are thirst and an urgent need to pass urine. De Vecchis et al. (2016) suggest that fluid restriction may not be necessary, and the tablets can be taken at a time to minimize the need to pass urine, e.g. at night or before going out. Patients are often tempted to restrict fluid intake further if they have urinary incontinence or poor mobility. Some diuretics can cause metabolic acidosis, and caution is advised for patients with comorbid COPD.

Anticoagulants such as warfarin reduce the risk of thromboembolism, stroke and myocardial infarct (Hopper et al. 2013). Opioids for SOB can be administered safely (Oxberry 2013).

Implanted devices include biventricular pacemakers, defibrillators and left ventricular assist devices, followed by rehabilitation (English & Speed 2013). Some patients benefit from revascularization. Transplantation may be considered if there are severe refractory symptoms or cardiogenic shock.

Patients with acute disease do not need to restrict their sodium and water intake (Aliti et al. 2013). They require assessment for risk before discharge (Stiell et al. 2013). Multidisciplinary palliative care should be initiated early (Smith 2013).

## CORONARY HEART DISEASE

Coronary heart disease (CHD), also called coronary artery disease, has a prevalence similar to chronic lung disease (Enriquez 2013) and along with vascular disease it is the leading cause of death globally (Coffeng et al. 2017), with over half of patients being virtually asymptomatic until the first fatal presentation (Yang & Vargas 2012).

### Causes

Contributors to CHD are hypertension, obesity, smoking, excess alcohol consumption, high intake of salt or sugar (Shi et al. 2016), air pollution (Hartiala et al. 2016), marijuana use (Franz 2016), sleep disturbance (Liu et al. 2016b), inactivity (Ding et al. 2016) and red meat consumption (Wong et al. 2013). Other predisposing factors are COPD (Rothnie et al. 2016b), rheumatoid arthritis (Sen 2014), shift work (Alefishat & Abu 2015) and early life stress such as maternal separation (Loria et al. 2014). The contribution of stress in adult life is thought to relate to increased amygdala activity (Tawakol 2017). An outburst of anger can double the chance of triggering a myocardial infarct (Mostofsky 2013).

### Pathophysiology

#### Atherosclerosis

Atherosclerosis underpins CV disease but takes decades to produce symptoms (Coffeng et al. 2017). Fatty streaks may form early in life but only become significant if they develop into atheromatous plaques. Plaques tend to develop where arteries branch because there is more stress on the vessel wall. Injured endothelium allows low density lipoprotein (LDL or 'bad cholesterol') to enter the vessel wall, where it is oxidized and attracts white blood cells, which differentiate into macrophages. These ingest the LDL and become part of the atheromatous plaque. Inflammatory mediators released by the macrophages stimulate smooth muscle cells in the artery wall to migrate towards the damaged tunica intima. Here they multiply and synthesize collagen, forming a fibrous cap on the arterial wall. This projects into the lumen of the artery and obstructs blood flow. Even at this stage, maintaining cardiovascular fitness by regular exercise helps to reduce LDL (Yoshikawa et al. 2013).

The innate antithrombotic effects of normal vascular endothelium are disabled by atherosclerotic plaques. The damaged artery wall attracts platelets and triggers the formation of thrombi (blood clots). A small thrombus, or any material which leaks from the plaque, can be carried in the bloodstream as an embolus and block smaller vessels downstream, resulting in ischaemia of the tissues supplied by the artery.

## Myocardial ischaemia

Much coronary blood flow occurs during ventricular diastole (relaxation), because the deep coronary arteries are compressed during systole. When exercising, increased HR raises myocardial oxygen demand while shortening diastole, leaving less time for myocardial perfusion. To meet the shortfall, the coronary arteries dilate in response to metabolites. In CHD, oxidized LDL molecules in atherosclerotic coronary arteries inhibit this vasodilation so that on exercise or under stress, areas of myocardium may be deprived of oxygen.

## Myocardial infarction

Severe or prolonged ischaemia leads to tissue death or infarction. MI is caused by blockage of blood flow through a coronary artery, usually caused by a thrombus in an artery narrowed by atherosclerosis, i.e. coronary thrombosis.

## Classification and Clinical Features
### Stable angina

Myocardial ischaemia leads to the crushing chest pain of angina pectoris. This is due to anaerobic respiration in ischaemic tissue, which releases chemicals such as adenosine and lactic acid, sometimes worsened by vasospasm. It may be brought on by exertion, cold weather, stress or even eating, and can radiate to the neck, jaw and arms. Patients may describe the sensation as tightness or pressure rather than pain, sometimes using a clenched fist to help them explain. It resolves on rest.

### Acute coronary syndrome

Acute coronary syndrome (ACS) is triggered by rupture or erosion of an atherosclerotic plaque, leading to activation of the coagulation cascade and formation of a platelet–fibrin thrombus, which can grow rapidly and obstruct coronary blood flow, causing myocardial ischaemia or infarction. Chest pain that occurs at rest and is more severe and long-lasting than stable angina indicates ACS. It may radiate from the chest but is not relieved by rest or medication. ACS is classified as follows:

- **Unstable angina**, caused by coronary occlusion but not associated with infarction; this is temporary but can progress to MI. Any new onset angina is considered unstable in the first few weeks since it suggests a new problem in a coronary artery.
- **Non-ST-segment elevation MI** (NSTEMI), relating to the ECG trace and caused by coronary occlusion sufficient to affect the innermost layers of the heart wall (NICE 2013b).
- **ST-segment elevation MI** (STEMI), resulting from coronary occlusion, which causes full thickness cardiac necrosis.

In addition to chest pain, MI can cause dyspnoea, pallor, lightheadedness, nausea, sweating and sometimes loss of consciousness. Elderly people may present more subtly with fatigue, nausea, sweating or syncope. A 'silent MI' causes no symptoms and is only picked up if the patient has an ECG. Arenja et al. (2013) found that one in four people with suspected CHD had already had a silent MI.

Complications include stroke, and arrhythmias such as atrial fibrillation. Fatalities occur if a large proportion of muscle is damaged or if severe arrhythmias are triggered. Patients without hypoxaemia should not be given oxygen because it can cause coronary vasoconstriction (Decalmer & O'Driscoll 2013).

### Tests

Acute chest pain requires a 12-lead resting ECG. Chest pain provoked by exercise requires an exercise ECG. In neither case does a normal ECG exclude ACS. A blood test can pick up biomarkers such as troponin, released by damaged myocardium within hours. This lingers for 1–2 weeks and helps to detect ACS, evaluate its severity and distinguish MI from angina. Computed tomography coronary angiography identifies patients likely to benefit from revascularization, and other imaging techniques can detect subclinical atherosclerosis (Yang & Vargas 2012).

## Prevention and Treatment

Before any CV signs are evident, recommendations are for regular exercise, smoking cessation and a Mediterranean diet (Shi et al. 2016). Exercise training and drug management are considered superior to surgery for stable disease (Uhlemann et al. 2012) and appear to mitigate disease progression (Boden 2013). Major depressive disorder is present in approximately 20% of patients (Thombs 2013) and should be treated because it increases mortality (Stenman et al. 2013). Over half of patients hospitalized for CHD also have musculoskeletal problems, which place them at greater cardiovascular risk, so these will need attention (Marzolini et al. 2012).

### Drugs

Aspirin and statins are used for primary and secondary prevention (Qato et al. 2016). The statins bring a bonus of reducing COPD exacerbations (Wang et al. 2013b) but also the risk of peripheral neuropathy (Novak et al. 2015). Stable angina is usually managed with nitrates. If ACS occurs, antiplatelets or anticoagulants to reperfuse the myocardium are required, usually within hours, along with measures to prevent the risk of bleeding. β-Blockers benefit patients with acute coronary syndrome (Allen et al. 2017), but if these are not tolerated, calcium channel blockers may be given (Pascual et al. 2016).

### Angioplasty

Coronary angioplasty, or percutaneous coronary intervention, involves the passage of a catheter, using a femoral or radial approach, into the blocked vessel, where a balloon at its tip inflates to crush the atheroma. A stent is usually left in place to keep it open (Fig. 4.4). Patients then lie flat for several hours to prevent bleeding, and after a period of observation are discharged with minimal activity restrictions. The procedure has shown better clinical outcomes than thrombolytic drugs and a lower risk of stroke than bypass grafting (Kappetein et al. 2016).

### Surgery

Coronary artery bypass grafting (p. 317) is used for multivessel disease or after failed angioplasty. A hybrid

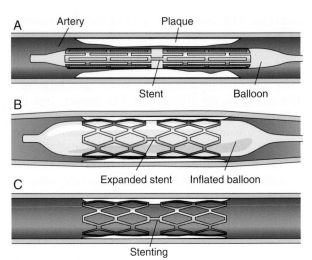

**FIGURE 4.4** Angioplasty, showing (A) placement of deflated balloon, (B) balloon inflation and (C) stent in place after removal of balloon.

technique combines surgery and angioplasty (Hong et al. 2016).

## ARRHYTHMIAS

An abnormal HR or irregular rhythm is due to a change in electrical conduction. Arrhythmias may be short-lived or long-lasting, permanent or reversible, harmless or life-threatening. The type of arrhythmia is dependent on the origin of the defect, e.g. sinoatrial node fault, disruption of the normal atrial or ventricular conducting pathway, or another part of the myocardium taking over as pacemaker.

The effect on CO or BP is key to determining its significance. Trends are also important, a constantly changing HR or rhythm creating its own risk.

### Tests

The body's high water content makes it a good electrical conductor, allowing electrodes on the skin to detect electrical potentials generated by the heart. A 12-lead ECG produces a waveform that has five main components (Fig. 4.5). Each component represents the electrical activity during a specific phase of the cardiac cycle:

- The P wave represents atrial depolarization, leading to atrial contraction.
- The PR interval represents the time taken for the impulse to travel from the sinoatrial node (the

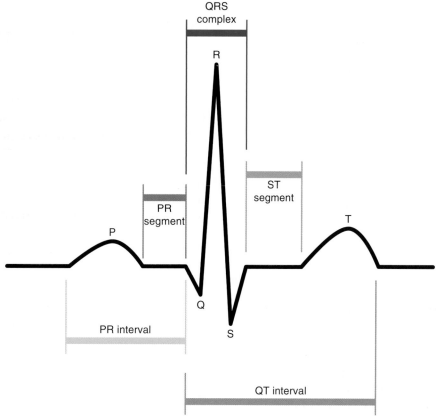

**FIGURE 4.5** Components of a normal electrocardiogram trace.

onset of atrial depolarization) through the atrio-ventricular (AV) node and into the ventricles (the onset of ventricular depolarization).

- The QRS complex represents depolarization of the ventricles, causing ventricular contraction.
- The ST segment represents the interval between ventricular depolarization and repolarization.
- The T wave represents ventricular repolarization in preparation for next cycle.

## Clinical Implications of Arrhythmias

Arrhythmias may affect CO if the ventricular rate is low or the stroke volume is decreased due to reduced ventricular filling time or ineffective ventricular contraction. Arrhythmias that reduce CO cause hypotension, dizziness and syncope (Fu 2015), contraindicating exercise.

Arrhythmias that produce a variable stroke volume such as atrial fibrillation (AF) do not accurately reflect the actual HR, i.e. there is a pulse deficit, so measurement of the radial pulse is inaccurate. The larger the difference between the radial pulse and apex beat, the less inefficient are cardiac contractions.

The role of the autonomic nervous system in controlling HR means that stimulation of the vagus nerve results in a drop in HR. This principle is used in the Valsalva manoeuvre (Smith et al. 2015) and in carotid sinus massage (Collins and Higgins 2015) to assess and treat some types of tachycardia. Endotracheal suctioning may also reduce HR, which may be due to this mechanism.

The most common sustained arrhythmia is AF, which increases with age. Poor ventricular filling in AF and atrial flutter is associated with pooling of blood in the atria, risking thrombus formation, embolism and a 5-fold increase in stroke (Martin et al. 2017). Preventive anticoagulation therapy may be required. Patients on the antiarrhythmia drug amiodarone should be regularly monitored because adverse effects occur in 75% of patients, including pulmonary toxicity (Vigário & Mendonça 2016). Yoga may reduce BP and HR (Wahlström et al. 2016).

If a cardiac device such as a pacemaker is implanted, transcutaneous electrical nerve stimulation, diathermy and interferential electrical current are best avoided, but laser therapy, traction and ultrasound do not appear to present a risk (Digby et al. 2009).

## PERIPHERAL ARTERIAL DISEASE

PAD, sometimes called peripheral vascular disease, is due to atherosclerosis of any arteries other than the coronary arteries, but most usually affects those of the lower limbs. PAD may or may not be symptomatic, but about 20% of the UK population aged over 60 have evidence of the disease (NICE 2012b). It is not directly life-threatening but treatment helps reduce the risk of secondary events such as MI or stroke (Muller et al. 2013).

### Causes

In common with CHD, predisposing factors include smoking, obesity, hypertension, diabetes (Newman et al. 2017) and depression (Columbo et al. 2016).

### Clinical Features

Intermittent claudication, a fiendish cramplike calf pain caused by ischaemia, occurs in 10%–15% of patients, set off by walking and ceasing on rest. It may also occur in the buttock, thigh or arch of the foot, depending on the location of the blockage (Muller et al. 2013). Pain at rest (Table 4.5) indicates progression of the disease towards critical ischaemia. Repeated ischaemic episodes damage the muscles and nerves (McDermott 2015).

Objective examination may reveal cool skin, altered skin colour, loss of hair and poor toe nail growth.

### Tests

A comprehensive history is needed to exclude musculoskeletal causes of leg pain. Good foot pulses are insufficient to exclude PAD, and a specialist clinic is required to compare systolic pressures in the upper and lower limbs (Koch et al. 2016b), apply walking tests and questionnaires, and sometimes administer a heel rise test (Monteiro et al. 2013) or assess calf oxygenation (Miranda et al. 2012).

To accurately localize the narrowed segments, noninvasive imaging such as ultrasound, magnetic resonance angiography or computed tomography angiography may be used (Oda et al. 2016b). The abdomen is also palpated to check for a pulsatile abdominal mass that could indicate an aortic aneurysm.

### Treatment

> **KEY POINT**
>
> The principles of management are stopping smoking and keeping moving.

Limb ischaemia and cardiovascular complications can be reduced by controlling smoking, BP, cholesterol, blood sugar and weight (Hussain et al. 2016a) and the

| TABLE 4.5 | Classification of peripheral arterial disease | | | | |
|---|---|---|---|---|---|
| **FONTAINE** | | **RUTHERFORD** | | | |
| **Stage** | **Symptoms** | **Grade** | **Category** | **Symptoms** | |
| I | Asymptomatic | 0 | 0 | Asymptomatic | |
| IIa | Mild claudication | I | 1 | Mild claudication | |
| IIb | Moderate to severe claudication | I | 2 | Moderate claudication | |
| | | | 3 | Severe claudication | |
| III | Ischaemic rest pain | II | 4 | Ischaemic rest pain | |
| IV | Ulceration or gangrene | III | 5 | Minor tissue loss | |
| | | | 6 | Major tissue loss | |

Norgren L., Hiatt W.R., Dormandy J.A., et al., 2007. Inter-society consensus for the management of peripheral arterial disease (TASC II). Eur. J. Vasc. Endovasc. Surg. 33 (suppl 1), 51–570.

sleep apnoea from which 85% of patients suffer (Utriainen et al. 2013). Drugs include statins, antiplatelets and ACE inhibitors or angiotensin receptor blockers (Montminy et al. 2016).

Revascularization is by localized angioplasty and/or bypass grafting (Grandjean et al. 2016). Patients who have had an aortofemoral graft should avoid hip flexion on the affected side for 3 days. They may get up before they are allowed to sit, and can start gentle mobilization 2–3 days postoperatively, depending on graft patency and the surgeon's instructions. Spinal cord stimulation may beneficial for late-stage disease (De Caridi et al. 2016) but if critical limb ischaemia has developed, amputation of the affected limb is required.

# ANEURYSMS

An aneurysm is a permanently dilated section of a blood vessel to more than 150% of its normal diameter (Lavall et al. 2012), occurring most commonly in a cerebral artery or the aorta and often associated with hypertension (Takagi & Umemoto 2016) and other risk factors (Table 4.6).

## Causes

Weakness of elastin and collagen fibres in the vessel wall predispose to an aneurysm. Atherosclerosis is usually the culprit, with connective tissue disorders also posing a risk because of loss of elastic and muscle fibres. Once formed, aneurysms progressively enlarge and the diameter is a strong predictor of rupture, which brings high mortality.

## TABLE 4.6  Risk factors for thoracic and abdominal aortic aneurysms

| Thoracic | Abdominal |
|---|---|
| Marfan syndrome | Smoking |
| Bicuspid aortic valve | Age |
| Syphilis | Hypertension |
| Tuberculosis | High cholesterol |
| Genetic/familial history | Male gender |
| Atherosclerosis (descending aorta) | Atherosclerosis |
| Trauma | Family history |

Adapted from Isselbacher 2005.

## Clinical Features

An intact aortic aneurysm is often asymptomatic and the first indication of its presence may be when it ruptures. Occasionally patients develop pain in the chest, abdomen, or, of interest to musculoskeletal physiotherapists, the back. Aneurysm of the ascending aorta may cause aortic valve regurgitation which can progress to congestive cardiac failure.

## Complications

Thrombus formation inside the aneurysm is common and may be a source of emboli. Aortic dissection occurs if the aortic layers separate longitudinally, progressing within the vessel wall in either direction, leading to pain, ischaemia and sometimes rupture. A ruptured aortic aneurysm presents with severe chest or abdominal pain, hypotension and tachycardia, for which urgent surgery or endovascular stent graft is required. Comorbid COPD increases the risk of rupture (Takagi & Umemoto 2017).

## Tests

Ultrasound screening may be offered to people at risk (Morioka et al. 2016). Thoracic aneurysms might be detected on a chest X-ray, but most aneurysms require specialized imaging (Apostolakis et al. 2016). Risk scores and diagnostic algorithms are available for early detection of dissection (Suzuki et al. 2013).

## Treatment

Patients with a known aneurysm are advised on the management of risk factors, and antihypertensive medication and statins may be prescribed. Moderate physical activity is thought to reduce progression of atherosclerosis-related aneurysms (Lavall et al. 2012) and is considered safe if the aneurysm is <5 cm in diameter (Myers et al. 2011). Regular ultrasound screening monitors its growth.

Once over 5.5 cm, elective surgical repair is considered because the likelihood of rupture begins to overtake the risks of surgery. Laparoscopy is possible, but open procedures are more common. Elective repair has an operative mortality of 1%–5%, which contrasts with the 80% mortality associated with the emergency surgery that is required for a rupture (Gawenda 2012).

Aortic aneurysm is a contraindication for head-down postural drainage.

# THROMBOEMBOLISM

Thrombosis is the development of a clot in the vascular system. Embolism occurs if the clot breaks away and is swept off in the blood stream.

## Thrombosis

Arterial thrombosis is most commonly associated with atherosclerosis. Venous thrombosis is usually caused by Virchow triad: slow blood flow, damaged or abnormal vessel walls and altered blood chemistry. The veins of the legs are the most common site of deep vein thrombosis (DVT), which may present as pain, tenderness, swelling, redness, warmth and sometimes pain on dorsiflexion (Homan's sign), any of which must be reported. Diagnosis is by tomography and ultrasound (Viana et al. 2017). Predisposing factors include surgery, cancer, obesity (Liew et al. 2016) and mechanical ventilation, especially in patients with central lines or on vasoconstrictor drugs (Minet et al. 2015).

Prevention of DVT is by adequate hydration, avoidance of immobility including prolonged sitting (Howard et al. 2013) and anticoagulants if there is no bleeding risk. Thromboembolus deterrent (TED) stockings promote blood flow from superficial to deep veins, so long as there is no PAD, neuropathy, leg oedema or skin disorder. They apply graduated compression that is greater in the lower calf and diminishes up the leg, and must be individually measured, fitted and monitored (Macintyre et al. 2013). The physiotherapist's main task is to advise patients or their family to smooth out the omnipresent tourniquet-like wrinkles in TED stockings, which reduce blood flow and can themselves cause thrombosis (Byrne 2001). Better still are pneumatic compression devices (Liew et al. 2016).

## Pulmonary Embolism

A fragment of thrombus may escape to form an embolus which is carried in the circulation until it becomes lodged in a smaller vessel. The natural resting place of an embolus which has originated from a DVT is a pulmonary arteriole. The relationship between DVT and pulmonary embolism. (PE) has given rise to the term venous thromboembolism, which is the most common preventable cause of hospital death (Yasui et al. 2017), bringing a mortality of 10%–30% within a month (Hillegass et al. 2016).

PE is a blockage in the pulmonary vasculature, usually by a blood clot. It is the third most common cardiovascular disorder after CHD and stroke, may cause chronic pulmonary hypertension and is the leading preventable cause of death in hospital patients (Franchini 2016). It is commonly not diagnosed or suspected until after the patient dies, and close to 40% of patients with a DVT have an asymptomatic PE (Berman 2003). Death occurs if the clot leads to pulmonary hypertension severe enough to cause unmanageable right ventricular afterload and right HF (Tapson 2012).

Suspicions are raised if a patient complains of dyspnoea and a sharp localized pleuritic pain, occasionally complicated by haemoptysis. Pallor may be apparent, peripheral arterial oxygen saturation ($SpO_2$) is usually reduced and a pleural rub can sometimes be heard on auscultation. Diagnosis is by specialist magnetic resonance pulmonary angiography (Hu et al. 2016).

Prevention is by avoidance of DVT or implantation of a filter in the inferior vena cava in high-risk individuals. Immediate management of PE is by giving oxygen and placing the patient supine, which boosts venous return to the left heart, which has been deprived of pulmonary artery flow. Treatment is by thrombolytic therapy to dissolve the clot, followed by heparin. If there is a reversible risk factor, treatment is continued for 3 months, but with active cancer or a second unprovoked PE, treatment is indefinite (Lapner 2013). Embolectomy may be needed for a PE that is chronic (Polastri 2013) or massive (Mazur et al. 2013).

Mobilization is considered safe when therapeutic threshold levels of anticoagulants have been reached (24–48 h for heparin, 2–5 h for other drugs) (Hillegass et al. 2016).

## CASE STUDY: MS GF

*Consider the management of this 87-year-old patient from Muscat admitted with a chest infection and deteriorating mobility.*

### Background

- Lives alone
- Independently mobile prior to admission
- No relevant medical history

### Nurse report

- Patient needs assistance to mobilize

## Subjective

- Pain in right leg

## Objective

- Calf swollen and hot
- Doppler ultrasound confirms DVT

Started on subcutaneous heparin and TED stockings

## Questions

1. What is the most likely cause of DVT in this case?
2. Will mobilizing increase the likelihood of a PE?
3. Would bed rest prevent a PE?
4. Would bed rest or ambulation be more effective in reducing pain and swelling?
5. Goals?
6. Plan?

---

### CLINICAL REASONING

*Postoperative noninvasive ventilation (NIV) was extolled in a study in which the active NIV group received 50% oxygen but the control group (without NIV) received unspecified oxygen using a 'venturi mask at an adjusted oxygen flow of 6 L/min'.*

*BMC Anesthesiol* (2011) 11, 10

---

## Response to Case Study

1. Immobility.
2. Early ambulation, combined with compression and anticoagulants, does not significantly increase the incidence of new PE with uncomplicated acute DVT (Pashikanti & Von 2012, Galanaud & Kahn 2013, Clark et al. 2013, Vali et al. 2015).
3. Prescribing bed rest for patients with acute DVT does not reduce their risk of developing a new PE (Trujillo-Santos et al. 2005).
4. Pain and oedema resolve faster in patients treated with early ambulation and compression than those 'treated' with bed rest (Partsch et al. 2004).
5.
   - Relief of pain and swelling
   - Independent mobility and ADL
6.
   - Education on hydration and exercise
   - Liaise with nursing staff rehydration and mobility
   - Provide exercise tick chart and stretchy bands

- Mobilize frequently, with mobility aid at first if required
- Encourage getting dressed in the daytime
- Liaise with occupational therapist and domiciliary team

---

### RESPONSE TO CLINICAL REASONING

*For the control group, there is no explanation of what the oxygen was adjusted for, and what was adjusted.*

*BMC Anesthesiol* (2011) 11, 10

---

## RECOMMENDED READING

Al-Ansary, L.A., Tricco, A.C., Adi, Y., et al., 2013. A systematic review of recent clinical practice guidelines on the diagnosis, assessment and management of hypertension. PLoS ONE 8 (1), e53744.

Alastalo, H., 2012. Cardiovascular morbidity and mortality in Finnish men and women separated temporarily from their parents in childhood. Psychosom. Med. 74, 583–587.

Becattini, C., Cohen, A.T., Agnelli, G., et al., 2016. Risk stratification of patients with acute symptomatic pulmonary embolism based on presence or absence of lower extremity DVT: systematic review and meta-analysis. Chest 149 (1), 192–200.

Berardi, C., 2013. Heart failure performance measures: eligibility and implementation in the community. Am. Heart J. 166 (1), 76–82.

Bergh, C., Udumyan, R., Fall, K., et al., 2015. Stress resilience and physical fitness in adolescence and risk of coronary heart disease in middle age. Heart 101 (8), 623–629.

Blazek, A., 2013. Exercise-mediated changes in high-density lipoprotein. Am. Heart J. 166 (3), 392–400.

Brusselle, G., Bracke, K., Pauw, M., 2017. Peripheral artery disease in patients with chronic obstructive pulmonary disease. Am. J. Respir. Crit. Care Med. 195 (2), 148–150.

Buber, J., Rhodes, J., 2014. Exercise physiology and testing in adult patients with congenital heart disease. Heart Fail. Clin. 10 (1), 23–33.

Burg, M.M., Soufer, R., 2016. Post-traumatic stress disorder and cardiovascular disease. Curr. Cardiol. Rep. 18 (10), 94.

Chase, S.C., Wheatley, C.M., Olson, L.J., et al., 2016. Impact of chronic systolic heart failure on lung structure–function relationships in large airways. Physiol. Rep. 4 (13), e12867.

Chesbro, S.B., 2013. Reliability of ankle-brachial index measurements. Top. Geriatr. Rehabil. 29 (3), 195–202.

Curtis, A.B., 2013. Practice implications of the Atrial Fibrillation Guidelines. Am. J. Cardiol. 111 (11), 1660–1670.

Davies, G., Aurora, P., 2017. The use of multiple breath washout for assessing cystic fibrosis in infants. Expert. Rev. Respir. Med. 11 (1), 21–28.

Ellulu, M.S., 2016. Atherosclerotic cardiovascular disease: a review of initiators and protective factors. Inflammopharmacology 24 (1), 1–10.

ESC, 2016. European Society of Cardiology Guidelines for the diagnosis and treatment of acute and chronic heart failure. Eur. J. Heart Fail. 18 (8), 891–975.

Felhendler, D., Lisander, B., 1999. Effects of non-invasive stimulation of acupoints on the cardiovascular system. Complement. Ther. Med. 7, 231–234.

Forslund, A.S., 2013. Risk factors among people surviving out-of-hospital cardiac arrest and their thoughts about what lifestyle means to them. BMC Cardiovasc. Disord. 13, 62.

Heit, J.A., Spencer, F.A., White, R.H., 2016. The epidemiology of venous thromboembolism. J. Thromb. Thrombolysis 41 (1), 3–14.

Hornik, C., Meliones, J., 2016. Pulmonary edema and hypoxic respiratory failure. Pediatr. Crit. Care Med. 17 (8 Suppl. 1), S178–S181.

Karapanagiotis, S., 2017. Ventilatory limitation and dynamic hyperinflation during exercise testing in cystic fibrosis. Pediatr. Pulmonol. 52 (1), 29–33.

Kitchen, L., 2016. Emergency department management of suspected calf-vein deep venous thrombosis. West. J. Emerg. Med. 17 (4), 384–390.

Koelsch, S., Jäncke, L., 2015. Music and the heart. Eur. Heart J. 36 (44), 3043–3049.

Lucchetti, G., 2013. Rare medical conditions and suggestive past-life memories. Explore (N.Y.) 9 (6), 372–376.

Miller, N.H., 2012. Adherence behavior in the prevention and treatment of cardiovascular disease. J. Cardiopulm. Rehabil. Prev. 32 (2), 63–70.

Monroe, V.D., 2013. Blood pressure lability. Crit. Care. Nurs. Q. 36 (4), 425–432.

Ndanuko, R.N., Tapsell, L.C., Charlton, K.E., et al., 2016. Dietary patterns and blood pressure in adults. Adv. Nutr. 7 (1), 76–89.

Nedeljkovic, I., 2016. The combined exercise stress echocardiography and cardiopulmonary exercise test for identification of masked heart failure with preserved ejection fraction in patients with hypertension. Eur. J. Prev. Cardiol. 23 (1), 71–77.

NICE Guideline, 2013. Lower limb peripheral arterial disease [CG147].

NICE Guideline, 2013. Myocardial infarction with ST-segment elevation [CG167].

NICE Guideline, 2013. Secondary prevention in primary and secondary care for patients following a myocardial infarction [CG172].

NICE Guideline, 2013. Venous thromboembolic diseases [CG144].

NICE Guideline, 2014. Atrial fibrillation [CG180].

O'Connor, C.M., 2017. Developing breakthrough drugs for heart failure: lessons learned from the cystic fibrosis experience. JACC. Heart Fail. 5 (1), 71–72.

Oechslin, E., 2015. Congenital heart disease: management of adults with cyanotic congenital heart disease. Heart 101 (6), 485–494.

Perera, P., 2014. Cardiac echocardiography. Crit. Care Clin. 30 (1), 47–92.

Saint-Criq, V., Gray, M.A., 2017. Role of CFTR in epithelial physiology. Cell. Mol. Life Sci. 74 (1), 93–115.

Sands, S.A., Mebrate, Y., Edwards, B.A., et al., 2016. Resonance as the mechanism of daytime periodic breathing in patients with heart failure. Am. J. Respir. Crit. Care Med. 195 (2), 237–246.

Shen, L., 2013. Role of diuretics, β-blockers, and statins in increasing the risk of diabetes in patients with impaired glucose tolerance. Br. Med. J. 347, f6745.

Siervo, M., Fewtrell, M.S., Wells, J.C.K., 2013. Acute effects of violent video-game playing on blood pressure and appetite perception. Eur. J. Clin. Nutr. 67, 1322–1324.

Stansby, G., Berridge, D., 2013. Venous thromboembolism. Br. J. Surg. 100, 989–990.

Stevens, D., 2017. Clinical value of pulmonary hyperinflation as a treatment outcome in cystic fibrosis. Respirology 22 (1), 12–13.

Tanaka, K., Kamada, H., Shimizu, Y., et al., 2016. The use of a novel in-bed active Leg Exercise Apparatus (LEX) for increasing venous blood flow. J. Rural. Med. 11 (1), 11–16.

Tung, A., 2013. Critical care of the cardiac patient. Anesthesiol. Clin. 31 (2), 421–432.

White, A., Broder, J., Campo, T.M., 2012. Acute aortic emergencies. Adv. Emerg. Nurs. J. 34 (3), 216–229.

# General Management

## LEARNING OBJECTIVES

*On completion of this chapter the reader should be able to:*
- understand the indications and precautions for oxygen therapy and apply this knowledge to the practicalities of oxygen administration;
- contribute to the teamwork required to ensure that patients are optimally nourished and understand the relevance of this to rehabilitation;
- discuss appropriate medication for respiratory conditions and use clinical reasoning to identify suitable drug delivery devices for each individual;
- summarize the diagnostic and therapeutic purposes of bronchoscopy.

## OUTLINE

Physiotherapists liaise with doctors for oxygen therapy, dieticians for nutrition, and pharmacists or nurses for medication. The main input with patients is educational.

## OXYGEN THERAPY

*If used appropriately, oxygen can be a great friend.*
**Decalmer & O'Driscoll 2013**

Oxygen is a colourless, odourless drug with side effects and risks, but with rational prescription, precision of administration and objective monitoring, it can be a potent therapy for the respiratory patient. However, it is notorious for inadequate prescription and monitoring, various studies finding that:
- the majority of patients with respiratory failure have their oxygen wrongly prescribed (Ganeshan et al. 2006);
- less than one-third have their oxygen prescribed at all, only 10% have a target saturation specified and only 5% have it signed off (Kane et al. 2013);
- for acute patients with chronic obstructive pulmonary disease (COPD), only 16% achieve their target peripheral arterial oxygen saturation ($SpO_2$) (Chow et al. 2016).

### Indications and Limitations

**KEY POINT**

*Oxygen is a treatment for hypoxaemia, not breathlessness.*

BTS 2017

The UK guidelines begin with the wise words above. There is no evidence that supplemental oxygen reduces dyspnoea in a normoxaemic patient (Decalmer & O'Driscoll 2013), and education is more helpful than the psychological crutch of an expensive drug. Most people cannot feel hypoxaemia, although some veteran patients know that a certain fuzzy feeling in the head indicates reduced oxygen levels (Uronis et al. 2011), in which case this should be objectively confirmed by oximetry and supplemental oxygen titrated to their target saturation. Shortness of breath (SOB) and hypoxaemia often coexist, but they are caused by different mechanisms and require different management.

Supplementary oxygen is normally prescribed for a resting partial pressure of oxygen in arterial blood ($PaO_2$) of <8 kPa (60 mmHg) or $SpO_2$ <94%. This includes temporary hypoxaemia such as:

- after suction;
- during exercise, if demonstrable benefit is shown;
- at night, if desaturation is identified;
- postoperatively, even after routine surgery (Maity et al. 2012).

Oxygen may also be required for potential hypoxaemia, e.g. after premedication for some cardiorespiratory patients, and for first-time administration of bronchodilator drugs or hypertonic saline.

Oxygen for patients who are not hypoxaemic can be damaging for some patients, e.g. it can increase infarct size with acute coronary syndromes, increase oxygen free radicals with stroke and damage the foetus in pregnancy (BTS 2017):

- Kane et al. (2013) state that after normoxaemic stroke, oxygen can raise mortality by increasing oxygen free radicals.
- Cabello et al. (2013) state that following normoxaemic myocardial infarction, oxygen therapy may increase infarct size by reducing coronary artery blood flow, increasing coronary vascular resistance and causing reperfusion injury from oxygen free radicals.

Assessment for both acute and long-term oxygen includes nocturnal monitoring because of the risk of respiratory failure in some patients (Fig. 5.1) and the lack of correlation between day and night requirements (Fig. 5.2). Desaturation at night is associated with cognitive impairment (Yamout 2012).

Other limitations are the following:

1. Directing oxygen into the throat does not guarantee its arrival at the mitochondria. Tissue oxygenation depends not just on inspired oxygen but also on gas exchange at the alveolar–capillary membrane, lung perfusion, haemoglobin levels, cardiac output, vascular sufficiency and tissue perfusion.
2. If hypoxaemia is due to a large shunt, benefit is limited because shunted blood does not 'see' the added oxygen (p. 13).

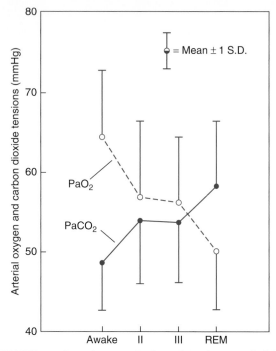

**FIGURE 5.1** Drop in mean $PaO_2$ and rise in mean $PaCO_2$ during sleep stages in patients with severe stable chronic obstructive pulmonary disease, showing damaging episodes of ventilatory failure. (From Criner 2000.) *II*, Stage II; *III*, stage III; *REM*, rapid eye movement stage.

## Complications

1. For patients depending on their hypoxic drive to breathe (p. 5), high concentrations of inspired oxygen can impair this drive. These patients should have their own venturi mask, wristband and 'alert card' (Fig. 5.3) which provides information on their target saturation for ambulance and other health staff (BTS 2017).
2. Discomfort can be caused by dry mucous membranes, eye irritation, a sense of being smothered, difficulty expectorating, or excess work of breathing (WOB) due to inadequate flow. A patient oxygenating their forehead is a familiar sign of these problems. Aqueous cream may prevent dry lips, and increased flow may reduce WOB so long as this does not affect oxygen percentage, in which case a different device may be indicated. Humidification is required if the patient has thick secretions or feels uncomfortably dry, which is more likely at flows over 4 L/min (Chidekel et al. 2012).

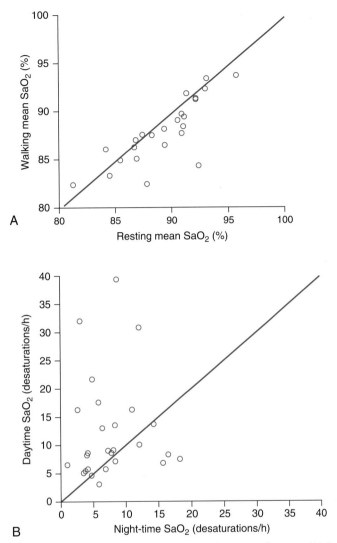

**FIGURE 5.2** SpO$_2$ in people with chronic obstructive pulmonary disease: (A) linear relationship between rest and exercise, (B) lack of relationship between day and night. (From Schenkel 1996.)

3. Oxygen is not physically addictive, but dependency occurs when patients rely on it unnecessarily.
4. Prolonged exposure to pure O$_2$ may cause inflammatory lung toxicity. This has been demonstrated in animals and healthy volunteers, who have experienced substernal pain, cough and sore throat after between 4 and 110 h of 100% oxygen, but for patients it is difficult to distinguish the effects of the disease, the oxygen and other treatments (Kallet & Matthay 2013). High concentrations should not be withheld from patients when indicated (Crooks et al. 2012).

5. Oxygen creates a fire hazard by supporting combustion. Smoking cigarettes or electronic cigarettes is banned, home equipment must be kept away from heaters and open flames, and an advisory visit from the fire service is recommended.
6. For newborns, high concentrations can cause blindness (p. 347).
7. 'Absorption atelectasis' can occasionally develop if high concentrations of oxygen replace inert nitrogen (the main constituent of air) so that alveoli are no longer held open by a cushion of gas. This can occur

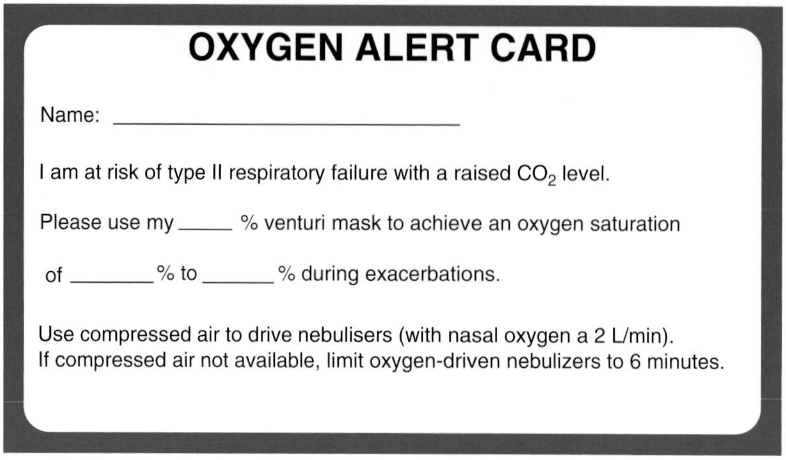

## OXYGEN ALERT CARD

Name: _____

I am at risk of type II respiratory failure with a raised $CO_2$ level.

Please use my _____ % venturi mask to achieve an oxygen saturation

of _____ % to _____ % during exacerbations.

Use compressed air to drive nebulisers (with nasal oxygen a 2 L/min).
If compressed air not available, limit oxygen-driven nebulizers to 6 minutes.

FIGURE 5.3  Oxygen alert card.

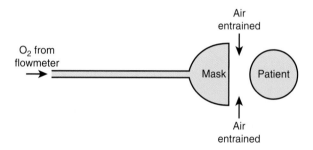

FIGURE 5.4 Dilution of oxygen by room air entrained through holes in an oxygen mask or around the edges of a mask or cannula.

during surgery (Randtke et al. 2015), or in mechanically ventilated patients receiving more than 70% oxygen at low tidal volumes (Cairo 2012, p. 339), but is not usually significant if a high fraction of inspired oxygen (FiO$_2$) is required. Absorption atelectasis can be used positively when oxygen is used to increase absorption of gas from a pneumothorax or subcutaneous emphysema (BTS 2017).

8. Tubing can be a trip hazard.

Individual devices may create their own complications, as discussed below.

## Delivery Devices

Oxygen emerges from the flow meter at 100% and is diluted by entrainment of room air (Fig. 5.4). After dilution, *high-flow* systems deliver a flow to the patient that usually matches their own peak inspiratory flow (PIF) and so are often preferred by breathless patients.

### KEY POINT

High- and low-flow systems relate to high and low accuracy, not to high and low concentration.

*Low-flow* systems deliver oxygen to the patient at a lower flow than their own.

### Low-flow (variable performance) mask

These simple masks deliver a flow that is less than the patient's own PIF, with room air sucked in through entrainment ports and the sides of the mask or cannula. The more breathless the patient, the more room air is entrained and the lower the FiO$_2$ they receive. FiO$_2$ therefore varies with the patient's own breathing pattern, as well as the flow selected on the flow meter. Low flow masks provide an uncontrolled oxygen percentage because of the variable FiO$_2$, but they are suitable for patients who do not require an exact concentration, e.g. with suction or after surgery.

The flow rate should be maintained above 5 L/min to avoid rebreathing carbon dioxide ($CO_2$) (BTS 2017). This flow can be marked on the flow meter with tape to remind staff of the correct setting.

### High-flow (fixed performance) mask

Known also as venturi masks (Fig. 5.5), these deliver a controlled oxygen concentration by forcing a jet of oxygen through a narrow orifice before it enters the mask, causing a shearing effect which draws room air into the gas stream through fixed-size entrainment ports. The speed of the resulting flow virtually

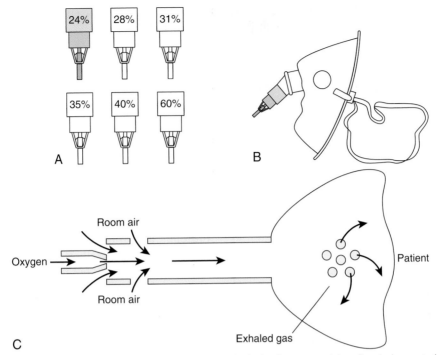

**FIGURE 5.5** High-flow venturi system: (A) colour-coded valves containing fixed-size entrainment ports, (B) blue 24% valve fitted to mask, (C) oxygen is delivered from the left, then driven through the narrow orifice which causes room air to be drawn through entrainment ports.

abolishes the rebreathing of room air via the mask, even if it is loosely fitted. It delivers the $FiO_2$ specified on the colour-coded venturi valve. The $FiO_2$ depends on the size of the entrainment ports on the valve, not the patient's PIF or the flow from the flow meter. The minimum flow from the flow meter is specified on the venturi valve and can be increased for comfort if the patient is breathless, because the concentration is fixed (Huffman et al. 2016).

A patient's PIF is on average 30–40 L/min, but breathless people may reach 70 L/min (Roca et al. 2016). Extra work is then required to entrain room air through the sides of the mask, causing increased WOB, sometimes inspiratory muscle fatigue and occasionally hypercapnia (Dodd et al. 1998). If the patient's respiratory rate is >30 breaths/min, the flow rate specified on the mask should be raised (BTS 2017), the correct level being ascertained by the following, in order of efficacy:
1. Ask the patient if they are receiving enough flow.
2. Observe the breathing pattern for signs of ↑ WOB (p. 37).
3. Check vital signs such as ↑ respiratory or heart rate, which may indicate severe fatigue.

Table 5.1 shows $FiO_2$ at different flow rates.

These masks cannot be humidified because moisture upsets the delicate balance of entraining the correct proportion of air. If humidification is required, large-volume nebulizing humidifiers can deliver a specific $FiO_2$ from 28% upwards (p. 203).

Venturi masks are used for patients needing an accurate $FiO_2$, e.g. hypercapnic COPD patients who are dependent on their hypoxic drive to breathe, and for breathless patients whose PIF is too high to tolerate a low-flow system. High capacity masks are available that can

### MINI CLINICAL REASONING

*'Numerous randomized controlled trials ... have documented the benefits of low-flow oxygen [for exacerbations of COPD]'*
                    ***Respir Care** (2004); 49(7):766–782*

**Response**
- Low flow does not mean low percentage.
- Most patients with an exacerbation are breathless and need high-flow oxygen. They may or may not need low percentage, depending on assessment.

**TABLE 5.1  Oxygen concentrations delivered from high-flow systems, showing how flow from the flow meter can be altered for different total flows to the patient according to need, while maintaining FiO$_2$**

| Concentration (%) | Oxygen flow (L/min) | Flow to patient (L/min) |
|---|---|---|
| 24 | 2 | 50 |
|  | 3 | 75 |
|  | 4 | 100 |
| 28 | 4 | 44 |
|  | 6 | 66 |
|  | 8 | 88 |
| 35 | 8 | 45 |
|  | 12 | 67 |
|  | 16 | 90 |
| 40 | 10 | 41 |
|  | 15 | 62 |
|  | 20 | 82 |
| 60 | 15 | 30 |
|  | 20 | 40 |
|  | 25 | 50 |
|  | 30 | 60 |

Adapted from Dodd et al. 1998.

maintain a steady percentage even with very breathless patients.

### Reservoir systems

Reservoir masks deliver high-percentage oxygen by means of a reservoir bag (Fig. 5.6). During exhalation, oxygen fills the bag instead of being lost to the environment, then during inhalation this oxygen enriches the inspired gas. A **non-rebreathing** system has valves at the reservoir bag and at one side vent of the mask to prevent the mixing of exhaled gases with the fresh gas, delivering up to 90% oxygen. A **partial rebreathing** system receives oxygen plus exhaled gas equivalent to the patient's anatomic dead space, delivering approximately 35%–60% oxygen on the next breath (Garvey et al. 2012).

Before applying the mask, the reservoir bag must be filled with oxygen by occluding the valve between the reservoir and the mask. The flow rate must be at least 15 L/min, or high enough to keep the bag at least partially inflated throughout the respiratory cycle, however

breathless the patient. Reservoir masks cannot be humidified.

### Tusk mask

High FiO$_2$ can be achieved by creating reservoirs out of two 20 cm lengths of wide-bore corrugated tubing, which are inserted into each exhalation port of a simple mask (Fig. 5.7) or partial rebreathing mask (Hnatiuk et al. 1998).

### Nasal cannula

These cannulae deliver oxygen to the nostrils so that patients can talk, cough, eat and drink unhindered. They are low-flow systems and the FiO$_2$ is not accurate, rapid breathing increasing the FiO$_2$ because less room air is entrained. Mouth-breathers receive a less accurate FiO$_2$ (Applegate et al. 2016) but not a lower FiO$_2$ because the pharynx acts as a reservoir for oxygen during expiration, which is drawn on during inspiration (Wettstein et al. 2005). High flow from the flow meter may cause irritation and sometimes nose bleeds. Nasal discomfort can be eased by aqueous cream, but not lanolin, in case of allergy, and not petroleum jelly (Vaseline) which is petrol-based and reacts with oxygen.

Indications for nasal cannulae are:

- home oxygen;
- patients who find masks uncomfortable;
- confused patients, especially if high concentrations are needed, when cannulae can be used with a mask in case the mask is pulled off;
- hypoxaemic patients using an incentive spirometer or inspiratory muscle trainer.

### High-flow nasal cannula (Fig. 5.8)

Oxygen at FiO$_2$ between 0.21 and 0.60 can be delivered through a heated humidifier via medium-bore tubing with flow rates up to 60 L/min (Kim 2016).

Advantages are the following:

1. It enhances oxygen delivery (Kim 2016), can reduce the need for intubation and, for breathless patients, the high flow may decrease SOB and improve thoracoabdominal synchrony (Nishimura 2016).
2. It is more comfortable than noninvasive ventilation (NIV), although NIV can achieve greater oxygenation (Roca et al. 2016).
3. Positive airway pressure is created from the resistance generated by the high gas flow, which, along with the washout of dead space gas, may help

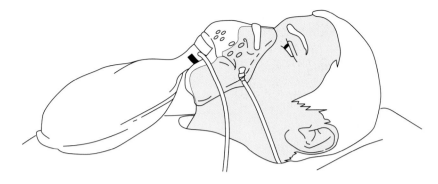

Partial rebreathing mask

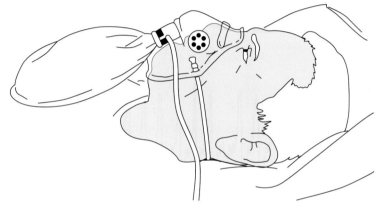

Non-rebreathing mask

**FIGURE 5.6** Partial rebreathe and non-rebreathe reservoir masks. (From Fisher & Paykel.)

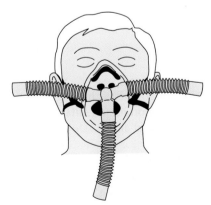

**FIGURE 5.7** Tusk mask.

prevent postoperative atelectasis (Suzuki & Takasaki 2014), improve $SpO_2$ and reduce $CO_2$, while the humidification increases mucociliary clearance (Roca et al. 2016).

4. The metabolic cost of warming and humidifying inspired gases, which normally consumes 156 calories/min, is conserved, and inspiratory effort reduced, which may be significant in hypermetabolic or cachectic patients (Roca et al. 2016).

5. Of particular interest to physiotherapists is the claim that it can increase exercise tolerance in people with advanced COPD when using an exercise bike or treadmill (Chatila et al. 2004).

Disadvantages are that it delivers a less accurate $FiO_2$ (Chikata et al. 2017) and facilitates transmission of infection (Yip 2013).

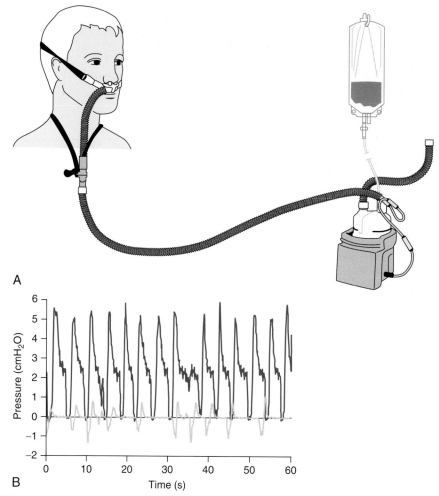

A

B

**FIGURE 5.8** (A) Optiflow high-flow system (From Fisher & Paykel). (B) Pressure exerted by a high-flow nasal cannula (dark trace), set at 2.7 cmH$_2$O pressure and 35 L/min flow, compared to a face mask (pale trace).

### Nasopharyngeal catheter

A specialized low-flow catheter can be lubricated and inserted into a nostril to reach just behind the uvula, then taped to the face. Several holes near the tip diffuse the flow, but patients often complain of a sore throat. These catheters are often not tolerated by children and are unsuited to infants because they occlude most of the nasal airway. They are sometimes used for short periods when a device is needed that must not become dislodged. A flow of 3–4 L/min usually delivers inspired concentrations of 30%–40%, but high flows have been known to cause barotrauma (Alifano 2010) or, rarely, gastric rupture (Yao et al. 2015).

### Transtracheal catheter

A small hole can be surgically created into the trachea, percutaneously or through a tunnelled route, through which a small oxygen catheter can be introduced to deliver long-term oxygen therapy (Fig. 5.9). These transtracheal catheters may reduce WOB and augment CO$_2$ removal (Garvey et al. 2012). They suit patients who

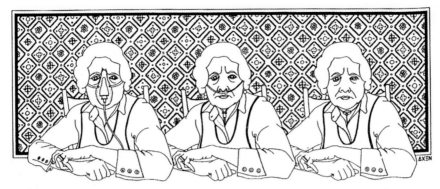

**FIGURE 5.9** Oxygen delivery systems. From left: simple mask, nasal cannula, transtracheal catheter. (From Haas & Haas 2000.)

prefer their relative invisibility and who can undertake measures to prevent encrustation and infection. Disadvantages relate to the need for surgical placement, with the accompanying risks of infection or subcutaneous emphysema.

### Head box

Clear plastic boxes over the heads of babies deliver high-flow humidified oxygen (p. 348). The flow must be directed away from the baby's face and care taken to ensure that the edges of the box do not rub the skin.

### T-piece

A T-piece delivers oxygen to an intubated, spontaneously breathing patient via the tracheal tube. Humidified oxygen is delivered through one end and exhaled gases leave through the other. So long as the flow rate is greater than the patient's PIF, it acts as a high-flow device.

### Acute Oxygen Therapy

In the acute setting, oxygen must be administered continuously (AARC 2002a) unless hypoxaemia has been demonstrated only in specific situations such as sleep or exercise. Patients should be informed that oxygen is not addictive, and some patients need reassurance that an oxygen mask is not a sign of terminal illness. Patients on acute oxygen therapy should only have their mask removed for expectoration or other brief reasons.

> **KEY POINT**
>
> *Prescription 'as required' is never appropriate for oxygen therapy.*
> BTS 2017

The UK guidelines stipulate that the target saturation should be prescribed on the drug chart and monitored on the observation chart (BTS 2017), and lack of prescription is defined as a drug error in some countries. Prescription should specify:
- the target saturation
- method of delivery
- nocturnal modifications

Some local protocols enable physiotherapists to prescribe oxygen.

Astute budget holders find it cheaper to supply their relevant beds with 24-h oximetry rather than waste unnecessary oxygen or deprive patients of oxygen at night. Inadequate oxygenation is not obvious because the brain is the most vulnerable organ (Karakontaki 2013) and a degree of confusion is not unusual in acutely unwell patients.

> **PRACTICE TIP**
>
> *Oxygen should be prescribed to achieve a target saturation of **94%–98%** for most acutely ill patients and **88%–92%** for those at risk of hypercapnic respiratory failure.*
> Decalmer & O'Driscoll 2013

### TABLE 5.2   Summary of recommendations for acute oxygen use

| | |
|---|---|
| 1. Critical hypoxaemia, cause not yet diagnosed | • Give 15 L/min via reservoir mask; once stable, reduce oxygen to achieve 94%–98% SpO$_2$. If patient is at risk of type 2 RF, begin as above, request urgent ABGs. |
| 2. Other acutely hypoxaemic patients | • Initially give 2–6 L/min via nasal cannulae or 5–10 L/min via simple mask, aiming for 94%–98% SpO$_2$. If SpO$_2$ cannot be maintained or initial SpO$_2$ is <85%, use a reservoir mask at 10–15 L/min. If at risk of type 2 RF, aim for 88%–92% SpO$_2$, adjusting to 94%–98% if ABGs show normal PaCO$_2$. Repeat ABGs after 30–60 min. |
| 3. COPD or other condition at risk of type 2 RF, i.e. requiring controlled oxygen | • Before ABGs, use 28% venturi mask, aiming for 88%–92%, adjusting to 94%–98% if the ABGs show normal PaCO$_2$. Repeat ABGs after 30–60 min. If patient has oxygen alert card, aim for target range specified. If patient is hypercapnic and acidotic after 30 min, consider NIV. |

ABG, Arterial blood gas; NIV, noninvasive ventilation; RF, respiratory failure.
Kane et al. 2013.

## Patients with chronic obstructive pulmonary disease

People with hypercapnic COPD vary in their response to oxygen. The major risk is giving too little oxygen, which leads to cardiac arrhythmias and tissue injury including damage to brain cells (Murphy et al. 2001). However, a proportion of COPD patients retain CO$_2$ habitually, and nearly half retain CO$_2$ during an exacerbation (Kane et al. 2013) because sustained hypercapnia has left them dependent on hypoxia rather than hypercapnia as their chemoreceptor ventilatory stimulus. Uncontrolled oxygen may prevent compensatory hypoxic vasoconstriction (Abdo & Heunks 2012) and cause hypoventilation, drowsiness and respiratory acidosis, which can be lethal. Suggested reasons are a quashed hypercapnic respiratory drive, the Haldane effect, alveolar ventilation to perfusion ($\dot{V}_A/\dot{Q}$) mismatching, an increase in dead space or a combination (Littleton 2015). A similar reaction has been found in people with neurological conditions (Chiou et al. 2016), and occasionally those with sleep disorders, asthma, cystic fibrosis, bronchiectasis, chest wall disorders and obesity hypoventilation syndrome (BTS 2017).

For these patients, a simple low-flow mask is inadequate, and nasal cannulae are unsatisfactory because exhausted patients may hypoventilate, entrain little room air and receive dangerously high FiO$_2$ levels. If nasal cannulae are necessary for patient comfort, arterial blood

gas (ABG) assessments are required until it is known whether or not they are retaining CO$_2$ (Table 5.2).

Patients dependent on their hypoxic respiratory drive require controlled oxygen therapy titrated to their individual response, to preserve their respiratory drive while nourishing their brain cells (BTS 2017):

• If the patient has acute hypercapnia, or if they have a history of hypercapnia when acutely unwell, or if they habitually retain CO$_2$ in the chronic state, or if none of this is known, controlled oxygen should be delivered by venturi mask, starting at 28% and titrated upwards or downwards to maintain SpO$_2$ at **88%–92%.** If a nebulizer is needed, this should be driven by compressed air, with supplementary oxygen supplied concurrently by nasal cannulae, using oximetry to maintain the target SpO$_2$.

• If a normocapnic patient is not drowsy and is known not to have had previous episodes of hypercapnia, oxygen should be given to a target SpO$_2$ of **94%–98%.**

• If the patient has severe hypoxaemia and their response to oxygen therapy is not known, their target saturation should be **94%–98%** but the patient kept under constant observation until ABG levels are obtained.

Sometimes the FiO$_2$ required to correct hypoxaemia still affects the respiratory drive. If partial pressure of CO$_2$ in arterial blood (PaCO$_2$) rises above 10.6 kPa (80 mmHg) or pH falls below 7.35, or if the patient becomes drowsy or fatigued, NIV should be initiated. If

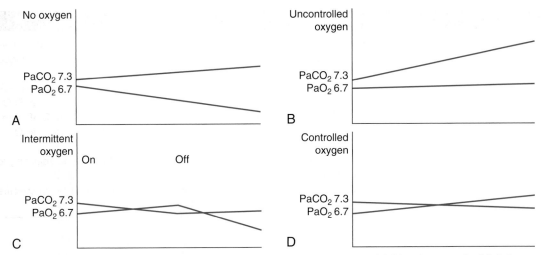

**FIGURE 5.10** Potential effects of oxygen administration on arterial blood gases (in kPa) for some COPD patients in ventilatory failure: (A) continued deterioration, (B) excessive FiO$_2$ leading to ↓ respiratory drive, hypoventilation and further ↑ PaCO$_2$, (C) intermittent removal of O$_2$, (D) normalization of blood gases.

PaCO$_2$ still continues to rise and pH to fall, a decision is required on whether to instigate mechanical ventilation and/or decrease FiO$_2$ further, bearing in mind that hypercapnia may not be a response to high FiO$_2$ but due to a deteriorating condition.

Worse than too-high or too-low FiO$_2$ is intermittent oxygen (Nadal 2013), which stirs up inflammation (Douglas et al. 2013) and is like intermittent drowning (Fig. 5.10C). The capacity of blood to hold CO$_2$ is approximately 10 times greater than oxygen (Wagner 2015) because abundant CO$_2$ is needed for acid–base balance and oxygen is only stored in the lungs and blood. If FiO$_2$ is allowed to fall, CO$_2$ crowds out the oxygen and causes a sharp drop in PaO$_2$ (Collins 1976).

In relation to timings:
- After FiO$_2$ has been changed, oxygen equilibration requires 10 min following an increase and 16 min following a decrease, after which ABGs can be reassessed (Weinreich 2013).
- Patients at risk who are given uncontrolled oxygen can be tipped into ventilatory failure in as little as 20 min (Chow et al. 2016).

A smart flow meter that automatically titrates oxygen flow to the target SpO$_2$ is available for acute patients (Lellouche & Erwan 2012) and for exercising patients (Cirio et al. 2011).

## Patients with other conditions

Patients with pneumonia or acute asthma may need generous levels of oxygen because they are often profoundly hypoxaemic. If they are also severely breathless, high flows are needed.

Postoperatively, hypoxaemia may be transient and low-risk patients usually require only a few hours' oxygen after surgery, but for people with lung disease or those undergoing heart, lung or other major surgery, several days and nights of supplementary oxygen may be required (p. 289).

## Home Oxygen

*'It's a fine line between helping me and being a blinking nuisance'*

**Pugh & Enright 2012**

### Long-term oxygen therapy

Long-term oxygen therapy (LTOT) can prolong life in people with COPD (Lahousse et al. 2016). Clinical reasoning and good communication are needed to ensure accurate assessment, prescription and acceptance.

LTOT has shown the following benefits:
- ↑ quality of life, sleep quality and survival (BTS 2015);

- ↑ exercise capacity (Hodgkin et al. 2009, p. 120), including for patients with heart failure (Koshy et al. 2016);
- ↑ $PaO_2$, ↓ $PaCO_2$, ↑ haemoglobin and possibly ↓ systemic inflammation (Howard 2012);
- ↓ pulmonary hypertension (Rowan et al. 2016);
- ↓ exacerbations and hospital admissions (Dunne 2009);
- ↑ cerebral blood flow, alertness and motor speed (Criner 2013).

Assessment for LTOT is mandatory, and at a time when the patient's condition is stable, using the equipment that is planned for their home. After resting for 30 min, $SpO_2$ is assessed. If it is >92% the patient is monitored at 6-monthly intervals. If it is <92%, a capillary blood gas (CBG) or ABG reading is taken on room air. LTOT is indicated if any of the following apply to people with COPD, interstitial lung disease, cystic fibrosis or heart failure (BTS 2015):

- chronic stable hypoxaemia with $PaO_2$ <7.3 kPa (55 mmHg) breathing air, on two samples taken at least 3 weeks apart;
- hypoxaemia <8 kPa (60 mmHg) if there is nocturnal hypoxaemia, peripheral oedema or pulmonary hypertension.

Patients should be initiated on a flow rate of 1 L/min and titrated up in 1 L/min increments every 20 min until $SpO_2$ is >90%. A CBG/ABG should then be taken to confirm that a target $PaO_2$ ≥8 kPa (60 mmHg) at rest has been achieved (BTS 2015).

Patients who develop respiratory acidosis and/or a rise in $PaCO_2$ of >1 kPa (7.5 mmHg) during the assessment on two occasions, while apparently clinically stable, should only receive LTOT in conjunction with nocturnal ventilatory support (BTS 2015). Any symptoms of $CO_2$ retention (headache, warm hands, flapping tremor) are noted so that the patient can recognize the symptoms.

Several nights' oximetry recording is required because of night-to-night variability (Lewis 2003) and the inability of predicting nocturnal requirements from daytime levels (Krachman et al. 2008 and Fig. 5.2). If this is not possible, nocturnal oxygen requirements can be identified by a CBG/ABG taken at 0700 (Tárrega et al. 2002) or the flow rate may simply be increased at night by 1 L/min if the patient is not hypercapnic (BTS 2015). Other causes of nocturnal desaturation, such as sleep apnoea, should be identified and treated first. The

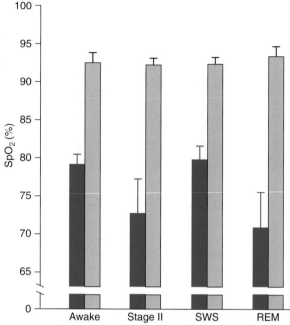

**FIGURE 5.11** $SpO_2$ during sleep without added oxygen *(purple bars)* and with oxygen *(grey bars)* in a patient with severe COPD. *REM,* Rapid eye movement sleep; *SWS,* slow wave sleep. (From Van der Schans 1996.)

significance of nocturnal oxygen therapy is shown in Fig. 5.11.

Oxygen should not be prescribed on hospital discharge unless hypoxaemia is severe, in which case it can be supplied temporarily, then the patient assessed objectively after a period of stability of at least 8 weeks (BTS 2015).

Follow-up is required at 3 months, to include assessment of CBG/ABG and flow rate to ensure that LTOT is still indicated. Thereafter follow-up visits at 6–12 months are needed, either at home or in combination with hospital visits, conducted by a specialist LTOT team (BTS 2015). Different activities may require different flow rates, e.g. eating, digesting, having sex or travelling (Nava 2011).

Patients are advised that oxygen should be used for as long as they can manage without unnecessary disruption to their lifestyle. 'The more the merrier' is their maxim. The minimum effective prescription is >15 h per 24 h, including always at night, but near-continuous

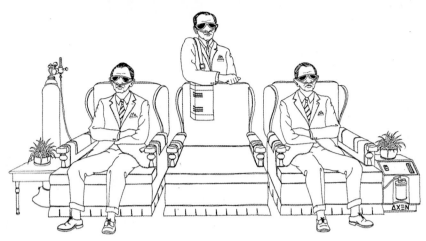

FIGURE 5.12 Home oxygen systems. From left: cylinder, portable liquid oxygen, concentrator. (From Haas & Haas 2000.)

oxygen is ideal (BTS 2015), one study reporting an increase in pulmonary vascular resistance when oxygen was stopped for just 3 h a day (Criner 2013). The goal is to achieve a $PaO_2$ of at least 8.7 kPa (65 mmHg) without a rise in $PaCO_2$ by more than 1.3 kPa (10 mmHg). The flow rate for this is generally 1.5 to 2.5 L/min, which can be increased by 1–2 L/min during exercise if indicated. Humidification is not required for non-tracheostomy patients (BTS 2015).

Three systems are available (Fig. 5.12):

1. Oxygen cylinders contain compressed oxygen, delivered through a regulator valve at flow rates of up to 4 L/min. They run out of oxygen rapidly and the pressure is inadequate for driving a nebulizer or if long tubing is required. They deliver cold, dry oxygen.
2. Oxygen concentrators separate oxygen from room air and deliver it at atmospheric temperature and humidity. The noise can be reduced by putting the machine on a towel and in a separate room. Small devices can be powered from a car battery.
3. Liquid oxygen is stored at near absolute zero in thermos containers. Advantages are that electricity is not required and light portable canisters can be filled from the container for easy mobility. Disadvantages include evaporation over time.

When being transported, cylinders should be secured with a seat belt or in the car boot. Liquid oxygen should be transported upright.

All patients need written (Appendix B) and verbal education. Domiciliary oxygen means that the disease is visible and can no longer be denied. Veteran patients on LTOT are often willing to talk to new patients and their carers, who may feel dismayed at the prospect of being tethered to bulky equipment for the rest of their lives.

Occasionally a patient stops needing their LTOT, either because it was needed temporarily after an exacerbation, or it was misprescribed, or because their condition has improved. In this case, they may find the prospect of losing their reassuring oxygen worrying. A suggested protocol for discontinuing LTOT is below (NHS 2011):

- First assessment: if $SpO_2$ is >94% after 15 min without oxygen, a further assessment is arranged in 1–2 weeks.
- Second assessment: if $SpO_2$ is >94% after 1 h without oxygen, the patient is given a diary to be kept for the next week. They record when and where they have used or felt they needed to use their oxygen, with telephone backup if required.
- If there is agreement with the patient and it is safe to do so, the diary is discussed and oxygen withdrawn.
- If the patient does not agree, the oxygen is continued and further support provided e.g. home visits, breathlessness management or consultant referral. The prescribed hours on oxygen can be reduced during this time, or only ambulatory oxygen advised.

## CLINICAL REASONING

'We use low-dose oxygen therapy, low-flow oxygen therapy, and long-term oxygen therapy as synonymous terms throughout this article.'

*Chest* (2016);149(2):303–306

(see p. 163)

### Ambulatory oxygen

'I love my ambulatory liquid oxygen—it's my best friend … [It] has taken me from being virtually housebound to adventures such as speeding down a zip–wire in Cornwall (with my oxygen on my back!)'

**Smith 2016**

Exercise-induced desaturation increases mortality (Andrianopoulos 2014), and portable oxygen is required if patients leave home regularly, desaturate on exercise, are motivated to use it and have been tested when stable and, if possible, have completed a pulmonary rehabilitation programme.

Exercise desaturation is not accurately predicted by baseline oxygen saturation but is likely if resting $SpO_2$ is <95% (Andrianopoulos 2014). Ambulatory oxygen (Ambox) is prescribed if patients desaturate by 4% or to <90% on exercise (LeBlanc et al. 2013). This may occur in the first minute and then stabilize, or it may be progressive. Postexercise desaturation occasionally occurs during subsequent sleep (Lanzi et al. 2014).

The benefits of Ambox include:
- ↑ cerebral oxygenation and exercise capacity (Vogiatzis et al. 2013)
- ↑ quality of life (Dyer et al. 2012)
- ↑ exercise tolerance
- ↓ hyperinflation and exertional SOB (O'Donnell et al. 2007).

Disadvantages can be avoided by education:
1. Morgan (2009) found that some patients reduce their activity rather than increase it because they feel anxious or hampered by the equipment.
2. Patients may use Ambox inappropriately for short bursts in an attempt to relieve SOB (Young 2005).

It is handy to combine assessment for Ambox with assessment for pulmonary rehabilitation. Ear oximetry is sometimes more accurate than finger oximetry due to movement artefact, so long as the ear is pink and well perfused (Barnett 2012). Assessment is in Table 5.3.

### TABLE 5.3 Assessment for Ambox

1. Rest for 30 min on room air or on added oxygen at the patient's resting $O_2$ prescription rate if they are on LTOT.
2. Record Borg score and $SpO_2$.
3. Perform baseline walk test on room air or at the patient's usual LTOT flow rate. Record distance, Borg and $SpO_2$.
4. Rest for 30 min (6MWT) or 40 min (ESWT) on room air or LTOT.
5. If $SpO_2$ is <90%, repeat walk test with an extra 2 L/min oxygen. Record distance, Borg and $SpO_2$.
6. If $SpO_2$ is still <90%, rest, repeat with an extra 2 L/min oxygen. Record distance, Borg and $SpO_2$.
7. Continue as above, adding oxygen until $SpO_2$ is >90%.
8. Record recovery time to baseline Borg and $SpO_2$ levels.

*6MWT*, Six-minute walk test; *ESWT*, endurance shuttle walk test; *LTOT*, long-term oxygen therapy.
Duck & Barnett 2004, Young 2005.

This protracted process is unacceptable to many patients but can be shortened by staff walking behind the patient and peering at the oximeter without disturbing their walking rhythm, then increasing the flow rate on the move if $SpO_2$ falls <90%.

If $SpO_2$ criteria are not met, Ambox can sometimes still be prescribed if it increases walking distance or decreases SOB by 10% (Young 2005). The risk of $CO_2$ retention is less on exercise because the extra ventilation washes out $CO_2$. If the flow rate is increased for exercise, patients must return it to their LTOT level afterwards.

Portable oxygen in lightweight cylinders or liquid canisters can be transported in a backpack or shopping trolley. Duration of use may be increased by an oxygen-conserving device, which releases a pulse of oxygen on inspiration. This should not be used at night when the breathing rate reduces, or for children, or for breathless patients needing a high flow, because their inspiratory flow will exceed the capability of the device. They are less efficient for mouth-breathers.

Length of tubing for an adequate flow is:
- liquid oxygen: 60 m (Cullen & Koss 2005);
- cylinders and concentrators: 30 m for flows up to 5 L/min (Aguiar et al. 2015).

These should be verified with the manufacturers.

Breathless patients with high respiratory rates, e.g. those with interstitial lung disease, may need a venturi mask, and should be supplied with oxygen equipment that is able to deliver the required high flow rates (BTS 2015).

For driving, self-assessment is advised. For flying, aircraft cabins contain the equivalent of 15% oxygen, so patients are advised to arrange for oxygen to be provided if their $PaO_2$ is below 9.4 kPa (70 mmHg) on $FiO_2$ of 0.15 (Dodd et al. 1998). The battery life of portable concentrators varies (Fischer 2013) as do airline charges, and masks or nasal cannulae may not be provided.

### Palliative oxygen therapy

People with SOB due to cancer or end-stage cardiorespiratory disease require physiotherapy (p. 231) and/or drugs (p. 169). If SOB continues to be intractable, assessment for home oxygen by a specialist team should include the effect of palliative oxygen on reducing SOB and improving quality of life (BTS 2015).

### Short-burst oxygen therapy

There is no evidence for using short-burst oxygen therapy, including before and after exercise or on discharge from hospital (BTS 2015). Short-burst oxygen is different from temporary oxygen (p. 150).

## Hyperbaric Oxygen Therapy

Hyperbaric oxygen is 100% oxygen delivered at pressures greater than atmospheric. Once haemoglobin is fully saturated, hyperbaric oxygen can push up the partial pressure of oxygen in the plasma, which increases the driving force of oxygen diffusion from blood into the tissues. Hyperbaric oxygen does not improve tissue oxygenation under normal circumstances but can stimulate healing in refractory wounds or irradiated tissues, and may reduce the risk of lower limb amputation two- to threefold in people with diabetes (Thom 2011). Other benefits have also been claimed for:

- acute brain injury (Geng et al. 2016)
- airway stenosis after lung transplant (Mahmood et al. 2016)
- some sports injuries (Barata 2011)
- stroke (Zhang 2010)
- complex regional pain syndrome (Katznelson et al. 2016)
- carbon monoxide poisoning (Liu et al. 2016c)

- tinnitus (Holy et al. 2016)
- autism (Rossignol et al. 2009)
- ischaemic limbs (Tin 2016), fistulae, gangrene (Feitosa et al. 2016) and necrotizing fasciitis (Marongiu et al. 2016)

Complications include middle ear barotrauma, dizziness, SOB, claustrophobia and chest pain (Hadanny et al. 2016). Undrained pneumothorax is a contraindication.

### Heliox

Helium is an inert gas with one-eighth the density of nitrogen. When blended with oxygen it is called heliox and can be used to bypass obstructed airways, e.g. with refractory asthma (Cavallaria et al. 2017), COPD (Varga et al. 2015), bronchiolitis (Seliem 2017) or vocal cord paralysis (Deckert 2010). It also allows lower driving pressures during lung-protective mechanical ventilation (Beurskens et al. 2016).

---

**RESPONSE TO MINI CLINICAL REASONING (from p. 162)**

*These terms are not synonymous. Results would be confusing at best and misleading at worst.*
**Kopp & Stavas 2016**

---

# NUTRITION

**Anorexia**: reduced desire to eat, usually related to physical or mental illness
**Malnutrition**: lack of specific nutrients, accompanied by undernutrition or sometimes obesity
**Undernutrition**: inadequate intake of dietary energy, leading to <90% ideal body weight
**Wasting**: loss of fat and muscle
**Cachexia**: severe loss of fat and muscle, including respiratory muscle, caused by excess protein catabolism and leading to <80% of ideal body weight
**Sarcopenia**: loss of muscle mass and strength, caused by cachexia or ageing

*Nutrition and hydration are often neglected in all types of healthcare.*

***Leach et al. 2013***

Breathing and eating are basic life processes that are intimately related in their mechanics, emotive associations and physiology. Air and food share common pathways for intake then separate for processing, and then their products join up in the blood for distribution to the tissues for the production of energy. Despite this interdependence, nutrition is still an overlooked area of respiratory medicine, even though malnutrition is the most common condition in hospitalized patients (Frew et al. 2010). A third of patients admitted to UK hospitals are malnourished or at risk of malnutrition, and half of elderly patients do not have adequate assistance with eating or access to fresh drinking water (Leach et al. 2013).

If malnutrition combines with disease and inflammation, it can reach the point of cachexia, which is associated with breathlessness, respiratory muscle atrophy and poor prognosis (Dudgeon 2016). Cachexia may be helped, but is not reversed, by nutritional support (Engineer & Garcia 2012). Muscle accounts for 60% of the body's protein stores, and inadequate nutrition increases the risk of falls (Elia et al. 2016).

Fatigue is a debilitating accompaniment to COPD, but Similowski (1991) found that for well-nourished people with stable COPD, chronic fatigue is abolished.

> **KEY POINT**
>
> Physiotherapy may be nullified if a patient is malnourished.

## Causes of Poor Nutrition in Cardiorespiratory Patients

- Eating becomes a chore rather than a pleasure for breathless people because the combined actions of eating and breathing are in competition.
- People with hyperinflated chests may feel full after a small meal, especially when accompanied by the air-swallowing associated with dyspnoea.
- Appetite may be reduced by smoking, depression, the taste of sputum and some inhaled drugs.
- Desaturation can be caused by the accessory muscles being diverted to assist with eating, the breath-holding required for swallowing, and the extra metabolic activity of digestion and assimilation.
- Increased WOB raises calorie requirements.
- Exercise limitation and fatigue discourage the preparation of healthy food and predispose to excess fat stores.

- Oxygen therapy or mouth-breathing can dry the mouth.
- 'Hospital malnutrition' increases mortality (Agarwal et al. 2013) and is exacerbated by unappetizing food, missed meals due to tests or procedures, patients' loss of access to their own kitchen and long overnight fasts. Hospitals and care homes tend to use processed high-salt foods to which elderly people may be unaccustomed, and which increase thirst (Verbrugghe et al. 2013).
- Other contributions are dysphagia, poor cognition and feeling ill (Leach et al. 2013).

## Effects of Poor Nutrition

Nutrition affects cardiorespiratory health from the womb onwards. Maternal malnutrition increases the risk of cardiovascular disorders in their offspring (Jackson et al. 2011) and a high sugar intake in youth predicts chronic disease risk (Hirshberg 2012). Caffeinated fizzy drinks, which tend to leach calcium from bone, are associated with fractures in teenage girls (Wyshak 2000), while energy drinks tend to increase blood pressure (Svatikova et al. 2016) and, in 40% of adolescents, cause side effects (Nordt et al. 2016). At all ages, excessive consumption of high-calorie processed foods can lead to systemic inflammation (Alissa & Ferns 2012).

Poor nutrition erodes muscle (Pierik et al. 2017), impairs ciliary motility, aggravates the emphysematous process, depletes surfactant, increases WOB (DeMeo 1992), impairs rehabilitation and physical function (Shiraishi et al. 2016), increases infection, length of stay, morbidity and mortality (Dizdar et al. 2016), and reinforces the whole unhappy process by blunting hunger. It increases hospital costs, and on discharge leads to poorer physical function and a greater need for residential care or readmission (Collins et al. 2016a). Malnourished surgical patients have three times more postoperative complications and four times greater risk of death than well-nourished patients having similar operations (Bairami et al. 2012). More cheerfully, a Mediterranean diet is associated with cardiovascular health (Casas et al. 2016) and optimum cognition (Hardman et al. 2016).

## Management

Attention to nutrition should be a routine preventive measure for preoperative patients and for those with acute or chronic illness, especially those with COPD or conditions associated with dysphagia. Nutritional supplements can improve quality of life and increase muscle strength in malnourished people with COPD. For those with hypercapnia, high-fat formulae may cause less metabolic $CO_2$ production than high-carbohydrate formulae (Hsieh et al. 2016). Supplements should not wait until protein has been cannibalized from the respiratory muscles.

For breathless patients, education includes the following:

1. It may be helpful to clear secretions before meals.
2. Try multiple small meals.
3. Teeth-cleaning or using a mouthwash before eating can reduce the lingering taste of inhaled drugs or sputum. This also helps reduce the periodontitis which is common in smokers and exacerbates the inflammation of COPD (Terashima et al. 2016).
4. If breakfast is difficult, try liquidizing it.
5. Have prepared meals ready in the freezer, to microwave when feeling too breathless to cook.
6. Ensure adequate vitamin E, required for optimum lung function (Hanson et al. 2016).
7. Ensure adequate vitamin C, which is needed daily because it is poorly stored in humans. Vitamin C reduces the respiratory oxidative damage caused by pollution (Jin et al. 2016), reduces blood pressure in people with hypertension (Ried et al. 2016), speeds mucous transport (Behndig et al. 2009), dampens down inflammation (Fukui et al. 2015), improves mood (Wang et al. 2013b) and helps preserve muscle strength (Cesari 2004).
8. Ensure adequate vitamin D, a lack of which has been found in approximately a third of the population and two-thirds of cardiac patients, and affecting physical fitness, cardiovascular and bone health (Ucay et al. 2017), rheumatoid arthritis and multiple sclerosis (Hirani et al. 2010). Vitamin D supplements improve exercise capacity (Kaul et al. 2016), and their antiinflammatory and antimicrobial properties benefit people with cardiac and critical illness (Venkatesh & Nair 2014). Sufficient vitamin D can be obtained from exposure of the hands and face to 10 min strong sunlight for light skin, or 60 min for dark skin (Love 2003).
9. Consider the antioxidant effects of garlic ('Russian penicillin'), said to help prevent cardiorespiratory disease and infection, aid expectoration and reduce hair loss (Petrovska 2012). Combining its ingestion with milk reduces its antisocial side effect (Persson & Persson 2012).
10. Make use of homemade drinks such as milk shakes and, if there is no sensitivity to the acid, fresh fruit juice.
11. Try taking liquids separately from meals, to reduce satiety.
12. Avoid hard or dry food, or add sauces such as gravy or custard.
13. Avoid gas-forming foods.
14. It is helpful if meals are leisurely, enjoyable and taken sitting up with elbows on the table to stabilize the accessory muscles.
15. If secretions are a problem, it may help to reduce milk intake because dairy products can increase the production of mucus (Bartley & McGlashan 2010). A month without dairy products may be needed to identify if this is helpful, in which case calcium-enriched substitutes are required.

Supplementary feeds orally or nasogastrically (NG) have shown cost savings (Elia et al. 2016). For patients with dysphagia who are intolerant of an NG tube or for those requiring long-term supplementary feeding, percutaneous endoscopic gastrostomy (PEG) feeding directly into the stomach is advised (Fig. 5.13). Oral feeds should be taken with a glass rather than through a straw to avoid excess WOB, and are supplementary to meals, not a replacement. Enteral feeds are best given at night to encourage daytime eating, with the head of the bed raised. For patients at risk of desaturation, insertion of NG or PEG tubes should be accompanied by oximetry (Rowat 2004).

For surgical patients, pre- and postoperative fasting should be avoided (p. 296) and specific nutrients with metabolic effects can help to modulate postsurgical stress (Braga 2016). For medical patients, nutrition screening should take place on admission, especially for cardiorespiratory patients who may show a complicated pattern of weight loss, fluid retention, obesity and masked malnourishment (Frew et al. 2010). For intensive care unit (ICU) patients, nutritional support can lead to better clinical outcomes and earlier discharge (Yeh et al. 2016). Happily for cardiovascular patients, moderate chocolate intake improves both cardiac and vascular function (Steinhaus 2017).

Physiotherapists may be the first to identify the need for nutritional support and request a dietician referral.

*Nutrition and physical activity are highly interrelated, complementary and synergistic.*
***Franklin et al. 2013***

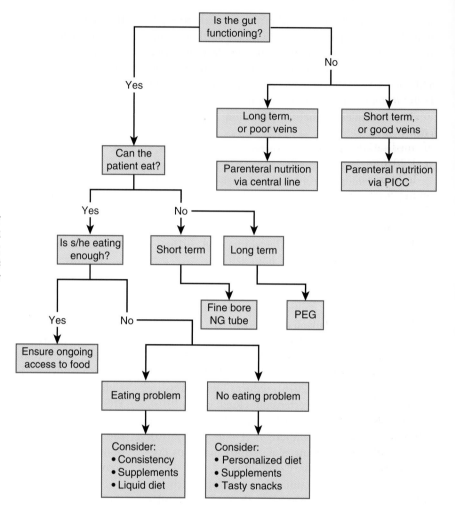

FIGURE 5.13 Flow chart for cardiorespiratory patients at risk of malnutrition. *NG*, Nasogastric; *PEG*, percutaneous endoscopic gastrostomy; *PICC*, peripherally inserted central catheter.

# RESPIRATORY DRUGS

*One of the first duties of the physician is to educate the masses not to take medicine.*

**William Osler**

---

**Agonists** activate a receptor response
**Antagonists** block a receptor response
**β₁-Receptors** stimulate heart rate and contractility
**β₂-Receptors** stimulate bronchodilation
**Half-life** indicates the time for plasma levels of a drug to drop to 50%; a drug is eliminated after five half-lives
**Drug metabolism** is determined by patient age, size and the drug's route of excretion; the very young and very old are slower to metabolize drugs

---

Diseases such as COPD are largely irreversible, but despite this (or maybe because of it) patients tend to be subjected to blind polypharmacy. Advanced countries are more likely to show this bias towards overtreatment (Katz 2013). Campbell (2014) claims that Americans take twice as many drugs as people in other countries and have the worst health of any industrialized nation, with medication-related problems being the fifth-most common cause of death.

Darbishire (2012) found that up to 50% of patients are non-adherent to their drugs, causing more than 10% of older-adult hospital admissions and 20% of preventable adverse drug reactions. With inhaled drugs, this is often due to difficulty in using the device, and the outcome may be over- or underdosing, which can double mortality (Ari 2015a).

It may be the pharmacist or nurse who educates patients about their medication, but this often needs to be reinforced by the physiotherapist, who should understand the indications, side effects and delivery systems of different drugs. For patients returning home from hospital, community physiotherapists need to check the drugs with their discharge summary and ensure that there is no unintentional continuation of medications prescribed for acute illness (Scales et al. 2016).

To fit in with the body's circadian rhythm, optimum timing for taking some drugs has been suggested by Kaur et al. (2016):

- steroids – morning;
- theophylline – evening;
- statins – evening;
- proton pump inhibitors – morning (if reflux occurs mostly during exercise), or evening (if it occurs at night);
- flu vaccinations – morning (Nurs Times 2016).

Medication for specific diseases is described in the relevant chapter, those for cardiovascular conditions in Chapter 4 and those for respiratory problems below.

## Drugs for Inflammation

Glucocorticosteroids (also called corticosteroids, and shortened to the term 'steroids' here) are potent and non-specific antiinflammatory agents. In the airways, they reduce the inflammation that can set off bronchospasm, oedema and hypersecretion of mucus. They reduce symptoms and exacerbations in COPD and asthma but do not slow disease progression (Raissy 2013). Side effects are listed in Table 5.4, with details below:

1. Immune suppression can be caused by mediation of the inflammatory response.
2. Fracture risk is greater even when steroids are inhaled (Sanel et al. 2016) and patients should have their bone mineral density monitored regularly.
3. Depression is a risk (Lehmann et al. 2013).
4. Oral steroids can cause myopathy (Shee 2003), which reduces exercise tolerance and can increase SOB. This may be ascribed mistakenly to deterioration of the disease and dosage can then be increased (Decramer 1994).

On top of the evidence-based side effects, both patients and staff are prone to 'steroid phobia', especially as patients may confuse corticosteroids with the anabolic steroids misused by some athletes.

Systemic side effects are reduced by using the inhaled route. Local side effects from inhalation can be minimized by using a spacer, inhaling slowly, and afterwards rinsing the mouth or gargling. If using a mask, the face should be wiped afterwards.

Concern about side effects tempts prescribers to nibble at the problem with low-dose therapy. This is fine for chronic asthma, but acute respiratory disease requires short sharp doses.

## Drugs for Bronchospasm

Response to a bronchodilator is usual in acute asthma, less so in chronic bronchitis and no more than a placebo in emphysema. However, few people with COPD have only emphysema, and combined long-acting bronchodilators have been found helpful in COPD (Spina 2014). Reversibility to a bronchodilator is defined as improved forced expiratory volume in one second ($FEV_1$) or forced vital capacity (FVC) by 12%–15% after a short-acting bronchodilator trial (Hanania et al. 2011). Measurements are taken 20 min after $\beta_2$-agonist administration or 40 min after an anticholinergic.

Both sympathetic (adrenergic) and parasympathetic (cholinergic) receptors have been identified in bronchial smooth muscle.

Sympathomimetics are versatile drugs which mimic the action of the sympathetic nervous system. Those which stimulate $\beta_2$-receptors in bronchial smooth muscle are known as $\beta_2$-stimulants, $\beta_2$-adrenergics or $\beta_2$-agonists. Examples are:

- short-acting drugs, e.g. salbutamol or terbutaline: onset of action 3–5 min, peak effect 20 min, duration of action 3–5 h;
- long-acting drugs, e.g. salmeterol: onset 15 min, peak effect 1 h, duration 12 h; formoterol: onset 3–5 min, duration 12 h;
- ultralong-acting drugs, e.g. indacaterol: duration 24 h.

With chronic asthma, short-acting or 'rescue' $\beta_2$-agonists should be taken symptomatically. Regular use is confined to those with acute or severe chronic disease, or as prophylaxis before exercise or allergen exposure. Regular $\beta_2$-agonists, if taken unnecessarily, may induce tolerance to their own bronchoprotective effects (Cazzola et al. 2013). With COPD, ultralong-acting $\beta_2$-agonists may be as effective as a long-acting $\beta_2$-agonist/steroid combination (Cope et al. 2011). $\beta_2$-Agonists are not suitable for adults or children with acute cough or acute bronchitis (Becker et al. 2015).

## TABLE 5.4   Medication for airflow obstruction[a]

| Drug | Delivery | Side effects |
|------|----------|--------------|
| **Cromones to prevent inflammation (asthma only, p. 85)** | | |
| Nedocromil sodium (Tilade) | Inhalation | |
| **Corticosteroids to treat inflammation** | | |
| Beclometasone (Qvar, Clenil), budesonide (Pulmicort), fluticasone (Flixotide), mometasone, ciclesonide | Inhalation | Hoarse voice, oropharyngeal candidiasis, dysphonia, pharyngitis, glaucoma, osteoporosis |
| Prednisone | Intravenous | Weight gain, muscle atrophy, infection risk, peptic |
| Prednisolone | Oral | ulceration, fragile skin, bruising, hyperglycaemia, diabetes, hypertension, mood change, adrenal suppression, delayed healing, retarded growth in children |
| **Antileukotrienes to treat inflammation (asthma only)** | | |
| Montelukast (Singulair), zafirlukast (Accolate). | Oral | Headache |
| **Bronchodilators to treat bronchospasm** | | |
| ***Short-Acting $\beta_2$-Agonists*** | | |
| Salbutamol (Ventolin) | Inhalation | Tremor, tachycardia, agitation, atrial fibrillation, muscle |
| Terbutaline (Bricanyl) | Oral | cramps and (with high doses) 'inner restlessness' |
| Fenoterol | Intravenous | |
| Levalbuterol | Subcutaneous | |
| ***Long-Acting $\beta_2$-Agonists*** | | |
| Salmeterol (Serevent) | Oral | |
| Formoterol (Foradil) | Inhalation | |
| Bambuterol (Bambec) | | |
| Indacaterol (Onbrez) | | |
| Arformoterol | | |
| Indacaterol | | |
| Tulobuterol | | |
| ***Short-Acting Anticholinergics*** | | |
| Ipratropium (Atrovent), oxitropium bromide | Inhalation | Dry mouth, blurred vision, constipation (or diarrhoea from laxatives), urine retention, glaucoma, possible cardiovascular risk |
| ***Long-Acting Anticholinergics*** | | |
| Tiotropium (Spiriva), clidinium bromide, glycopyrronium bromide, umeclidinium | | |
| ***Methylxanthines*** | | |
| Theophylline | Oral | Headache, gastric ulcer, insomnia, nausea and vomiting, |
| Aminophylline | Intravenous | tachycardia, osteopaenia and CNS effects such as dizziness and seizures |

| Drug | Delivery | Side effects |
|---|---|---|
| **TABLE 5.4    Medication for airflow obstruction—cont'd** | | |
| ***Combined Short-Acting Bronchodilators*** | | |
| Fenoterol and ipratropium, Ipratropium and salbutamol (Combivent) | Inhalation | |
| ***Combined Long-Acting Bronchodilators*** | | |
| Formoterol and aclidinium, indacaterol and glycopyrronium, vilanterol and umeclidinium | | |
| ***Combined Steroid and Bronchodilator*** | | |
| Fluticasone and salmeterol (Seretide), budesonide and formoterol (Symbicort), beclometasone and formoterol (Fostair) | Inhalation | |

<sup>a</sup>Brand/trade names are in brackets.

**Anticholinergic** (antimuscarinic) bronchodilators such as tiotropium block the effect of acetylcholine on autonomic nerve endings. They have a slow onset of 20–30 min and are most effective with COPD, sometimes reducing exacerbations and increasing exercise tolerance (Yoshimura et al. 2012). They may show an additive effect in combination with $\beta_2$-agonists. Individuals show different response patterns and may react better to $\beta_2$-agonists, anticholinergics or both. Side effects include a risk of falls (Marcum et al. 2016), a possible increase in cardiovascular morbidity and mortality (Matera et al. 2014), and, with the nebulized drug, glaucoma if a mask is used rather than a mouthpiece, especially if combined with a $\beta_2$-agonist (Ah-Kee et al. 2015).

**Theophylline** and its derivatives such as aminophylline or caffeine are part of the methylxanthine group of drugs which can bronchodilate, reduce inflammation, reverse steroid resistance (Barnes 2013), stimulate ventilation, enhance respiratory muscle function (Jagers et al. 2009) and improve exercise capacity (Voduc et al. 2012). Side effects are legion (Table 5.4) and stringent monitoring of blood levels is required, plus vitamin D supplements (Pal et al. 2016).

If an inhaled bronchodilator and steroid are prescribed, it is best to take the bronchodilator first to assist dissemination of the steroid, but complicated instructions can demotivate patients and it is more important that the drugs are taken than a sequence adhered to.

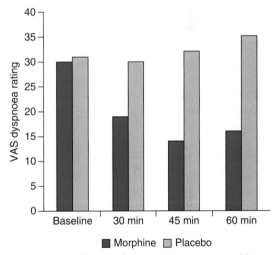

**FIGURE 5.14** Effect of subcutaneous morphine on dyspnoea in cancer. *VAS*, Visual analogue scale. (From Manning 2000.)

## Drugs for Breathlessness

Sometimes the cause of SOB can be treated, e.g. by diuretics, bronchodilators or steroids. For a direct effect on the symptom itself, the following have shown varying degrees of efficacy:

1. Opiates are the mainstay (Fig. 5.14), preferably via a patient-controlled device (Schmitz et al. 2016). Regular low doses of sustained-release morphine can safely reduce breathlessness without respiratory

depression (Currow et al. 2014). The side effect of respiratory depression does not appear to affect gas exchange except in severe cases (Boland et al. 2013), and it must be given in sufficient dosage (Uronis et al. 2006). The skills of a palliative team may be required to get the right balance.

2. Fentanyl is an opioid that can relieve SOB in as little as 5 min when given transmucosally as 'lollypops' (Hallenbeck 2008).

3. Bronchodilators may reduce SOB in some patients independent of their bronchodilating effect, probably by reducing hyperinflation.

4. Buspirone is an anxiolytic that can reduce breathlessness and increase exercise tolerance without causing sedation (Argyropoulou 1993, Gökben et al. 2012).

5. Sildenafil (Viagra) may reduce pulmonary hypertension in pulmonary fibrosis (Ryerson et al. 2012) and COPD (Vitulo et al. 2016).

6. The steroid dexamethasone can ease SOB in people with cancer (Hui et al. 2016a).

7. Selective serotonin reuptake inhibitor antidepressants either lift the depression that increases SOB, or the serotonin acts directly on the brainstem respiratory centres (Uronis et al. 2006).

8. Inhaled furosemide may ameliorate SOB in people with acute COPD (Vahedi et al. 2013).

## Drugs to Help Clear Secretions

If mucoactive drugs are needed, they should improve mucous transport, rather than irritate the airways to create more mucus. They should also optimize viscosity rather than over- or underhydrate the mucus because cilia prefer a viscoelastic gel rather than either extra-thin or extra-thick secretions.

The following may be beneficial for some patients:

1. Mucolytics such as carbocisteine (Mucodyne), acetylcysteine, erdosteine and lysozyme hydrochloride (Ohbayashi et al. 2016) reduce viscosity by degrading polymers in mucus. Some also have antiinflammatory and antioxidant properties (Zheng 2013).

2. $\beta_2$-Agonists may increase ciliary beat frequency in healthy subjects, but do not have a significant impact on clearance of mucus in people with lung disease (AARC 2015).

3. Aerosolized surfactant can decrease adhesion between the ciliary tip and mucous layer, inhaled anticholinergics reduce the hypersecretion stirred up by inflammation and, in chronic bronchitis or bronchiectasis, inhaled indomethacin may decrease hypersecretion (Rubin 2015b).

4. Nebulized saline (p. 203) may be beneficial if preceded by the diuretic amiloride (Sood et al. 2003).

5. Mannitol is a diuretic, but inhaled as a dry powder it creates an osmotic drive for water to move into the airway lumen. It is less irritating than hypertonic saline and can benefit people with bronchiectasis or cystic fibrosis (Rubin 2015b).

## Drugs for Smoking Cessation

Medication doubles a person's quit rate (Mulhall 2016). Nicotine replacement is available as patches, gum, lozenges, inhalers, nasal sprays (GOLD 2016) and a metered dose inhaler (Caldwell & Crane 2016). Drugs include bupropion (Zyban) and varenicline (Champix), although side effects, including a tendency to suicide, have been reported (Mulhall 2016). Users of e-cigarettes are exposed to nicotine, the addictive cigarette ingredient, but not to the more toxic ingredients (Göney et al. 2016). Vaccines offer promise (Jacob et al. 2016).

## Drugs for Infection

*The 'war on antimicrobial resistance' by escalation is about as likely as the chance of winning the 'war on terror'*

**Isaacs & Andresen 2013**

An antibiotic is indicated if a patient's condition is caused by bacterial infection, if the organism responsible is sensitive to the antibiotic prescribed, and if the infection is unlikely to resolve without assistance. It is administered orally, intravenously or by nebulizer.

Antibiotics often have to be given blind at first because 24 h are needed for microbiology results. Thereafter, antibiotics should be specific and time-limited, to inhibit the emergence of resistant organisms. The 'revenge of the microbe' has led to bacteria becoming resistant to antibiotics faster than new drugs are created, mostly due to their use in agriculture (Aitken et al. 2016), especially when used as growth promoters. For mild disease, antibiotics sometimes maintain a cycle of medicalizing a self-limiting illness in which patients attribute resolution to their antibiotics. For critically ill patients, ICUs have been called factories for creating resistance to antibiotics (Gonzalez et al. 2013). Prophylactic antibiotics are reserved for people with chronic sepsis such as in cystic fibrosis.

Interesting alternatives are essential oils (Yap 2013), probiotics for ICU-acquired pneumonia (Barraud et al. 2013) and maggot therapy for antibiotic-resistant wound infections (Linger et al. 2016).

## Drugs to Inhibit Coughing

To suppress a nonproductive and irritating cough, the order of efficacy is:

- identification and treatment of the cause, e.g. asthma;
- physical methods (p. 216);
- medication.

Most patients report limited or no effectiveness of drugs (Chamberlain et al. 2015), but protocols have been developed (Gibson et al. 2016). Drugs include antileukotrienes for asthma-associated cough, morphine for cough associated with malignancy, amitriptyline (Ryan 2016), pregabalin (Vertigan et al. 2016) or dextromethorphan for idiopathic cough, menthol or honey for cough associated with respiratory infections (Koskela 2016), and nicotine replacement, which explains the temporary increase in coughing with smoking cessation (Bolser 2010).

'Cough mixtures' often contain both expectorant and suppressant, but are strong placebos (Cohen 2015). It has been recommended that over-the-counter cough and cold remedies should not be used to treat children less than 2 years old (Goodman 2015).

## Drugs to Improve Ventilation

Respiratory stimulants are not recommended for ventilatory failure (GOLD 2016) because the respiratory muscles are already struggling and further stimulus may override the protective function of fatigue. However, an infusion of doxapram is sometimes tolerated by drowsy patients who hypoventilate following surgery, have taken a drug overdose, or who are awaiting noninvasive ventilation (Golder et al. 2013). This is at the cost of central nervous system stimulation, agitation, shaking, hallucinations, increased WOB, SOB and sometimes panic attacks (Wemmie 2011). These are less frightening if they have been explained to patients before the drug is administered.

## Drugs to Improve Sleep

Patients prefer to have a choice between behavioural or pharmacological treatments for insomnia (Cheung et al. 2016). Traditional sedatives and hypnotics tend to suppress the respiratory drive, but drugs that may be suitable for respiratory patients are melatonin receptor agonists (Greenberg & Goss 2009) or possibly zolpidem, although this carries infectious, malignant and central nervous system risks (Laia 2016) and occasionally brings suicidal tendencies (Sun et al. 2016a).

> **KEY POINT**
>
> *Drugs are tested by the people who manufacture them … Sometimes whole academic journals are owned outright by one drug company.*
>
> Goldachre 2012

## Delivery Devices

Are respiratory drugs best ingested or inhaled? Aerosolized medication has been delivered to the respiratory tract since 1500 BC (Colice 2009), and its advantages are the same today:

- rapid onset of action
- local delivery to maximize positive effects and minimize side effects
- delivery of drugs that are inactive by other routes

Disadvantages are:

- loss of much of the drug to the atmosphere, pharynx and stomach, although high doses compensate for this;
- less effective lung deposition with airflow obstruction, turbulent airflow or mucous plugging, leading to patchy and mostly central airway distribution in people with advanced COPD or acute asthma (Laube et al. 2011);
- localized side effects from deposition in the upper airways, especially with steroids (Nave & Mueller 2013);
- with nebulizers, infection risk (AARC 2002a).

### Inhalers (Fig. 5.15)

**Pressurized inhalers** such as the metered dose inhaler (MDI) deliver an aerosol by suspending an active drug in a propellant. The traditional MDI is portable and cheap, but inhaler technique has been found incorrect in 75% of people with COPD (Pothirat et al. 2015), in 50% of those with asthma and, somewhat embarrassingly, by in 5% of junior doctors (Price et al. 2013), while another study found that no pharmacists were able to demonstrate it successfully (Ali et al. 2014).

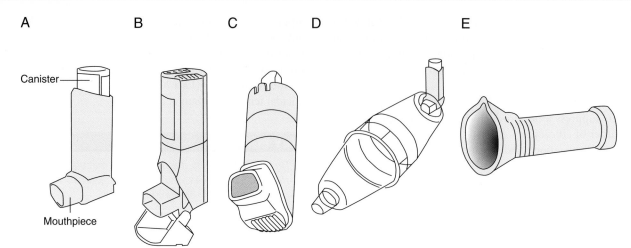

FIGURE 5.15 Pressurized inhalers and spacers: (A) metered dose inhaler, (B) Easi-breathe inhaler, (C) Autohaler, (D) Volumatic spacer, (E) Aerochamber spacer.

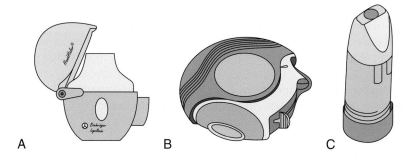

FIGURE 5.16 Dry powder inhalers: (A) Handihaler, (B) Accuhaler, (C) Turbohaler.

Accurate inhaler technique could prevent 45% of admissions for COPD, according to Mulhall (2016). Breath-actuated inhalers such as the Autohaler or the Easi-Breathe coordinate drug release with inhalation. Slow deep breathing is usually recommended to facilitate peripheral deposition (Sanchis et al. 2013).

A **spacer** (Fig. 5.15D & E) is a chamber between the patient and inhaler which acts as a reservoir from which the patient inhales the aerosol. Advantages are that:

- propellants and large particles drop out in the chamber and aerosol momentum is slowed, so that less is lost by impaction on the back of the throat, thus reducing local side effects and doubling pulmonary deposition (Vincken et al. 2010);
- less coordination is required because the drug remains suspended in the spacer until the patient inhales, although early inhalation is advised;
- high doses can be delivered during acute episodes.

Spacers should be used when possible for MDIs, and always for children taking steroids. Tidal breathing is recommended. For infants, a soft face mask can be attached to the spacer. Large pear-shaped spacers such as the Volumatic are cumbersome but efficient, simulating the aerosol cloud from an inhaler. These should be washed with detergent once a month without rinsing, then air-dried to reduce the static charge that attracts the drug to the walls of the spacer rather than the lungs (NICE 2012a). The Aerochamber gives a warning whistle if used incorrectly.

**Dry powder inhalers** such as the Handihaler, Accuhaler and Turbohaler (Fig. 5.16) require less coordination, but Schantz et al. (2016) found that only 16%–48% of patients used them correctly. Inhaling through the device draws air through powder to create an aerosol. A disadvantage is that children under 6 years, breathless people and those with bronchospasm may be unable to

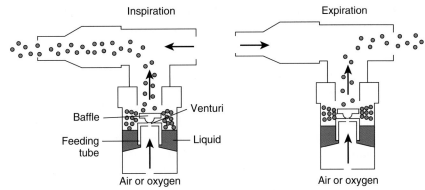

**FIGURE 5.17** Small-volume jet nebulizer for delivery of saline or medication. (From O'Callaghan et al. 1997.)

generate sufficient inspiratory flow. The powder is sensitive to moisture, so it is either stored in foil blisters or patients are warned against exhaling into the device. Tiotropium delivered via the Respimat inhaler has been associated with higher mortality than when delivered by the Handihaler (Jenkins & Beasley 2013).

Problems for all inhalers are:
- the need for coordination and/or manual dexterity;
- confusion about when to use which inhaler, or forgetting the number of puffs (patients can remember by lifting one finger as they take each puff);
- difficulty in understanding instructions, e.g. mistaken spraying of the drug up the nose, onto the chest, into the armpits or, after one patient was told that her asthma was caused by her cat, onto the unfortunate pet.

---

**KEY POINTS ON INHALER EDUCATION**

- Patients to try out and choose which device suits them
- One-on-one individualized training, plus family if agreeable to patient
- Reinforcement in writing (Appendix B)
- Follow-up to check technique (Ari 2015a)

---

### Small-volume nebulizers

Nebulizers deliver solutions of a drug dissolved in a liquid or suspensions of drug particles in a carrier liquid, using compressed air, oxygen or ultrasonic power.

**Jet nebulizers** (Fig. 5.17) run on air or oxygen and use the venturi principle (p. 153), which creates a variety of droplet sizes:
- large particles impact on a baffle and fall back into the nebulizer chamber;
- particles >6 µm diameter are lost in the upper airways;
- particles 2–6 µm target the bronchi and bronchioles and are used for bronchodilators and steroids;
- particles <2 µm deliver antibiotics to the alveoli (Darquenne 2012).

Breath-synchronized devices reduce some of the wastage.

The following technique is suggested:
1. The driving gas should be prescribed on the drug chart (Satya 2004). Acutely hypoxaemic asthmatic patients require high $FiO_2$ levels, which, paradoxically, may be best delivered by air-driven nebulization combined with nasal cannulae (Caille et al. 2009). People with acute hypercapnic COPD require the same combination but with monitoring of $SpO_2$, close observation with the first dose, and patients asked to report any symptoms of $CO_2$ retention (p. 160); if an air compressor is not available, oxygen-driven nebulization should be limited to 6 min (BTS 2008).
2. Select a mouthpiece if possible, unless patient preference or excessive dyspnoea precludes this. Nose-breathing filters the drug and reduces lung deposition, and aerosol escaping from a mask can affect the eyes.
3. If possible, patients should vary their position during nebulization, to maximize deposition (Dhanani et al. 2016), or sit upright.

4. Fill to between 2.5–6 mL, depending on the nebulizer. Set the flow rate to 6 L/min, unless a compressor is used, which has a preset flow rate.
5. Advise the patient:
   • to mouth-breathe if possible;
   • to intersperse tidal breaths with some slow deep breaths and some end-inspiratory holds to improve deposition (Bauer et al. 2009);
   • if using a mouthpiece, not to obstruct the air port;
   • to allow 10 min for completion;
   • after each use to empty and dry the nebulizer with a paper towel, or when in hospital, to follow infection control protocol.

A typical protocol is to disinfect, then rinse with sterile water or air-dry (Ida et al. 2016). Drying is the most important part of the cleaning process (Dodd 1996).

For home nebulizers, family education includes:
• the importance of cleaning the equipment as per the manufacturer's instructions;
• regular servicing; the compressor becomes less effective even though it continues to produce a mist;
• '4-hourly nebs' does not include the night.

As well as bronchodilators, nebulizers can be used to deliver antibiotics, surfactant, antiinflammatory drugs and analgesics. When exact dosage is required, the nebulizer can be tapped when the liquid is beginning to fizz, to minimize wastage. Some nebulizer solutions should not be mixed. When nebulizing via a tracheostomy, the inner tube should be removed (Pitance et al. 2013).

**Ultrasonic nebulizers** are popular with patients because the density of the mist speeds up the process, but they do not suit all drug suspensions.

For patients with chronic disease who remain symptomatic despite inhaler use, a nebulizer trial can be performed, with the first dose administered in hospital in case of side effects such as cardiac arrhythmias. Drug trials for home use should not be undertaken during acute illness. If patients use nebulizers at home, they require ongoing support and backup servicing.

Positive expiratory pressure (p. 211) can be combined with nebulizers but the dose may need adjustment (Berlinski 2014).

### Inhaler or nebulizer?

MDIs with spacers are at least as effective as nebulizers for children (Mitselou et al. 2016) and adults, but patients tend to prefer nebulizers (Smyth et al. 2001), possibly because they are automatically used on admission to hospital, so nebulizers 'must be best', or perhaps because nebulizers create an impressive mist and do not demand respiratory gymnastics for coordination. However, nebulizers come with disadvantages:
1. People at home with severe acute asthma may be over-reliant on repeated use when their airways are dangerously obstructed and they need to get themselves to hospital (Heslop & Harkawat 2000).
2. Nebulizers are expensive and require servicing and cleaning (Yawn et al. 2012).
3. 'Horrifying tales' of contamination have been reported, both in hospital (Botman 1987) and at home (Towle et al. 2016), which can lead to pneumonia (Ida et al. 2016).
4. Patient adherence is worse than with an MDI and systemic side effects are more likely (Rubin 2015b).
5. Less drug reaches the lung (Fig. 5.18), although this varies between devices and a higher dose compensates.

NICE (2012a) stipulates that nebulized therapy should only be prescribed at home if it leads to one or more of the following:
• ↓ symptoms
• ↑ ability to undertake activities of daily living

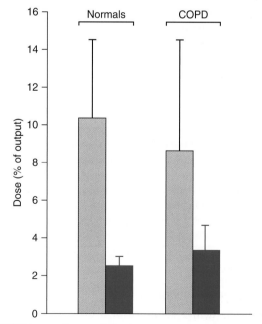

**FIGURE 5.18** Dose of drug delivered by metered dose inhaler *(grey columns)* compared to nebulizer *(purple columns)*. (From Dolovich et al. 1993.)

- ↑ exercise capacity
- ↑ lung function

The following may be suited to nebulizers:

- people who are too breathless or confused to use an inhaler;
- people who need large doses rapidly;
- antibiotic, antifungal or local anaesthetic drug delivery;
- patients for whom assessment has shown improved outcome compared with inhalers.

Deposition of the drug is improved by chest clearance beforehand, if indicated (Wolkove et al. 2001).

> *The young physician starts life with 20 drugs for each disease, and the old physician ends life with one drug for 20 diseases.*
>
> **William Osler**

## BRONCHOSCOPY AND LAVAGE

Access to the bronchial tree for diagnostic or therapeutic purposes is achieved by passing a fibreoptic bronchoscope through the nose and down into the subsegmental bronchi using local, nebulized or general anaesthesia. Complications include discomfort, laryngospasm, bronchospasm, bleeding, arrhythmias, infection, ↓ $PaO_2$, ↑ $PaCO_2$ (Sadot et al. 2016) and the complications of the suction pressure that is usually applied (Palazzo & Soni 2013). Hypoxaemia is reduced by using high-flow nasal oxygen (Papazian et al. 2016).

Diagnostically, bronchoscopy can be used for observation or biopsy. Brushings are used to obtain lower airway microbiology samples or identify parenchymal lung disease, and ultrasound assists diagnosis of peripheral lesions (Hayama et al. 2016). Lavage involves wedging the tube into a bronchus, washing 120–200 mL warm saline through a separate channel, then aspirating this along with fluid and cells from the lower respiratory tract and alveoli for diagnosing parenchymal lung disease.

Therapeutically, bronchoscopy can be used for lung volume reduction procedures, placing stents, identifying and resecting tumours, palliating upper airway cancers or removing foreign bodies. It may substitute for physiotherapy in clearing secretions if there is intractable sputum retention with no air bronchogram on X-ray, i.e. with blocked central airways. To re-expand atelectatic areas, it can be combined with selective insufflation of air, which needs to be followed by physiotherapy to prevent recurrence (Jelic et al. 2008).

Patients are usually told the 'why' of bronchoscopy, but not always the 'how'. Physiotherapists can check that patients understand the procedure and that they feel able to ask questions of their bronchoscopist, who tends to underestimate patients' level of tolerance (Hadzri et al. 2010). Distress is reduced by deep sedation (Haga et al. 2016b) or distraction techniques (Navidian et al. 2016).

## CASE STUDY: MR FJ

*A 32-year-old father from Eastbourne has been referred for 'twice weekly percussion and postural drainage'. He has polychondritis (chronic inflammation of the cartilage, including in the tracheobronchial tree), which has led to collapse of his tracheal and bronchial cartilages.*

### History of present complaint

Surgery on deformed chest and formation of tracheostomy 15 years ago

Discharged with instructions to change and clean tracheostomy tube twice weekly

### Medication

Prednisolone

### Social history

Lives with wife and three children, started office job 2 months ago, nonsmoker

### Subjective

- Occasional chest infections, last one 6 weeks ago, which has never quite resolved
- Always have a bit of phlegm, usually no problem clearing it but more difficult over the last 6 weeks
- Change tracheostomy tube 9-monthly
- Slightly breathless on exertion but not bothersome
- Tracheostomy tube sometimes causes a dry cough

### Objective

- Abnormal chest shape (Fig. 5.19)
- Respiratory rate normal
- Breathing pattern slightly laboured
- Clinically well hydrated
- Posture: round shoulders
- Auscultation: scattered crackles

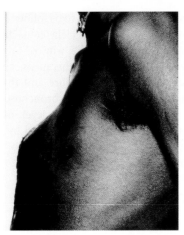

**FIGURE 5.19** Mr FJ.

## Questions

1. Why might Mr FJ have chest infections?
2. What could have prevented the last chest infection from being fully resolved, and what could be causing the difficulty in clearing his chest?
3. Is the breathlessness on exertion a problem?
4. Is the dry cough a problem?
5. Analysis?
6. Problems?
7. Goals?
8. Plan?

## Response to Case Study

1. Tracheostomy bypassing upper airway defences, infrequent tube changes.

2. Change in job 2 months ago: inactivity, dry office atmosphere.
3. It is not bothersome at present but may become so as Mr FJ ages and loses respiratory reserve.
4. It depends on whether it worries the patient.
5. No major disruption to lifestyle at present but potential for deterioration over time if chest infections recur.
6.
   • Risk of chest infections
   • Some sputum retention
   • Mild increase in WOB, probably due to chest shape
   • Potential for reduced exercise tolerance
7.
   • Reduce risk of infection
   • Increase exercise tolerance
8.
   • Negotiate more frequent tube changes. Twice weekly changes are unlikely to be adhered to and are probably not necessary at home (which is safer than the infection-prone hospital atmosphere). Motivate Mr FJ by explaining that a clean tube might reduce his dry cough.
   • Negotiate lifelong and achievable programme to prevent chest infections and maintain exercise tolerance, preferably based on enjoyable exercise, e.g. football with children, but offer variety of techniques for clearance of mucus (Chapter 7).
   • Discuss possible effects of office atmosphere.
   • Posture correction with advice on reminders, e.g. stickers on fridge.
   • Advise patient to ask general practitioner's advice on bone mineral density scan to check for steroid-induced osteoporosis.
   • Review 6-monthly by phone and yearly face-to-face.

# RECOMMENDED READING

Beaudart, C., Dawson, A., Shaw, S.C., et al., 2017. Nutrition and physical activity in the prevention and treatment of sarcopenia: systematic review. Osteoporos. Int. 28 (6), 1817–1833.

Berlinski, A., 2015. Assessing new technologies in aerosol medicine: strengths and limitations. Respir. Care 60 (6), 833–849.

Blakeman, T.C., 2013. Evidence for oxygen use in the hospitalized patient. Respir. Care 58 (10), 1679–1693.

Bossard, M.K., 2013. Help with metered dose inhalers. J. Asthma Allergy Educ. 4 (5), 237–239.

Braillon, A., Bewley, S., Herxheimer, A., et al., 2012. Marketing versus evidence-based medicine. Lancet 380 (9839), 340.

Bush, A., Pavord, I.D., 2013. Hot off the breath. Omalizumab: NICE to USE you, to LOSE you NICE. Thorax 68, 7–8.

Cates, C., 2013. Inhaled corticosteroids in COPD: quantifying risks and benefits. Thorax 68 (6), 499–500.

Chang, J., Erler, J., 2014. Hypoxia-mediated metastasis. Adv. Exp. Med. Biol. 772, 55–81.

Charlton, M., Thompson, J., 2017. Adverse drug reactions. Anaesth. Int. Care. Med. 18 (4), 205–209.

Chikhani, M., Hardman, J.G., 2013. Pharmacokinetic variation. Anaesth. Int. Care Med. 14 (3), 126–128.

Dai, B., Kang, J., Yu, N., et al., 2013. Oxygen injection site affects $F_IO_2$ during noninvasive ventilation. Respir. Care 58 (10), 1630–1636.

Delvadia, R.R., Longest, P.W., Hindle, M., et al., 2013. In vitro tests for aerosol deposition. J. Aerosol. Med. Pulm. Drug Deliv. 26 (3), 145–156.

Domenico, S., 2014. Current and novel bronchodilators in respiratory disease. Curr. Opin. Pulm. Med. 20 (1), 73–86.

DTB, 2017. An update on LAMA/LABA combinations for COPD. Drug Ther. Bull. 55 (1), 2–5.

Dyer, F., Callaghan, J., Cheema, K., et al., 2012. Ambulatory oxygen improves the effectiveness of pulmonary rehabilitation in selected patients with COPD. Chron. Respir. Dis. 9 (2), 83–91.

Esposito, S., 2017. Inhaled antibiotic therapy for the treatment of upper respiratory tract infections no access. J. Aerosol. Med. Pulm. Drug Deliv. 30 (1), 14–19.

Fink, J.B., 2013. Inhaler devices for patients with COPD. COPD 10 (4), 523–535.

Gariballa, S., Alessa, A., 2013. Sarcopenia: prevalence and prognostic significance in hospitalized patients. Clin. Nutr. 32 (5), 772–776.

Gomes, C.A., Jr., Lustosa, S.A., Matos, D., et al., 2012. Percutaneous endoscopic gastrostomy versus nasogastric tube feeding for adults with swallowing disturbances. Cochrane Database Syst. Rev. (3), CD008096.

Hatley, R.H.M., 2017. Variability in delivered dose from pressurized metered-dose inhaler formulations due to a delay between shake and fire. J. Aerosol. Med. Pulm. Drug Deliv. 30 (1), 71–77.

Heunks, M.A., Abdo, W.F., 2012. Oxygen-induced hypercapnia in COPD: myths and facts. Crit. Care 16, 323–326.

Jahedi, L., 2017. Inhaler technique in asthma: how does it relate to patients' preferences and attitudes toward their inhalers. J. Aerosol. Med. Pulm. Drug Deliv. 30 (1), 42–52.

Kamin, W., 2014. Inhalation solutions – which ones may be mixed? Physico-chemical compatibility of drug solutions in nebulizers – update 2013. J. Cyst. Fibros. 13 (3), 243–250.

Kane, B., Decalmer, S., O'Driscoll, R., 2013. Emergency oxygen therapy: from guideline to implementation. Breathe 9, 246–253.

Lafond, J., 2016. Pharmacovigilance implemented by patients. Therapie 71 (2), 245–247.

Levy, M.L., Dekhuijzen, P.N.R., Barnes, P.J., et al., 2016. Inhaler technique: facts and fantasies. NPJ Prim. Care Respir. Med. 26, 16017.

Longest, P.W., 2013. High-efficiency generation and delivery of aerosols through nasal cannula during noninvasive ventilation. J. Aerosol. Med. Pulm. Drug Deliv. 26 (5), 266–279.

Morley, J.E., 2014. Cognition and nutrition. Curr. Opin. Clin. Nutr. Metab. Care 17 (1), 1–4.

Mulhall, A.M., Zafar, M.A., Record, S., et al., 2017. A tablet-based multimedia education tool improves provider and subject knowledge of inhaler use techniques. Respir. Care 62 (2), 163–171.

Myers, T.R., 2013. The science guiding selection of an aerosol delivery device. Respir. Care 58 (11), 1963–1973.

Nedel, W.L., 2017. High-flow nasal cannula in critically ill subjects with or at risk for respiratory failure. Respir. Care 62 (1), 123–132.

Olivieri, D., Chetta, A., 2014. Therapeutic perspectives in vascular remodeling in asthma and chronic obstructive pulmonary disease. Chem. Immunol. Allergy 99, 216–225.

Peel, D., 2013. Evaluation of oxygen concentrators for use in countries with limited resources. Anaesthesia 68, 706–712.

Pinto, T., 2017. Mouthpiece ventilation and complementary techniques in patients with neuromuscular disease. Chron. Respir. Dis. 14 (2), 1–7.

Pitance, L., Reychler, G., Leal, T., et al., 2013. Aerosol delivery to the lung is more efficient using an extension with a standard jet nebulizer than an open-vent jet nebulizer. J. Aerosol. Med. Pulm. Drug Deliv. 26 (4), 208–214.

Ramadan, W.H., Sarkis, A.T., 2017. Patterns of use of dry powder inhalers versus pressurized metered-dose inhalers devices in adult patients with chronic obstructive pulmonary disease or asthma. Chron. Respir. Dis. 14 (3), 309–320.

Sanford, A.M., .5Flaherty, J.H., 2014. Do nutrients play a role in delirium? Curr. Opin. Clin. Nutr. Metab. Care 17 (1), 45–50.

Schols, A.M., 2013. Nutrition as a metabolic modulator in COPD. Chest 144 (4), 1340–1345.

Spina, D., 2014. Current and novel bronchodilators in respiratory disease. Curr. Opin. Pulm. Med. 20 (1), 73–86.

Stass, H., 2017. Ciprofloxacin dry powder for inhalation in patients with non-cystic fibrosis bronchiectasis or chronic obstructive pulmonary disease, and in healthy volunteers. J. Aerosol. Med. Pulm. Drug Deliv. 30 (1), 53–63.

Suissa, S., Dell'Aniello, S., Ernst, P., 2017. Long-acting bronchodilator initiation in COPD and the risk of adverse cardiopulmonary events: a population-based comparative safety study. Chest 151 (1), 60–67.

Vargas, O., 2013. The use of metered-dose inhalers in hospital environments. J. Aerosol. Med. Pulm. Drug Deliv. 26 (5), 287–296.

Yawn, B.P., Colice, G.L., Hodder, R., 2012. Practical aspects of inhaler use in the management of chronic obstructive pulmonary disease in the primary care setting. Int. J. Chron. Obstruct. Pulmon. Dis. 7, 495–502.

# Physiotherapy to Increase Lung Volume

## INTRODUCTION TO CARDIORESPIRATORY PHYSIOTHERAPY

*When applying evidence-based care, clinicians should ensure that each of their individual patients is involved in decision making.*

**Lodewijckx et al. 2012**

What is cardiorespiratory physiotherapy? And does it work? The aims are to facilitate oxygen delivery to the tissues and improve a patient's quality of life. Methods to achieve this include education, manual and mechanical techniques, accurately targeted exercise, reflective practice and response to patients in distress. It is ineffective to intervene with a process as personal as breathing without attention to the person as a whole.

Patients have described a physiotherapist's sensitivity and attentiveness as the most important part of the intervention; this includes praise, honesty, and encouraging patients' own ideas (Wood et al. 2013). Involving patients in goal-setting improves outcomes (Arnetz et al. 2004), and our strongest tool is how we listen, validate and respond to patients. Humane care can save time (Mansfield 2013) and is compatible with evidence-based practice (Box 6.1).

A suggested approach is to:
- assess the patient
- identify problems
- clarify expectations and negotiate SMART goals (see next paragraph)
- agree a management plan and time frame
- apply education and treatment

**179**

## BOX 6.1   Challenging Dogma (1)

*'Suffering, apparently, is not evidence based. Does this mean that we should discourage or shun evidence-based studies? Certainly not. Does it mean that it is so impossible to understand the subjective experience of another person that we shouldn't try? Absolutely not. It does mean that evidence-based methodologies are just one set of tools, useful for understanding certain aspects of reality, but not necessarily the best for understanding others.'*

Hallenbeck (2008)

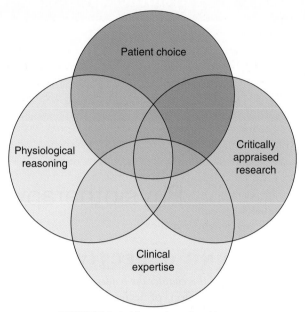

**FIGURE 6.1** Hierarchy of evidence.

- re-assess
- discuss and modify the plan according to ongoing assessment
- check if goals are met

Using the preceding approach and the ICF (p. 29), education should be reinforced in writing in order to improve adherence. Patient handouts should be explicit, short, clear and copied for the physiotherapy notes. For hospital patients, these can be kept on memory sticks and slotted into ward computers so that they can be individualized for each patient. In the community, standard handouts (Appendix B) may be used, or they can be individualized back in the office and sent to patients, to include their name, exercises to suit their home environment, and advice on where to put reminder sticky notes or tie stretchy bands.

Autonomy is facilitated by working with patients to set their own SMART goals, which are:

- specific
- measurable
- achievable
- relevant
- time-based (Bowman et al. 2016)

These should be regularly reviewed and involve the family if appropriate.

Evidence-based practice is facilitated by Fig. 6.1. This is a reminder that, for a profession backed by limited research, 'absence of evidence is not evidence of absence'.

An example of the physiological reasoning component is in Box 6.2.

Chapters 7–10 facilitate accurate treatment by distinguishing the three respiratory problems of reduced lung volume, increased work of breathing and sputum retention. They include the experience of patients so that

## BOX 6.2   Challenging Dogma (2)

*'Is IPPB a useful modality or a dangerous weapon in CF? We are told that IPPB is contraindicated in CF for risk of causing a pneumothorax. Is this a real or theoretical risk? Does anyone have proof of pneumothorax? The intrathoracic pressures generated during coughing (a frequent forced expiratory manoeuvre in CF) must surely exceed the pressures produced by IPPB? I have used IPPB—cautiously— and have found it invaluable when the patient is exhausted during chest infection and finding it difficult to cooperate. I would like to hear a well-reasoned argument against this practice and if one cannot be produced perhaps we should remove it from the contraindications and place it amongst the precautions.'*

Bastow (2006)

*CF,* Cystic fibrosis; *IPPB,* intermittent positive pressure breathing.

empathy can be nurtured, without which the effectiveness of physiotherapy is limited.

*Science is validating what humans have known throughout the ages: that compassion is not a luxury; it is a necessity.*

***Halifax 2011***

# WHAT IS LOSS OF LUNG VOLUME AND DOES IT MATTER?

Normally, lung volume is maintained by position change, mobility and sighs taken 9–10 times an hour (Hartland et al. 2015), but some patients are not able to sustain this.

The following conditions involve a degree of lost lung volume, anatomically or functionally or both, and with varying degrees of responsiveness to physiotherapy.

1. Atelectasis is collapse of anything from a few alveoli to the whole lung. Segmental, lobar, and lung collapse are evident on X-ray (Cortés & Martínez 2013), or by reduced breath sounds/bronchial breathing, depending on size (p. 45). Causes include prolonged periods of shallow breathing, pleural disorder, surfactant depletion, diaphragm inhibition from poor positioning, pain, compression from abdominal distension or neurological impairment, or a mucous plug large enough to obstruct an airway above the level of collateral ventilation (Qanneta 2016). Some of these causes are responsive to physiotherapy. All are relevant to physiotherapy. Hypoxic vasoconstriction (p. 13) can compensate for a degree of atelectasis, but significant lost volume decreases lung compliance (see Fig. 1.6), impairs oxygenation (van Aswegen & Eales 2004), risks alveolar injury (Duggan & Kavanagh 2005) and, if due to a blocked airway, interrupts mucociliary clearance and facilitates bacterial growth distal to the blockage (Wanner et al. 1996). Physiotherapy is indicated to treat or prevent atelectasis if it is caused or anticipated by immobility, poor positioning, mucous plug or diaphragm dysfunction.

2. Consolidation, indicated by opacity on X-ray and bronchial breathing, reduces functioning lung volume. Physiological reasoning indicates that it is not possible to break down this inflammatory process by physical means, but the effects may be ameliorated by positioning or mobilization.

3. Pleural effusion, pneumothorax and abdominal distension compress the lung but are themselves inaccessible to physiotherapy. Positioning may improve comfort or gas exchange, and sometimes the patient may need assistance to re-expand the lung after the cause has been resolved.

4. Other restrictive disorders of the lung or chest wall (pp. 100–113) reduce lung volume. The conditions themselves may not respond to physical treatment, but physiotherapy will usually be required for the patient as a whole.

Does atelectasis matter? Loss of lung volume is a problem if it causes a significant degree of:

- reduced surface area for gas exchange, leading to ventilation/perfusion ($\dot{V}_A/\dot{Q}$) mismatch and ↓ peripheral oxygen saturation ($SpO_2$);
- reduced lung compliance;
- increased work of breathing.

Choice of technique to resolve these, as with other problems, is best achieved by reflective practice, listening to the patient, and clinical reasoning, the latter incorporating practical, intuitive and ethical reasoning (Jensen & Greenfield 2012).

## CONTROLLED MOBILIZATION

The most fruitful technique for lung recruitment is getting up and walking (Dean 2006). When accurately targeted, this combines the upright posture, which reduces pressure on the diaphragm, with natural deep breathing. It is the first-line treatment for patients who can get out of bed.

To ensure accuracy, the level of activity is controlled so that patients become slightly breathless, but not enough to cause muscle tension. They are then asked to lean against a wall to get their breath back, while being discouraged from talking, which would upset the breathing rhythm. Relaxing against a wall minimizes postural activity of the abdominal muscles, allowing the diaphragm to descend more freely. The controlled 'slight breathlessness' can then become deep breathing, rather than wasted as shallow apical breathing. Nonsurgical patients can hold their hands behind their back while leaning against the wall, which stabilizes the chest and facilitates diaphragmatic descent.

Patients who are not able to walk can use controlled activity by simply transferring from bed to chair, then getting their breath back by relaxing against the back of the chair. Even less ambitiously, when bed-bound patients have rolled onto their side, they can be encouraged to relax with their nondependent arm resting on a pillow, which facilitates deep breathing as they recover their breath.

Once patients understand these principles and can identify the feeling of 'slight breathlessness' and 'getting their breath back', they can practice on their own, using walking and their normal functional activities as a medium for improving lung volume. Regular graded exercise can then be facilitated.

The body's reaction on moving from supine to standing (p. 25) is inhibited after prolonged immobility, requiring a longer time sitting over the edge of the bed before standing up. Other safety precautions when mobilizing patients are the following:

- check the patient's notes for risks, e.g. if haemoglobin is low, this may be a contraindication to walking, but usually patients can be mobilized with caution if they are asymptomatic and do not need transfusion;
- check brakes on beds, chairs and wheelchairs;
- place chairs strategically in advance, supported against a wall;
- for stairs, place chairs on landings;
- safeguard intravenous lines;
- avoid holding any arm that is using a walking aid;
- ensure patients keep their hands out of their pockets; if dyspnoea obliges them to facilitate accessory muscle function by stabilizing their arms, they can hook just their thumbs into their pocket or a belt;
- for the first 24 h after surgery, watch the patient's face for colour change, which might indicate postural hypotension caused by preoperative fluid restriction and perioperative fluid shifts;
- discourage breath-holding;
- when sitting a patient in a chair or wheelchair, add stability by tucking a foot behind the chair leg or wheel;
- stand below the patient when going up or down stairs.

For patients who are unstable or have been immobile for an extended period, further safety precautions are on p. 503.

## POSITIONING

Positioning is incorporated into the treatment of patients with any of the three respiratory problems. It can be used in its own right or in conjunction with other techniques. This chapter covers patients who have lost lung volume, and, as this affects ventilation, how mismatch with perfusion affects gas exchange. Other aspects of positioning are mentioned when relevant.

> **PRACTICE TIP**
>
> No treatment should be carried out without consideration of the position in which it is performed.

## The Physiology of Positioning

1. Functional residual capacity (FRC) increases progressively from supine, to sitting, to standing (Fig. 6.2A). Overall it doubles from supine to upright (Harris 2005). This is due to a reduction in pressure from the viscera against the diaphragm and reduced thoracic blood volume as gravity draws blood away from the chest.
2. FRC increases from supine to side-lying (Fig. 6.2B) or prone (Fink 2002).
3. Slumped lying can sometimes be worse than supine due to pressure from the abdominal contents (Olsén 2005).
4. Lung compliance increases and work of breathing (WOB) decreases, from supine, through sitting, to standing. WOB is 40% higher in supine than sitting (Wahba 1991), partly because of the load against the diaphragm and partly because small airways collapse and push the lungs down the compliance curve (see Fig. 1.6).
5. Compliance, FRC and $SpO_2$ tend to be higher in side-lying than supine (Frownfelter & Dean 2006). $SpO_2$ is worse in supine than in a comfortable upright position (BTS 2017).
6. Side-lying significantly increases the proportion of ventilation directed to dependent lung regions, compared to upright (Wettstein et al. 2014), although this varies with age. At the same time, the upper lung has the greatest volume (Duggan & Kavanagh 2005) because it is pulled open by the weight of the mediastinum and the other lung dragging down on it (see Fig. 1.9C). Although lungs consist of mostly air by volume, they are relatively heavy because of the weight of their circulating blood.
7. In right-side-lying, rolling the patient forward into semi-prone further increases basal lung volume in the upper lung because it is even less compressed by the heart (Mase et al. 2016).

### Positioning for Lung Volume

The following principles apply to immobile or relatively immobile patients who have atelectasis or potential atelectasis.

1. *Sitting upright* in a comfortable chair improves lung function (Nielsen 2003) so long as the patient is relaxed, which allows the diaphragm to descend. The benefit is limited if the patient is obese or has a distended abdomen (Fig. 6.3). A foot stool tends to encourage the slumped position, and may also stretch

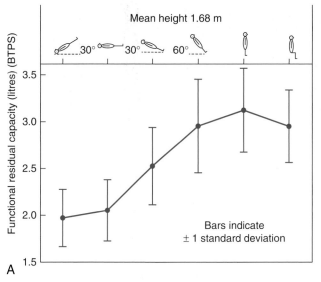

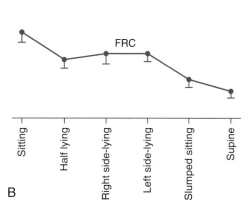

**FIGURE 6.2** (A) Functional residual capacity (FRC) in different positions (From Lumb 2010). *BTPS,* body temperature and pressure, saturated. (B) FRC as a percentage of the sitting value. 'Sitting' means sitting upright with legs dependent (From Jenkins et al. 1998).

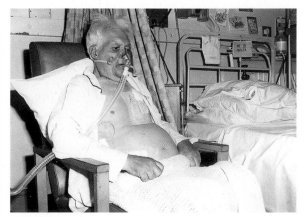

**FIGURE 6.3** Sitting. Mr C has an acute abdomen, which is too rigid to move with respiration. He is sitting upright and with supported arms, but breathing is still restricted by pressure from the abdominal contents.

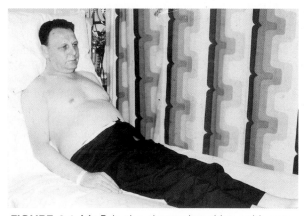

**FIGURE 6.4** Mr B in the slumped position, with pressure from the abdominal contents restricting diaphragmatic descent.

the sciatic nerve and overload lumbar disc pressures, but some patients need it for comfort, ankle oedema or a recent vein graft. Sitting for prolonged periods risks pressure sores (Ribeiro et al. 2015), especially with the feet up because this tilts the pelvis backward onto the sacrum, but patients will be uncomfortable long before this and need to be returned to bed when they ask.

2. *Half-lying* rapidly becomes the *slumped position* for most patients as they slide down the bed (Fig. 6.4). Time in half-lying should be limited for patients with reduced lung volume, unless necessary for a specific medical reason, or to minimize pain, or if the patient finds it the most comfortable position.

3. Time should be spent in *side-lying*, well forward so that the diaphragm is free from abdominal pressure (Fig. 6.5). Side-lying can also be encouraged for

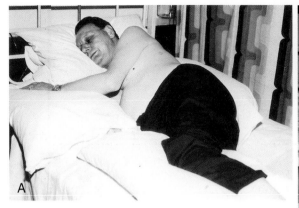

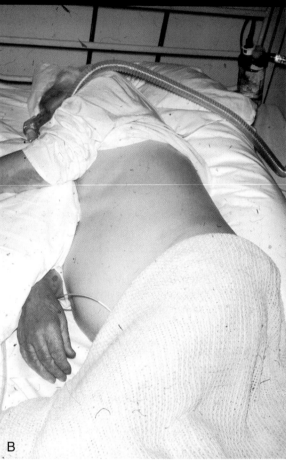

FIGURE 6.5 (A) Mr B in side-lying position. The abdominal contents are now free to fall away from the diaphragm but the left arm is not supported (thus recruiting abdominal muscle activity) and the head is slightly too high (exerting some pressure on the left lower lobe). (B) Mr C in side-lying position. The patient is rolled well forward, has a supported left arm and only one pillow, so the diaphragm is free from pressure.

sleeping. Relatively immobile patients should turn, or be turned, 2-hourly in order to maintain comfort, lung volume and skin integrity.

---

**PRACTICE TIP**

Compare breath sounds over your patient's lower lobes in different positions.

---

4. The supine position is unhelpful for gas exchange (O'Driscoll et al. 2008), and lying down for lengthy periods is best avoided, especially for patients who have a high closing volume, e.g. those who smoke or are elderly or obese. Obese people lose 50% of their vital capacity in supine: Allman & Wilson (2011), and McCallister et al. (2010) describe improved lung function for this group of patients with the whole bed tilted head up by 45 degrees.
5. Walking is ideal.

## Positioning for Gas Exchange

Positioning for lung volume and for gas exchange usually go hand in hand, but to optimize $\dot{V}_A/\dot{Q}$ matching in people with unilateral lung disorders, specific considerations apply. Reduced ventilation on the affected side overrides any physiological ventilation gradient

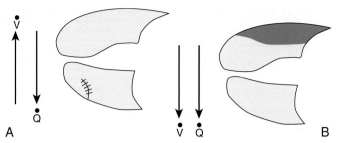

**FIGURE 6.6** Effect of positioning with one-sided pathology, e.g. thoracotomy or unilateral pneumonia. With the affected lung dependent (A) the better-ventilated upper lung does not match the better-perfused lower lung. With the affected lung uppermost (B) the lower lung is both better ventilated and better perfused. $\dot{V}$, Ventilation; $\dot{Q}$, perfusion.

(p. 11) and lying with the affected lung uppermost leads to better ventilation of the dependent normal lung, which is matched with its better perfusion (Fig. 6.6).

However, patients vary and clinical reasoning suggests the following order of preference when positioning patients for optimum lung volume and gas exchange:
1. patient comfort (patients do not breathe well if uncomfortable);
2. oxygen saturation (this may take precedence over patient comfort if $SpO_2$ is compromised);
3. The physiological reasoning above.

As well as optimizing gas exchange, the 'affected lung up' rule promotes comfort following thoracotomy or chest drain placement, facilitates postural drainage, and helps improve lung volume when atelectatic lung is positioned uppermost to encourage expansion (Tucker & Jenkins 1996).

Exceptions to the 'affected lung up' rule are:
- recent pneumonectomy (p. 313);
- large pleural effusion (p. 105 and Fig. 2.18);
- bronchopleural fistula, in case unsavoury substances drain into the unaffected dependent lung;
- occasionally if there is a large tumour in a main stem bronchus (Fig. 6.7), because, with the affected side uppermost, the tumour may obstruct the bronchus and cause breathlessness;
- any situation in which the oximeter or patient comfort contradicts the above.

These are guidelines only and patients need individual assessment.

For people without unilateral disease, the prone position delivers the most homogenous ventilation (Riera

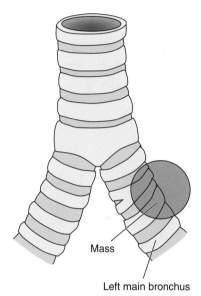

Mass

Left main bronchus

**FIGURE 6.7** Tumour in left main bronchus, which may obstruct the airway if the patient is positioned with this side uppermost.

et al. 2013), which is normally impractical except for some people with acute respiratory distress syndrome (p. 547).

After treatment, the physiotherapist should clarify to nursing staff why the patient has been left in a specific position, explaining that this should be maintained until the patient wants to move or it is time to turn. Night staff should be included in training on positioning. Oximetry is useful to demonstrate the effectiveness of positioning to patient, family and staff.

# BREATHING EXERCISES TO INCREASE LUNG VOLUME

Deep breathing to increase lung volume may be required for patients who have demonstrable atelectasis and are relatively immobile. There is no evidence for a preventive effect, but clinical reasoning suggests that prophylactic deep breathing may be beneficial for high risk patients, e.g. following oesophagectomy, so long as it is done accurately. It should be performed in cycles of no more than three to four breaths so that maximum effort is put into each breath, dizziness from overbreathing is avoided and shoulder tension inhibited.

## Deep Breathing

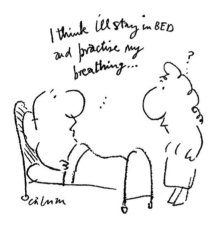

Mel Calman.

Optimum conditions are needed to ensure that the deep breaths reach peripheral lung regions, i.e.:
- minimum pain, nausea, dry mouth, discomfort, fatigue, anxiety or tension;
- accurate positioning, usually alternate side-lying inclined toward prone, to facilitate expansion of the base of the uppermost lung (Nozoe et al. 2014);
- avoidance of distractions;
- minimum breathlessness, e.g. patients having time to get their breath back after turning;
- taking a slow steady breath to maintain laminar flow (Fig. 6.8).

Breathless people should not be asked to breathe slowly.

If side-lying is undesirable, upright sitting is the next option. Long-sitting might be necessary in some circumstances but limit diaphragmatic descent.

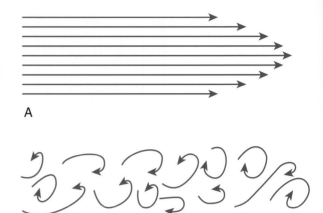

FIGURE 6.8 (A) A slow smooth breath facilitates laminar flow and peripheral distribution of inhaled gas. (B) A fast breath encourages unhelpful turbulence.

When patients are relaxed and have got their breath back, they are asked to breathe in through their nose, deeply and slowly to ensure optimal distribution of ventilation, then sigh out. A demonstration is usually required. Breathing through the nose warms and humidifies the air but doubles resistance to airflow, and patients may need to mouth-breathe if they are breathless or have a nasogastric tube. Some respond better when asked to take a long breath rather than a deep breath, or when asked to 'breathe in your favourite smell'. Monitoring is by observation that abdominal and rib cage excursion are maximal but without counterproductive tension. Subtle changes in instruction can help this balancing act of a breath that is both deep and relaxed.

Distribution of ventilation is related to position, flow and pathology. The physiotherapist's hands may be placed over the basal area for monitoring purposes and for patient reassurance, but not with any assumption that this magically redistributes ventilation to the underlying lung. Similarly, 'localized' breathing exercises do not make physiological sense because humans are unable to deform individual portions of the chest wall. Even so, patients can still be found obediently performing 'unilateral breathing' and 'basal costal breathing'. If localized breathing were physically possible, as in some yogi masters, the way in which the two layers of pleura slide over each other means that the lung responds generally rather than locally to a deep breath.

After every few breaths, the patient should relax and regain their rhythm. Breathing rate and pattern should be observed at this time, and the patient may need praise or a change in instruction before proceeding. Patients should not be engaged in conversation between cycles.

> **PRACTICE TIP**
>
> Sometimes patients are more relaxed and breathe more effectively between a cycle of deep breaths than during the deep breathing itself, in which case attention should be paid to minimizing tension during the next cycle.

Deep breathing has shown the following benefits:
- ↑ diaphragmatic displacement and basal ventilation (Brasher et al. 2003);
- ↓ atelectasis, ↑ oxygenation, preferential gas distribution to dependent regions (Westerdahl 2015);
- ↑ lung compliance and $\dot{V}_A/\dot{Q}$ matching (Agostini & Singh 2009);
- ↓ airway resistance (Hillman 2013);
- ↑ mucociliary clearance (Button & Boucher 2008).

Slow deep breathing can reduce stress, anxiety, chronic pain and depression (Woo 2016), and can help stabilize alveoli (Tomich et al. 2010). Relaxed slow deep breathing may reduce heart rate, blood pressure (Fig. 6.9) and oxygen consumption (Dick et al. 2014).

Rhythmic breathing has the effects described on p. 237. The benefits for postoperative patients are on p. 302.

The term 'thoracic expansion exercises' is synonymous with deep breathing but care must be taken to ensure that more than the thorax is expanding. The art of deep breathing is to allow the abdominal muscles to relax and the diaphragm to descend.

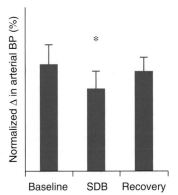

**FIGURE 6.9** Reduction in mean arterial blood pressure *(BP)* caused by slow deep breathing *(SDB)*. (From Dick et al. 2014.)

Ten deep breaths every waking hour are considered necessary to maintain lung volume (Westerdahl 2015). This is a tall order for those who are distracted by the events and uncertainties of hospital life, and a tick chart or incentive spirometer (p. 189) can be useful reminders.

Controlled mobilization (p. 181) is a more functional way of increasing lung volume, but some patients need deep breathing as well as mobilization because the former increases tidal volume, whereas the latter mainly increases respiratory rate (Durrant & Moore 2004).

### End-Inspiratory Hold

Air can be coaxed into poorly ventilated regions by including a breath-hold for a few seconds at the end of a full inspiration. This boosts collateral ventilation, distributes air more evenly between lung segments and is thought to be as important as the volume inspired (Tomich et al. 2010). Observation will identify if the end-inspiratory hold is effective, comfortable or, conversely, disturbs the breathing pattern. Accurate instruction is needed to prevent shoulder girdle tension. The end-inspiratory hold is unsuited to breathless people because it upsets their breathing pattern.

### Abdominal Breathing

When used in an appropriate position, abdominal breathing (p. 237) can increase lung volume if used with an emphasis on the depth of the breath (Fig. 6.10) and may improve lung inflation and oxygenation in postoperative patients (Alaparthi et al. 2016).

### Sniff

Even after a full inspiration, it is often possible to squeeze in a wee bit more air and further augment collateral ventilation by taking a sharp sniff at end-inspiration, which facilitates diaphragmatic action (Cahalin et al. 2002). Sceptical patients can be won over by a reminder that however packed a rush-hour underground train is, an extra person can usually squeeze in.

### Neurophysiological Facilitation of Respiration

Lung volume may be increased by indirect stimulation, for example:
- perioral stimulation, applied for 10 s just above the top lip;
- intercostal stretch, applied unilaterally or bilaterally on exhalation (Fig. 6.11).

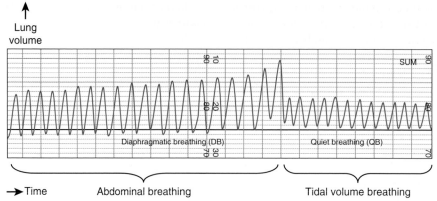

FIGURE 6.10 Increased lung volume with abdominal breathing. (From Fernandes et al. 2011.)

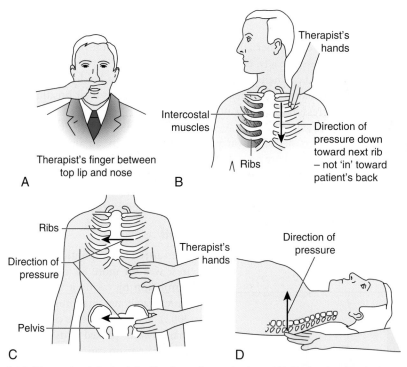

FIGURE 6.11 Neurophysiological facilitation of respiration. (A) Perioral stimulation: moderate pressure inwards and downwards. (B) Intercostal stretch: firm pressure downwards on ribs 2 and 3. (C) Co-contraction: pressure against lower ribs and pelvis, applied at right angles on alternate sides and maintaining pressure for up to 2 min or until desired effect. (D) Vertebral pressure: finger pressure against vertebrae between T2 and T10. (Adapted from Davis 1996.)

The mechanism of these techniques may relate to stimulation of the suckling reflex and intercostal muscle stretch reflex respectively (Chang et al. 2002).

Other effects are yawning, coughing and abdominal contraction (Jones 1998). Some patients vary in their response from breath to breath and day to day. It is worth trying slightly different finger positions and pressures can be tried, and sometimes finger vibrations. Effects may be cumulative.

The technique is useful for some drowsy patients, those with neurological conditions, in whom excess tone may decrease (Bethune 1994) and patients on assisted ventilation, especially if they are unable to turn.

## Rib Springing

Rib springing is chest compression during expiration, with overpressure downward and inward in the bucket handle direction of rib movement, then a quick release at end-expiration. This may cause a deeper subsequent inspiration.

## INCENTIVE SPIROMETRY

A sustained deep breath can be facilitated by an incentive spirometer, which gives visual feedback on volume and flow, and when used regularly can both prevent and reverse atelectasis (AARC 2011). The Coach, Voldyne and Respivol (Fig. 6.12) are **volume** devices that encourage slow and controlled inhalation by maintaining a marker (indicating flow) between two marks, and encourage a deep breath by raising a disc (indicating volume) to the level of the clip, which is raised as the patient improves. The end-inspiratory hold is maintained while the disc descends. These devices impose half the work of breathing of the other incentive spirometers, encourage abdominal rather than ribcage

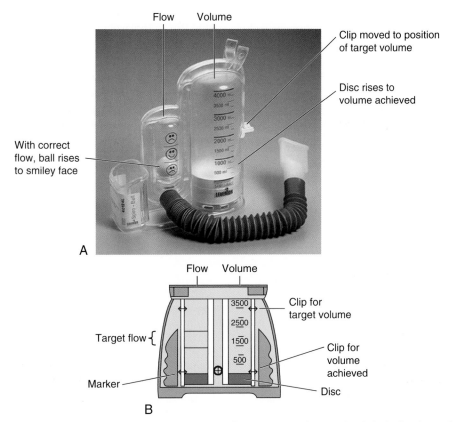

**FIGURE 6.12** Volume incentive spirometers: (A) Spiroball, the disc on the right indicating volume and the ball on the left indicating flow; (B) Respivol (Henleys).

motion (Agostini & Singh 2009), lead to slower, deeper breathing (Tomich et al. 2010) and increase chest wall volume (Paisan 2013).

**Flow** devices are slightly less patient-friendly. The Triflo (Fig. 6.13A) controls flow by the patient inhaling so that two out of three plastic balls are raised, the third being a control, which should not move because this indicates excess flow and therefore turbulence. An end-inspiratory hold is maintained for 3–5 s while the balls are suspended. It is possible to cheat by taking short sharp breaths, and some patients enjoy turning it upside down and blowing.

The Mediflo Duo (Fig. 6.13B) is cheap and cheerful, and can also be used as a PEP device (p. 214). For incentive spirometry, the tubing is inserted into the side and the top hole blocked. The pointer is turned to the target number on the blue scale and the patient breathes in until the ball floats, then holds his or her breath for the end-inspiratory hold by keeping the ball floating.

Suggested technique is the following:

1. A demonstration is given using a separate device kept for teaching purposes.
2. Patients should be relaxed and positioned as for deep breathing, either side-lying (particularly if extra

volume is required for one lung) or sitting upright, preferably in a chair with their feet down.

3. With lips sealed around the mouthpiece, the patient inhales slowly and deeply. He or she watches the flow indicator while the physiotherapist monitors the patient's breathing pattern.
4. An end-inspiratory hold is sustained if possible.
5. After exhalation, normal breathing is resumed and shoulder girdle relaxation rechecked.

Patients are advised to take ten incentive spirometry breaths per waking hour. Those on oxygen can use nasal cannulae or an incentive spirometer that entrains oxygen. People with a tracheostomy stoma can use a connection via a paediatric face mask (Garg & Dutta 2016).

The same effect can be obtained by deep breathing without the incentive spirometer, but the incentive of using a device often creates greater inhaled volume, a more controlled flow and more enthusiasm to practice. However, individuals vary, as does the research, which is either positive (Wren et al. 2010) or neutral (Makhabah et al. 2013). In particular, benefits have been found after abdominal surgery (p. 308). Observation of expansion and breathing pattern is therefore required to identify whether the patient takes a deep breath more effectively with or without the device.

Incentive spirometry can be learned by demonstration and is suitable for children, including those with cerebral palsy because it can assist breath control for speech production (Choi et al. 2016b). It is not suited to breathless people, and those with fragile lungs should not use it too vehemently because a pneumothorax has been recorded in a person with emphysema (Kenny 2013).

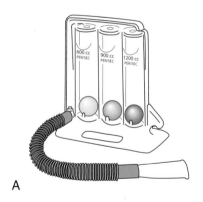

A

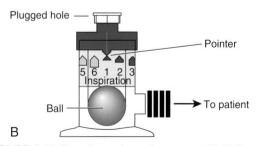

B

**FIGURE 6.13** Flow incentive spirometers: (A) Triflo and (B) Mediflo (Henleys).

**MINI CLINICAL REASONING**

Q. Is there logic in the following arguments?

*'There is little evidence to support the use of incentive spirometry in airway clearance...'*
      *Eur. Respir. J.* (1999), 14, 1418–1424

*'Incentive spirometry is not a sensitive method for the study of pulmonary function'*
      *Am. Assoc. Osteopathy J.* (1995), Fall, 9–13

A. Incentive spirometry is not intended for airway clearance or for pulmonary function testing.

# CONTINUOUS POSITIVE AIRWAY PRESSURE (CPAP)

For spontaneously breathing patients who cannot muster the breath for incentive spirometry, FRC can be improved by a device that delivers continuous positive pressure by face mask. This improves gas exchange by pneumatically splinting open the alveoli. The same effect is achieved with the grunting adopted by infants in respiratory distress and the yelp used by some tennis players.

Compared to noninvasive ventilation, CPAP delivers the same flow of gas throughout inspiration and expiration, exceeding the flow rate of patients even when they are breathless. It is like a person putting their head out of the window of a speeding car, and, along with the tight-fitting mask (Fig. 6.14), is not comfortable. A full face mask or a helmet (Luo et al. 2016) may be better tolerated. Alternatively, modest positive pressure can be achieved by a high-flow nasal cannula (p. 154) or a cheap 'bubble-CPAP' device (Walk et al. 2016).

## Effects and Indications

When comfort is optimized, CPAP increases FRC (Fig. 6.15) and has been found useful for people with the following:

- pneumonia (Brambilla et al. 2014) or pulmonary oedema (Luiz et al. 2016);
- flail chest (Pettiford et al. 2007), which can be stabilized more comfortably with the steady pressure of CPAP than with the varying pressures of assisted ventilation (Fig. 6.16), so long as there is no barotrauma;
- postoperative patients (Ireland et al. 2014).

Raising the FRC is primarily aimed at improving gas exchange rather than recruiting lung volume. Atelectasis may be prevented by CPAP, but resolution of established atelectasis requires an increase in tidal volume rather than FRC.

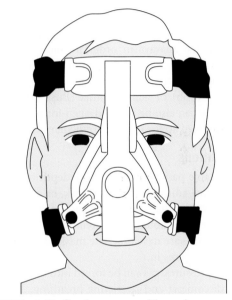

**FIGURE 6.14** Continuous positive airway pressure mask.

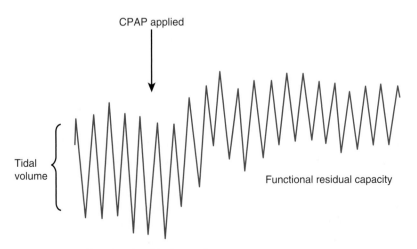

**FIGURE 6.15** Effect of continuous positive airway pressure (CPAP) on lung volumes, showing the rise in FRC.

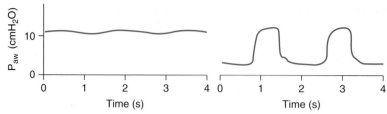

**FIGURE 6.16** Pressure–time waveforms for CPAP (left) and noninvasive ventilation, which delivers reduced pressure on expiration (right). $P_{aw}$, Airway pressure.

As well as splinting open the alveoli, CPAP may also splint open the airways in order to allow escape of trapped gas and reduce hyperinflation in people with severe chronic obstructive pulmonary disease (COPD) (Sun et al. 2016b) or acute asthma (Busk 2013). The upper airway can also be splinted open for people with obstructive sleep apnoea, using domiciliary CPAP.

## Complications

Uncomfortable patients restrict their depth of breathing. Individual adjustment of the mask, or a change of mask, can prevent chafed skin, sore ears or dry eyes. The bridge of the nose should be covered before rather than after a pressure sore develops. The mask seal is assisted by keeping dentures in.

At high pressures, gas can be forced into the stomach, causing discomfort and restricting breathing. The risk is reduced by using a nasogastric tube, although this may interfere with the mask seal. CPAP also depresses the swallowing reflex (Nishino 2012) thus risking aspiration.

Coughing requires removal or adjustment of the mask to avoid high pressures that may damage the ears or, with emphysema or late-stage cystic fibrosis cause a pneumothorax. CPAP should only be used on wards with access to chest drain equipment.

High pressures may compress alveolar vessels, redistribute blood from the chest to the abdomen, increase right ventricular afterload and reduce cardiac output.

$CO_2$ retention can occur if a hypercapnic patient breathes with a small tidal volume against a high pressure setting.

## Contraindications and Precautions

CPAP should not be used in the presence of:
- barotrauma: undrained pneumothorax, subcutaneous emphysema or large bulla

- inability to protect the airway from aspiration
- facial trauma including surgery (Chebel et al. 2010)
- excessive secretions
- haemoptysis of unknown cause
- type II respiratory failure.

It should be used with caution in the presence of:
- major hemodynamic instability;
- intracranial pressure >15 mmHg;
- a bronchopleural fistula;
- a large tumour in the proximal airways, because gas under pressure may be able to enter but not exit past the obstruction.

A nasogastric tube is required if CPAP is used:
- following oesophageal surgery, to prevent positive pressure jeopardizing the anastomosis;
- in the presence of nausea because vomiting into a sealed mask against a rush of positive pressure risks aspiration, and is not a happy experience.

CPAP for people who do not need it tends to overdistend the lungs and increase oxygen consumption (Soilemezi et al. 2016).

## Technique

The high flows of CPAP require an efficient heated humidifier to safeguard the cilia (Sommer et al. 2013), but a heat–moisture exchanger may be adequate for short periods.

A suggested procedure is the following:
1. Patients should be in a high-dependency area or close to the nurses' station on a dedicated respiratory ward.
2. After explanations and consent, a pressure is chosen that is low enough to be tolerable but high enough to maintain adequate gas exchange, usually 5–10 $cmH_2O$.
3. The flow is turned on.
4. The patient assists with putting on the mask in order to reduce anxiety. The mask should not be strapped

on until the patient has felt the flow and says that they are ready.

5. Flow, pressure and fraction of inspired oxygen ($FiO_2$) are readjusted for patient comfort and the target $SpO_2$.

6. Regular checks are required on $SpO_2$, comfort and the mask seal.

7. After use, the mask should be removed before turning off the flow.

---

**MINI CLINICAL REASONING**

Q. Do we need to read further than the title of this article?

*'CPAP has no Effect on Clearance, Sputum Properties, or Expectorated Volume in Cystic Fibrosis'*
         *Respir. Care* (2012), 57, 1914–1919

A. Physiological reasoning banishes any sense that CPAP could be expected to clear secretions.

---

# INTERMITTENT POSITIVE PRESSURE BREATHING (IPPB)

The slings and arrows of fashion have not been kind to IPPB, and attitudes have oscillated between hero-worship and ostracism. The technique has been scrutinized mercilessly in the literature and found wanting, usually because it has been used in the wrong way for the wrong patients. IPPB is simply pressure-supported inspiration without positive end-expiratory pressure (PEEP) (Fig. 6.17) using a machine such as an in–exsufflator (p. 217) without the expiratory component, or the Bird (Fig. 6.18).

Unlike CPAP, positive pressure is intermittent and triggered by the patient, followed by passive expiration.

## Indications

IPPB is theoretically noninvasive ventilation but is not normally referred to in this category because it is not used to rest the respiratory muscles. Those who may benefit are:

- patients with atelectasis who are drowsy, weak or exhausted, but not those who are unwilling, restless or in pain; postoperative pain is not a contraindication in itself, but if atelectasis is caused by pain, it is best to deal first with the pain because muscle splinting may prevent the patient accepting the positive pressure;
- patients with sputum retention who are drowsy, weak or exhausted;
- people with neuromuscular disorders who require assisted lung insufflation to improve peak cough flow (Mellies & Goebel 2014).

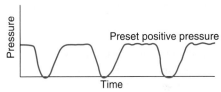

**FIGURE 6.17** The pressure–time waveform of IPPB, showing the slight negative pressure of each patient-triggered breath.

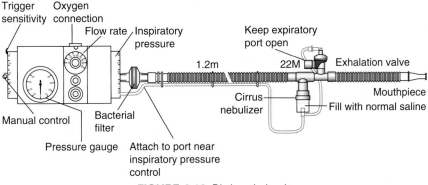

**FIGURE 6.18** Bird and circuit.

## Effects

If the patient is relaxed, comfortable and well positioned, and with controls accurately adjusted, IPPB recruits lung volume (Chen et al. 2016f), this increase lasting for about an hour (AARC 2003), or longer if followed by accurate positioning. Compared to CPAP, positive pressure reaches higher pressures and raises tidal volume rather than FRC, thereby helping open up collapsed lung. In practical terms, IPPB is best for opening up collapsed alveoli, and CPAP is best for maintaining the increased volume.

IPPB is less effective than spontaneous deep breathing in patients able to do so, and the extra air is delivered less homogenously to diseased lungs (Banks et al. 2010).

## Complications

With the Bird, it is possible that hypercapnic COPD patients may lose their hypoxic respiratory drive because 40% oxygen is delivered by most machines. This may not be a problem if adequate tidal volumes are delivered (Starke et al. 1979), but it would be advisable for patients at risk to be kept under observation after treatment. An option is to use air as the driving gas instead of oxygen, with supplemental oxygen added via either a nasal cannula (if a mouthpiece is used), or entrained directly into the tubing. More accurate adjustments are achieved with machines that have an oxygen blender.

Air swallowing may occur, especially if bulging cheeks are noticed or the patient burps.

A side effect that can sometimes be used to advantage is that techniques such as IPPB, incentive spirometry or deep breathing can make patients slightly breathless, even though this is not the aim. These patients can then be positioned for optimum distribution of ventilation and allowed to get their breath back. If undisturbed, this encourages comfortable deep breathing using the same 'slight breathlessness' as that used with controlled mobilization.

## Contraindications and Precautions

These are similar to CPAP, except for type 2 respiratory failure, which is not a contraindication for IPPB.

## Technique for the Bird

Patients are normally positioned comfortably in side-lying with the affected lung uppermost. If the aim is to increase lung volume, this directs the positive pressure preferentially to this nondependent lung (Guérin et al.

2010). If sputum retention is the problem, this acts as modified postural drainage, which does not load the diaphragm.

The machine is plugged into the oxygen outlet. The **apnoea switch** should be kept off to prevent automatic triggering. The **nebulizer** is filled with sterile isotonic saline and tested by activating inspiration with the red manual button.

The **air-mix switch** is maintained in the out position by a clip, which ensures that air is entrained to dilute the oxygen. For occasional patients who require high levels of oxygen, 100% can be delivered by pushing in the air-mix button.

The inspiratory **sensitivity** determines how much negative pressure the patient must generate in order to trigger a breath, a low number indicating that little effort is required. It is set so that the patient can trigger inspiration with ease ('Is it easy to breathe in?').

The **flow rate** determines how fast the gas is delivered, a low number being used for a slow long breath and a high number for a fast short breath. It is set as low as comfortable to encourage laminar flow and optimum distribution of ventilation (see Fig. 6.8). Breathless patients need a higher flow for comfort ('Is that enough air?').

The **inspiratory pressure** is set according to patient comfort ('Is that blowing too hard?'). The pressure gauge should show a smooth rise to the preset pressure at each breath to indicate patient coordination with the machine. It is sometimes helpful to start with sensitivity, flow and pressure all at no. 10.

The patient then takes a small breath in to trigger the Bird and the machine does the rest, so long as the patient does not prematurely stop inspiration by active exhalation. The flow and pressure dials may need adjusting until the patient's breathing pattern settles ('allow all that fresh air to fill your lungs'). Then:

1. If volume loss is the problem, the pressure is gradually increased until maximum expansion is obtained without disturbing the breathing pattern; these increases may need to be in tiny increments, and stopped as soon as the breathing pattern looks the slightest upset, then turned down marginally until the breathing pattern settles.
2. If sputum clearance is the aim, it is less important to maximize lung expansion with the inspiratory pressure button and the aim is optimum comfort.

Percussion may be included for chest clearance if it does not upset the breathing pattern, but measures that decrease lung volume, such as the head-down tip or vibrations, may distract the patient from the delicate process of allowing the air in.

The physiotherapist's job is to:
- adjust the pressure, and occasionally adjust the flow rate to compensate because flow governs the speed with which the preset pressure is reached;
- reassure and advise the patient to allow the air to fill the lungs, and not to blow out;
- observe the abdomen for unwanted active expiration;
- observe the face for discomfort;
- observe rib cage and abdominal movement to ensure that expansion is improving.

Usually the objective is achieved within 5–10 min for lung volume and 5–15 min for sputum clearance. If there is no change in auscultation or sputum production in this time, it can probably be judged ineffective, though another attempt later may be successful. The patient should be positioned appropriately afterwards, to maintain any benefit. The nebulizer is then cleaned according to hospital policy.

Occasionally well-practiced and alert patients can use IPPB independently and are sometimes reassured by having it available by their beds at night.

Options include a retard cap to create a slight PEEP, and a mouth flange to assist the mouth seal. A mask can be held on the face of semiconscious people, but this can be frightening, and patients need explanations and the freedom to say no. IPPB can also be used via a tracheal tube with inflated cuff; this might suit spontaneously breathing patients with a tracheostomy, but for ventilated patients, manual hyperinflation is more adaptable.

Fig. 6.19 shows how IPPB increases lung volume. It also shows how the sitting position does not facilitate ventilation to the lower lobes.

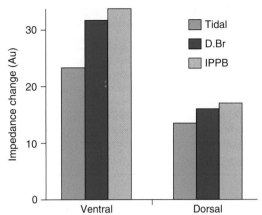

**FIGURE 6.19** Increased volume with tidal breathing, deep breathing and intermittent positive pressure breathing *(IPPB)* in sitting, showing preferential ventilation to the anterior (ventral) lung compared to the dorsal (posterior) lung, which contains mostly the lower lobes. *Electrical impedance tomography*, measurement of lung volume. *Tidal*, Tidal volume breathing, *D.Br*, deep breathing. (From Banks et al. 2010.)

## Problems

1. Prolonged inspiration, and preset pressure not reached: check for leaks in the circuit or at the mouth; if these are not the cause, try reducing pressure and/or increasing flow; if unsuccessful, try a nose clip.
2. Preset pressure reached too quickly: check that the patient is not actively breathing out, blocking the mouthpiece with the tongue or letting pressure generate in the mouth only; if a semiconscious patient blocks their airway, the head should be slightly extended and the jaw protracted.
3. Machine triggers into inspiration too early: turn up the sensitivity, check that the apnoea knob is off.
4. Machine repeatedly triggers during inspiration: check that servicing is up to date.

IPPB will become obsolete as noninvasive ventilators evolve, but at present it is very useful for a very small number of acutely unwell patients.

Table 6.1 compares the different mechanical aids to increase lung volume.

## OUTCOMES

Success in the treatment of patients with reduced lung volume can be identified by the following:
- ↑breath sounds or elimination of bronchial breathing;
- resonant percussion note;

### MINI CLINICAL REASONING

Q. Do we need to read further than the title of the following article?

*'Efficacy of chest physiotherapy and intermittent positive pressure breathing in the resolution of pneumonia'*
  *New Engl. J. Med.* (1978), 299, 624–627

A. Neither 'chest physiotherapy' nor IPPB could logically influence the pathology of pneumonia, which is an inflammatory process and not amenable to physical intervention.

**TABLE 6.1    Characteristics of devices to increase lung volume**

| Incentive spirometry | CPAP | IPPB |
|---|---|---|
| • Full patient participation | • Positive pressure is continuous | • Positive pressure on inspiration only |
| • End-inspiratory hold | • Face or nasal mask | • Mouthpiece or face mask |
| • Physiological distribution of ventilation | • Can accommodate breathless or tired patient | • Can accommodate breathless or tired patient |
| • Minimal supervision | • Usually uncomfortable | • Can accommodate semiconscious patient |
| • Minimal infection risk | • Used for raising functional residual capacity and increasing gas exchange | • Used for raising tidal volume and opening collapsed alveoli |
| • Quiet | | • Used for sputum clearance |
| • Cheap | | |

*CPAP*, Continuous positive airway pressure; *IPPB*, intermittent positive pressure breathing.

- opacity cleared radiologically (see Fig. 23.3);
- ↑ chest expansion;
- ↑ $SpO_2$, with allowance for other variables which affect oxygenation, e.g. increased $FiO_2$;
- lung ultrasonography or electrical impedance tomography (Wallet et al. 2013);
- achievement of SMART goals and ↑ function, e.g. stair climbing or activities of daily living.

## CASE STUDY: MS MB[a]

*Identify the problems of this 72-year-old postoperative patient from London, then answer the questions.*

### Social history
- Sheltered accommodation; uses walking frame

### History of present complaint
- OA knee → total knee replacement
- Two days later: transferred to intensive care due to respiratory distress; intubated and ventilated
- One day later: extubated and returned to ward

### Subjective
- Sleepy, wakeful night
- Little pain

### Objective
- Apyrexial
- Good fluid balance

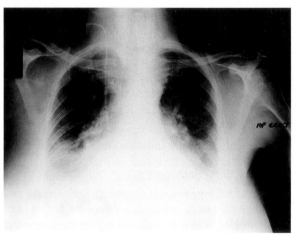

**FIGURE 6.20** Ms MB.

- Obese
- Slumped in bed
- Restless
- Rapid asymmetric breathing pattern
- Feeble nonproductive coughs
- Frequently falls asleep → mask slips → $SpO_2$ drops
- PN dull both lower lobes
- Auscultation: ↓ breath sounds RLL, ML and LLL; scattered coarse crackles
- $SpO_2$: 52% on air, 60% on $FiO_2$ of 0.6
- Radiograph as in Fig. 6.20

### Questions
1. Analysis?
2. Problems?
3. Goals?
4. Plan?

[a]*FiO_2*, fraction of inspired oxygen; *LLL*, left lower lobe; *ML*, middle lobe; *OA*, osteoarthritis; *PN*, percussion note; *RLL*, right lower lobe.

## CLINICAL REASONING

*Comment on the physiology and logic of the following:*

*'...in patients with suspected pulmonary emboli there is no evidence that IPPB would increase alveolar ventilation more than deep breathing...'*

*'From the term 'deep breathing', it is understood that by voluntarily moving regions of the wall of the thoracic cage, underlying lung tissue is appropriately aerated.'*

S. Afr. J. Physiother. (1991), 41, 63–67

*IPPB,* Intermittent positive pressure breathing.

## Response to Case Study[b]

1. Analysis
   - Radiograph indicates ↓ lung volume bibasally
   - Possible causes of disorientation: hypoxia, ICU experience, lack of sleep
   - Immobility, poor position and shallow breathing are exacerbating ↓ lung volume
   - Disorientation and immobility exacerbating sputum retention
2. Problems
   - Inability to fully cooperate
   - Poor gas exchange
   - Atelectasis
   - Sputum retention
   - Knee weak and immobile
3. Goals
   - Short term: orientate, optimize gas exchange, mobilize
   - Long term: rehabilitate for sheltered accommodation
4. Plan
   - Liaise with team about obtaining ABGs and improving gas exchange; consider CPAP if oxygen therapy inadequate, or NIV if ventilation inadequate
   - Communicate with patient, family and team to assist orientation
   - Liaise with team and family about optimizing environment for autonomy, familiarity, rest and sleep

---

[b]*ABG,* arterial blood gas; *ACBT/AD,* active cycle of breathing and/or autogenic drainage; *CPAP,* continuous positive airway pressure; *ICU,* intensive care unit; *NIV,* noninvasive ventilation.

- Position for gas exchange, mobilization of secretions, knee comfort and function
- Attempted deep breathing (ineffective)
- Attempted ACBT/AD (ineffective)
- IPPB
- Percussion and vibrations
- Daily written programme of knee exercises, plus maintenance trunk and arm exercises, communicated to relatives
- Progress to incentive spirometry and ACBT/AD as patient becomes more alert.
- Sit out, mobilize with walking frame, progress

(Neither CPAP nor NIV were needed due to success of orientation, positioning and IPPB.)

## RESPONSE TO CLINICAL REASONING

The physiology defies logic. Increasing alveolar ventilation would not break up a pulmonary embolus.

The logic defies logic. The only way of 'moving regions of the wall of the thoracic cage' is to fracture the ribs.

The premise defies logic. IPPB is not intended to increase alveolar ventilation more than deep breathing. It is for patients who are unable to deep breathe voluntarily.

## RECOMMENDED READING

AARC, 2003. Clinical practice guideline: intermittent positive pressure breathing. Respir. Care 48 (5), 540–546.

Agostini, P., Naidu, B., Cieslik, H., et al., 2013. Effectiveness of incentive spirometry in patients following thoracotomy and lung resection including those at high risk for developing pulmonary complications. Thorax 68 (6), 580–585.

Bott, J., Blumenthal, S., Buxton, M., et al., 2009. Guidelines for the physiotherapy management of the adult, medical, spontaneously breathing patient, Joint BTS/ACPRC Guideline. Thorax 64 (Suppl. 1), i1–i52.

Cammarota, G., Vaschetto, R., Turucz, E., et al., 2011. Influence of lung collapse distribution on the physiologic response to recruitment maneuvers during noninvasive continuous positive airway pressure. Int. Care Med. 37 (7), 1095–1102.

Chiou, M., Bach, J.R., Jethani, L., et al., 2017. Active lung volume recruitment to preserve vital capacity in Duchenne muscular dystrophy. J. Rehabil. Med. 49 (1), 49–53.

Chung, L., Tsai, P., Liu, B., et al., 2010. Home-based deep breathing for depression in patients with coronary heart disease: a randomised controlled trial. Int. J. Nurs. Studies 47 (11), 1346–1353.

Kalisch, B.J., Dabney, B.W., Lee, S., 2013. Safety of mobilizing hospitalized adults. J. Nurs. Care Qual. 28 (2), 162–168.

# Physiotherapy to Clear Secretions

## SPUTUM IN PERSPECTIVE

Airway mucus is normally swallowed once it reaches the throat. If expectorated, it is called sputum. **Sputum retention** is suspected in a patient with excess secretions who is dehydrated, semicomatose or with an ineffectual cough due to weakness or inhibition. Sputum retention is considered a problem, by definition. **Excess secretions** are identified subjectively by the patient or objectively by crackles heard at the mouth or on auscultation.

### Are Excess Secretions a Problem?

*The production of large amounts of sputum does not necessarily mean that the patient is experiencing difficulty clearing sputum.*

*Hess 2002*

In the short term, if excess secretions are seen or heard to obstruct breathing, or if they cause distress or oxygen desaturation, they are a problem and need to be cleared.

In the long term, excess secretions in chronic obstructive pulmonary disease (COPD) cause some airflow obstruction but, unlike inflammation or bronchospasm, the excess mucus is patchy. People with nonacute COPD tend to complain more about breathlessness than sputum, and the evidence that excess secretions affect lung function in stable COPD is underwhelming, although they may predispose to infection (Vliet 2005). If patients are not troubled by a cough and are able to cough out their sputum when required, it is probably unnecessary for them to include routine chest clearance in their daily lives, but with an exacerbation they may need advice or assistance on chest clearance.

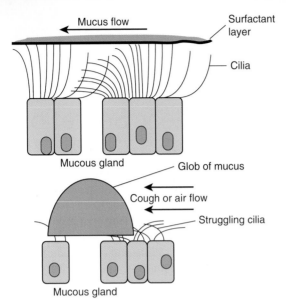

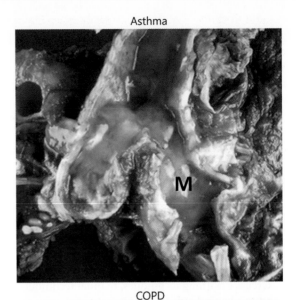

Asthma

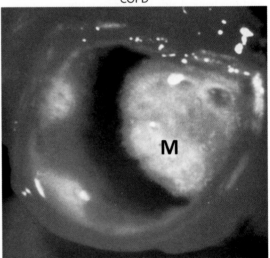

COPD

**FIGURE 7.1** Top: normal mucociliary clearance mechanism. Bottom: thick mucus impairing ciliary function. (From Rubin 2002.)

However, patients with bronchiectasis, cystic fibrosis (CF) or primary ciliary dyskinesia have a damaged mucociliary escalator (Fig. 7.1) and are locked into a vicious cycle of excess secretions and inflammation (see Fig. 3.10). The thickness of the mucus causes more damage than impaired mucociliary clearance (Livraghi et al. 2017), but excess secretions cause local pockets of anoxia and increased temperature, both of which selectively favour the growth of certain microbes (Dickson et al. 2017). Excess secretions are therefore assumed to be a problem for these patients in the long term, and they are advised on a daily regimen of chest clearance. This can be a chore, with adherence rates between 33% and 91% (Peek et al. 2016) so a choice of techniques is advised.

**FIGURE 7.2** Excess mucus (M) partially occluding the large airways in acute asthma and chronic obstructive pulmonary disease.

### What is the Specific Problem?

1. Mucociliary clearance may be the problem, impaired by thick secretions (Fig. 7.2), hypoxia, infection, damaged airways, dehydration, cigarette smoke, immobility, anaesthetic agents or pollution (Randell et al. 2006, Houtmeyers 1999).
2. Coughing may be the problem, impaired by weakness or pain.
3. Expectoration may be the problem, impaired by a dry mouth or embarrassment.

## HYDRATION AND HUMIDIFICATION

The mucociliary escalator provides a frontier against the onslaught of 25 million inhaled particles per hour, or 50 million for the average smoker (Rogers 2007). Its function relies on optimum viscosity of the mucus and optimum thickness of the sol layer so that the cilia tips can reach the mucus (p. 2). Normally the upper airway warms and moistens the inspired air such that, from the level of the carina downwards, airway secretions are bathed in 100% relative humidity at 37°C, the average core temperature of humans (Tucci & Costa 2015). This 'saturation boundary' is moved deeper into the lungs by mouth-breathing, rapid breathing, dry medical gases or bypass of the natural airway with a tracheal tube, making it more difficult to maintain the integrity of the mucous blanket. Systemic dehydration compounds this problem.

Hydration helps maintain the correct viscosity of mucus systemically, while humidification enables fluid to be absorbed into the mucous layer, causing it to swell and maintain the connection between cilia and mucus (Randell et al. 2006).

## Classification
### Hydration
Water is the main constituent of the body, which is intolerant of even a 1% loss (Holdsworth 2012), and systemic hydration is the dominant variable governing mucus clearance. It is more important than ciliary activity, as shown by the following:
- The airway dehydration of CF leads to more rapid and severe airway destruction than the dysfunctional cilia of primary ciliary dyskinesia.
- Neutrophils struggle to kill bacteria that are enmeshed in thick mucus (Randell et al. 2006).

Mucus has the viscoelastic properties of both liquids (viscosity) and solids (elasticity), and hydration optimizes this balance (Button & Boucher 2008).

Adequate daily fluid intake is thought to be approximately 2 L, 80% of which comes from fluids and 20% from the water in food (Holdsworth 2012). Thirst is an adequate guide for most adults (Benton 2011), but elderly people and some patients need advice to drink their 1.5 L a day (Fig. 7.3), although requirements vary with ambient temperature, fever and exercise.

People normally drink because of thirst, for enjoyment, to keep cool or warm, or for a drink's energy content. Patients may restrict their intake because of anxieties about stress incontinence, frequency due to diuretics or, in hospital, not being near the toilet. One study found that over a third of hospitalized patients were unable to drink as often as needed, and over half were thirsty due to an inability to reach their drink and unwillingness to bother busy staff (Blower 1997). Dehy-

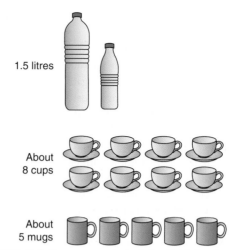

**FIGURE 7.3** Recommended daily fluid intake for a healthy adult.

dration is associated with urinary tract infection, unstable blood pressure, coronary heart disease and venous thromboembolism (Popkin et al. 2010).

Caffeine drinks such as tea, coffee and cola have some diuretic action but are adequate as fluid intake, preferably not taken with meals as they tend to bind with iron. Juices and canned drinks are not as efficient as water and should be taken with meals because of their acid content. Pineapple and papaya contain bromelain, a protein-digesting enzyme that some patients find helps loosen their mucus. Milk is included as fluid intake and has been shown to be more effective for rehydration than a sports drink (Desbrow et al. 2014). Alcohol does not count as fluid intake (Mentes & Kang 2011).

Fluid regulation may be complicated by acid–base or electrolyte disturbance, kidney dysfunction, pulmonary oedema or diuretic therapy (Popkin et al. 2010).

> **PRACTICE TIP**
>
> A glass of water kept beside the patient, in hospital or at home, is a useful reminder to maintain hydration.

### Hot water humidification
The capacity to hold moisture is increased when gas is heated. A **hot water humidifier** or hot water bath creates vapour by passing gas over sterile water, which is maintained at 45–60°C. This is allowed to cool along a

specific length of tubing to reach the patient at 37°C and relative humidity of 100%.

When used with non-intubated patients, the nose and larynx cause much of the vapour to condense into drops, which are too large to navigate the airways. Hot water humidifiers are therefore most effective for intubated patients and for small children to keep their narrow upper airways clear. However, for adults with an intact upper airway, enough humidity may reach the airways, e.g. for those at home with chronic hypersecretory lung disease, for whom 2 h a day can reduce exacerbations (Rea et al. 2010), and hot water humidifiers improve comfort and adherence when patients use a positive pressure device (Soudorn et al. 2016).

The humidifier must be heated continuously to minimize colonization with bacteria. If the wide-bore tube contains no hot wire to reduce condensation, the humidifier should be kept below the patient to prevent condensed water tipping into their airway, and the tubing needs regular emptying manually or by water traps in the circuit.

**Steam inhalation** uses the same principle by delivering vapour from near-boiling water to the patient via a mouthpiece or with a towel over their head. Some patients find it beneficial, but the temperature of the water is not controlled and the container is easily knocked over. It is contraindicated for hospitalized patients and children (Himdani et al. 2016). Patients at home may prefer a steamy cup of tea or hot shower.

### Cold water bubble humidification

Cold gas bubbled through cold water (Fig. 7.4A) shows no objective benefit (Ward 2013) except as a placebo. These devices were condemned as 'dangerously inadequate' over four decades ago (Graff & Benson 1969), and are castigated in the British guidelines as being without evidence and for bringing a risk of infection (BTS 2017). The untiring enthusiasm of sales representatives has kept up sales in the form of 'diffuser' humidifiers (Fig. 7.4B), which create smaller bubbles, but for which research is lacking.

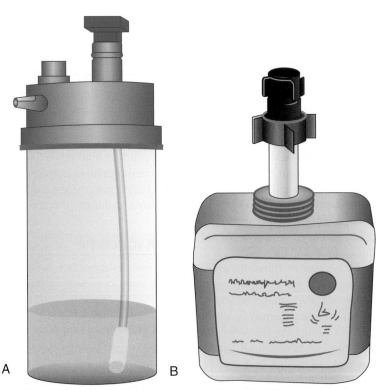

A B

**FIGURE 7.4** (A) Bubble-through humidifier. (B) Diffuser humidifier.

## Nebulized humidification

Large-volume nebulizers convert a sterile liquid into an aerosol whose droplets are small enough to navigate the nasal passages and vocal cords to reach the airways.

**Large-volume jet nebulizers** (Fig. 7.5) commonly use sterile cold water because heat is not necessary for this mechanism, although heated nebulizers are available which combine both vapour and aerosol. When used continuously they increase mucous transport (Sood et al. 2003).

**Small-volume jet nebulizers**, used periodically before physiotherapy, are the same as those used for drug delivery (p. 173). These 'saline nebs' deliver typically 2 mL normal saline, also known as physiological saline or isotonic saline, and are of the same osmolarity as the body. They wet the throat and upper airway, but efficacy has not been established (Rubin 2015b) and neither research nor physiological reasoning has suggested that this small amount improves mucociliary clearance, or that the benefit outweighs the infection risk. However, patients often find them helpful (Khan & O'Driscoll 2004), possibly because they contain saline rather than water, so they can be justified under the hierarchy of evidence (p. 180).

It is therefore suggested that:
- If the patient's problem is a dry mouth or throat, mouth care may be sufficient.
- If the problem is thick secretions, and systemic hydration has been optimized, continuous large-volume nebulization is required.
- If the patient finds a small-volume nebulizer helpful, or if it produces more secretions than the large-volume nebulizer alone, it can be used as often as required, but not in place of continuous large-volume nebulization.

Small-volume saline nebulizers may also be useful in the community, where bacteria are less venal than the hospital varieties, but patients must be given information on infection control (Bonilla et al. 2014).

An **ultrasonic nebulizer** is a self-contained electrical device that transmits vibrations through a liquid to atomize its particles. Oxygen can be added with a nasal cannula. Advantages are its silence, speed and efficiency. Disadvantages are expense and the density of the aerosol, which may cause bronchospasm in people with sensitive

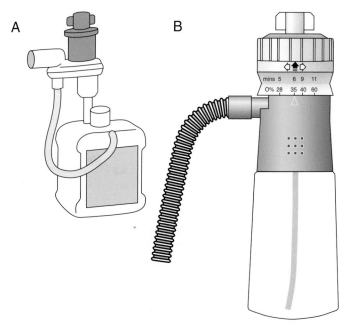

**FIGURE 7.5** Large-volume nebulizers: (A) is similar to Fig. 7.4B but incorporates a venturi device to deliver fixed percentage humidified oxygen; (B) requires the venturi system to be screwed into a prefilled jar of sterile water (Intersurgical).

airways. For patients who have difficulty clearing their own secretions, a physiotherapist should be on hand because of the increased volume of secretions that may be produced.

### Heat–moisture exchange

Heat–moisture exchangers (HMEs) are normally used with a tracheal tube or noninvasive respiratory support. They provide passive humidification by trapping a patient's expired heat and moisture during expiration and returning it on the next inspiration (Fig. 7.6). They are classified as:

- a **condenser** HME, also known as a Swedish nose (p. 330), which traps expired water vapour and some body heat, and fits over a tracheostomy tube.
- a **hydrophobic** HME, which has a large surface area by using pleated material. It is water-repellent and conducts heat poorly, thus causing a temperature gradient, leading to evaporation, cooling and conservation of water on expiration (Table 7.1).
- a **hygroscopic** HME, which is the most efficient (Branson et al. 2014). It is impregnated with a chemical that absorbs expired moisture and uses this to humidify the subsequent inspiration. If used for more than 24 h, it may become saturated and increase airflow resistance.

HMEs are not as efficient as the natural nasal passages and become less effective over time. They are inadequate for patients on oxygen therapy (Chikata et al. 2013) or for those with thick secretions (Branson 1996) but are convenient for mobile patients, for use with manual hyperinflation (p. 490) or for limited periods of assisted ventilation. They usually incorporate a bacterial and viral filter.

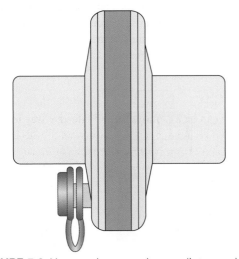

**FIGURE 7.6** Heat–moisture exchanger (Intersurgical).

## Complications

Hospital bacteria enjoy nothing more than stagnant humidifier water, especially at room or lukewarm temperatures. Bacteria have been found in 78% of oxygen cylinder humidifiers and 47% of small-volume nebulizers (Jadhav et al. 2013), and *Legionella pneumophila* has been found in CPAP humidifiers (Stolk et al. 2016). Hot water baths are less risky than nebulizing systems, partly because they are hot and partly because vapour molecules are too small to carry organisms (Pilbeam 1998 p. 161). HMEs are the least hazardous, unless clogged with mucus.

Bronchospasm can be caused in susceptible patients by a dense ultrasonic mist or hypertonic saline.

Hypercapnic COPD patients may lose their respiratory drive if uncontrolled oxygen is used as the driving gas. However, large-volume nebulizers can be set to run from 28% oxygen upwards.

A mask may cause a wet face.

| TABLE 7.1 | Comparison of humidification systems | | |
|---|---|---|---|
| | **Hot water humidifier** | **Nebulizing humidifier** | **Heat–moisture exchanger** |
| Moisture output (g/m³) | 35–50 | 20–1000 | 25–35 |
| Infection risk | Reservoir and circuit | Reservoir, circuit and aerosol | Low risk |
| Advantages | Bacteria not transmitted with vapour | Good for tenacious secretions | Simple Cheap |
| Disadvantages | Labour intensive Bulky | Labour intensive | May block with mucus May be inadequate |

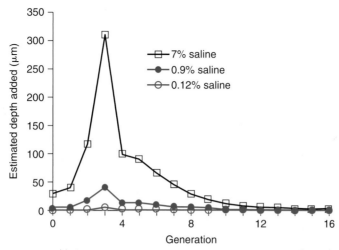

**FIGURE 7.7** Increase in depth of airway surface liquid at different airway generations with hypertonic saline (7%), normal saline (0.9%) and hypotonic (0.12%) saline. (From Sood et al. 2003.)

## Indications

Humidification is advisable for:

- patients using noninvasive mechanical assistance such as CPAP or noninvasive ventilation (an HME may be adequate if the patient is comfortable);
- people with thick secretions;
- babies at risk of airway blockage with secretions;
- people on oxygen therapy who (1) have hyperreactive airways (heated system required) or (2) are using a mask for prolonged periods with high flow rates and find this uncomfortable (BTS 2017), or (3) are mouth-breathing, nil-by-mouth or have a dry mouth and find expectoration difficult, a high-flow nasal cannula providing the greatest humidification (Chikata et al. 2016);
- people whose upper airway is bypassed with a tracheal tube.

Humidification is not required for people with permanent tracheostomies because adaptation occurs over time (p. 330).

## Technique

A mask or mouthpiece can be used, depending on patient comfort. For a hot water humidifier, the manufacturer's instructions specify the correct length of tubing, how to maintain gas flow and how to ensure the reservoir does not dry out.

Large nebulizers normally use sterile water to avoid salt deposition. Small nebulizers use isotonic saline. Hypertonic saline may be used therapeutically (Fig. 7.7) or diagnostically (Appendix A, Chapter 2).

## EXERCISE

Exercise can be an enjoyable and effective way to speed up mucociliary clearance (Ramos et al. 2015). The increased minute ventilation augments shear stresses on mucosal surfaces and helps regulate mucus hydration (Kim & Criner 2013), and the accompanying catecholamine release stimulates cilia (Randell et al. 2006). Benefits have been identified for people with bronchiectasis (Main et al. 2015), COPD (Langer et al. 2009) and CF, in whom it increases peripheral arterial oxygen saturation ($SpO_2$) as well as clearing secretions (Kriemler et al. 2016). It is used cumulatively with other techniques.

## BREATHING TECHNIQUES

Both of the following techniques are flexible, efficient and effective when taught correctly. They foster independence because once taught they can be used without assistance. They are particularly suited to people with chronic lung disease, but are adaptable to those with acute conditions, autogenic drainage being preferable

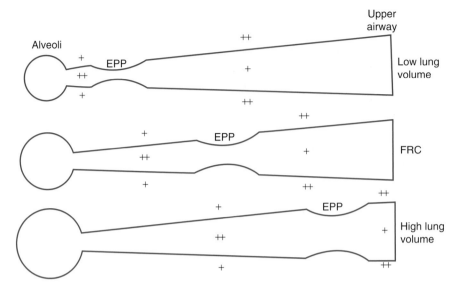

**FIGURE 7.8** The equal pressure point *(EPP)* moving from distal airways (top) to central airways (bottom). *FRC,* functional residual capacity.

for fatigued patients. They are described separately but are based on the same principles and can be adapted and combined to suit each patient.

## Active Cycle of Breathing Techniques

The active cycle of breathing techniques (ACBT) consist of a cycle of huffs at various lung volumes interspersed with relaxed abdominal breathing and deep breathing. Relaxed abdominal breathing reduces the risks of bronchospasm, desaturation or coughing fits. Deep breathing counteracts airway closure, augmented by end-inspiratory breath-holds to further open airways via collateral ventilation.

### Mechanism

Airflow from the huff interacts with the liquid-lined surface to develop a shear force, which, if fast enough, propels mucus in the direction of flow (Graf & Marini 2008). The location at which this occurs depends on the lung volume at the start of the huff. During the huff, pleural pressure becomes positive and equals airway pressure at a point called the equal pressure point (EPP). Towards the mouth from this point, the normal pressure gradient is reversed so that pressure outside the airway is higher than inside, squeezing it by a process known as dynamic airway compression. This limits airflow, but the squeezing of airways mouthwards of this point mobilizes secretions. At low lung volumes, the EPP is

furthest from the mouth because pleural pressure is higher and lung elastic recoil pressure lower, so that huffing facilitates more peripheral airway clearance. Huffing at higher lung volumes is thought to mobilize secretions from the more central airways nearer the mouth (Fig. 7.8).

### Technique

Patients take up their position of choice. This is often sitting, but some find postural drainage positions helpful, e.g. alternate side-lying, or head-down if they are not at risk of a headache when they do the huff. If the patient is sitting, the following sequence is best demonstrated while facing them:

relaxed abdominal breathing at tidal volume (breathing control) to facilitate relaxation
↓
1–3 deep breaths (thoracic expansions) with end-inspiratory hold
↓
relaxed abdominal breathing
↓
one or two huffs, from low lung volume at first, to mobilize secretions
↓
relaxed abdominal breathing

Cycles continue until the chest is subjectively or objectively clear, or the patient tires.

Huffing usually starts from low lung volume, i.e. the patient takes only a tiny breath before the huff. Once the patient feels their secretions move proximally, the huff starts from a medium-sized inhalation. When secretions are felt or heard to move to the central airways, a deep breath from a higher lung volume may be used. Many patients can identify when secretions are shifting, or they can simply move the starting point of their huff from a low to higher lung volume after several cycles.

If secretions are heard or felt at the start, they should be cleared from the upper airway with a cough or huff from high lung volume, before beginning the cycle.

**PRACTICE TIP**

Huffing from low lung volumes may be easier for some patients if they take a normal breath in, partially breathe out, then huff near the end of the exhalation.

Maintaining an open throat during the huff is facilitated by patients keeping their mouth and throat relaxed, rolling their tongue, imagining they are either steaming up a mirror or pushing a tennis ball out of their open mouth, or huffing through a paediatric peak flow mouthpiece (so long as they know not to do the short sharp blow needed for a peak flow test).

Flexibility is encouraged. The number of deep breaths and huffs varies, and the force of the huff can vary greatly to balance efficacy with avoidance of adverse effects. Rests between cycles may be required, and for those who are tense or sensitive to bronchospasm, more abdominal breaths can be taken. The sequence is flexible so long as the principle of alternate stretching and squeezing is maintained, interspersed with relaxed breaths. If patients cannot breathe abdominally, they can just allow their breathing to become relaxed and rhythmic during that part of the cycle.

The patient will make their own adaptations and the physiotherapist can check whether these are helpful. Unhelpful examples include:
- huffing at too high a lung volume at first;
- taking too sharp an inhalation, thus pushing the secretions back down or stirring up bronchospasm;
- not relaxing between cycles;
- coughing before secretions are accessible;
- huffing without doing the full cycle, which can cause more airflow obstruction than coughing (Fig. 7.9).

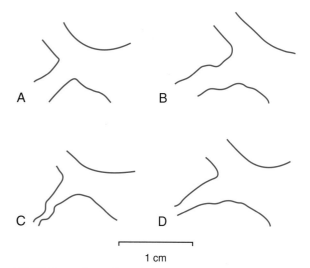

**FIGURE 7.9** A section of the bronchial tree (A) at functional residual capacity, (B) at full inspiration, (C) at full expiration and (D) during coughing. (From Marshall & Holden 1963.)

Patients with undiagnosed hyperventilation syndrome may develop symptoms when they take the deep breath, in which case the technique needs to be modified.

Huffing should be delayed or modified if it causes bronchospasm, fatigue or spasms of coughing. Some patients prefer to do several cycles of deep and abdominal breathing before the huff. Technique must be checked regularly.

Compared with other clearance techniques, outcomes appear to be similar (McKoy et al. 2016) or superior (Lewis et al. 2012). Compared with manual techniques, patients tend to prefer ACBT (Syed 2009) or autogenic drainage (AD) (McIlwaine et al. 2010). If patients find it complicated to learn three components, the principles can be applied using two components only, i.e. the deep breath can be combined with the abdominal breath by taking 'a nice, big, comfortable, relaxed sigh'. This stretches the airways but maintains relaxation.

**Autogenic Drainage**

AD creates high airflow in different generations of bronchi (Fig. 7.10) without allowing airway collapse, using control of the rate and depth of the breath. This clears secretions from small to large airways by gradually increasing functional residual capacity (FRC) from low to high volume.

For people with CF or bronchiectasis, the full sequence can take 30–45 min, but it is less burdensome when combined with activities such as nebulizing drugs or watching TV. For other patients, the length of treatment is shorter and flexible. Control of FRC, and the speed of inhalation and exhalation, are the keys.

## Indications

AD is particularly suited to people with chronic hypersecretory disease, but selected components can be used, e.g. with postoperative patients who are anxious about pain and stitches, people with haemoptysis or bronchospasm or those at risk of panic attacks. For breathless people, short sessions are required, with modifications to avoid upsetting the breathing pattern, e.g. no breathhold, and maintenance of an adequate respiratory rate. Adolescents appreciate that AD may reduce their hyperinflated chests, so long as they do not start inhalation before fully breathing out.

## Effects

AD improves airflow in the small airways, clearing secretions that are not easily accessible. Compared with ACBT, it may show faster mucous clearance (Miller et al. 1995), a greater increase in $SpO_2$ and, for chronically hypercapnic patients, a greater reduction in $PaCO_2$ (Savci et al. 2000). However, patients are best able to identify which suits them.

## Technique

Patients choose their position. Most sit upright, though some prefer supine, side-lying or prone. Facial muscles, shoulders and arms should remain relaxed throughout and the throat and glottis kept open, with the neck maintained in slight extension to avoid obstruction to airflow.

Patients may need to blow their nose if it is obstructed, and the upper airway cleared of secretions to reduce resistance to airflow. The AD cycle is then followed:

Relaxed abdominal breathing to steady
the breathing pattern
↓

Inhalation through the nose to 1½-to-twice tidal volume, slow enough for the breath not to be heard and using an abdominal breathing pattern if possible. Slow inspiration prevents secretions moving distally and encourages equal filling of all areas of lung
↓

End-inspiratory pause for 2–3 s with an open glottis
↓

Exhalation at maximum flow without collapsing the airways, and to a low enough volume (Fig. 7.10) to access the mucus, i.e. until the rattle of secretions is felt by the patient.

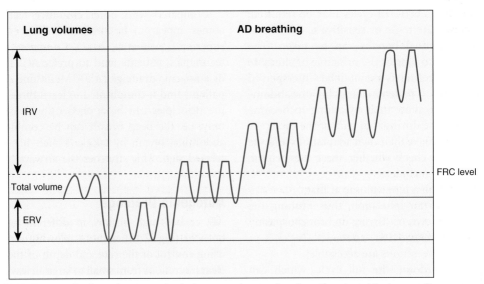

**FIGURE 7.10** Cycles of autogenic drainage at increasing functional residual capacity as secretions move centrally. *AD,* Autogenic drainage; *ERV,* expiratory reserve volume; *FRC,* functional residual capacity; *IRV,* inspiratory reserve volume. (From Paula Agostini.)

An open glottis and/or a paediatric peak flow mouth-piece help to keep the upper airway open. But if there is a wheeze or evidence of hyperinflation, exhalation can be through the nose, pursed lips, a paediatric peak flow mouthpiece or bubble PEP (p. 211), to support the airways. Feeling the expiratory flow at the mouth will identify if there is sufficient flow and if the temperature of the air is warm enough to indicate that the small airways have been reached.

To access the most distal secretions, a wide Velcro strap can be applied firmly around the chest at the end of a tidal expiration to achieve low lung volumes. When the patient then inspires, this helps facilitate relaxation of the inspiratory muscles, allowing a further reduction in lung volume. Going for a walk with the strap in situ encourages ventilation at distal airway level.

The location of secretions is identified by the patient exhaling until they can feel a rattle. The later the rattle, the more peripheral are secretions, as confirmed by palpation. When secretions move mouthwards, i.e. the rattle is felt or palpated earlier on exhalation, breaths are taken at a higher FRC. Cycles at low FRC may need to be repeated several times before the rattle of secretions is felt. Cycles at higher FRC then move the mucus to the upper airways, from where it can be expectorated by a huff or gentle cough.

Patients at risk of bronchospasm can exhale as gently as when a receding wave ripples down the beach. Others can exhale against a tissue held at arm's length or by misting up spectacles, to encourage maximum airflow and discourage noise in the throat, which indicates upper airway closure. Cupping a hand over one ear accentuates the sound of airflow and enables the patient to keep it low.

AD is best interspersed with relaxation, and PEP (p. 211) may be incorporated.

A technique of slow expiration with an open glottis, 'ELTGOL', uses side-lying with the affected lung downwards. The patient is asked to breathe out to residual volume, while the physiotherapist compresses their abdomen to reduce lung volume further. Patients with stable COPD and bronchiectasis have shown increased clearance of secretions from the periphery of the dependent lung (Martins et al. 2012), leading to less need to cough for the rest of the day (Herrero et al. 2016).

## POSTURAL DRAINAGE

Research into the traditional techniques of postural drainage (PD), percussion and vibrations often does not distinguish each component, but the combination appears to improve mucous transport (Ramos et al. 2015), lung function and oxygenation (Andrews et al. 2013). They tend not to be popular with patients (Sontag et al. 2010), but for those who are not physically able and alert enough to use ACBT/AD or the devices discussed later, these passive techniques may be suitable.

---

**MINI CLINICAL REASONING**

*Postural drainage and chest percussion in patients without sputum production is not indicated*
*Chest; 78:559–564 (1980)*

Response on p. 211.

---

### Effects

Using gravity to propel secretions mouthwards has shown benefit (Vliet 2005) but not if patients find it uncomfortable, e.g. sometimes with acute disease, or inconvenient, e.g. sometimes with chronic disease. The movement of changing into a PD position may provide some of the benefit because expectoration sometimes occurs immediately after changing position. Some patients also find this when cleaning the bath or gardening.

### Technique

PD is usually combined with other techniques. For patients needing to clear individual lobes, 3–15 min may be spent in each position (AARC 1991). If a disease affects the whole lung, each lobe requires drainage, but a maximum of three positions per session keeps it tolerable. If bronchodilators are prescribed, these are best taken 15 min beforehand.

Patients are positioned with the area to be drained uppermost (Appendix E), bearing in mind that these positions may need modification for patient comfort or if lung architecture has been distorted by surgery, fibrosis, a large abscess or bullae. The most affected area is drained first to prevent infected secretions spilling into healthy lung. Patients on monitors should be checked for arrhythmias or desaturation before, during and afterwards. The procedure is discontinued if the patient complains of headache, discomfort, dizziness, palpitations, breathlessness or fatigue.

Modifications include:
- alternate side-lying only, the most commonly used positions for patients with generalized secretions;

- sleeping in a modified PD position, e.g. by using thick books to prop up the foot of the bed, so long as this does not stir up coughing at night.

## Indications

PD is used for people who find it preferable or more effective than other techniques. For patients with acute problems, modified positions are often required to accommodate dyspnoea. With chronic conditions, poor compliance is understandable and a week's trial should include motivating patients to find ways to fit the programme into their daily routine.

## Contraindications to Head-Down Postural Drainage

- Cerebral oedema, e.g. recent stroke or acute brain injury
- Trauma to the head or neck, including burns or recent surgery
- Recent pneumonectomy or surgery to the eyes, spine, aorta, oesophagus or cardiac sphincter of the stomach
- Risk of aspiration, e.g. unprotected airway
- Recent meal
- Symptomatic hiatus hernia
- Epistaxis or haemoptysis
- Hypertension or aortic aneurysm

## Precautions to Head-Down Postural Drainage

- Headache
- Undrained pneumothorax or subcutaneous emphysema
- History of seizures
- Abdominal distension, including pregnancy or obesity
- Acute spinal cord lesion
- Bronchopleural fistula or empyema
- Gastro-oesophageal reflux (p. 125)
- Confusion
- Breathlessness
- Reduced cardiac reserve, e.g. pulmonary oedema, arrhythmias or cardiovascular instability

## MANUAL TECHNIQUES

Percussion or vibrations are usually performed in a PD position. It is thought that they cause oscillations that increase ATP release and thereby hydrate mucus (Button & Boucher 2008), but research is hampered by the inconsistency with which these techniques are performed.

Manual techniques reinforce patient dependency but are suited to people who find them subjectively helpful. They may be useful for young children, patients with learning difficulties or those with neurological disease. They may also suit patients who are too exhausted to use a more independent technique, e.g. if they have an exacerbation of disease.

## Effects

When combined with PD, manual techniques can boost airway clearance in patients with COPD or bronchiectasis (Jones & Rowe 2000) and slow lung function decline in people with CF (Oermann et al. 2000). Individual components have shown the following:

- Percussion at 4 Hz increases upper airway mucociliary clearance (Ragavan et al. 2010).
- Vibrations shear secretions off the airway wall by increasing expiratory flow by an average 50% (McCarren et al. 2006), although this is less effective in people with COPD because of expiratory airflow obstruction (Fig. 7.11), suggesting that percussion might be preferable in these patients.

Self-percussion may be beneficial subjectively but can cause desaturation in patients with marginal reserve, and oximetry is advisable for the first session.

## Technique

**Percussion** consists of rhythmic clapping on the chest wall throughout the respiratory cycle with a loose wrist and cupped hand, creating an energy wave that is transmitted to the airways. A sheet or pyjama top should cover the patient, but thick covering dampens transmission through the chest wall (Frownfelter & Dean 2006 p.345), and correct cupping of the hand ensures that the procedure is comfortable. Indeed, when performed correctly it can soothe children and sometimes give relief to people who are acutely breathless. Patients choose whether they prefer a slow, rhythmic single-handed or a rapid double-handed technique. Carers can use adult Palm Cups (p. 355).

**Vibrations** consist of a fine oscillation of the hands against the chest, down and inwards against the direction of the bucket handle act of breathing (p. 5),

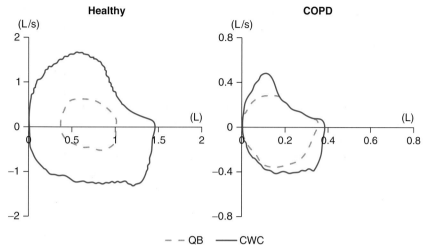

**FIGURE 7.11** Flow–volume curves during quiet breathing and chest wall compression in a healthy control group and in COPD patients. *COPD*, Chronic obstructive pulmonary disease; *CWC*, chest wall compression; *QB*, quiet breathing. (From Nozoe et al. 2016.)

performed throughout exhalation after a deep inhalation. **Shaking** is a coarser movement in which the chest wall is rhythmically compressed. Both are less effective on a squashy mattress.

Vibrations, shaking and percussion should be interspersed with relaxed deep breathing to prevent airway closure, desaturation or bronchospasm.

## Contraindications

- Osteoporosis
- Rib fracture, or potential rib fracture, e.g. metastatic carcinoma
- Loss of skin integrity, e.g. surgery, burns or chest drains
- Recent epidural
- Lung contusion
- Recent pacemaker placement
- Recent or excessive haemoptysis, e.g. following lung contusion or an abscess

## Precautions

- Local pain such as pleurisy or post-herpetic neuralgia
- Potential bleeding, e.g. platelet count <50,000 mm$^{-3}$
- Undrained pneumothorax or subcutaneous emphysema

- Active pulmonary tuberculosis
- Unstable angina or arrhythmias

### RESPONSE TO MINI CLINICAL REASONING

No chest clearance technique is indicated in patients without sputum production.

## MECHANICAL AIDS

### Positive Expiratory Pressure

PEP is the application of positive pressure at the mouth during expiration. Breathing out against resistance is thought to stabilize airways, prevent airway closure, reduce gas trapping, homogenize the distribution of ventilation, counteract early airway closure (Wettstein et al. 2014) and force air through collateral channels so that it can get behind the mucus (Fig. 7.12). It also helps prevent airway closure caused by floppy airways or coughing (Fig. 7.13).

Via a mask or mouthpiece, resistance to expiration is provided by a narrow orifice or tube, the spring of a threshold resistor, a floating ball or a wind instrument, the latter being short on research but long on positive patient feedback.

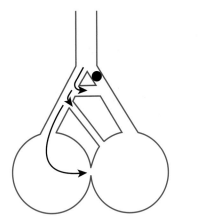

**FIGURE 7.12** Ventilation finding its way through collateral channels to get behind a mucous plug.

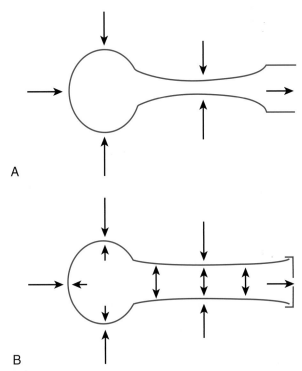

A

B

**FIGURE 7.13** (A) Forced exhalation compressing the airway and predisposing to airway collapse. (B) Exhalation against positive expiratory pressure, stabilizing the airways and preventing collapse. (From Fink 2002.)

## Indications

PEP is mostly used by people with CF who have been able to improve their lung function and $SpO_2$ (Darbee et al. 2004) or those with bronchiectasis. Some people with COPD have found short-term gain (Olsén & Westerdahl 2009). Most children can use PEP from 4 years old.

## Contraindications

Positive pressure techniques are inadvisable in the presence of:
- an undrained pneumothorax, which might lead to air being forced into the pleura;
- haemoptysis, which might be exacerbated by the positive pressure;
- raised intracranial pressure.

## Technique

1. Patients take up their position of choice, but for those with advanced disease, sitting with their elbows resting on a table may protect the lungs from over-distension.
2. After relaxing their breathing, the patient inhales slowly to slightly greater than tidal volume, holds their breath briefly at end-inspiration, then exhales actively but not fully or forcefully through the resistance. They should experience a comfortable effort, as if giving way to the resistance. Exhalation should last no more than 4 s. About 10 PEP breaths are alternated with several relaxed breaths.

When secretions have been mobilized, they can be cleared by a huff or cough. The location from which secretions are mobilized may be altered by breathing from different lung volumes (p. 206). Patients with large quantities of mucus may need to add ACBT/AD. For mask PEP, the manometer can be removed once the patient knows the feel of the correct pressure. A mouthpiece device may need a higher pressure (Larsson & Olsén 2006).

During stable disease, most patients find that two 15-min or three 10-min sessions a day are adequate, which can be done while watching a not-too-diverting television programme. The physiotherapist should check the resistance every fortnight for 6 weeks, then every month for 3 months.

## Variations

1. The **PEP tube** (Fig. 7.14A) creates airflow resistance from the turbulence of blowing into thin tubing cut to a length of about 30 cm. The technique is research-light but can be clinically reasoned to create PEP, and patients will confirm if it helps them. The positive pressure created by airflow resistance depends on the

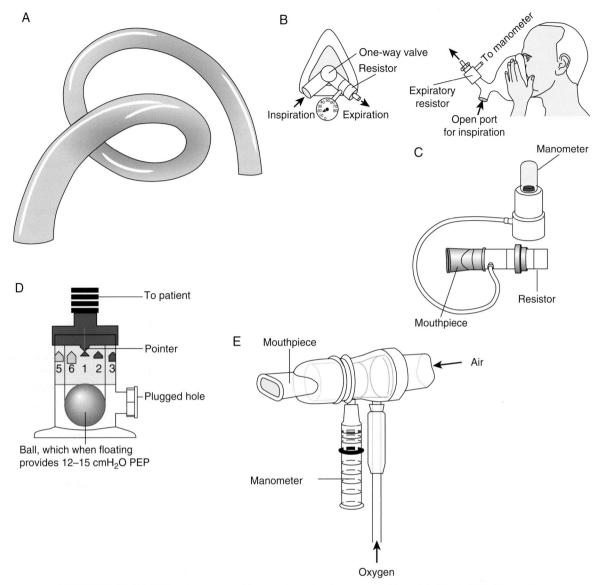

**FIGURE 7.14** (A) PEP tube, created from a length of oxygen tubing. (B) Mask PEP. The patient breathes out against the resistance of a narrow tube, which connects to a manometer to measure the resistance. (C) TheraPEP (Henleys). (D) Mediflo PEP device, in which the pointer is turned to a value on the 'expiration' scale that allows the patient to continue for 2 min without undue effort (Henleys). (E) EzPAP (Henleys).

length of tubing and how hard patients blow, both of which they are usually able to judge and modify. The tube is cleaned in hot soapy water.

2. For **mask PEP** (Fig. 7.14B) and **TheraPEP** (Fig. 7.14C), a resistance is chosen that the patient can use comfortably for 2 min, usually 10–20 cmH$_2$O during mid-exhalation. The manometer is observed by the physiotherapist but not the patient at first, who might otherwise try to reach the target pressure by altering their breathing pattern.

3. With the **Mediflo** (Fig. 7.14D), a pointer is turned to the value on the 'expiration' scale that allows the patient to continue for 2 min without undue effort.

4. **EzPAP** (Fig. 7.14E) connects to a flow of air or oxygen to create the positive pressure. Claims have been made that it can also reduce dynamic hyperinflation in people with severe COPD (Iberl et al. 2014).

## Oscillatory Positive Expiratory Pressure

These devices are suited to anyone who can blow bubbles. Oscillations are added to positive pressure, which further aids mucociliary clearance by means of ATP-mediated secretion of airway surface liquid (Button & Boucher 2008), leading to improved ventilation, symptoms, exercise capacity and quality of life (Svenningsen 2007). Patients breathe in to above tidal volume, then breathe out through the oscillatory device, hard enough to create the optimum vibrations. This may be less tiring than ACBT and is often preferred by patients (Lee et al. 2015). Contraindications and technique are as for PEP, with extra details below and in Appendix B.

### Bubble PEP

A cheap way of creating positive pressure and oscillations is by blowing out through water (p. 382).

### Flutter

The Flutter (Fig. 7.15A) resembles a short fat pipe and has shown benefit for people with COPD (Gastaldi et al. 2015), bronchiectasis (Figueiredo et al. 2012), CF (Guimarães et al. 2014) and for patients following surgery (Zhang et al. 2016c). By exhaling into the device, the patient creates a positive vibrating pressure which appears to alter secretion transport properties (Tambascio et al. 2011).

Patients inhale through their nose, then exhale through the mouthpiece. They must keep their cheeks taut on exhalation and avoid blocking the holes on the device with their fingers. The aim is for maximum oscillation, not maximum force. This is achieved by adjusting the angle at which the Flutter is held, assessed subjectively by the patient and objectively by the physiotherapist palpating for vibrations over the chest. Positive inclinations tend to optimize the PEP effect, and negative inclinations the huff effect (Alves et al. 2008). The device is used for between 5 min (e.g. COPD) and 15 min (e.g. CF) per session, in batches of 8–10 breaths. The steel ball should be kept away from toddlers.

### Acapella

The Acapella (Fig. 7.15B) is popular because it does not require heroic efforts and can be used at any angle, being dependent on magnetic attraction rather than gravity. Exhaled gas causes oscillations by interaction of magnets and a counterbalanced lever, the proximity between the two being adjusted by a dial to alter frequency and amplitude. An inspiratory valve allows patients to inhale through the device as well as exhale.

Patients are advised to start at the lowest frequency, then experiment with what they feel is most effective, one study finding frequency number 4 to be the most effective (Mueller et al. 2014). If they cannot maintain exhalation with vibrations for 3–4 s, they adjust the dial clockwise. A green device usually suits patients with expiratory flows >15 L/min and a blue one for those with flows <15 L/min.

Patients with poor respiratory effort often find it beneficial (Narula 2014), and for exhausted patients, e.g. during an exacerbation of disease, the device can be slotted onto the expiratory port of an IPPB device.

The Flutter and Acapella are usually available on prescription in the UK, depending on local policy.

---

**MINI CLINICAL REASONING**

*Article title: 'A randomized controlled trial comparing incentive spirometry with the Acapella...'*

Cho et al. (2014)

Do we need to read further than this? See p. 216.

---

### Shaker

The Shaker (Fig. 7.15C) is cheaper than the Flutter or Acapella and can generate a similar level of PEP (Santos et al. 2013).

### Cornet

The Cornet (OHTAS 2009) creates vibrations by means of a flexible hose inside a curved plastic tube (Fig. 7.15D). Its moveable mouthpiece provides variable flow and pressure. There is limited research but it comes with its own microwaveable bag and it suits some patients.

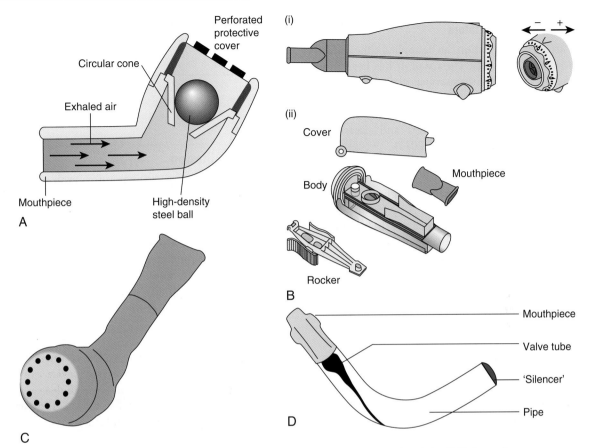

**FIGURE 7.15** (A) Flutter. B(i) Acapella, with the frequency dial on the right. B(ii) Acapella parts, the rocker containing magnet and lever. (C) Shaker (PowerBreathe). (D) Cornet.

## Lung Flute

The Lung Flute is similar to the Cornet. A study finding it beneficial for people with COPD did not describe treatment for the control group (Sethi et al. 2014).

## Machines

The following devices allow patients to be passive and sometimes take nebulized drugs at the same time.

### High-frequency chest compressors

The 'Vest' delivers pulsatile compressions through an inflatable jacket round the torso, with adjustments for frequency and pressure to create expiratory flow bias (p. 496) and 'mini-coughs'. It can be started from age 2 years, and is convenient for families and popular with patients, who can use their social media at the same time. Compared to oscillatory PEP, which is particularly beneficial for excess secretions, the Vest appears suited to thick secretions (Ragavan et al. 2010).

### Intrapulmonary percussors

High gas flows at 60–400 cycles/min send vibrations directly into the airway via a mouthpiece, mask or tracheal tube, along with nebulized saline or medication (Toussaint et al. 2012). The device may also recruit collapsed alveoli (Rand et al. 2013).

## High-frequency oscillators

High-frequency oscillation can be applied either directly to the airway or via the chest wall. It has been found beneficial for people with neurological disease (Lechtzin et al. 2016), those on ventilators (Huang et al. 2016c) and for postoperative patients (Park 2012). For some children it has caused discomfort and occasionally oxygen desaturation (Rand et al. 2011).

## Intermittent positive pressure breathing

Some weak or drowsy patients with sputum retention may respond to IPPB (Chen et al. 2016f), which brings the added advantage of aerosol delivery. In-exsufflators (p. 217) have a vibratory mode that delivers intrapulmonary percussion.

## Hydroacoustic therapy

Lying in a bath of vibrating water for 30 mins is an enjoyable alternative (Jarad et al. 2010).

---

**RESPONSE TO MINI CLINICAL REASONING**

Incentive spirometry is for recruiting lung volume. The Acapella is for clearing secretions.

---

# COUGH

## Cough Facilitation

Causes and suggested remedies for problems with coughing are shown in Table 7.2.

Inhibition of expectoration may be caused by embarrassment or disgust. As physiotherapists, we learn to become comfortable around sputum (indeed are often delighted to see it), and may forget that patients need curtains drawn and reassurance that we are not repelled by it.

Patients should sit up to cough if possible, and avoid repetitive coughing, which reduces effectiveness (Hegland et al. 2014).

---

### TABLE 7.2  Difficulties with coughing

| Problem | Management |
| --- | --- |
| Pain following surgery | Pain relief |
| | Manual assistance |
| Thick secretions | Hydration |
| | Humidification |
| Dry mouth | Hydration |
| | Hot steamy drink |
| | Sips of water, juice or soda water |
| | Ice or semifrozen pineapple or lemon juice |
| | Mouth care |
| Poor technique | Positioning upright |
| | Demonstration |
| Inhibition due to anxiety | Information (e.g. postoperative stitches, stress incontinence, fits of coughing) |
| Unstable airways | Autogenic drainage for bronchospasm, positive expiratory pressure for floppy airways |
| Upper airway obstruction, e.g. tumour | Try different positions |
| Weakness | Manual or mechanical assistance (p. 217) |
| Semiconsciousness | Abdominal co-contraction (see Fig. 6.11) |
| | Gentle skin pressure upwards over the trachea, just above the suprasternal notch |
| Last resort (1) | Blow out through straw into glass of water |
| Last resort (2) | Gentle stimulation at entrance to one or other outer ear canal to stimulate Arnold's nerve response (p. 4), but without using any instrument |

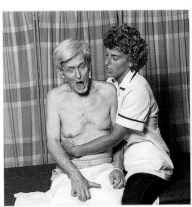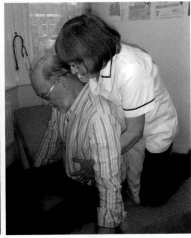

**FIGURE 7.16** Manually assisted cough.

## Manually assisted cough

Patients with neurological disorders demand a resource-ful physiotherapist. All measures should first be taken to bring the secretions proximally. Physical assistance is then given by helping the patient sit over the edge of the bed if possible. The abdomen is then compressed manu-ally, inwards and upwards, while either sitting beside or kneeling behind the patient (Fig. 7.16). Abdominal thrusts are coordinated with the patient making an expiratory effort and leaning forward, assisted by the physiotherapist. If the patient cannot sit up, it is done in supine.

Abdominal pressure should be avoided or modified in patients with the following:

- unstable angina or arrhythmias;
- rib fracture: if pain is controlled with a nerve block, manual assistance may be acceptable with modified hand positions;
- high muscle tone: the patient may require antispas-modic drugs;
- spinal fracture;
- gastro-oesophageal reflux disease (GORD);
- paralytic ileus or abdominal injury/surgery.

Some patients can assist themselves by sitting with a pillow pressed against their abdomen, then after a deep breath, bending forward while exhaling sharply.

## Mechanically assisted cough

Mechanical insufflation–exsufflation (MIE) is provided by the Nippy Clearway (Fig. 7.17) or CoughAssist (Appendix A). They apply positive pressure to the upper airway, usually via a mask held by the physiotherapist or carer, then rapidly shift to negative pressure, creating a high expiratory flow to simulate a cough.

It is best to start on manual mode and talk the patient through what to expect. Beginning with a low inhale flow, inspiratory and expiratory pressures may start equally at 10–20 cmH$_2$O, with 1–2 s each for inhale time, exhale time and pause time. The expiratory pres-sure can be gradually increased up to 40–45 cmH$_2$O. By watching the breathing pattern, the exsufflation 'cough' can be switched on at the end of the patient's exhala-tion. Three to five cycles of in–exsufflation (with or without an abdominal thrust during exsufflation) are followed by about 30 s rest, during which the patient is asked about timing and pressure, and the machine adjusted accordingly. The automatic mode can then be used.

Potential complications include abdominal disten-sion, aggravation of GORD, discomfort, increased blood pressure and, rarely, haemoptysis or pneumothorax. Bradyarrhythmias can occur in people with high spinal cord injury. The risk of complications is reduced by adequate rest between applications and avoidance of hyperventilation.

Insufflation alone acts as a form of breath-stacking (p. 112), and Jones et al. (2012) found the full MIE cycle to be more effective than a manually assisted cough. MIE can also be used with a mouthpiece or tracheal tube. It is not suited to patients with floppy airways, as can occur with advanced COPD or CF.

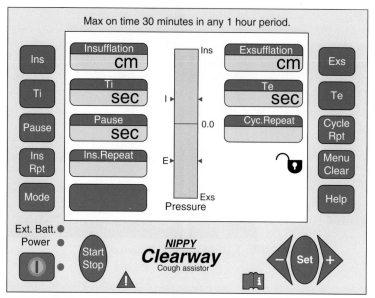

**FIGURE 7.17** Nippy Clearway insufflator–exsufflator (B&D Electromedical).

MIE should be avoided in patients with:

- inadequate bulbar function
- undrained pneumothorax or subcutaneous emphysema
- bullous emphysema
- nausea
- chest pain of unknown origin
- severe acute asthma
- recent lung surgery
- raised intracranial pressure
- inability to communicate
- haemodynamic instability

It is most effective for patients who are able to muster a weak cough.

Both manual and mechanical assistance should be avoided after meals.

## Cough Control

> **KEY POINT**
>
> Unnecessary coughing can cause bronchospasm, desaturation, distress and a vicious cycle of paroxysms of coughing.

Coughing is subject to more voluntary control that other respiratory reflexes such as sneezing, and may need to be inhibited in the following situations:

- during ACBT/AD, before secretions are accessible;
- after eye or cranial surgery, or recent pneumonectomy;
- if there is an aneurysm or subcutaneous emphysema;
- sometimes after hernia or aneurysm repair, depending on the surgeon;
- if the cough is dry and irritates the airways, or is unnecessary.

Unnecessary coughing may disrupt sleep, work and social life, and cause musculoskeletal chest pains, a hoarse voice, vomiting, blackouts and stress incontinence (Seo et al. 2016), which is best managed by pelvic floor exercises (Ostle 2016). Controlling needless coughing can improve quality of life (Patel et al. 2011), but inappropriate cough suppression, e.g. for social reasons, can lead to 'Lady Windermere syndrome', a form of bronchiectasis caused by retention of secretions and inflammation of the long, narrow airways of the middle lobe and lingula, both of which are served meagrely by collateral ventilation (Reich 2014). The need for this type of cough suppression may be reduced by patients clearing their chest before a social event.

The first step when dealing with a dry, unproductive cough is to identify the cause (p. 35). A cough caused by asthma should disappear once inflammation is controlled, unless the actual cause is comorbid hyperventilation syndrome (HVS). Coughs and throat-clearing due to HVS will melt away once the syndrome is treated.

A smoking-related cough usually subsides 3–4 weeks after smoking cessation.

Excess coughing tips the patient into a vicious spiral so that it is triggered by smaller stimuli. Consciously suppressing the cough dampens down cough receptors so that afferent input summates to a less sensitive threshold (Vertigan 2007).

Suggestions for patients to control their cough include the following:

- identify whether the cough is wet or dry; if dry, the cough is unnecessary;
- swallow;
- try a Valsalva swallow, i.e. swallow hard with neck flexion and while tightening the muscles of the neck and shoulders;
- take sips of water or cold grape juice;
- drink fizzy water;
- take slow and/or shallow breaths;
- breathe in through the nose, breathe out through pursed lips;
- keep the throat relaxed;
- take repeated short sniffs;
- use AD techniques to control airflow;
- suck nonmedicated lozenges, ice pops or frozen seedless grapes;
- chew gum;
- inhale the steam from hot water poured over root ginger, then drink the warm solution (with honey, cinnamon and/or lemon);
- for a nocturnal cough, avoid supine;
- for fentanyl-induced cough, acupressure below the medial ends of the clavicles (Solanki et al. 2016);
- honey has been found moderately beneficial in children (Oduwole et al. 2014), and maintaining an adequate fluid intake is helpful for all ages (Chamberlain et al. 2013b).

Sometimes a dry cough may be helpful and need not be suppressed, e.g. if a patient finds that one brief cough will settle it, as if scratching an itch.

## MINI CLINICAL REASONING

*Behaviour modification is appropriate for a subset of the total population with chronic cough represented by those people whose cough is deemed to be refractory to medical treatment*
*Chr Respir Dis (2007) 4:89–97*

Behaviour modification should come before medication.

# SUCTION

*'The worst part is the initial introduction of the catheter into the nostrils. Once past the turn at the back of the nose, it is not too unpleasant until a cough is stimulated; then it feels like hours as the catheter is brought back up. It felt as if I was choking'*
**Ludwig 1984**

These remarks come from a physiotherapist who found herself at the wrong end of a suction catheter, and they illustrate why most clinicians are, rightly, reluctant to put their patients through the ordeal of pharyngeal suction, which is usually distressing and sometimes painful. It is also dirty, risky and limited in effectiveness, but there are occasions when it is necessary. Suction for intubated patients is described on p. 497.

## Indications

Suction is performed if all the following criteria are met:

- secretions are accessible to the catheter, as indicated by crackles in the upper airway on auscultation;
- secretions are detrimental to the patient;
- the patient is unable to clear the secretions by other means.

Patients who are semiconscious, weak or neurologically impaired may require suction, but those who are fatigued rarely do so because, unless fatigue is extreme enough for the patient to need ventilatory support, coughing is usually possible. Risks are increased in a combative patient, and those who need physical restraint for suction rarely need to undergo the procedure because they are usually strong enough to cough effectively, even if they choose not to. Suction against a patient's wish is unethical, illegal in the UK and acceptable only if the patient is deemed to lack capacity to give consent and their health will otherwise suffer significantly.

## Catheters

Catheters have an end hole through which the mucus is suctioned and side eyes to relieve the vacuum if the end hole becomes blocked (Fig. 7.18). The side eyes should not be too large (Fig. 7.18C) or they will reduce suction efficiency, and their total size should be less than that of the end hole so that they do not become suction channels. The ideal catheter is flexible, with a smooth rounded tip, small multiple countersunk side eyes and, if possible, a curved tip (Grigoriadis et al. 2015).

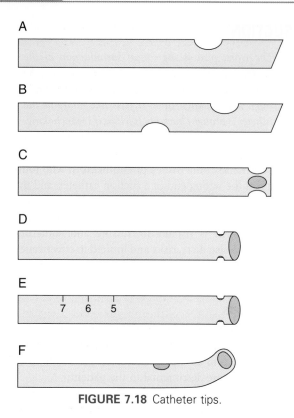

A

B

C

D

E

      7   6   5

F

**FIGURE 7.18** Catheter tips.

## Complications

Untoward effects of suction include the following:

- pain, uncontrollable coughing, infection, haemoptysis, atelectasis, hypoxaemia (Arcuri et al. 2016);
- hypoxia due to atelectasis, suction of oxygen from the airways, enforced apnoea or increased oxygen demand;
- haemodynamic instability;
- bronchospasm;
- airway damage because mucosa is exquisitely sensitive to both passage of the catheter and pull from the vacuum, exacerbated by poor technique (Branson et al. 2014);
- vomiting, in which case the patient should be helped to sit up but suction continued to avoid aspiration (AARC 2004);
- for elders, increased risk of aspiration pneumonia (Manabe et al. 2015).

Laryngospasm is rare but may cause the catheter to become stuck and the patient unable to breathe, in which case the following steps should be taken:

- press the crash button and call for help;
- ask the patient to sniff (Sandhu 2013);
- press hard into both postcondylar notches behind the earlobe (between the base of the skull, the mastoid process and the mandible) while displacing the mandible forward in a jaw thrust, and give 100% oxygen with a tight-fitting mask (Miles & Cook 2017).

### MINI CLINICAL REASONING

Pneumothorax has been described as a complication of suction, but it is difficult to find original studies for this in adults, and it would require rather enthusiastic suction to poke a catheter through the airway wall, through a lung, then through the visceral pleura.

## Contraindications

1. Stridor indicates a dangerously narrowed airway, which could become obstructed if pharyngeal suction is attempted.
2. After basal skull fracture, nasopharyngeal suction is contraindicated in case there is cerebrospinal fluid leak, which could become infected if jabbed with a suction catheter.
3. Oesophageal varices may bleed (p. 539).

## Precautions

1. Unexplained haemoptysis is a warning to avoid suction unless essential.
2. If a patient has pulmonary oedema, suction does not help the condition and may remove surfactant if performed repeatedly.
3. Suction aggravates bronchospasm (but so too does excess mucus).
4. Following recent pneumonectomy or lung transplant, the catheter should not be taken beyond the pharynx in case it impinges on the bronchial stump or anastomosis.
5. After recent oesophagectomy with a high anastomosis, or with a tracheo-oesophageal fistula, the catheter should not go beyond the pharynx in case it enters the oesophagus. A minitracheostomy may be required.
6. Raised intracranial pressure is exacerbated with suction.

7. If the patient has a clotting disorder (INR >3.0, platelets <50,000/mm$^{-3}$) or is receiving heparin or thrombolytic drugs, suction may cause bleeding (Grigoriadis et al. 2015).

## Technique

The patient should be talked through each step. The following are suggested:

1. Explain to the patient how it will feel, how long it will last and that they may ask for a pause at any time, a request that must be responded to. Obtain consent. Unconscious patients also need an explanation.
2. Check resuscitation status.
3. Choose a size 10 FG catheter, or occasionally size 12. Large sizes are more uncomfortable and increase the damaging negative pressure (Branson et al. 2014).
4. Ensure the patient is upright or side-lying, in case of vomiting.
5. Preoxygenate for 2 min if this is not contraindicated. The oxygen mask should then be kept close to the patient's face throughout.
6. Ask the patient to take a few rapid breaths, if they can. There is no evidence that reducing $PaCO_2$ prolongs tolerance to suction, but it enables patients to feel a little more in control. Reassure them that their oxygen status is being monitored.
7. Put on a visor, or mask and goggles.
8. Set the suction pressure to no more than −20 kPa (−150 mmHg) (Branson et al. 2014). The pressure should be set with the machine turned on and the end of the suction tubing occluded.
9. Partially unpeel the catheter pack, and attach to the suction tubing, while keeping the rest of the catheter in the pack, tucked under the arm.
10. Put a sterile glove on the dominant hand. This hand must now not touch anything except the sterile catheter.
11. Remove the catheter from the pack and lubricate the tip with lignocaine jelly (Grigoriadis et al. 2015) or, if not available, water-soluble jelly, while maintaining sterility of catheter and glove.
12. With the suction port open, slide the catheter gently into the nostril, directing it parallel to the floor of the nose. If resistance is felt at the back of the pharynx, rotate the catheter slowly between the fingers and ease very gently forward.
13. To reduce the risk of entering the oesophagus, ask the patient to tilt their head back, stick out their tongue and cough. If coughing is not possible, slide the catheter down during inspiration, when the glottis is open. If the patient swallows, the catheter has slipped into the oesophagus, in which case it should be slightly withdrawn, the head repositioned and the procedure continued. The catheter is usually in the airway if the patient coughs spontaneously.
14. When resistance is felt, the catheter should be withdrawn slightly before applying vacuum pressure, to limit trauma.
15. Block the catheter port with the non-dominant hand to apply suction, though not too suddenly, at the same time bringing up the catheter slowly and smoothly, avoiding catheter rotation or sudden intermittent suction. Slow withdrawal reduces the need for a second attempt, but total apnoeic time should not exceed 10 secs. If the patient appears distressed, the catheter should be partially withdrawn until distress stops, then the vacuum removed, again not too suddenly, and oxygen applied with the catheter still in situ until the patient is ready to continue.

Rotation is unnecessary, and intermittent suction involving the sudden on/off application of vacuum pressure may damage mucosa (Day et al. 2002) while reducing effectiveness because the flow can be reduced from 19 to 8.5 L/min (Brown 1983), making further suction passes more likely. Protection of mucosa is best maintained by continuous withdrawal, without stopping to change the position of the dominant hand on the catheter. If suction pressure rises unacceptably, the rocking thumb technique should be used, which is the smooth and partial removal of the non-dominant thumb from the control port of the catheter to reduce negative pressure gently.

---

**PRACTICE TIP**

Obtain an endotracheal tube and catheter. Insert the catheter, then withdraw it while rotating. Observe the tip to identify that rotation does not transmit to the tip of the catheter.

---

If, during withdrawal, it becomes apparent that a second suction pass will be required, i.e. crackles continue to be heard, it is best to withdraw the catheter until the patient can breathe, then stop suction with the catheter in situ.

The patient is then helped to sit forward and given oxygen, then once $SpO_2$ has returned to normal and the patient has got their breath back, consent is obtained for a further suction pass. Keeping the same catheter in situ avoids repetition of the sometimes painful process of passing a new catheter through the bend in the throat, and clinical reasoning suggests that passing another catheter through the nostril (whose job is to catch dirt) increases infection risk. If the catheter is removed and further suction is required, a fresh catheter must be used.

Afterwards, wind the catheter around the sterile glove, remove the glove inside out over the catheter and discard. Rinse out the suction tubing using tap water in a jug. Give the patient oxygen and comfort, check monitors and auscultate. Discard the water in the jug.

If the nasal route is uncomfortable, the other nostril can be tried or the oral route used. For this, the catheter is inserted into a Guedel airway, which is a plastic tube shaped to conform to the palate with a flange to prevent it slipping into the throat (Fig. 7.19A). A size 4–6 airway is average, but it is best sized by holding it against the side of the face and measuring it from the corner of the mouth to the angle of the jaw below the ear.

After explanations and obtaining consent, the catheter is first inserted into the Guedel airway. With the tip protruding just beyond the end of the airway, both airway and catheter are passed into the mouth (after removal of dentures) with the curve upwards to avoid pushing the tongue towards the throat. The patient is then advised to 'breathe it in', and the catheter is rotated so that the curve is downwards and then passed gently into the throat. During insertion it should be pressed downwards onto the tongue so that it does not impinge on the soft palate and cause gagging. Introducing the airway is not painful but may be distressing, and the patient should be talked through the process and reassured that it will not stop them breathing (the clinician can demonstrate first with a separate airway passed into their own throat). Passage of the catheter then proceeds through the airway, as described above. The airway can only be used in a patient who is able to maintain consent and not resist, or who is unconscious, because biting may cause it to splinter.

---

### PRACTICE TIP

Hold your breath throughout the time the patient is unable to breathe.

---

### Nasopharyngeal Airway

A nasopharyngeal airway (Fig. 7.19B) can be used for patients who need frequent suction, but insertion is painful and sinus infection is a risk. A size 6 mm is usually suited to women and 7 mm to men, or about the diameter of the patient's little finger. After local anaesthetic spray (Chang 2014, p. 129), it is lubricated with aqueous or lignocaine gel before insertion, passed gently into the straightest (often the right) or largest nostril, then directed backwards along the floor of the nose parallel to the hard palate until the flange is flat with the

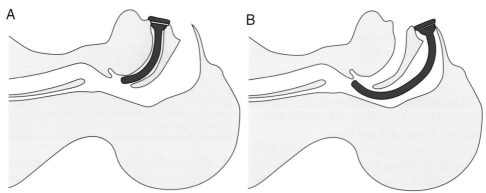

**FIGURE 7.19** (A) Oral Guedel airway and (B) nasopharyngeal airway.

nostril. The size is correct if the airway can be moved slightly inside the nose. The tip rests behind the tongue just above the epiglottis. A safety pin across the top, outside the nostril, prevents it disappearing into the patient.

Suction can then proceed through the airway, which avoids the discomfort of passing a catheter each time through the bend at the back of the throat. The airway can be left in place for a maximum 24 h, after which, if necessary, it can be cleaned and reinserted. It should not be used in patients who have polyps, congenital deformities, old nose fractures, cerebrospinal fluid leak or bleeding from the nose or ear.

## Minitracheostomy

A minitracheostomy (Fig. 7.20) allows access for safe and comfortable suction. It is usually performed under local anaesthesia on the ward and left in place for as many days as necessary. Suction with a size 10 catheter can then be performed through the aperture, with the patient breathing normally throughout. Some secretions are too thick for a minitracheostomy, although saline instillation may be helpful. A spigot protects the airway when the tube is not in use.

A minitracheostomy tube is uncuffed and preserves the function of the glottis so that natural humidification is maintained and the patient can cough, speak, eat and breathe normally. It is often performed later than optimal, so the physiotherapist can act as instigator to ensure that it is used early enough to be effective or obtain training in minitracheotomy themselves. Prophylactic placement during surgery may be useful for patients at high risk of postoperative sputum retention (Beach et al. 2013).

---

**MINI CLINICAL REASONING**

Is the following statement logical (or kind)?

*Indications for tracheal suction include ... to assess endotracheal or tracheostomy tube patency* **Cardiopulmonary Physiotherapy**, Oxford (2002)

It is unclear why a patient should be put through this procedure to identify what could be ascertained by asking them to breathe or observing the ventilator screen.

---

## Home Suction

The carers of patients requiring domiciliary suction should be taught how to suction, or, when possible, the patient can be taught to suction themselves. This is first

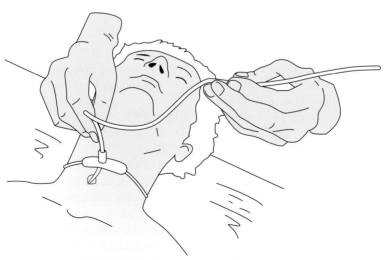

**FIGURE 7.20** Suction via minitracheostomy.

assessed in hospital in case oxygen is required. The discharge summary should indicate individual modifications for the patient and their subjective and objective responses. Detailed guidelines are in AARC (1999a).

## OUTCOMES FOR AIRWAY CLEARANCE

*Lacking evidence that any technique is superior to another, patient preference is an important consideration.*

**Hess 2002**

The following can be used to evaluate effectiveness:
- the patient's opinion;
- ↓ crackles on auscultation or by sound analysis (Marques et al. 2012);
- ↑ volume of sputum cleared;
- ↑ $SpO_2$, so long as other variables are excluded;
- ↑ independence of patients to manage their own secretions.

Physiotherapists can evaluate their manual techniques through a bronchoscope, if their patient is to undergo this procedure. The effect can be impressive.

For patients with hypersecretory disease, functional outcome measures are detailed in Chapter 3.

Using the literature to identify effective techniques is a minefield. Studies *in vitro* or in people with normal lungs bear limited relation to clinical practice. Studies that do not correct for cough alone are suspect because most techniques include coughing. Studies that do not follow up secretion clearance for several hours after treatment are of limited use. Studies that measure sputum volume or sputum weight do not compensate for saliva or swallowed secretions. Sputum volume is adequate for outcome measurement but is not valid for research. Cabillic et al. (2016) found that only AD, ACBT and ELTGOL showed evidence to level B.

On the assumption that mucociliary clearance benefits the patient, it can be assessed for research purposes by delivering a radio-isotope as an inhaled aerosol. This is caught by the mucus and the subsequent decline in radioactivity measured (Bennett et al. 2013). Coughing should be excluded because this affects the clearance rate.

For people with hypersecretory disease, research tracking the change in forced expiratory volume in 1 s

($FEV_1$) over time could indicate that clearing mucus from the larger airways is beneficial, on the assumption that stagnant secretions lead to damage that causes airflow obstruction. However, the procedure itself alters bronchial status quo by shearing secretions off the airway wall, and it does not appear to be responsive to airway clearance (Sontag et al. 2010). Using the same assumption about secretions and airway damage, it might be more useful to measure lung clearance index, which detects changes in the small airways (Rodriguez et al. 2016a), gas mixing efficiency (Robinson et al. 2013) or mid forced respiratory flow ($FEF_{25-75\%}$) (Sontag et al. 2010).

## CASE STUDY: MS

*A 17-year-old patient is admitted with an exacerbation of advanced CF.*

### Social history
- MS lives with his parents and is about to start college.

### Home management
- Brief morning session and longer evening session using ACBT, Flutter and PD;
- Exercise mainly by biking to school; little exercise in holidays;
- Regular reviews with community physiotherapist;
- Frequent admissions.

### Subjective
- Bored
- Not feeling ill
- Not clearing phlegm
- Not hungry or thirsty

### Objective
- Hyperinflated chest
- Thin
- Top-up feeding by gastrostomy at night
- Intravenous antibiotics
- Clinically dehydrated
- $SpO_2$ 95%
- Spiking temperature
- Auscultation: widespread crackles
- Frequent small nonproductive coughs
- Radiograph as Fig. 7.21

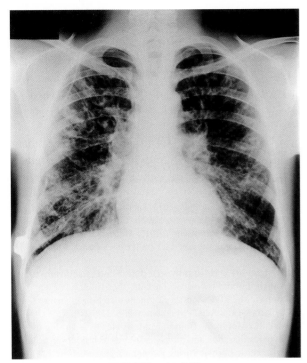

**FIGURE 7.21** MS.

**CLINICAL REASONING (1)**
Do you need to read further than the title of this study?

*A comparison of the Acapella and a threshold inspiratory muscle trainer for sputum clearance in bronchiectasis*
                                    Naraparaju et al. (2010)

**CLINICAL REASONING (2)**
*Are the following statements problem-based and/ or evidence-based?*
1. *Deep breathing exercises have been proposed to assist the tachypnoeic patient.*
2. *IPPB is claimed to be useful in delivering aerosolized bronchodilators.*
3. *Available evidence suggests that postural drainage and controlled coughing or FET may be the most effective components.*
                                *Eur Resp J* (1993) 3, 353–355

*FET,* Forced expiration technique (predecessor to active cycle of breathing techniques [ACBT]); *IPPB,* intermittent positive pressure breathing.

## Questions

1. Analysis?
2. Problems?
3. Goals?
4. Plan?

## Response to Case Study

1. Analysis
   - Radiograph shows widespread cystic shadowing.
   - Lack of eating may indicate depression because MS's anorexia is not related to feeling ill, and although he is undoubtedly bored, his use of this term might also indicate depression because a 17-year-old is unlikely to admit to this.
   - Lack of fluid intake may be contributing to sputum retention.
   - Frequent small nonproductive coughs are ineffective and may cause fatigue or strain the pelvic floor.
2. Problems
   - Depression → inactivity → sputum retention
   - Depression → dehydration → sputum retention
   - Depression → poor nutrition → immunocompromise → slow resolution of infection
   - Ineffective cough → sputum retention
   - Long term: lack of exercise in holidays
3. Goals
   - ↓ Depression
   - Control cough
   - Clear chest
   - Long term: review chest clearance regimen
4. Plan
   - Liaise with team including community physiotherapist regarding (1) management of depression, to include possible discussion on end-of-life care and (2) increasing fluid intake intravenously
   - Re-educate cough: suppress ineffective coughs, cough only when secretions are accessible
   - Check ACBT technique, suggest gym
   - If patient is tired or weak, discuss which passive techniques might suit him, e.g. PD, manual techniques, IPPB
   - Consider mask for biking to college

None of the conventional techniques were effective until hydration took effect. However, the patient enjoyed IPPB because he was shown how to administer it himself, then used it frequently to good effect. He was coaxed down to the gym, chose which equipment to use and was then able to use it whenever the gym was staffed. Both these techniques, chosen by him, facilitated autonomy. He was discharged to the care of the community team.

---

**RESPONSE TO CLINICAL REASONING (1)**

The Acapella is for sputum clearance.

The inspiratory muscle trainer is for training the inspiratory muscles (surprise).

The outcome was that the Acapella was better for sputum clearance (shock).

**RESPONSE TO CLINICAL REASONING (2)**

1. Tachypnoea indicates increased work of breathing, not loss of lung volume.

   If deep breathing exercises 'have been proposed', by whom?

   Deep breathing is counterproductive for breathless patients.

2. The words 'claimed to be' are unreferenced.

   IPPB is an expensive and inefficient way of delivering medication.

3. The 'available evidence' is unreferenced.

---

# RECOMMENDED READING

Al-Hajjaj, M.S., 2017. Management of chronic unexplained cough. Ann. Rehab. Med. 40 (2), 1–2.

Andersen, T., Sandnes, A., Hilland, M., 2013. Laryngeal response patterns to mechanical insufflation-exsufflation in healthy subjects. Am. J. Phys. Med. Rehabil. 92 (10), 920–929.

Bach, J.R., 2013. A historical perspective on expiratory muscle aids and their impact on home care. Am. J. Phys. Med. Rehabil. 92 (10), 930–941.

Bennett, W.D., Laube, B.L., Corcoran, T., et al., 2013. Multisite comparison of mucociliary and cough clearance measures using standardized methods. J. Aerosol. Med. Pulm. Drug Deliv. 26 (3), 157–164.

Brusasco, C., 2013. In vitro evaluation of heat and moisture exchangers designed for spontaneously breathing tracheostomized patients. Respir. Care 58 (11), 1878–1885.

Cross, J., Elender, J., 2012. Findings from the MATREX study: a treatment protocol for the delivery of manual chest therapy in respiratory care. Respir. Care 57 (8), 1263–1266.

Iyer, V.N., Lim, K.G., 2013. Chronic cough: an update. Mayo Clin. Proc. 88 (10), 1115–1126.

Laghia, F., 2017. Determinants of cough effectiveness in patients with respiratory muscle weakness. Resp. Physiol. Neurobiol. 240, 17–25.

Lai, S.K., Wang, Y.-Y., Wirtz, D., et al., 2010. Micro- and macrorheology of mucus. Adv. Drug Deliv. Rev. 61 (2), 86–100.

Lv, J., Wu, J., Guo, R., et al., 2013. Laboratory test of a visual sputum suctioning system. Respir. Care 58 (10), 1637–1642.

Munkholm, M., Mortensen, J., 2013. Mucociliary clearance: pathophysiological aspects. Clin. Physiol. Funct. Imag 34 (3), 171–177.

Nadel, J.A., 2013. Mucous hypersecretion and relationship to cough. Pulm. Pharmacol. Ther. 26 (5), 510–513.

Nikinmaa, M., 2013. Control of mucus secretion in airway inflammation. Acta. Physiologica. 208, 218–219.

O'Neill, K., Moran, F., Tunney, M.M., et al., 2017. Timing of hypertonic saline and airway clearance techniques in adults with cystic fibrosis during pulmonary exacerbation. BMJ Open Respir. Res 4 (1), e000168.

Osadnik, C.R., McDonald, C.F., Jones, A.P., 2012. Airway clearance techniques for chronic obstructive pulmonary disease. Cochrane Database Syst. Rev. (3), CD008328.

Rush, E.C., 2013. Water: neglected, unappreciated and under researched. Eur. J. Clin. Nutr. 67, 492–495.

Sears, P.R., 2013. Human airway ciliary dynamics. Am. J. Physiol. Lung Cell. Mol. Physiol. 304 (3), L170–L183.

Tambascio, J., de Souza, H.C.D., Baddini, M., et al., 2013. The influence of purulence on ciliary and cough transport in bronchiectasis. Respir. Care 58 (12), 2101–2106.

Yiallouros, P.K., Papadouri, T., Karaoli, C., et al., 2013. First outbreak of nosocomial Legionella infection in term neonates caused by a cold mist ultrasonic humidifier. Clin. Infect. Dis. 57 (1), 48–56.

# Physiotherapy to Decrease the Work of Breathing

## INTRODUCTION

> 'There is nothing worse than not being able to breathe'
>
> **Patient, quoted by Simon et al. 2013**

Increased work of breathing (WOB) may manifest objectively as a disturbance in the breathing pattern (p. 37) and subjectively as breathlessness. Breathing usually occurs subconsciously, but **breathlessness** occurs when there is awareness of the intensity of breathing (Fig. 8.1). **Dyspnoea** is breathlessness that is distressing and occurs at a level of activity where it would not normally be expected. In practice, the words breathlessness and dyspnoea are used interchangeably, along with **shortness of breath** (SOB). These should be distinguished from the objective terms:

- tachypnoea: rapid breathing;
- hyperpnoea: increased ventilation in response to increased metabolism;
- hyperventilation: ventilation in excess of metabolic requirements.

Breathless patients are caught in a pincer of decreased ventilatory capacity and increased ventilatory requirements. The basic principle of management is therefore to balance supply and demand, as summarized in Table 8.1.

Training and rest, whether systemic or limited to the inspiratory muscles, are not mutually exclusive, indeed they are complementary. The principles of training and rest form the basis of clinical reasoning when treating the breathless patient.

Increasing energy supply requires multidisciplinary teamwork. Reducing energy demand is the domain of physiotherapy and occupational therapy.

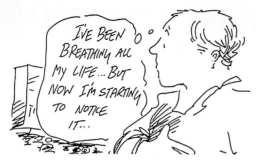

**FIGURE 8.1** Breathlessness. (From Leboeuf 2000.)

| TABLE 8.1 **Measures to optimize the balance between energy supply and demand** | |
|---|---|
| Measures to ↑ energy supply | Measures to ↓ energy demand |
| • Oxygen therapy<br>• Nutrition<br>• Fluid and electrolyte balance<br>• Optimum cardiac output<br>• Vascular sufficiency<br>• Adequate haemoglobin | • Stress reduction<br>• Sleep, rest and relaxation<br>• Positioning<br>• Breathing re-education<br>• Paced exercise<br>• Inspiratory muscle training and rest |

There is overlap between this chapter and Chapter 9. Assessment for breathlessness is on p. 34.

# BREATHLESSNESS

*'It's very difficult not to panic when you're fighting for breath … you feel as if a vacuum is sucking the air out of you … you're quite literally fighting for your life'*

**Patient, quoted by Williams 1993**

Breathlessness is one of the most frightening and distressing symptoms that a person can experience. It is associated with anxiety, panic, helplessness and fear of dying (Simon et al. 2013), and affects all domains of the ICF, including isolation for the family. It shares certain neural networks with pain (Dangers et al. 2015) and, like pain, shows wide variation between individuals because it includes reactions to the symptom as well as the symptom itself. Like pain, it has affective (emotional)

and sensory (intensity) mechanisms and shares the four components of physical, psychological, interpersonal and 'other distress' (Kamal et al. 2012). Unlike pain, it commonly goes unmeasured and untreated (Ekström et al. 2016). The experience is difficult for others to fully understand because normal breathlessness, such as when running for a bus, is of known duration, under control and without the fear component.

## Causes

> **KEY POINT**
>
> Breathlessness is a major link between disease and disability.

Breathlessness is a recurrent and intrusive symptom across acute, chronic, critical and terminal illness. Two-thirds of the causes are cardiorespiratory (Lai 2011), the symptom occurring in over 94% of people with chronic lung disease, more than 78% with lung cancer, and 50% with heart disease in the last year of life (Reilly et al. 2016). Other causes are neuromusculoskeletal disorders, hyperventilation syndrome, hyperthyroidism, anxiety, renal failure, anaemia, cancer, distended abdomen and pain (Gui 2012). The quality of SOB may help identify its cause (Table 8.2), and biomarkers can assist diagnosis in acute disease (Stokes et al. 2016a). Dyspnoea may also occur at the end of life, and in 30% of elderly people during their activities of daily living (ADL) (O'Donnell et al. 2007).

'Air hunger' describes an uncomfortable urge to breathe, as if at the end of a long breath-hold. Patients may describe not getting enough air or they may use emotionally charged descriptors such as a fear of dying.

## Physiology

*A respiratory physiologist offering a unitary explanation for breathlessness should arouse the same suspicion as a tattooed archbishop offering a free ticket to heaven.*

**Campbell & Howell 1963**

Dyspnoea cannot be predicted from physiological data (Ambrosino 2004). The experience is a private phenomenon, inaccessible through the traditional understanding of physiology. It incorporates both

**TABLE 8.2    Some characteristics of dyspnoea with different disorders**

| Disorder | Breathlessness | Other signs and symptoms |
| --- | --- | --- |
| Chronic obstructive pulmonary disease | Slow onset | Sometimes productive cough<br>Fatigue |
| Asthma | Episodic<br>Especially on exhalation | Chest tightness<br>Wheeze |
| Interstitial lung disease | Progressive<br>Especially on inhalation | Rapid shallow breathing<br>Dry cough |
| Pneumonia | On movement | Sometimes pleuritic pain |
| Pneumothorax | Sudden | Pleuritic pain |
| Hyperventilation syndrome | Air hunger<br>Not relieved by rest | Symptoms of $\downarrow$ $PaCO_2$ |
| Pulmonary oedema | Positional<br>Suffocating | Bilateral crackles on auscultation |
| Myocardial infarction | Sudden | Pain<br>Nausea |
| Neuromuscular | Exertional | Rapid shallow breathing |

sensory physiology and perceptual psychology, with the mechanics and emotional experience being inseparable. Like pain, it varies with the meaning of the sensation to the individual and shares afferent pathways and cortical regions, but the respiratory motor system is unusual in having both automatic (brainstem) and voluntary (cortical) sources of motor command. Like pain and coughing, it originates in afferent nervous systems that detect and signal real or impending threats (Banzett & Moosavi 2001).

Breathing is monitored by multiple sensory systems including muscle afferents, lung receptors, airway receptors and chemoreceptors (Fig. 8.2). When excessively stimulated, these provide sensory feedback via vagal, phrenic and intercostal afferents to the medulla and central nervous system, which processes it as a sense of effort, perceived as dyspnoea (Parshall et al. 2012). This perception incorporates both intensity and distress, the latter processed in the prefrontal cortex and midbrain (Horton 2010). Mechanical, cortical and chemical inputs are described below.

**Mechanical inputs**

Activation of proprioceptive pathways may be caused by an increase in workload or drive to breathe:

- $\uparrow$ WOB: mechanical abnormalities such as hyperinflation are sensed by receptors in the joints and muscles of the chest wall (Ahmedzai et al. 2012, p. 84).
- $\uparrow$ Drive: peripheral receptors respond to stimuli from the lung parenchyma, e.g. in pneumonia, while receptors in the airway respond to inhaled irritants, e.g. with asthma.

In health, the perception of increased effort does not usually elicit distress, the extra respiratory drive being rewarded by increased mechanical output and ventilation. However, when increased inspiratory muscle force becomes 10%–20% greater than the muscle force needed for unloaded inspiration, a mismatch between medullary respiratory motor discharge and peripheral afferent feedback gives rise to SOB (Burki & Lee 2012). This 'inappropriate length–tension relationship' means that a change in respiratory muscle length does not equate to tension developed by the muscle. The causes of this mismatch between incoming information and outgoing motor control are:

- $\uparrow$ resistive load, e.g. airflow resistance caused by obstructive airways disease;
- $\uparrow$ elastic load, e.g. reduced compliance caused by a rigid chest, distended abdomen, fibrotic lungs or increased alveolar surface tension due to surfactant depletion;
- $\downarrow$ energy supply, e.g. malnutrition or shock states in which perfusion to the diaphragm is impaired;

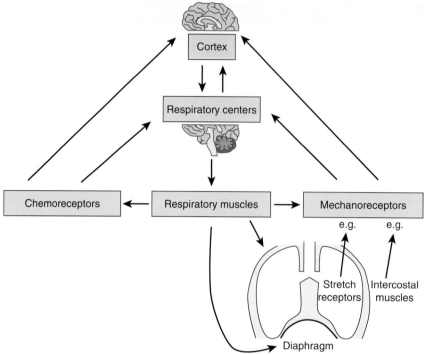

**FIGURE 8.2** Mechanism of dyspnoea. If input and output are balanced, whether at rest or on exercise, there is neuromechanical coupling and no shortness of breath. If the system is out of balance, there is neuromechanical dissociation and the patient feels breathless.

- ↑ drive to breathe, e.g. parenchymal disorders (such as fibrosis or pneumonia, which stimulate nerve impulses from interstitial receptors), acidosis or anaemia;
- ↓ power, which reduces the ability to cope with normal WOB, e.g. neuromuscular deficiency, disadvantaged diaphragm due to hyperinflated lungs, or fatigue, the latter magnifying the perception of effort in the same way that a weight feels heavier the longer it is carried.

In chronic obstructive pulmonary disease (COPD), airflow resistance is the main contributor to SOB at rest and hyperinflation the main contributor on exercise (Chen et al. 2016b).

### Cortical inputs

*Past and present experiences shape an individual's understanding and it is important to be able to piece together with the patient what meaning the symptom holds for them.*

*Syrett & Taylor 2003*

Cortical and subcortical inputs affect any subjective sensation, and the wide variation in the experience of SOB relates to interactions between physiological, psychological and behavioural responses, in particular anxiety (Garcia 2016) and, via the limbic system, fear (Kuroda 2012). These feed into a vicious cycle:

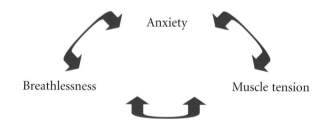

Other factors such as uncertainty and frustration exacerbate SOB, leading to variations in how the symptom is experienced. Education is therefore the first step in management, especially by reattribution using desensitization (p. 232).

*'My anxiety had taken away any power that I might have to cope with my breathlessness'*
**Patient, quoted by Syrett & Taylor 2003**

### Chemical inputs

Central chemoreceptors are limited in their contribution (Mahler et al. 2003), as illustrated by some patients with abnormal arterial blood gases (ABGs) not feeling breathless, while many breathless patients have normal ABGs (Uronis et al. 2006). The chemical contribution is mostly through sensing a rise in partial pressure of $CO_2$ in arterial blood ($PaCO_2$), mediated through pH. Reduced partial pressure of oxygen in arterial blood ($PaO_2$) plays little part in the drive to breathe and contributes only slightly to SOB, which explains the limited effectiveness of oxygen therapy for dyspnoea. Excess stimulation of chemoreceptors can also result from lactic acidosis.

The above mechanical, cortical and chemical processes send afferent impulses to the respiratory centres, from where a deluge of efferent impulses are discharged to the muscles, perceived as a sense of effort:

Receptor (mechanoreceptor or chemoreceptor)
↓
Afferent impulse
↓
Integration in the central nervous system,
including contextual and cognitive influences
↓
Efferent impulse
↓
SOB

### Effects on the Patient

*'It's the worst feeling in the world … it's like smothering to death … to lose control of your breathing'*
**Patient, quoted by DeVito 1990**

The conscious experience of excess motor output can vary from feeling that breathing is no longer automatic, to total preoccupation and unremitting fear. Fear itself makes breathing more difficult, and mechanical loads stimulate neural fear centres (O'Donnell et al. 2007), with patients feeling that they have lost control of their most basic physiological need. This is often compounded by isolation for the patient and family, especially when SOB limits the patient's ability to converse. Carers themselves have reported feelings of helplessness, isolation and frustration (Bailey et al. 2010).

A degree of imaginative skill is needed when working with people who are breathless, to identify with the experience of, for example, spending night after night in a chair unable to sleep, dreading the effort of going to the toilet, or anticipating the inexorability of death.

---

**PRACTICE TIP**

Hold your nose and breathe through a straw rapidly until you feel breathless. Invite colleagues to do the same then discuss your experiences, which will vary widely.

---

### Management

Treatment is by addressing the cause when possible, using medication when suitable (p. 169), multidisciplinary care through pulmonary rehabilitation for people with chronic SOB, and a breathlessness clinic for those with severe (Fig. 8.3) or end-stage disease (Higginson et al. 2014). Physiotherapy management in this chapter covers both acute and chronic SOB.

## HANDLING BREATHLESS PEOPLE

*'At every breath I felt: was it going to be enough? I thought life was over, even though I knew that was irrational. I didn't want to have to be polite, I didn't want the effort of please and thank you. I didn't mind how much phlegm was there, it could just stay there. The thought of a physio coming near me made me feel even more ill'*

Clare is a physiotherapist whose description, above, of the dyspnoea that she experienced with pneumonia is a reminder of the sensitivity with which breathless people must be handled.

Most patients need acknowledgement of the reality of their experience, not empty phrases like 'don't worry', which can be counterproductive (Booth et al. 2008). If patients know that we are aware that breathlessness can be frightening or even panic-inducing, this can be affirming and enables them to feel that we have some understanding of their experience. This is reinforced by asking patients how they manage the symptom themselves, e.g. a drink, chewing gum, distraction, pacing or the examples in Fig. 8.4.

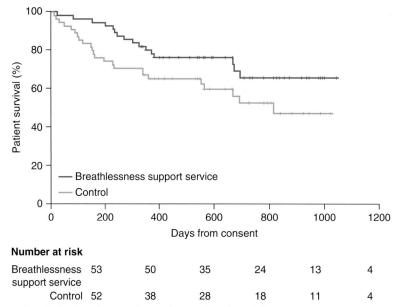

**FIGURE 8.3** Survival of patients who took part in a breathlessness clinic (top) and those who did not (bottom). (From Higginson et al. 2014.)

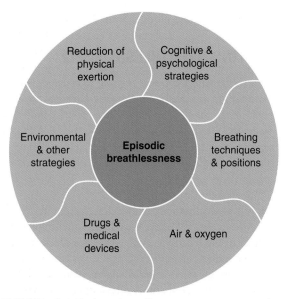

**FIGURE 8.4** Patients' self-management strategies. (From Simon et al. 2016.)

For severely breathless people, questions should require only a yes/no answer, or a thumb up or down, and patients should not have their sentences finished for them unless we know that this is what they want. They need to take their time and not be expected to talk unless they want to. For long-term breathless patients, as with anyone who is chronically disabled, it is important to respect their knowledge. They know more than we do about the experience of their disease and we learn much by listening to them.

The physical handling of acutely breathless patients requires maximum support, minimum speed and a rest between each movement. When patients are getting their breath back after activity, they should not be asked questions.

> **PRACTICE TIP**
>
> More than with any other respiratory problem, patients who are breathless need some control of their treatment.

*'It's such a relief not to be told 'keep calm' and 'just take a really deep breath'. Neither works when I panic'*

**Patient, quoted by Syrett & Taylor 2003**

## Desensitization to Breathlessness

*'Will I get much shorter of breath? Can I manage it? Is something terrible going to happen?'*

**Patient, quoted by Booth et al. 2008**

To reduce the anxiety that may inhibit activity and contribute to panic, patients are encouraged to disengage fear from their dyspnoea. First and foremost, they are told that breathlessness itself is not harmful. This is a revelation to some patients, who feel that it must be causing damage and that every breathless attack further progresses their disease. They are more likely to believe us if we acknowledge that, although the disease is harmful, breathlessness is a symptom of the disease and not damaging in itself. Any other feelings associated with SOB are checked, along with thoughts, beliefs and habitual responses associated with the sensation (e.g. avoiding physical activity), then misconceptions corrected.

Once this is understood, patients are encouraged in activities that increase SOB in a way that they control, and then gently regain their breath, no longer fearful that they are damaging themselves. Patient and physiotherapist start by walking together, at a speed to cause a slight increase in SOB but not distress, the patient being reminded to maintain relaxed rhythmic movement, relaxed rhythmic breathing, a good posture and to stop and get their breath back whenever they want. Patients who are deconditioned and fearful might simply walk around the bed and sit down. They are then praised for their success in increasing and controlling their breathlessness, and desensitization is reinforced by reminders that they have done themselves good rather than harm. This encourages them to switch from fear of SOB to confidence in their ability to control it.

Desensitization is progressed by increased exposure to gradual increases in SOB on exertion, then integrating this with other activities, using the same rhythmic breathing, steady movement and reinforcement of the message. Attention to pacing is required for those who tend to rush at activities.

## Fan

*'… you could get the fans on, get the doors open'*
**Patient, quoted by Simon et al. 2013**

Dyspnoea, including postexertion dyspnoea, may be reduced by air blowing across the dermatomes of the trigeminal nerve on the face (Fardy 2016), either from an open window or a fan. Patients with sensitive airways may need a bladeless fan. A hand-held fan (Fig. 8.5) needs a strong flow and soft blades because patients like

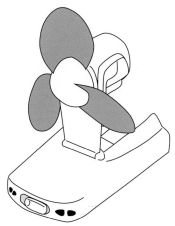

**FIGURE 8.5** Hand-held fan which sits on a table or can be kept on a loop around the neck.

to hold it close to their face. Some patients prefer a water spray.

## Positioning

Many breathless people automatically assume a posture that eases their breathing, but others need advice to find the position that best facilitates their inspiratory muscles. Patients with a flat diaphragm may benefit from forward-lean positions which create pressure from the abdominal contents to push the muscle back towards its normal dome-shaped position and provide some stretch to its fibres so that it can work more efficiently. The following may be helpful:

1. Forward-lean sitting (Fig. 8.6) or forward-lean standing, e.g. with elbows on a mantlepiece. Arms should be relaxed and supported to stabilize and increase the efficiency of the accessory muscles (Ogino et al. 2015). When out shopping, patients can lean on their supermarket trolley or, to get their breath back, lean on the supermarket freezer. When watching television or reading, they can lean on their table for as long as they are comfortable. Fig. 8.7 shows the benefit of this position.
2. For some patients with a hyperinflated chest, lying flat or occasionally even a head-down tilt (Bott 1997). Pressure from the abdominal contents helps to further dome the diaphragm in these positions.
3. High side-lying (Fig. 8.8).
4. Sitting upright in a chair with supported arms. For many patients, it is easier to breathe in this position

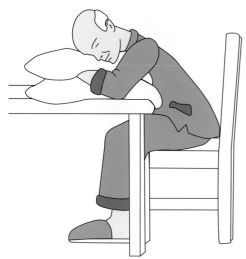

FIGURE 8.6 Relaxed forward-lean sitting, suitable for most patients with a hyperinflated chest and for some other patients with respiratory disease. (From Taylor 2007.)

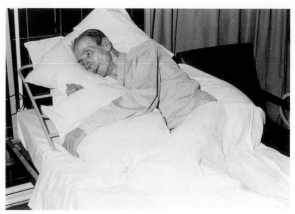

FIGURE 8.8 High side-lying. The head rest is relatively low to prevent the patient slipping down the bed and to avoid kinking the spine.

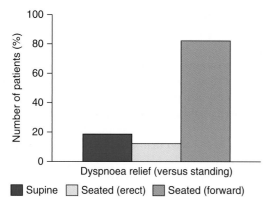

FIGURE 8.7 Proportion of patients finding benefit in forward-lean sitting. (From Gosselink 2004.)

than in bed. Some like to lean back for support, others prefer to lean slightly forward to put some stretch on the diaphragm.

5. Standing relaxed leaning back against a wall, with arms in pockets if support is needed for the accessory muscles. If patients are walking outside and need to stop to rest, they can put their phone to their ear so as not to feel self-conscious about standing still.

6. For patients who are breathless due to pulmonary oedema or a distended abdomen, upright positions are usually preferred.

Individuals can experiment with different positions. Some find the forward-lean positions claustrophobic, others unpredictably desaturate in different positions. Oximetry is useful as biofeedback and reassurance.

## Mechanical Input

Vibration over the chest appears to reduce breathlessness by augmentation of afferent feedback from the parasternal intercostal muscle spindles. Burki and Lee (2012) suggest that this is best done in phase with breathing, i.e. over the external intercostal muscles during inspiration and the internal intercostals during expiration. However, this is fiddly and the patient is best placed to say what is effective. Vibrations can be manual or with a mechanical vibrator, applied more gently than when clearing secretions so that they do not disturb the breathing pattern. The family can be shown this, as well as gentle rhythmic percussion. Oscillatory vibrations can also be delivered directly to the airway by a hand-held device (Morris et al. 2014). Neuromuscular electrical stimulation can reduce dyspnoea (Marciniuk et al. 2011) as well as increasing muscle strength (Maddocks et al. 2016).

## Quality of Movement

Patients can be advised that breathing is affected by talking, eating, moving, posture and muscle tension. Many know this, but it is difficult for some to adapt if, for example, they have spent a lifetime being hyperactive. Regularly pointing out how this disturbs their breathing, with reminders from carers to reinforce the message, enables patients to pace themselves and modify their quality of movement.

## Thoracic Mobility

Thoracic mobility may be impaired by chronic muscle tension, shortened anterior chest and shoulder muscles, abnormal mechanics of breathing, a forward head posture or tension due to a misplaced attempt to 'store' air. This can add a restrictive element to an obstructive condition and cause pain, sometimes misdiagnosed as pleurisy. Claims that mechanical impairment of the chest wall affects prognosis in COPD have not been backed up by research (Engel & Vemulpad 2011) but the following may improve posture, increase mobility or ease pain:

- myofascial release of sternomastoid, trapezius, intercostal, paravertebral muscles and the diaphragm, and mobilization of scapulothoracic and vertebral joints (Yilmaz et al. 2016);
- in forward-lean sitting, mobilizations to vertebral and scapular joints (Jones & Moffat 2002), which may reduce chest wall rigidity and dyspnoea in COPD (Engel & Vemulpad 2011);
- sitting astride a chair to fix the pelvis: active or passive thoracic rotation;
- crook lying with a roll under the thorax: thoracic extension, assisted by passive arm elevation (particularly helpful for people with cystic fibrosis);
- for some participants who have developed a stiff hyperinflated chest: manual compression on exhalation in a bucket-handle direction;
- muscle stretches (Carr 1993), which can increase vital capacity, reduce SOB (Kakizaki et al. 1999) and decrease hyperinflation (Matsumoto 2004);
- thoracic rotation and anterior compression with stretching in sitting; trunk extension and rib torsion in supine; lateral stretching in side-lying: the combination has shown improvement in SOB and chest expansion, although CPT was added for good measure, which slightly tarnishes the results (Leelarungrayub et al. 2009).

Precautions include checking for steroid-induced osteoporosis, and ensuring that handling and positioning do not exacerbate dyspnoea. Patients are encouraged to do their own stretching exercises, including side flexion, rotation and extension over the back of a chair, and hand-over-head exercises.

## Other Respiratory Problems

### Loss of lung volume

If a breathless person also has a problem of reduced lung volume, positioning is the first-line treatment because it is least disruptive to the breathing pattern. If patients are relaxed, lung expansion is facilitated as they get their breath back after turning to a position that facilitates both lung expansion and efficient breathing, e.g. high side-lying.

If further measures such as deep breathing are necessary, the respiratory rate should be maintained throughout. When asked to take a deep breath, breathless patients sometimes respond by holding their breath. This can be avoided by advising them to 'keep breathing in and out', or telling them when to breathe in and out, until they find their own rhythm. No more than two deep breaths should be taken at a time.

### Sputum retention

If a breathless person has a problem of sputum retention, the vibrations from oscillatory partial expiratory pressure devices (p. 214) are transmitted into the airways and can help reduce SOB (Fridlender et al. 2012) as well as clearing the secretions. If manual vibrations are used, they should not disturb the breathing pattern. Percussion can be relaxing if a slow, rhythmic technique is used. The head-down postural drainage position is usually unsuited to breathless people, except occasionally for those with a flat diaphragm.

> *Breathlessness cannot be treated in isolation from its complex physiological, psychological and environmental components.*
>
> *Reilly et al. 2016*

## SLEEP, REST AND RELAXATION

> *'There's no peace, no let up with this thing, it's with you 24 h a day'*
>
> *Patient, quoted by Williams 1993*

The only treatment for acute fatigue is rest. This can be achieved most satisfactorily by sleep. One of the cruel ironies of SOB is its effect on sleep. Fragmentation of sleep brings complications (pp. 24 and 432) and tips patients into another vicious cycle:

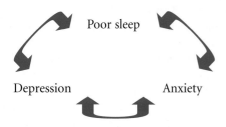

Sleep deprivation in respiratory patients may be due to SOB, coughing or anxiety, aggravated in hospital by noise, an unfamiliar environment or being woken for nebulizers.

Physiotherapists should avoid waking patients unnecessarily, ensure that their treatment does not cause excess fatigue, and contribute to, or initiate, the teamwork required for a good night's sleep. It is a continuing puzzle that there is so little emphasis in the health care system on promoting the healing power of sleep.

Relaxation is facilitated by positioning, sensitive handling and information to reduce anxiety. Deeper relaxation may be achieved by using a relaxation technique. For this, patients should be warm, comfortable and have adequate fresh air. The physiotherapist's bleep should be rerouted and they should sit beside the patient rather than directly in front, to minimize self-consciousness. A technique such as the Mitchell method may be chosen that does not entail breath-holding or strong muscle contraction (Payne 2010). Other methods can be used that incorporate breathing itself, such as yoga techniques, which may also reduce stress and improve immune function (Zope & Zope 2013).

Patients should be reassured that there is no right or wrong way of relaxing and that they can follow what feels right for them. Although it does not matter if they fall asleep (and relaxation can be a helpful technique for this when required), the purpose is to enjoy a hypometabolic conscious state and experience the tranquillity, so that they can recreate them as desired and integrate them into their ADL.

The aim of relaxation is not to add another burden to the patient's daily routine, but for them to find brief moments in the day to check for tension and choose any aspect of relaxation that suits them, e.g. Appendix B.

The effects of relaxation are:
- ↓ SOB (Mahler et al. 2010);
- a more focused mental state (Kobayashi 2016);
- ↓ heart rate and respiratory rate, ↑ sleep onset (Omlin et al. 2016);
- ↓ anxiety and airway obstruction (Gift 1992);
- with meditation: ↓ respiratory rate, heart rate and blood pressure (Melville et al. 2012).

The key to relaxation is ongoing maintenance.

## BREATHING RE-EDUCATION

The previous measures may be adequate, but some patients find structured breathing re-education helpful. The aims are to reduce WOB and give patients confidence in their ability to control breathless attacks.

When intervening in a person's breathing pattern, a minimalist approach is advised, and patients' individual compensatory mechanisms should not be interfered with mindlessly. Even if their breathing appears unnatural, it may be optimum for them. For example:
- If a patient relies on their accessory muscles to breathe, relaxing their shoulders is not always helpful.
- Hyperinflation increases SOB but may also be assisting the airways to stay open, so asking patients to reduce this by prolonging exhalation may or may not be helpful.

But if breathing is irregular, paradoxical or unnecessarily tense, re-education to improve breathing efficiency is usually helpful.

There is no clear evidence that a voluntary act can become automatic, but practice can enable a breathing technique to be used more easily when required. Patients tend to find that the techniques are most useful when getting their breath back after exertion.

### Preliminaries

Each of the following steps is best taken one at a time. Close observation will then determine whether this has been helpful and/or if the next step should be initiated.
1. The position is chosen by the patient, but the physiotherapist might suggest any of the positions described previously.
2. Awareness of breathing is encouraged by bringing the person's attention to their breathing pattern. Are they breathing apically, abdominally, paradoxically, asynchronously, using pursed lips and prolonged expiration, or breathing through their nose or

mouth? The physiotherapist can sit in front of the patient and mirror their breathing pattern, then minor corrections can be suggested, but the aim is simply awareness at this stage.

3. If the patient shows localized tension, e.g. of their hands or facial muscles, they can be advised to let that part feel heavy and relaxed.

4. Breathing patterns and body movements are contagious (Kuroda 2012) and the physiotherapist's own relaxed posture, steady breathing and quiet voice will help reduce the patient's tension.

5. Encouraging comments such as 'well done' and 'take your time' help facilitate relaxation.

Breathing then usually becomes slower and deeper naturally. Shallow breathing wastes energy because of ventilating dead space, and rapid breathing wastes energy because of turbulence. However, it may be counterproductive to encourage slow deep breathing beyond that developed naturally through the above, because it can fatigue the diaphragm (Gosselink 2004). This is particularly relevant for people with interstitial lung disease, who tend to adopt rapid shallow breathing, a logical breathing pattern because of their high elastic recoil and low lung compliance.

## Rhythmic Breathing

> *'I walked a mile the other week without any problems, then over the weekend I got out of my car and immediately became breathless'*
> **Patient, quoted by Simon et al. 2013**

Breath-holding increases tension and upsets the fine balance of steady breathing, which further disturbs the breathing pattern. It is common in anxious people, especially when changing activity or making an effort. If breath-holding is pointed out to the patient at each opportunity, with advice to 'keep the rhythm going', patients are often able to bring it under control. Patients find this easier to change than other manifestations of anxiety such as rapid talking or body tension. The physiotherapist, patient and family members can compete to be the first to notice each instance of breath-holding.

In patients without excessive SOB, nose-breathing may be helpful, facilitated by suggesting that they keep their lips together, while keeping their jaw loose to maintain relaxation. Once breathing is rhythmic, patients may be able to gently develop an abdominal pattern of breathing, as described below.

## Abdominal Breathing

An emphasis on abdominal movement during inspiration may lead to naturally slower deeper breathing, less turbulence, reduced dead space and shoulder girdle relaxation. Other terms are:

- 'diaphragmatic breathing', which is often understood by patients who have learnt it during singing or childbirth classes, though it is not strictly accurate because, in the absence of phrenic nerve malfunction, all breathing patterns involve some diaphragmatic activity (Bruton et al. 2011);
- 'breathing control', which is abdominal breathing at tidal volume.

The depth of the abdominal breath is immaterial (unless the aim is to increase lung volume) and the focus should be on a relaxed, efficient breathing pattern.

Abdominal breathing may visibly break through a patient's wall of tension and has shown the following benefits:

- $\downarrow$ oxygen consumption ($\dot{V}O_2$) (Hodgkin et al. 2009, p. 51)
- $\uparrow$ gas exchange (Cahalin et al. 2002)
- $\uparrow$ functional capacity and exercise tolerance (Yamaguti et al. 2012)
- $\uparrow$ quality of life (Borge et al. 2016)

However, patients vary in how they respond and Fernandes et al. (2011) found that for patients with asynchronous thoracoabdominal motion who are dependent on their upper chest accessory muscles, abdominal breathing can actually increase SOB. This may be minimized by emphasizing rhythmic breathing, or using demonstration, visual feedback with a mirror or a spirogram and verbal feedback, the combination of which may reduce exertional SOB (Gimenez 2010). Some patients are uncomfortable with mirrors.

Clinical reasoning therefore suggests that the breathing pattern should be stabilized beforehand by facilitating rhythmic breathing. The following is then suggested, with close observation of the breathing pattern to ensure that synchrony is maintained.

1. The patient finds a comfortable and symmetrical position such as upright sitting or forward-lean sitting.

2. The manoeuvre is explained and demonstrated unhurriedly, avoiding words like 'push', 'pull', 'try' and 'harder'.

3. The patient rests their dominant hand on their abdomen, with elbows supported; then, keeping their

shoulders relaxed, they breathe in through the nose, allowing their hand to rise gently, while visualizing air filling their abdomen like a balloon (the word 'stomach' can be substituted for abdomen).

4. They sigh the air out and then check that their shoulders remain relaxed and heavy, unless this upsets the breathing pattern.

5. If appropriate, they progress to forward-lean standing and other positions.

Patients may respond to the physiotherapist's hands placed on their lower abdomen to encourage breathing 'in and down', but overpressure does not appear to increase abdominal displacement (Tomich et al. 2010) and may inhibit abdominal relaxation.

Variations include:

• putting the other hand on the quiet upper chest to compare it with movement of the abdomen;
• advising the patient to imagine a piece of elastic round their waist that stretches as they breathe in;
• trying a sniff at end-inspiration, which specifically recruits the diaphragm (Cahalin et al. 2002) so long as this does not destabilize the breathing pattern;
• if supine, placing a box of tissues on the abdomen to visually reinforce the movement;
• incorporating incentive spirometry, to encourage a steady flow.

Some patients find that other positions facilitate abdominal movement, e.g. standing with hands on hips and elbows pushed backwards, or, for the agile, four-point kneeling.

Efficacy is not always identifiable subjectively because of the unfamiliarity of a different way of breathing. If observation of the breathing pattern indicates that it appears more efficient, the patient can be advised to practice at home. Subsequently, if the patient finds it helpful, they will be motivated to continue. If they do not find it helpful despite mastering the correct technique, then it is not worth persisting.

## Square Breathing

As both distraction and an aid to steadying the breathing, patients can focus on an imaginary square, or on a real square such as a window, picture or (blank) screen. They breathe in (through the nose if possible) as they focus on the corner of the square and breathe out (through pursed lips if required) as they move along the borders. A few minutes in the morning and evening may enable them to feel more in control and then use it as

required. Distraction has been shown to reduce SOB (Von Leupoldt et al. 2007), and patients might like to choose their own strategies.

## Yoga Breathing

'Grounding the energy' is the simplest and quickest of relaxation techniques. Patients sit with their feet flat on the floor and visualize breathing air 'in through your head and out through your feet into the floor'. This is not exactly anatomical but usually facilitates relaxation during exhalation. Patients are encouraged to maintain a steady breathing pattern and to 'sink into the chair' on the out-breath.

## Prolonged Exhalation

A reduction in the inspiratory:expiratory ratio may help to decrease lung hyperinflation, which can diminish SOB. This may be assisted by counting, e.g. 'in/one, out/one/two/three', sometimes integrated with walking, so long as this does not stiffen the gait.

## Pursed Lips Breathing

Prolonged exhalation may be incorporated into pursed lips breathing, which involves breathing out actively through pursed lips, keeping other facial muscles relaxed if possible. With the floppy airways of emphysema, the positive pressure reduces airway collapse (Jiang et al. 2008). Patients who have not learnt it spontaneously may benefit, and it can be taught via Skype (Nield & Hoo 2012). The following effects have been identified:

• ↓ SOB (Nield & Hoo 2012);
• ↓ dynamic hyperinflation during physical activity in people with COPD (de Araujo et al. 2016);
• ↑ exercise capacity (Bhatt et al. 2013);
• ↑ $SpO_2$, speedier recovery after exercise (Garrod & Mathieson 2013);
• ↓ panic attacks (Uronis et al. 2006).

The majority of people with COPD find pursed lips breathing beneficial and continue to use it long-term (Roberts et al. 2016a).

## EXERCISE AND PACING

Exercise can itself improve the breathing pattern (Collins 2001), especially in how it improves spinal stability (Kweon et al. 2013). Exercise is discussed with patients at the first encounter, along with desensitization to breathlessness and the link to their SMART goals and ADL. Exercise should be simple and written down on tick charts (Appendix B), along with advice to exercise little and often.

For chronic SOB, exercise is best provided in a pulmonary rehabilitation programme (Chapter 9). Patients who prefer to stay home can put a static bike in front of their television. Using it just thrice weekly is sufficient to increase exercise tolerance (Guzun et al. 2012). For acute SOB, quadriceps exercises or T'ai Chi (Leung et al. 2013) are beneficial. However breathless a patient, there is always a brief exercise that they can do, before building it up into exercise training.

Patients who have not learnt to pace themselves may rush at their exercise, which can be counterproductive. Walking alongside the patient, steadily and sometimes more slowly than they are used to, enables them to achieve control, stop when they need to, and understand the benefit of energy conservation. Recreating and managing situations that increase SOB for each individual will improve confidence.

## NONINVASIVE VENTILATION

Noninvasive ventilation (NIV) provides inspiratory muscle rest for people in ventilatory failure. This may be because of reduced mechanical efficiency from a hyperinflated chest, increased load from obstructed airways or decreased force from weak or fatigued muscles.

NIV delivers a predetermined pressure or volume in response to patient effort, delivered by mask or other interface. Compared with continuous positive airway pressure (CPAP), it is used for ventilatory (type II) respiratory failure rather than oxygenation (type I) respiratory failure. Compared to invasive mechanical ventilation, NIV brings fewer complications and reduced mortality (Baird 2012), and is usually more comfortable. Intensive care is not required and patients can participate in their own management. However, NIV does not protect the airway, allows no direct access to the trachea for suction and cannot provide complete inspiratory muscle rest (Kallet & Diaz 2009).

### Noninvasive Ventilation for Acute Disorders

For the 75% of patients who tolerate it (Liu et al. 2016c), NIV can unload the inspiratory muscles, relieve SOB (Mahler et al. 2010), improve oxygenation and ventilation, prevent intubation and decrease mortality (Allison & Winters 2016). Patient handling skills are required to talk anxious patients through the process so that they allow the machine to assist their breathing.

Benefits have been found for people who have:

- acute COPD, leading to lower mortality and length of stay (Peng et al. 2016) and reduced need for mechanical ventilation (Rettig 2016);
- acute asthma, pneumonia, a need for palliative care or after surgery (Mas & Masip 2014);
- neurological disease (Vandoorne et al. 2016);
- cystic fibrosis (Bargellini 2013);
- acute respiratory distress syndrome (Patel et al. 2016);
- pulmonary oedema, if CPAP is not suitable (Dres & Demoule 2016);
- patients needing controlled oxygen therapy when the target $SpO_2$ cannot be maintained without hypoventilation and acidosis (p. 158).

High concentrations of oxygen can be entrained if necessary, even with hypercapnic COPD patients, so long as there is a safety backup of mandatory breaths irrespective of respiratory drive.

A plan is required which addresses how potential failure of NIV will be dealt with, i.e. whether NIV is the ceiling of treatment or whether escalation is appropriate. If the latter is likely, the patient should be in a high dependency area where intubation is available, otherwise a respiratory ward is acceptable.

### Noninvasive Ventilation for Chronic Disorders

*'From our very first night she made a quite startling difference to my life. Just one night converted me to the joys and thrills of home ventilation. For the first time in months I felt reasonably clear-headed, I no longer fell asleep in mid-sentence, my headaches disappeared … my posture and balance noticeably improved'*

**Brooks 1990**

NIV should be considered for people with chronic hypercapnia and may be set up at home using an autotitrating system (Mandal et al. 2017). Benefits include:

- ↑ exercise tolerance, ↑ $PaO_2$, ↓ $PaCO_2$, slower decline in lung function and ↓ mortality in people with stable COPD (Tang & Qin 2016);
- ↓ WOB for people with fibrosis (p. 103);

- ↑ wellbeing and survival for people with neurological disease (p. 112) or cystic fibrosis (p. 95).

## Criteria

The indications for acute NIV are pH <7.35 and $PaCO_2$ >6 kPa (45 mmHg) (RCP 2008).

Mixed acid–base and lactate disorders during hypercapnic COPD exacerbations are a strong indication (Terzano et al. 2012). Patients with other chronic disorders may also benefit, e.g. those with neuromuscular disease or scoliosis, or those awaiting lung transplantation (Fuehner et al. 2016). Glottic control must be adequate to prevent aspiration.

## Contraindications, Precautions and Complications

Exclusion criteria are the following (BTS/RCP/ICS 2008):
- life-threatening hypoxaemia, i.e. the patient needs to go straight to intubation;
- haemodynamic instability requiring inotropes or vasopressors (unless in the ICU);
- confusion or agitation;
- upper gastrointestinal surgery or bowel obstruction, in case of air swallowing;
- as with CPAP and IPPB: risk of vomiting, excessive secretions, facial trauma, barotrauma or haemoptysis of unknown origin.

Barotrauma can itself be caused by NIV (Fig. 8.9), especially with acute asthma and lung fibrosis (Fukushima et al. 2008).

Discomfort and mask leaks are managed by trying different sizes and types of mask. Pressure sores are prevented by using forehead spacers or changing the interface. Other options are customized masks or different masks used in rotation. Some masks contain an inner lining which improves the seal by inflating on inspiration and lessens skin pressure by deflating on expiration. Skin irritation is also lessened by daily washing of the mask, spacer and the patient's skin, and by using minimal strap tension. If the straps feel too tight, a smaller mask may allow them to be loosened or a skull cap can be used.

Gastric distension sometimes occurs with volume-controlled machines or in patients with a stiff chest wall. Options are:
- experimenting with different positions;
- considering a fine bore nasogastric tube;

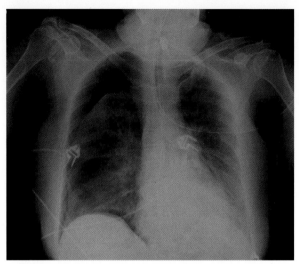

**FIGURE 8.9** Right pneumothorax following noninvasive ventilation. (From Carron et al. 2007.)

- using the lowest effective pressure;
- changing from volume to pressure control (p. 441), or trying a different ventilator.

Nasal dryness may be helped by nasal drops. Mouth dryness usually responds to reducing air leaks through the mouth. Some machines have a button to switch off insufflations during swallowing (Terzi 2014).

The main causes of intolerance are distress, SOB or a too high flow/pressure (Liu et al. 2016c), which underlines the need for sensitive application of the device to a well-informed patient.

## Mode of Action

NIV is more comfortable than CPAP because of individually controlled inspiratory and expiratory pressures superimposed on the patient's spontaneous breathing, i.e. bilevel positive airway pressure (BiPAP). The pressures are termed inspiratory positive airway pressure (IPAP) and expiratory positive airway pressure (EPAP) (Fig. 8.10). In relation to the terminology for invasive ventilation:
- EPAP is equivalent to positive end-expiratory pressure (PEEP) (p. 451)
- IPAP minus EPAP ≡ pressure support ventilation (p. 443)

The term 'BiPAP' has been patented as a brand name for the Respironics models. The word is therefore

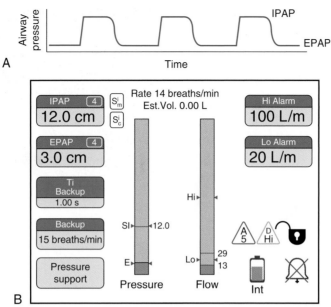

**FIGURE 8.10** (A) BiPAP waveform. (B) Nippy ventilator showing IPAP set at 12 cmH$_2$O and EPAP at 3 cmH$_2$O. The patient's respiratory rate is 14 breaths/min, with a safety backup rate set at 15 breaths/min. *Backup*, Respiratory rate if patient fails to trigger inspiration; *EPAP*, expiratory positive airway pressure; *IPAP*, inspiratory positive airway pressure; *Pressure support*, equivalent to BiPAP; *Ti*, inspiratory time.

synonymous with either the Respironics machine or this mode of ventilation on any machine. Other manufacturers may use different terms for the BiPAP mode, but it is used here in its generic sense.

Most machines are flow-triggered, flow-cycled and pressure-controlled (p. 440). *Pressure control* limits peak pressure, reducing the risk of pneumothorax and compensating for minor leaks so that ruthless tightening of headgear is not required. People with COPD might require the cycling criterion to be set above the default setting of 20%–30% of peak inspiratory flow, for comfort (Moerer et al. 2016). *Volume-control* machines may be suited to people with high or fluctuating airway resistance or lung compliance. The feel of different machines varies and patients have their own preferences.

The spontaneous mode relies on the patient to trigger every breath. The spontaneous/timed mode adds mandatory breaths if the patient does not breathe after a set time interval, with a backup respiratory rate (RR) set at about 10 breaths/min. The timed mode provides fully controlled ventilation for patients who have central sleep apnoea, or for some exhausted and sleep-deprived patients during their first night.

Although the natural airway is intact, high flows may overwhelm the usual airway humidification mechanism, and hot water humidification is advised (AARC 2012), especially if there is a mouth leak. The heated wire inside this tubing is best built into the wall or wrapped around the outside so that it does not interfere with the gas flow. Passive humidification by heat–moisture exchanger can increase airflow resistance, impair CO$_2$ elimination in hypercapnic patients (Lellouche et al. 2012) and may interfere with patient triggering (Cairo 2012 p. 388), but low dead space models are sometimes suitable (Boyer et al. 2010).

People with acute disease normally need entrained oxygen titrated to their target SpO$_2$. Both oxygen flow and humidification may affect the pressure settings. A nasogastric tube is required if the patient is at risk of vomiting or if high IPAP is used.

### Interface

Oronasal or full face masks (Fig. 8.11) are useful for the first 24 h when patients are likely to be breathless and mouth-breathing. If nasal masks are used, they should be small enough to fit from halfway down the bridge of

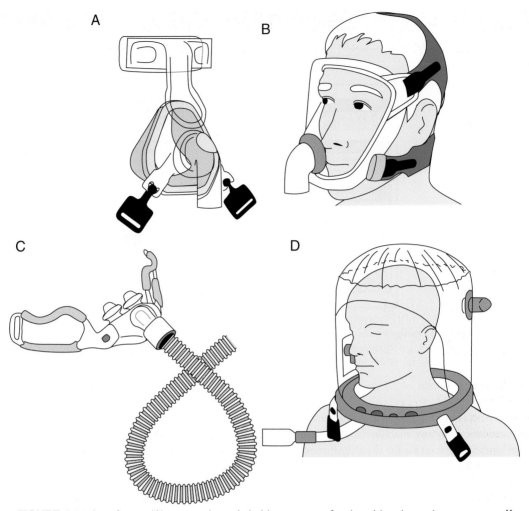

**FIGURE 8.11** Interfaces: (A) oronasal mask (with spacer at forehead level to take pressure off the bridge of the nose); (B) full face mask; (C) nasal pillows; (D) helmet.

the nose to just below the nose, without impinging on the nostrils. A mask sizing gauge is helpful. A helmet is a transparent plastic hood attached to a soft neck collar (Olivieri et al. 2016), and appears to be more successful in people with obstructive disease than restrictive disease (Oda et al. 2016a). Devices that cover both nose and mouth require quick-release straps that the patient can use, and anti-asphyxia valves in case of ventilator malfunction. Some ventilator-dependent people prefer a mouthpiece in the daytime and customized mask at night, while others favour a tracheostomy. Most interfaces affect eating, for which protocols are advised (Reeves et al. 2014). Characteristics are shown in Table 8.3.

## Technique

Patients need to be told the rationale of NIV and, when obtaining consent, what the other options are, including intubation or palliation. The following sequence is advised:

1. If the patient cannot take off the mask independently they must be in a high dependency unit.
2. Exhalation ports are designed to exhaust $CO_2$ and must not be blocked, except initially to test that flow is present. They should be directed away from the patient's face.
3. The patient takes up the position they prefer, within reach of their call bell.

**TABLE 8.3   Interfaces for noninvasive ventilation**

| Name | Position | Advantages | Disadvantages |
|---|---|---|---|
| Oronasal/face mask | Covers nose and mouth | No problem if air leaks through mouth | Pressure on bridge of nose |
| Full face mask | Covers nose, mouth and eyes | As above | Drying of eyes<br>Humidification impractical because of condensation |
| Nasal mask | Covers nose | Allows speech, expectoration, inhaled drugs, eating and drinking<br>Suited to patients who may vomit | Nasal irritation<br>Mouth leak with some patients |
| Nasal pillows | Plugs into nostrils | As above<br>Avoids pressure on the bridge of the nose or cheeks<br>↓ Dead space<br>Less claustrophobic<br>Allows spectacles | As above |
| Mouthpiece | Held by patient's mouth | Useful if pressures >25 cmH$_2$O are needed | |
| Helmet | Covers head and neck | Less claustrophobic for some patients | Pressure in axillae due to armpit straps<br>Humidification impractical because of condensation<br>May lead to CO$_2$ rebreathing |

4. IPAP is usually started at about 10 cmH$_2$O and titrated until a therapeutic response is achieved, using 2–5 cmH$_2$O increments every 10 min for acute patients. The maximum tolerated is normally 25 cmH$_2$O, but IPAP at 15 cmH$_2$O and EPAP at 5 cmH$_2$O brings most measures of WOB towards normal (Kallet & Diaz 2009). If inspiratory and expiratory pressures are equal, CPAP is delivered, which is not usually the intention.

5. The machine is turned on and the patient allowed to feel the air blowing against their hand, and then on their face, before the mask is strapped on. The straps should then be tightened equally on both sides and with enough space for two fingers under the straps, to protect the skin (Nava et al. 2009).

6. Patients are asked to keep their mouth shut if they can. Some may voluntarily do this once they feel the relief of their breathing being supported, but others are committed mouth-breathers, in which case a chin strap or collar may be used, or the patient may prefer side-lying with a pillow supporting their chin. Small leaks are acceptable with pressure-controlled machines if they do not interfere with triggering into inspiration or cycling into expiration, and so long as tidal volumes and ABGs are adequate.

7. Improvement in RR and pH in the first hour is a predictor of success. If PaO$_2$ does not rise adequately, IPAP and EPAP should be increased equally, and/or fraction of inspired oxygen (FiO$_2$) increased. If PaCO$_2$ does not reduce sufficiently, IPAP is increased, but PaCO$_2$ should not be forced down too quickly if there is high bicarbonate, otherwise metabolic alkalosis may supervene. SpO$_2$ should be checked after any alteration in IPAP or EPAP. A decision to proceed to intubation, if indicated, needs to be made within the first 4 h (BTS/RCP/ICS 2008).

8. For acute patients, SpO$_2$ is monitored continuously. One repeat ABG is required at 30–60 min, or transcutaneous capnography can be used alongside oximetry (Stieglitz et al. 2016). Vital signs, symptoms of hypercapnia, patient–ventilator synchrony and mask comfort are monitored quarter-hourly for the first hour, then, if stable, hourly for 4 h, then 2–4 hourly. Analysis of the waveforms helps optimize management (Di Marco et al. 2011). The 'rise time' is the time taken to reach the IPAP, and needs to be high for breathless patients.

9. Acutely ill patients are best given continuous NIV for 24 h, with a face mask if tolerated, removing the

mask only to talk, drink, eat, cough and use their nebulizer if required. Questions to the patient need to be specific and require a yes or no answer.

10. The mask should be removed before turning the machine off.

Nebulizers and pressurized inhalers, but not dry powder inhalers, can be used, except when using a full face mask or helmet, and after removal of the humidifier or heat–moisture exchanger (Soroksky et al. 2013). The active cycle of breathing or autogenic drainage can be performed during NIV (Inal-Ince et al. 2004); the mask is removed for the huff phase, and pressure or volume may need to be increased during the thoracic expansion phase.

Whether the NIV service is nurse-led, physiotherapist-led or doctor-led, relevant staff must be specifically trained, including the medical team to provide timely ABGs. Weaning takes the form of increasing periods of daytime spontaneous breathing, then the same process at night.

Quality of life outcomes for people receiving long-term NIV can be measured by the Severe Respiratory Insufficiency Questionnaire (Walterspacher et al. 2016).

## Other Ventilators

Some ICU ventilators have noninvasive modes, but ventilators designed specifically for NIV have better leak compensation (Hess 2013).

Negative pressure ventilation entails the application of negative pressure externally via a machine which encloses part of the patient's body, sucking air into the lungs through the natural airway. The machines are bulky but suit some individuals who require long-term support. Advantages are avoidance of the complications of positive pressure or mask, easier communication and the opportunity to use glossopharyngeal breathing (p. 112). They can also be used for patients with barotrauma (Hino et al. 2016). Disadvantages are the cumbersome machinery and risk of sleep apnoea due to upper airway collapse. Options are the following:

- A **tank** ventilator encloses the entire patient except the head in an airtight iron lung. Disadvantages are size, noise, discomfort from the neck seal, immobility and inaccessibility of the patient. If the patient vomits, pressure must be equalized immediately by opening a porthole because of the danger of aspiration.
- **Jackets** and the rigid shell-like **cuirass** apply negative pressure over the chest and abdomen, and may be preferred by patients at home without the manual dexterity to use a mask (Ho et al. 2013).

- The **rocking bed** uses gravity-assisted displacement of the abdominal contents to augment diaphragm excursion, usually for people with isolated bilateral diaphragm weakness. For immobile patients, the variation in pressure reduces the risk of skin breakdown (Tsakiridis 2012).
- The **pneumobelt** is preferred by some wheelchair users but is not for use in supine. For expiration, it inflates a bladder around the abdomen at 50 $cmH_2O$ to push up the diaphragm. For passive inspiration, it deflates to allow diaphragmatic descent (Liu et al. 2012).
- **High frequency oscillators** deliver bursts of gas either through a mouthpiece, or externally by generating oscillating pressures through a cuirass. They reduce WOB by overriding spontaneous ventilation, and they may also assist clearance of secretions (p. 453).

### MINI CLINICAL REASONING

Consider the logic of the conclusion of Shapiro et al. (1992) that 'inspiratory muscle rest confers no benefit' after encasing patients in negative pressure body suits overnight. Patients were too uncomfortable to sleep and found a visit to the toilet an ordeal.

Perhaps they should have tried positive pressure noninvasive ventilation.

## OUTCOMES

Reduced WOB can be judged by the following:
- ↓ SOB
- ↓ fatigue
- ↓ RR
- more synchronous breathing pattern
- for patients with chronic disease, ↑ exercise tolerance and ADL

Outcome measures for SOB are:
- visual analogue scale for dyspnoea (Mishra et al. 2015);
- Chronic Respiratory Disease Questionnaire, which can be self-administered (Bausewein 2012);
- Dalhousie Dyspnea and Perceived Exertion Scale, which uses pictures for both adults and children (Pianosi et al. 2016);
- Medical Research Council Scale and Baseline Dyspnoea Index (Perez et al. 2015);
- Dyspnea 12 Questionnaire and Multidimensional Dyspnea Profile (Ekström et al. 2016);

- Breathlessness Catastrophizing Scale (Solomon et al. 2015);
- Borg scale (Fig. 9.2);
- Severe Respiratory Insufficiency Questionnaire, suited to patients using long-term NIV (Laakso 2009).

## DISCHARGE FROM PHYSIOTHERAPY

'… I come home and I'm so weak I can't do the exercises'

**Patient quoted by Lewis & Cramp 2010**

Discharge planning should begin at the outset and involve all team members including the patient and family (DoH 2010b). Communication with relatives, the patient and primary care or continuing care teams are the basis of a smooth transition and can reduce readmission rates by 12–75% (Harrison et al. 2011). Follow-up phone calls can reduce readmissions and increase patient satisfaction (Naffe 2012). Copies of all letters should be sent to the patient, with a reminder that he or she will need to take the initiative in chasing them up.

## CASE STUDY: MS AB

*A 72-year-old patient with a diagnosis of asthma and COPD is referred with worsening respiratory status.*

### Relevant medical history
- Pneumonia aged 11
- Recently resected colon cancer

### History of present complaint
- Asthma since flu aged 30, worse last few months

### Family history
- Two brothers 'died of emphysema'

### Social history
- Lives with husband
- Two flights of stairs, crawls up on all fours due to breathlessness
- Never smoked

### Subjective
- Can do shopping, nothing much else (I was able to do everything till last year)
- Headache on waking, sometimes at night
- Poor sleep, slide off pillows and wake with cricked neck, sleepy in daytime
- Coughing attack sometimes, frightened of choking, usually little phlegm
- Wet myself when coughing, try not to drink too much
- Used to be hyperactive, difficult to be now, husband tells me to slow down
- Frightened of having emphysema
- Doctor says I don't have emphysema
- Breathlessness eased by nebulizer, neck massage, cup of tea

### Objective
- Rapid talking
- Rapid moving
- Rapid shallow breathing
- Tense breathing pattern, mostly upper chest
- Clinically dehydrated
- Dry cough
- Auscultation: scattered faint crackles

### Questions
1. Comment on the diagnosis.
2. What could be the cause(s) of Ms AB's headaches?
3. What could be the cause(s) of Ms AB's insomnia?
4. Analysis?
5. Problems?
6. Plan?

### CLINICAL REASONING

Comment on the connection between the following statements. Does the conclusion fit?

'… perceived quality of life appears to be linked with peripheral muscle force in COPD patients.'
'Consequently, peripheral muscle training may be an important tool in improving quality of life.'
*Eur Resp J* (1996) 9, 23, 144s

### Response to Case Study

1. Diagnosis
   - SOB could be caused by asthma, cancer or COPD, possibly augmented by anxiety.
   - Indirect questioning confirmed that patient had not asked about outcome of cancer surgery.
2. Headaches
   - Possible causes are 'cricked neck' at night, poor sleep, anxiety, $\uparrow PaCO_2$.

3. Insomnia
   - Possible causes are anxiety, SOB, sleeping position, headaches.
4. Analysis
   - Deterioration probably too consistent for asthma and too rapid for COPD, although there is a family history of COPD and maybe passive smoking. Possible return of cancer.
   - Anxiety could be related to SOB, stress incontinence, fear related to coughing attacks, fear of possible return of cancer, or linking brothers' deaths to Ms B's own condition.
   - Hyperactivity is counterproductive.
5. Problems
   - Ms AB's lack of clarity about diagnosis
   - Headaches
   - Stress incontinence
   - Inefficient use of energy by rapid talking, moving and breathing
   - SOB and reduced exercise tolerance
   - Possible sputum retention
6. Plan
   - Obtain clarification of diagnosis, including respiratory function tests, drug history, radiology and prognosis from cancer surgery
   - Explain COPD, emphysema and asthma to Ms AB
   - Sleep: position, butterfly pillow, sleep hygiene (Appendix B, Chapter 17)
   - Discussion on relaxation strategies. Ms AB chose sewing
   - Acknowledge difficulty of changing a lifetime's habit of a tendency to rush at things, provide advice
   - Exercise programme, energy conservation and pacing, including stairs
   - Breathing re-education, to be practised at intervals during the day
   - Explain that likely reason for stress incontinence is unnecessary coughing, explain pelvic floor exercises, refer to continence physiotherapist
   - Discussion on fluid intake
   - Cough control, including differentiation between dry and wet cough
   - Ensure that Ms AB has a selection of sputum clearance techniques and an effective cough
   - Discuss pulmonary rehabilitation
   - Discuss future unless Ms AB prefers not to
   - Follow up

> ## RESPONSE TO CLINICAL REASONING
>
> Chicken and eggs. The second statement may be a correct conclusion, but the first statement does not prove that weak peripheral muscles *cause* impaired quality of life. Peripheral muscles may weaken as a *result* of exercise limitation or malnutrition. Both are common in COPD, as is impaired quality of life.

## RECOMMENDED READING

Bambi, S., Peris, A., Esquinas, A.M., 2016. Pressure ulcers caused by masks during noninvasive ventilation. Am. J. Crit. Care 25 (1), 6.

Cano, G., 2013. Dyspnea and emotional states in health and disease. Respir. Med. 107 (5), 649–655.

Caroci, A.S., Lareau, S.C., 2004. Descriptors of dyspnea by patients with chronic obstructive pulmonary disease versus congestive heart failure. Heart Lung 33 (2), 102–110.

Delzell, J.E., 2013. Common lung conditions: acute dyspnea. FP Essent 409, 17–22.

Dwarakanath, A., Elliott, M.W., 2013. Noninvasive ventilation in the management of acute hypercapnic respiratory failure. Breathe 10, 338–348.

Gagliardi, E., Innocenti, B.G., Presi, I., et al., 2014. Thoraco-abdominal motion/displacement does not affect dyspnea following exercise training in COPD patients. Respir. Physiol. Neurobiol. 190, 124–130.

Gimenez, M., Saavedra, P., Martin, N., et al., 2012. Bilevel exercise training and directed breathing relieves exertional dyspnea for male smokers. Am. J. Phys. Med. Rehabil. 91 (10), 836–845.

Gregoretti, C., 2013. Choosing a ventilator for home mechanical ventilation. Breathe 10, 394–408.

Keenan, S.P., Sinuff, T., Burns, K.E.A., et al., 2012. Clinical practice guidelines for the use of noninvasive positive-pressure ventilation and noninvasive continuous positive airway pressure in the acute care setting. CMAJ 183 (3), E195–E214.

Luckett, T., Disler, R., Hosie, A., et al., 2016. Content and quality of websites supporting self-management of chronic breathlessness in advanced illness. Primary Care Respir. Med. 26, 16025.

Mercadante, S., Fusco, F., Caruselli, A., 2016. Background and episodic breathlessness in advanced cancer patients followed at home. Curr. Med. Res. Opin. 33 (1), 155–160.

Mularski, R.A., Reinke, L.F., Carrieri-Kohlman, V., et al., 2013. An official American Thoracic Society workshop report: assessment and palliative management of dyspnea crisis. Am. J. Respir. Crit. Care Med. 10 (5), S98–S106.

Simon, S.T., Kloke, M., Alt-Epping, B., et al., 2016. EffenDys – Fentanyl buccal tablet for the relief of episodic breathlessness in patients with advanced cancer: a multicenter, open label, randomized, morphine-controlled, crossover, phase II trial. J. Pain Symptom Manage. 52 (5), 617–625.

Spahija, J., 2010. Factors discriminating spontaneous pursed-lips breathing use in patients with COPD. COPD 7 (4), 254–261.

# Pulmonary Rehabilitation

## INTRODUCTION

*'It's really been such a breakthrough in being able to mix with people and not being so afraid. All … the new people that come, they're all in the same boat'*
**Gysels & Higginson 2009**

Rehabilitation for people disabled by breathlessness is one of the most rewarding aspects of physiotherapy. Irreversible disease does not mean irreversible loss of function, and multidisciplinary pulmonary rehabilitation (PR) is now mandated in all national and international guidelines (Steiner & Roberts 2016). People who have become entangled in a web of inactivity and helplessness are able to improve their independence and quality of life (QoL) through the following:
- understanding their disease, treatment options and coping strategies;
- reducing symptoms;
- improving exercise tolerance and activities of daily living (ADL);
- reducing dependence on family and medical resources.

The need is greater now that patients are being discharged from hospital 'quicker and sicker', and postexacerbation PR should begin within a month of discharge (BTS 2013), taking advantage of the 'teachable moment' when patients are their most receptive.

### Effects

*Pulmonary rehabilitation is the only approach to chronic lung disease short of lung transplantation that improves the long-term outlook for these patients.*
**Tiep 1991**

Participants report a sense of well-being from gaining control over symptoms, especially the fear of breathlessness. It is one of the most cost-effective treatments for people with chronic lung disease (Vogiatzis et al. 2016), with benefits independent of age, lung function or disability (Morgan 2009), and, for COPD, a larger effect than can be obtained with any other medical therapy (Morgan 2017), e.g.:

- ↓ shortness of breath (SOB) (Schroff et al. 2017);
- ↑ oxygenation, exercise capacity and QoL, ↓ depression, anxiety and emergency referrals (Sahin et al. 2016);
- ↓ hospitalization (Fig. 9.1) and length of stay, ↑ survival and participation in everyday activities (GOLD 2016);
- ↓ exacerbations, anxiety and depression, ↑ functional status (Figueiredo et al. 2016);
- ↑ quadriceps strength, ADL ability and health status (BTS 2013);
- ↓ fatigue (Lewko et al. 2014), ↑ sleep quality (Soler 2013), ↑ cognition (ACCP 2007), ↓ panic (Williams & Bruton 2010);

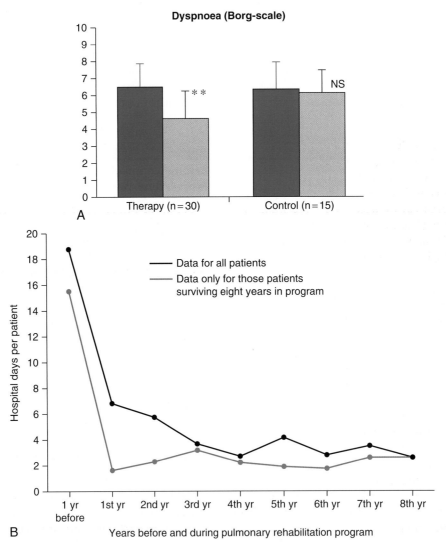

**FIGURE 9.1** (A) Borg ratings of SOB before and after pulmonary rehabilitation (PR) comprising breathing retraining, relaxation and exercise training, compared with no PR. (B) Reduced hospital admissions after PR. (From Hodgkin et al. 2009.)

- ↓ cardiovascular risk factors (Reis et al. 2013);
- for people with comorbid heart failure, ↑ exercise capacity and QoL (Man et al. 2016);
- ↑ balance (Smith et al. 2016b), ↓ frailty (Maddocks et al. 2016b);
- ↓ smoking (ACCP 2007);
- with severe chronic obstructive pulmonary disease (COPD), ↑ $\dot{V}O_2$ and ↓ $VCO_2$, i.e. a true training effect, plus a more efficient slow deeper breathing pattern (De Albuquerque et al. 2016);
- if inspiratory muscle training and rib cage mobilization are included: ↓ hyperinflation (Yoshimi et al. 2012).

## Participants

*No patient is 'too sick' or 'too well' to benefit from pulmonary rehabilitation.*

*Menier 1994*

For people with COPD, PR is not an optional extra (BTS 2013). There is also value for people with bronchiectasis (Lee et al. 2017), interstitial lung disease (Vainshelboim et al. 2016), cystic fibrosis, lung cancer (Wang et al. 2016b), neuromuscular disorders, and pre- and postsurgery (Hodgkin et al. 2009). People with heart failure fit in well, cardiac rehabilitation being usually for people who are younger and fitter (Man et al. 2016).

Patients can benefit if they are very elderly (Corhay et al. 2012) or at the end stage of disease (Ngaage 2004). Participants have described the value of being in a group of mixed severity and how this motivated them to persevere (Mein et al. 2007). For people with interstitial lung disease, hypoxaemia rather than respiratory mechanics usually limits exercise (Markovitz & Cooper 2010) and close monitoring is required.

The programme normally includes 8–10 participants. Selection criteria are the following:
- SOB limiting activity;
- medical management optimized;
- adequate ability to hear or otherwise communicate;
- motivation towards self-help and lifestyle change;
- ability to attend the full programme, apart from during exacerbations.

Patients who are unable or unwilling to attend the programme benefit from a multidisciplinary breathlessness service (Reilly et al. 2016).

## The Setup

The options are:
- an outpatient programme in a physiotherapy gym;
- a community programme in a day or leisure centre, which has equivalent outcomes (Neves et al. 2016) and aids transition to independent exercise;
- a home-based programme, which also shows equivalent outcomes, even with minimal resources (Holland et al. 2017);
- an inpatient programme in a dedicated rehabilitation ward;
- a seamless discharge programme after exacerbation, in- or outpatient based.

Predischarge wards are an ideal environment for PR, especially with frail elderly people who might otherwise remain in an acute medical ward, becoming deconditioned and prey to hospital infection.

Home-based programmes are becoming popular because, although they lack peer support, the exercise and energy conservation components can be adapted to an individual's environment, the family are easily involved and telehealth is becoming more sophisticated.

For group PR, the options are a cohort programme, when everyone starts and finishes at the same time, and a rolling programme, with one or two new patients each week, which means that patients who miss an education session due to illness can make it up easily and numbers can be made up immediately if patients drop out.

### KEY POINT

Group programmes should incorporate precautions against the risk of cross infection, especially when including people with cystic fibrosis or bronchiectasis.

### Resources

*'As soon as I get cold I lose my breath ...'*
*'The warmer the air ... the better ... it is for me'*
***Different patients, quoted by Simon et al. 2013***

The following are preferable for group PR:
- large warm room with easily-opened windows, cheerful atmosphere, wall space and nonslip floor, free from dust-collecting furniture;
- treadmill, exercise bike, steps, mini trampoline, quoits, weights, stretchy bands and any available gym equipment;

- comfortable chairs for family members, and comfortable upright chairs for participants;
- name labels;
- fans;
- sputum pots and tissues;
- high walking frame;
- teaching aids;
- demonstration inhalers;
- handouts, exercise booklets, diaries, writing materials;
- refreshments;
- door-to-door transport, e.g. volunteer drivers, to avoid the stress and delays of public or ambulance transport.

The following are essential:
- oxygen
- oximeters and blood pressure monitors
- crash trolley and team members trained in life support
- accessible toilet

Financial planning needs to take account of staffing, venue, equipment, stationery and administration time.

The team typically comprises a physiotherapist, occupational therapist, respiratory nurse, physician, dietician and clinical psychologist or social worker.

### Structure and timing

Twice weekly supervised sessions are required, and 8 weeks are optimal (Andrews et al. 2015). The initial session involves assessment and goal setting, and provides the foundations for motivation. A group session prior to assessment can increase success by improving knowledge, reducing fear of failure and correcting concerns about exercise (Fischer et al. 2012). Other aids to motivation are to avoid early morning programmes, or participants having to travel in rush hour or in the dark.

Each session is typically based on exercise, brief relaxation, a break for a drink and socialising, and an education component. A halfway review helps participants to take stock. Many of the components from Chapter 8 are incorporated into the programme.

## ASSESSMENT

Assessment incorporates the ICF domains:
1. Respiratory impairment: ↓ lung function, e.g. $FEV_1$.
2. Activity limitation: the effect of this impairment, e.g. ↓ exercise capacity.
3. Participation restriction, e.g. anxiety.

There is much variation between degree of impairment and how much patients are restricted in their participation. Lung function tests are checked to confirm diagnosis but are not used as outcome measures.

Participants are assessed as in Chapter 2, with factors relating specifically to rehabilitation in this chapter.

## BACKGROUND INFORMATION

The case notes are scrutinized to check that exercise training is safe. Contraindications include:
- unstable cardiac disease e.g. symptomatic angina, recent myocardial infarct, uncontrolled arrhythmias or hypertension, and second or third degree heart block;
- deep vein thrombosis, recent embolism or other unstable vascular condition;
- abdominal aortic aneurysm >5.5 cm (BTS 2013).

Relative contraindications include:
- resting systolic blood pressure >180 mmHg or diastolic >100 mmHg;
- disabling stroke or arthritis, if exercises cannot be adapted;
- haemoptysis of unknown cause;
- unstable asthma;
- impaired cognition to the extent of being unable to follow instructions;
- abdominal aortic aneurysm <5.5 cm (where surgery has been deemed inappropriate), indicating the need to avoid high intensity or resistive exercise (BTS 2013);
- underweight, until nutrition supplementation is established (Günay et al. 2013).

Liaison with the physician is suggested if partial pressure of $CO_2$ in arterial blood ($PaCO_2$) is above 8 kPa (60 mmHg).

People with comorbid stable cardiovascular disease benefit, with appropriate safeguards (Chapter 11), and those with osteoporosis gain from impact exercise (Mazokopakis 2011). People with insulin-dependent diabetes require specific precautions (p. 126) and referral for treatment of other comorbidities may be required (BTS 2013).

The following drug history is relevant:
- β-blockers render the blood pressure (BP) and pulse unreliable for monitoring purposes.
- If prescribed and indicated, bronchodilators and antianginal drugs should be taken before exercise.

• Steroids should be at the lowest effective dose, to minimize muscle weakness.

Body mass index should be measured before and after rehabilitation, and education adjusted accordingly (Vestbo et al. 2006).

## SUBJECTIVE

Participants tend to stop 'wanting' to do what they cannot do and often underestimate the effect of their symptoms, e.g. Jones et al. (2016c) found that over a third of patients who described their symptoms as being mild-to-moderate admitted to being too breathless to leave the house. Breathlessness must be explained to participants so that they distinguish it from sensations such as chest tightness.

Questionnaires, scales and outcome measures are on pp. 34, 264 and in Fig. 9.2.

### Exercise Tests

Assessment for exercise desaturation (p. 162) requires an oximeter which has been validated under exercise conditions.

### Six-minute walk distance

The 6-min walk distance (6MWD) is an endurance test that is more reflective of daily life activities than cardiopulmonary exercise tests (Meriem et al. 2015). It also helps predict prognosis, mortality and morbidity in adults and children with lung or heart disease (Watanabe et al. 2016). Participants are asked to walk for 6 min as fast as reasonably possible, along a corridor or around two cones, following standardized instructions:

1. You have 6 minutes to complete as many laps as you can.
2. You can stop or sit down as often as you like but these will be part of the 6 minutes.
3. Walk around each cone.
4. Say if you feel any pain, giddiness or other unexpected symptom.

The patient should be told when each 2 min has been completed. Encouragement is fine but must be standardized. Two tests are required, with patients resting as long as they need in between (Osadnik et al. 2016).

Participants should feel at the end that they have performed to their maximum capacity, but for those

| Modified Borg scale | | |
|---|---|---|
| 0 | Nothing at all | |
| 0.5 | Very, very slight (just noticeable) | |
| 1 | Very slight | |
| 2 | Slight | |
| 3 | Moderate | |
| 4 | Somewhat severe | Training zone |
| 5 | Severe | |
| 6 | | |
| 7 | Very severe | |
| 8 | | |
| 9 | Very, very severe (almost maximal) | |
| 10 | Maximal | |

| Medical Research Council dyspnoea scale | |
|---|---|
| 1 | Not troubled by breathlessness except on strenuous exercise |
| 2 | Short of breath when hurrying or walking up a slight hill |
| 3 | Walks slower than contemporaries on level ground because of breathlessness, or has to stop for breath when walking at own pace |
| 4 | Stops for breath after walking about 100 m or after a few minutes on level ground |
| 5 | Too breathless to leave the house, or breathless when dressing or undressing |

**FIGURE 9.2** Modified Borg and Medical Research Council scales.

with severe disease, it is best that they walk as fast as they like, rather than at their maximum, to avoid excessive symptoms, tachycardia or oxygen desaturation (Mattia et al. 2004).

The data to record are the distance, symptoms, heart rate (HR) and oxygen saturation ($SpO_2$). Repeat tests should be performed at the same time in relation to bronchodilator drugs. Normal 6MWD is 571±90 m (Casanova et al. 2011). Patients who desaturate by 4% or to below 88% in the first half of the test are likely to desaturate during their activities of daily living (ADL) (García-Talavera 2016).

A 2-min walk test shows comparable validity in detecting exercise-induced oxygen desaturation (Gloeckl et al. 2016), and a 6-min stepper test is useful for small spaces (Grosbois et al. 2016).

### Incremental shuttle walk test

The incremental shuttle walk test (ISWT) is more reproducible and less dependent on motivation than the 6MWT, being externally paced. Participants are asked to walk around a 10 m oval circuit with a cone at each end. The speed of walking is dictated by a taped bleep which increases in line with walking, gradually rising from 1 to 5 mph. Instructions are standardized and no verbal encouragement is given. The physiotherapist walks alongside the patient for the first minute to discourage them from exceeding the initial speed. Thereafter, if the cone is reached early, the patient waits for the beep before continuing. The test ends when the patient cannot complete a circuit before the beep. A practice walk is required before the programme, with a rest of 15 min between the practice walk and test walk (Hodgkin et al. 2009, p. 135/336).

The minimal clinically important improvement is 54 m for the 6MWT (for people with COPD) and 47.5 m for the ISWT (BTS 2013). The 6MWT correlates with $\dot{V}O_2$ and the ISWT correlates with maximum oxygen consumption ($\dot{V}O_2max$) (Stroescu et al. 2012).

### Endurance shuttle test

This is thought to be more responsive than the ISWT (Eaton et al. 2006). It uses the same 10 m shuttle course and is a paced walk at 85% of $\dot{V}O_2max$, as assessed by a prior ISWT. No practice walk is needed (Revill et al. 2009) but the three tests required make this too exhausting for many patients.

### Other tests

Simpler tests include:

- the Sit-to-Stand test, using a chair without arms, which counts standing up and sitting down over 1 min and can be used as an alternative to the 6MWT (Meriem et al. 2015);
- the Stair-Climbing test, which counts the steps climbed up and down in 2 min (Kon 2013);
- the Timed Up & Go test, which is a measure of functional mobility requiring little time or space: the patient rises from a chair, walks 3 m, walks back and sits down, a change of 0.9–1.4 s being clinically relevant (Mesquita et al. 2016).

Walking tests take little notice of upper limb capacity and do not assess ADL. Arm exercise capacity can be measured by arm ergometry (Janaudis et al. 2012) or an unsupported arm-lift test (Datta et al. 2013).

Observation of the participant during exercise tests indicates tension and fatigue. SMART goals (p. 179) are reassessed throughout the programme to assist motivation.

## EDUCATION

Education underpins all other components of PR. It facilitates adherence (ACCP 2007), improves self-management (Mousing 2012) and provides a non-threatening atmosphere for discussion and mutual support, especially with a buddy system of 'expert' patients (Hancock & Cox 2008).

Hypoxia can impair memory, and retention of information is optimal if:

- the room is free of distractions;
- the teaching plan is set out clearly;
- the most important points are made first;
- language is jargon-free;
- advice is specific rather than general;
- information is reinforced regularly throughout the programme;
- booklets and handouts are included.

The physiotherapist's job is to teach the management of breathlessness, the rationale of exercise training, chest clearance and, if included, inspiratory muscle training. The respiratory nurse or pharmacist covers drugs, inhalers and the importance of pneumococcal and flu vaccinations (NICE 2012a). The occupational therapist discusses stress management, welfare benefits and relaxation. The dietician suggests six-meals-a-day menus, advises on healthy eating and explains which foods are constipating or gas-forming.

The practicalities of oxygen therapy are explained by the physiotherapist, nurse or physician, who also discusses advance directives, which allow patients, while they still have capacity, to refuse specific treatment in the future if they may lack capacity. Less than 5% of patients are given the opportunity to discuss their options about life-prolonging treatment ahead of time (Curtis 2000), even though most value this (Burge et al. 2013). Group discussion is often less threatening than individual discussion for delicate subjects such as sex, stress incontinence and death. However, about 10% of patients do not want to know about advance directives and 4% do not want to participate in end-of-life discussions (Heffner 2000) and patients from varied cultures will have different preferences. It is therefore useful to advise patients of the content of the next educational session so that they can absent themselves if they prefer. Curtis et al. (2000) describe approaches to communicating with patients who have life-limiting illnesses.

A final session might include a question and answer discussion with the physician or all team members, and plans for the future. Participants with concomitant heart failure should be provided with disease-specific education or referred to the heart failure team (Triest et al. 2016).

### KEY POINT

Pulmonary rehabilitation is not a course of treatment to make patients better, but more of a life plan.

Education topics are listed in Appendix A.

## Motivation

*The therapist–patient relationship can succeed or fail depending on the care that the therapist takes in understanding the needs and circumstances of her patients.*

*Hay-Smith et al. 2016*

Motivation is the best predictor of success (Brannon et al. 1998, p. 346). Patients may be accustomed to the hierarchical hospital environment, which can encourage the sick role and an assumption that experts know best. This is counterproductive in the rehabilitation process, where education is more than just feeding information into an empty vessel and pressing the right buttons.

Factors that increase motivation are:
- clear advance information;
- customizing and simplifying learning, and reinforcing self-efficacy and confidence (Blackstock et al. 2016);
- patients taking responsibility for their self-management;
- realistic expectations and patients setting their own goals (Hay-Smith et al. 2016);
- active participation, e.g. self-monitoring, and encouraging questions and contributions;
- praise, warmth, humour, honesty and responsiveness from the rehabilitation team, including acknowledgement of patients' experiences;
- family involvement;
- focus on health rather than disease;
- early success, reinforced by progress charts;
- access to medical notes if required;
- continuity of personnel;
- participants swapping ideas, sharing transport and exercising together outside classes;
- certificate of completion.

Motivation is dampened by advice that is inconvenient or difficult to follow, boredom (e.g. repetitive exercise or waiting for transport), fatigue, fear of injury and not understanding the relationship between physical activity and health.

Reassurance, if used blandly or indiscriminately, can increase anxiety and reduce motivation if it does not supply new information (Warwick & Salkovskis 1985).

Most participants are enthusiastic learners, and liberal use of teaching aids can explain the disease process in a way that is enjoyable. A large-print diary is useful to log daily exercise, symptoms, feelings, diet, drugs and side effects. The diary can record negotiated functional goals, the time to achieve them, and obligations of the patient and the PR team. Achievement of the first goal gives participants a motivating boost.

Memory aids include stickers at home on kettles and the fridge, and the use of dead time for exercises, e.g. TV.

Most smokers want to stop (Mulhall 2016) and cessation advice is best provided before the programme starts because smoking has been found the sole independent predictor of dropout (Brown et al. 2016a). Cessation advice should avoid telling participants that they should stop (they know this) but acknowledge how difficult it is, provide patient-friendly literature, check that they know about local resources and offer positive information, e.g.:

- after 48–72 h cessation – improved ciliary function;
- after 1–2 weeks – ↓ sputum production;
- 6–8 weeks – immune function and metabolism normalized;
- 8–12 weeks – ↓ postoperative morbidity and mortality (NICE 2015a).

Smoking cessation can include behavioural interventions such as the 5As (ask, advise, assess, assist, arrange) (Schauer et al. 2016), drugs (p. 170), exercise, mindfulness practice or falling in love (Xu et al. 2012a). E-cigarettes are not recommended for pregnant women because the nicotine can leave their children with cardiorespiratory, neurologic, academic and behavioural problems (Holbrook 2016).

*There's nothing to giving up smoking. I've done it hundreds of times.*

**Mark Twain**

## Understanding Reactions to the Disease

*COPD is a family disease.*

***Figueiredo et al. 2016***

Participants can be advised that feelings are closely connected with breathing and that it is natural for breathless people to feel depressed and anxious, these being expressions of humanity, not weakness. Anxiety is exacerbated by fears, e.g. that they might 'forget' to breathe during sleep, or that death will be by suffocation, a common misconception that can contribute to panic attacks. Most respiratory patients, if they die from their disease, will do so after lapsing into a coma. When depression and anxiety coexist, depression may not be recognized, and when it is, this is often accepted as a manifestation of the disease and not addressed, even though the depressive symptoms of poor appetite, social isolation, low energy and insomnia can sabotage PR. The contribution of mental well-being to SOB is considered as important as disease severity (Man et al. 2016), and unexpected feelings have been identified such as shame and low self-compassion (Harrison et al. 2017).

Care should be taken with language because the word 'psychological' may be interpreted as psychiatric, and the word 'disabled' is difficult for people who have not thought of themselves in this context. To use emotionally charged words without preparation is like using the word 'stump' unexpectedly to a new amputee.

Family relationships may be affected by lack of spontaneity because breathless people often cannot waste breath in expressing anxiety, anger, love or happiness. This emotional straightjacket can isolate partners from each other, sometimes worsened by guilt or the bitterness of dependence, and relationships may change during PR. Denial may also complicate relationships, but some level of denial may be a necessary coping strategy.

Relationships with others may require a patient to explain about their need to walk slowly or use oxygen, to ask that adequate time is allowed for speaking, and to find strategies if the legitimacy of their invisible condition is doubted.

It is natural for chronically disabled people to harbour resentment at the loss of their dreams, and anger may be projected onto their family or any of the PR team. Allowing patients to talk gives them an opportunity to understand this process. If there is no outlet, resentment turns inward and can augment depression. People who are depressed usually respond to a receptive ear. Time is always needed when working with troubled people, but this is time well invested by a member of the team with whom the participant feels comfortable.

Self-esteem and sexuality are closely linked, and loss of sexual expression reinforces low confidence. Education can clarify the benefit of building up exercise tolerance and help discriminate between the effects of myth, illness and drugs on sexual activity. Myths perpetuated by society include the expectation that elderly people cannot have, do not want or should not want sexual relations, and that disabled people are sexually neutered. The reality is that:

- dyspnoea may limit the duration of kissing;
- during sex it may be useful to have a fan, oxygen or inhalers to hand;
- alternative positions may be helpful (Appendix B);
- libido can be affected by steroids, anticholinergics, antihypertensives, theophyllines, antidepressants, sedatives or alcohol, so a drug review may be helpful;
- sometimes a partner may think that abstention is in the patient's interest, whereas the opposite may be the case;

• hypoxaemia, smoking and exercise limitation contribute to the 67% of patients with varying degrees of erectile dysfunction (Turan et al. 2016b).
Practical information is provided by Steinke et al. (2016).

Some physiotherapists are comfortable to listen to patients talking about their feelings, but referral to other agencies may be required. The relevance of participants' feelings is shown by evidence that attitudes and beliefs bear more relation to exercise tolerance than ventilatory capacity (Morgan et al. 1983).

*The concept that best captures the experience of breathlessness is 'invisibility'.*
**Gysels & Higginson 2008**

## EXERCISE TRAINING

*'You've gotta be joking … I can't walk, I can't talk, how do you think I can do exercise?'*
**Gysels & Higginson 2009**

Patients are usually surprised that not only can they 'do exercise', they can also build up exercise tolerance and improve their QoL. This occurs whether exercise is limited by:
• breathlessness
• fear of breathlessness
• leg fatigue, which is common in people with COPD (Singer et al. 2012)
These contribute to a vicious circle of SOB and deconditioning (Fig. 9.3). An exercise programme enables patients to extricate themselves from this, but it must show tangible benefits and be designed so that it can be maintained unsupervised at home. Long-term commitment is needed because detraining occurs faster than training.

## Effects

> **KEY POINT**
>
> *Physical inactivity is the strongest predictor of all-cause mortality in patients with COPD.*
> Waschki et al. 2011

The benefits of exercise for people with normal lungs are well known (p. 25). Extra benefits are found for people with respiratory disease:
• ↓ SOB (Gagliardi 2014), ↓ gas trapping (Vogiatzis & Zakynthinos 2013);

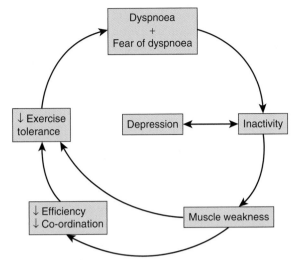

**FIGURE 9.3** Vicious circle that contributes to reduced exercise tolerance in breathless people.

• ↑ exercise tolerance and ventricular function (Brønstad et al. 2013);
• ↓ age-associated oxidative stress in muscle cells (Silva et al. 2016);
• ↑ balance and QoL, ↓ falls, cholesterol and BP (Kortianou 2010);
• ↑ cognition due to increased blood flow (Aquino et al. 2016);
• ↓ fatigue and ↓ smoking (Tödt et al. 2016);
• ↓ symptoms, lung function decline, exacerbations and mortality (Troosters et al. 2016);
• ↓ insulin resistance in the 59% of patients with advanced COPD who exhibit this (Cebron et al. 2016);
• ↓ lung inflammation, remodelling and pulmonary arterial hypertension in emphysema (Henriques et al. 2016).

## Mechanism of Training

Half of patients with moderate-to-severe COPD cannot reach their anaerobic threshold (Thirapatarapong et al. 2013) and their improved exercise tolerance is thought to be due to greater mechanical skill, which reduces the oxygen cost of exercise, a more efficient ventilatory pattern and desensitization to dyspnoea (Cooper 2009). This desensitization can be reinforced by assisting patients to explore their beliefs and validate them as useful or harmful, a form of cognitive behaviour therapy that is effective when embedded in exercise training (Williams et al. 2015).

## Safety

Dyspnoea may prevent exercise from stressing the cardiovascular system, but the relevant precautions are covered under assessment (p. 250) and below (AARC 2001):

- scrutiny of the notes following comprehensive medical screening;
- treatment of comorbidities such as anaemia;
- drug review, optimum nutrition and fluid intake;
- steady exercise with no rushing at the start or finish;
- discouragement of competition;
- adequate rest, with placement of chairs at intervals;
- emphasis on isotonic rather than isometric exercise, to reduce the risks of hypertension, impaired blood flow, and, with COPD, possible muscle damage (Rooyackers et al. 2003);
- oximetry to ensure that $SpO_2$ stays above 90% (Langer et al. 2009);
- in hot weather, extra fluids; when it is excessively hot, especially for those fasting during Ramadan, exercise may need to be stopped.

Exercise or exercise testing should be stopped if there is (AARC 2001):

- angina, cyanosis, pallor, cold clammy skin, unusual fatigue, confusion, headache, dizziness, nausea or palpitations;
- BP rise to >250 mmHg systolic or >120 mmHg diastolic;
- failure to raise systolic BP by at least 20 mmHg above its resting level;
- after the normal rise with exercise, a fall in systolic BP to below preexercise level or a fall of >20 mmHg;
- failure to increase HR;
- arrhythmias;
- for people with heart failure, increased ankle oedema, dizziness or cough.

## Technique

> **Strength:** capacity of muscle to generate force
> **Endurance:** capacity of muscle to maintain a certain force over time

Even if a conventional training response is not anticipated, the three principles of training are followed:

- overload: intensity must be greater than the muscle's normal load;
- specificity: only the specific activities practised will normally show improvement;
- reversibility: cessation of training loses the benefits gained.

**Endurance training**, comprising low-resistance, high-repetition exercise such as walking, forestalls the onset of inefficient anaerobic metabolism and enhances the use of oxygen.

**Strength training** brings similar benefits (Iepsen et al. 2015) and includes quadriceps exercises and arm weights or Theraband (Fig. 9.4), leading to reduced SOB during ADL, especially with unsupported arms (Romagnoli 2013). People with interstitial lung disease sometimes find strength training easier than endurance training.

**Interval training** brings similar benefits (Rodríguez et al. 2016) and resembles a patient's ADL, alternating 15–60 s episodes of exercise with rest (Fig. 9.5). This allows exercise to be sustained at an intensity that would otherwise be intolerable, and prevents lactic acidosis, along with the extra SOB that this causes. Patients with severe disease can also obtain a physiological training effect without ventilatory limitation, leading to a near tripling of the total exercise duration with lower metabolic and ventilatory responses (Kortianou 2010).

## Preliminaries

> 'You need to be taught to overcome the fear of exercise'
>
> ***Lewis & Cramp 2010***

Participants are reassured that exercise is not synonymous with pumping iron. Inpatients are best dressed in their day clothes, and all participants should have cleared their chests before exercising. Participants can bring their favourite music, which can itself reduce their dyspnoea (Kazuya et al. 2015).

Warming up (Box 9.1) in a group allows participants to enjoy movement for its own sake and helps distract them from preoccupation with their SOB. Five minutes is usually sufficient for respiratory patients, and for those who are severely breathless, warm up may simply mean starting their exercise slowly. Participants are

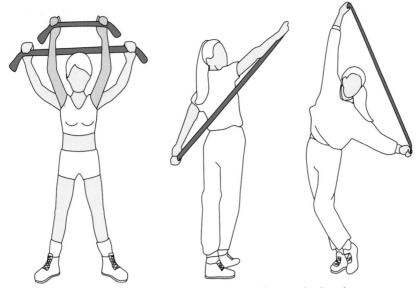

**FIGURE 9.4** Upper limb exercise with stretchy bands.

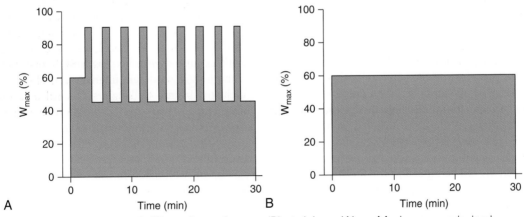

**FIGURE 9.5** Interval (A) and continuous (B) training. $W_{max}$, Maximum work load. (From Coppoolse et al. 1999.)

encouraged to maintain rhythmic quality of movement and avoid breath-holding.

## Exercise prescription

*'I … could do a little bit more and a little bit more and a little bit more, instead of giving up'*
**Witcher et al. 2015**

Four components make up the exercise prescription: mode, intensity, duration and frequency.

The **mode** of exercise depends on the patient. Some prefer the stationary bike or treadmill because they feel in control, can use oxygen easily and have support for their arms. Others enjoy activities that can be continued at home such as walking and stair-climbing. Upper limb exercises should include strength and endurance components (McKeough et al. 2012).

The leg fatigue that can limit the benefits of exercise training is reduced by alternating exercises between upper and lower limbs, and alternating those

---

## BOX 9.1   A Selection of Warm-Up and Stretching Exercises

Look up slowly, then look down slowly, keeping breathing steadily.

Keeping shoulders still, turn head slowly to look over each shoulder.

Facing forward, bring each ear down towards each shoulder.

Roll shoulder girdle up, back, down and forward, slowly and with a good stretch.

In sitting, raise alternate heels and toes.

With arms crossed and keeping hips facing forward, turn to each side while breathing out and return to the front while breathing in. Feel the spine stretch. Repeat with hands on shoulders. If sitting, finish by pulling on the back of the chair to get an extra stretch.

In standing or sitting, with hands on hips, push chest forward and shoulders back while breathing in, then relax while breathing out.

Lock hands, stretch arms forward at shoulder level while breathing out, feel the stretch between shoulder blades, then relax while breathing in.

Bend forward, breathing out on going down and breathing in on coming up.

Hands on hips, tilt pelvis forward on breathing in and back on breathing out. Feel stretch in lower back.

In standing, march on the spot, keep breathing rhythmic.

Hold the back of a chair, go up on tiptoes, and down. Repeat without holding the chair if possible.

Stretch arm out sideways, then circle in progressively increasing circles, keep breathing steady. Repeat with other arm.

Reach for the stars with right arm, stretch fingers, then bend to the left so that the arm goes up and over in order to side-flex the trunk. Repeat with left arm.

Hands on shoulders, circle elbows forward and then backwards.

Sideways walking.

Raise an arm, then bend elbow and drop hand behind back so upper arm feels stretched, then bring hand back down and move it to small of the back. Repeat with other arm.

Breathing out, lunge forward so that the calf of the back leg feels a good stretch. Repeat with the other side. Keep near something to hold onto.

Swimming action with arms, in time with breathing.

---

that cause aching muscles and those that cause SOB (De Albuquerque et al. 2016). Patients are advised to exhale during the most effortful part of an exercise ('blow as you go') such as arm raising. Balance exercises and fall prevention strategies should be included for people with COPD because of their impaired postural control (Roig et al. 2011).

Instructions can be pinned to the walls, and participants record their scores and progress on their clipboard with, if indicated from their assessment, their $SpO_2$ or HR. Participants are discouraged from becoming too focused on their oximeter and encouraged to maintain awareness of their subjective response to exercise. They rest between each exercise until their breathing returns to normal. Box 9.2 provides examples of exercises.

The **intensity** of exercise is recommended to be symptom-based, for both respiratory and heart failure patients (Man et al. 2016), using, for example:
- the feeling 'breathless but not speechless';
- rating of perceived exertion (Zainuldin et al. 2016);
- grades 3–5 on the Borg scale (Jenkins et al. 2011);
- grades 2–4 on a breathless scale (Box 9.3).

Other patients may be prescreened with symptom-limited cardiopulmonary exercise testing, from which

training intensity can be prescribed (Man et al. 2016). Examples are moderate intensity at 50% of $\dot{V}O_2max$, calculated from a walking test (Langer et al. 2009), or higher intensity at 70% (Zainuldin et al. 2012). Short exercise bouts or sprightly patients allow higher intensity.

For upper limb resistance training, patients with severe disease may fare best by working at <50% of maximum workload, measured by arm ergometry, because high intensity exercise can lead to hyperinflation, reduced efficiency and shortened endurance time (Colucci et al. 2011). For the lower limbs, Langer et al. (2009) suggest working in 2–5 sets of 8–15 repetitions at 60–80% of one repetition maximum.

The balance of **duration** and **frequency** depends on individual preference because the result is similar if total work is the same and one or both increase. For severely compromised patients, leg strength and QoL can be improved by a low intensity programme lasting a year and comprising repetitive standing, walking, relaxation, breathing re-education and ADL practice, although this needs follow-up support if it is to be maintained (Endo et al. 2016).

Supervised training sessions usually last for 30–60 min, but for home practice, respiratory patients are

## BOX 9.2   Circuit Exercises

Each Exercise is Continued for Between 15 s and 2 min.

**Biceps curls**. Sitting with elbows supported: lift and lower a weight. Repeat with other arm.

**Squats**. With back to wall, slide down the wall while breathing out, breathe in gently, then push back up while breathing out. Progress by increasing depth of squat.

**Ball**. Throwing and catching in pairs, or bouncing on floor or wall, without breath-holding.

**Quadriceps exercises**. In sitting, while breathing out, straighten one knee slowly until it is completely straight, hold for a count of three while breathing steadily, lower leg slowly. Repeat with other leg. Graduate to weights.

**Lift-ups from sitting**. Push down with both hands and lift pelvis off seat, or just take some weight through arms, then let yourself down slowly.

**Steps**, then graduate to carrying 'shopping'.

**Wall press-ups**. Stand with feet shoulder width apart, put hands on wall, lean forward and bend elbows while breathing out, breathe in gently, then push back while breathing out. Graduate to increasing distance from wall.

**High knee marching**. Lift alternate knees high without breath-holding. Progress to high knee walking. Keep near something to hold.

**Arm raise**. Sitting or standing, raise alternate arms above head, progress to weights.

**Sit to stand**. Using a firm chair, breathe out on standing up, breathe in while standing, breathe out on sitting down. Repeat without using arms of chair. Graduate to holding a ball.

**Equipment**. Static bike, hula-hoops, trampette, treadmill, gym ball, multigym.

**Pectoral stretch** (Fig. 9.6). Place elbows at shoulder height on either side of a doorway, then lean forward until a stretch (but no pain) is felt across the front of the upper chest. Alter position of elbows as required.

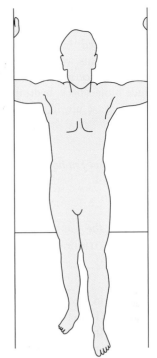

**FIGURE 9.6** Pectoral stretch.

## BOX 9.3   Breathless Scale

| Rating 1 | Comfortable breathing throughout |
|---|---|
| Rating 2 | During exercise: deeper breathing |
| | After exercise: recovery 2–5 min |
| | Day after exercise: comfortable |
| Rating 3 | During: harder breathing |
| | After: recovery 4–7 min |
| | Day after: comfortable |
| Rating 4 | During: breathless but not speechless |
| | After: recovery 5–10 min |
| | Day after: not tired |
| Rating 5 | During: breathless and speechless |
| | After: recovery >10 min |
| | Day after: tired |

advised on up to 15 min two to three times a day or >20 min once a day (Watchie 2010, p. 304), with a brief warm up and cool down, e.g. by slow walking. Patients need to exercise every day except on the days they come for PR or if they feel ill. People who tend to rush at their exercise in an attempt to get it over quickly may find that counting breaths with their steps helps them to pace themselves in the early stages, e.g. *in/one out/one*, or *in/one out/one-two*, including on the stairs. For others this disturbs their rhythm and distracts them from focusing on awareness of their breathing and level of effort. If a position or breathing technique (p. 236) has been found beneficial, individual patients may need reminding of this when getting their breath back.

Some participants find that breathing out against positive pressure during exercise eases their SOB by reducing exercise-induced hyperinflation (Monteiro et al. 2012). For many this would be impractical, but for some it might enhance motivation. Other accompaniments include biofeedback, hydrotherapy (Jenkins et al. 2011) and for those unwilling to do active exercise, neuromuscular electrical stimulation (Maddocks et al. 2016).

*'I can walk 10 min and I'm not going to die'*
**Witcher et al. 2015**

## Progression

*'Once you get over the fear of not being able to breathe if you're exercising, then you're off and running …'*
**Witcher et al. 2015**

Progression is usually in weekly increments, either by frequency or duration (Hill et al. 2012), or by intensity (Stroescu et al. 2012). Improvement usually continues for 4–6 months and when a plateau is reached, moderate exercise should be maintained.

# RESPIRATORY MUSCLE TRAINING

The concept that strengthening respiratory muscles would allow a patient to sustain increased exercise tolerance is an attractive one, but does it stand up to scrutiny?

## Rationale

The respiratory muscles may be either strengthened or weakened by lung disease. Weak muscles are due to systemic inflammation, especially in COPD or bronchiectasis, and sometimes hypoxia, malnutrition, steroid-induced weakness, deconditioning, drugs or, with hyperinflation, mechanical disadvantage (Gea et al. 2015). Strong muscles are due to the training effect of working against the extra resistance of stiff lungs or obstructed airways (Vendrusculo et al. 2016). Therefore for weak inspiratory muscles, the cause should first be addressed when possible, after which respiratory muscle training may be beneficial. For strong inspiratory muscles, it is probably unnecessary to add a further load.

If the problem is fatigue rather than weakness, training can cause 'overuse atrophy' and muscle damage

(Orozco-Levi et al. 2001) but this should not occur if we listen to the patient.

## Effects

When used appropriately, inspiratory muscle training (IMT) in rested and well-nourished patients improves inspiratory muscle strength and endurance, but this is only relevant if it relieves SOB, improves exercise tolerance or enhances QoL. The following outcomes have been reported:

- in people with COPD: ↑ QoL, ↓ SOB and fatigue (Borge et al. 2016);
- compared to exercise training alone, ↑ exercise capacity (Markovitz & Cooper 2010) and QoL (Majewska et al. 2016);
- compensation for respiratory muscle weakness caused by steroids (Weiner 1995) or statins (Chatham 2009);
- for ventilated patients, facilitation of weaning (Göhl et al. 2016);
- for people with early stage interstitial disease, ↑ exercise capacity, ↓ severe fatigue and SOB perception (Karadallı et al. 2016).

Specifically training the expiratory muscles can improve exercise performance in patients with COPD, and in other patients it may improve cough and reduce SOB during exercise (Beckerman 2003).

## Indications and Precautions

Most studies have investigated people with COPD, but benefits have been reported for other medical and surgical patients, as reported in the relevant chapters. Patients likely to respond are those who:

- find breathing re-education difficult, in which case using the device might familiarize them to an altered breathing pattern before progressing to self-regulation of their breathing;
- are fearful of exercise or unable to take up PR, in which case IMT can be used to desensitize them to breathlessness prior to venturing into exercise training;
- are unable to participate fully in whole-body exercise training due to surgery, injury, debility from cardiopulmonary or neurological disease, or obesity (Göhl et al. 2016).

A history of spontaneous pneumothorax is a relative contraindication (McConnell 2005).

## Technique

A pressure threshold device (Fig. 9.7) incorporates a spring-loaded one-way valve that allows patients to exhale without resistance but requires them to reach a preset load to inhale, set at 30–80% of their maximum inspiratory pressure (p. 64). If the aim is desensitization to breathlessness, resistance should be at a level that leaves the patient more breathless than normal but not speechless. In the UK, the PowerBreathe is available on prescription. An electronic flow-resistive device that stores data is also available (Langer et al. 2015).

As with systemic training, exercise should be alternated with rest and distressing levels of fatigue avoided, assessed subjectively by the patient, and objectively by the physiotherapist if there is overactivation of the accessory muscles. Ramsook et al. (2016) found that emphasizing abdominal movement favoured activation of the diaphragm. If they are able, patients should work at different volumes to prevent muscle fatigue, but hyperinflation should be avoided. Oxygen can be delivered by nasal cannula if required.

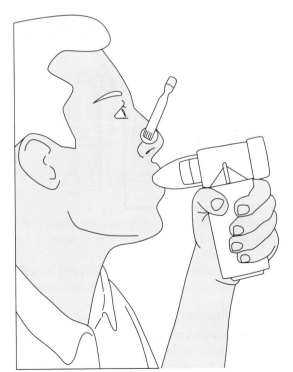

**FIGURE 9.7** Inspiratory muscle trainer (PowerBreathe).

Training should be at least daily (McConnell 2005) and preferably little and often, e.g. from about 5 min bd to about 15 min tds. Interval training creates the highest training loads (Hill et al. 2006). Excessive overloading, as reported by patient discomfort, should be avoided in people with COPD (Puente-Maestu et al. 2012).

When patients have mastered the art, IMT can be combined with watching television or reading. It must be maintained once a plateau is reached (Weiner et al. 2004), assisted by training diaries. For patients who find IMT boring, swimming has shown similar improvements in respiratory muscle strength (Santos et al. 2012).

## ENERGY CONSERVATION

*'They tell you: 'Don't use a towel, use a towelling dressing gown', it's fantastic, it's such a simple thing'*
**Gysels & Higginson 2009**

Strategies to conserve energy tend to be used in the later stages of disease, but they are best taught early to give participants greater control over how they achieve a balance of rest and exercise. Energy conservation is compatible with exercise training and indeed is integral to it. Once patients have learnt to listen to their bodies, they can decide when to make an extra trip up the stairs as an exercise, or when to follow the first tip below.

### Activities of Daily Living

Participants can be advised to selectively allocate their energy, e.g.:
- organise chores by location to avoid multiple trips;
- coordinate breathing with activities, e.g. exhale with pushing or bending;
- move smoothly, avoid extraneous movements or breath-holding;
- prioritize activities, plan in advance, use pacing and work in stages, including on the stairs;
- notice where there is muscle tension and release it;
- organize work space to reduce clutter and minimize reaching and bending;
- keep heavy items on worktops, slide rather than lift them;
- prepare large one-dish meals and freeze leftovers to use on breathless days;

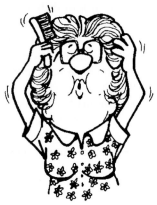

**FIGURE 9.8** Pursed lip breathing while doing unsupported upper limb activities. (From Ries et al. 2001.)

- soak washing up, drain dishes instead of towel drying;
- use a stool in the kitchen and bathroom, rest elbows on worktop or basin;
- reduce bending by crossing one leg over the other to put on socks, trousers and shoes;
- place chairs at strategic locations;
- use pursed lips breathing for upper limb activities (Fig. 9.8);
- use a rollator rather than a zimmer because it stabilizes the accessory muscles and reduces SOB (Ogino et al. 2015), or use other energy-efficient walking aids (Fig. 9.9).

Individuals vary:
- Some may find it more important to use their energy to get to the shops than to be independent with dressing.
- Some prefer to sleep downstairs rather than suffer the 'stigma' of a stairlift.
- Some find sitting in a shower (Fig. 9.10) easier than using a bath, while others find that water on their face upsets their breathing.
- Some are not happy to have their spouse bathe them.

Participants can share their strategies such as using inconspicuous 'puffing stations' during shopping trips or leaning on shopping trolleys. Activity analysis with the occupational therapist helps break down their ADL and identify problem areas. Many patients have tried to counteract fatigue with prolonged rest, which tends to do the opposite (Radbruch 2008). The benefit of balancing rest and exercise was shown by Zhou et al. (2016b) who provided alternating IMT and noninvasive

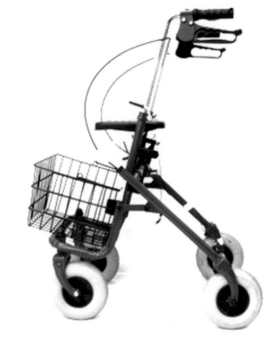

**FIGURE 9.9** Mobility aid that increases walking distance compared with a rollator. (From Vaes et al. 2012.)

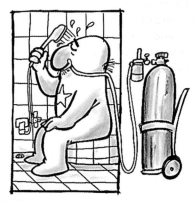

**FIGURE 9.10** Energy conservation in the shower. (From Ries et al. 2001.)

ventilation to people with advanced COPD, which led to improved exercise tolerance and reduced SOB.

## Stress Reduction

*Voluntary control of respiration is perhaps the oldest stress reduction technique known. It has been used for thousands of years to reduce anxiety and promote a generalized state of relaxation.*

***Everly 1989***

Stress is physiologically detrimental (p. 23), and putting a tense person through a physical training programme without advice on stress management is silly. People with chronic lung disease suffer muscle tension from breathlessness and the body positions needed to ease their breathing. A continually active muscle such as the diaphragm is in particular need of relative relaxation by returning to its resting position after contraction, especially when it is being overused as in hyperinflation. Some patients have become accustomed to muscle tension as their default position and forget how it feels to be relaxed. Stress is reduced by education, occupational therapy and the measures below.

### Relaxation

*'I was amazed how [relaxing my shoulders] had this calming effect … it helps my lungs to expand'*
**Wood et al. 2013**

Relaxation (Payne 2010 & Appendix B) should be taught early and reinforced throughout, often in brief snippets. Daily practice is then needed until the sensation is appreciated and the skill mastered, whereupon a degree of relaxation is integrated into everyday life by identifying stressful situations and practising mini-relaxation in different positions. Even walking can be maintained in a way that does not waste energy. Spot checks during the day help identify body tension.

Relaxation can be achieved in other ways, e.g. jigsaws, reading a poem or watching a lighted aquarium at night. Even looking at views of nature can reduce BP (Gladwell et al. 2012). Activities such as circle dancing provide rhythmic exercise with a meditative effect and also emphasize trunk rotation, posture and balance. Patients who have spent their working lives with the forward head postures of computer work may require extra attention (Kang et al. 2012).

*The best way to still the mind is to move the body*
**Roth 1990**

### Complementary therapies

Complementary therapies may help ease SOB and stress. It is useful to acquire knowledge of effective local resources for participants who request this information.

Described as 'cosmic rehabilitation' (Gilbert 1999b), **yoga** incorporates breathing techniques, meditation and postures that consume minimal energy and induce the physiological effects of deep relaxation. It can reduce SOB (Norweg & Collins 2013), increase adherence to exercise (Bryan 2012), decrease stress (Chong et al. 2011) and build bone mineral density (Fishman 2009). Meditation alone can reduce depression, insomnia (Thompson 2009), respiratory rate, HR, BP (Melville et al. 2012) and stress, and improve cognition (Singh 2012).

The **Alexander Technique** can inhibit muscle tension, reduce the work of breathing and improve objective measures such as peak flow and respiratory muscle strength (Austin et al. 1992). The **Feldenkrais** method is useful for balance control (Connors et al. 2010). **Biofeedback** to reduce muscle tension allows the sensation to be recognized and controlled (Hodgkin et al. 2009, p. 230). **Imagery** uses visualization of peaceful scenes and can increase relaxation and $SpO_2$ in people with COPD (Louie 2004). Dyspnoea can be reduced by **acupressure** (Maa et al. 1997), **acupuncture** (Suzuki et al. 2008), **acu-TENS** (Liu et al. 2015) or **reflexology** (Polat & Ergüney 2016). The rhythmic movements of **T'ai Chi** can reduce the distress of dyspnoea (Norweg & Collins 2013) or, at higher intensity, provide a similar stimulus to treadmill exercise (Qiu et al. 2016b).

Singing can improve QoL, possibly because of its control of breathing and posture (Lord et al. 2012), its I:E ratio being more akin to that of COPD (Salomoni et al. 2016), and can improve recruitment of latissimus dorsi, which is needed for active expiration and upper limb work (Watson et al. 2012). A local singing instructor may be available to take a session in the PR programme. Some patients may also like to take up a wind instrument, which reduces SOB, fatigue and depression (Canga et al. 2016) and brings the added perk of reducing the risk of obstructive sleep apnoea (Ward et al. 2012).

*'If I can … think, okay just drop your shoulders, mentally relax, calm everything down … Yeah I think it's just getting to a place of complete calm'*
**Patient, quoted by Simon et al. 2016**

## FOLLOW-UP

*Wellbeing needs to be understood not as the end point, but as a precarious balance needing skilful maintenance and hard work.*
**Gysels & Higginson 2009**

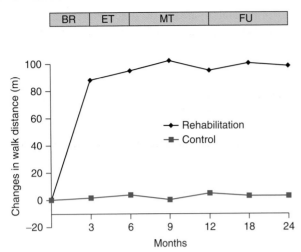

| BR | ET | MT | FU |

**FIGURE 9.11** Maintenance of exercise tolerance with 3 months of breathing retraining, relaxation, chest wall exercise and unsupervised exercise (BR), 3 months of supervised exercise (ET), 6 months of weekly group exercise (MT) and 6 months of unsupervised exercise (FU). (From Guell et al. 2000.)

A follow-up self-management programme has shown:

- ↑ motivation and adherence (Kruijssen et al. 2015);
- a universally positive attitude towards exercise (Spencer 2013);
- maintenance of continued exercise capacity (Fig. 9.11).

Maintenance needs to be stressed at the start of the programme. Some supervised training is best continued for a period after the initial programme, if possible, to prevent demotivation. Motivation is also helped by individuals choosing their own form of exercise, e.g. dance (Mejia-Downs 2011) or callisthenics (Duruturk et al. 2016), the use of paced music (Ho et al. 2012), activity-monitoring devices (Boeselt 2016) or phone apps (Vorrink et al. 2016), or walking in water, which engenders a higher metabolic rate than on land (Handa et al. 2016). Participants may not realise how hard they are working if the exercise is enjoyable and distracting, e.g. Wii exercise programmes (LeGear et al. 2016). Follow-up by phone or videoconference sessions can facilitate continued improvement (Zanaboni et al. 2016). Home visits provide the opportunity to check for safety hazards and support the family: a spouse may be stressed, neglect their own health, or feel guilty or fearful of sleeping lest their partner die at night.

Urban patients are advised to choose the least polluted times and places for outdoor exercise (Araneda et al. 2016). Those who walk by the sea usually find that they breathe more easily when the tide is coming in rather than going out. For leisure centres, fitness instructors can be reassured that patients bringing oxygen are responsible for this themselves, as with any other drug.

Half an hour of exercise five times a week is advised (BTS 2013). Once a week, participants should put themselves back on the same programme as on the final day of their training. If this is difficult, they have lost fitness and will need to increase their maintenance exercise. If training is interrupted by illness, their programme is restarted at a lower level. Attending a further PR programme is beneficial if resources allow (BTS 2013).

Half of COPD exacerbations go unreported, and telemedicine enables patients to electronically track daily symptoms so that if a set threshold is breached, alerts can be sent to the care team (Mulhall 2016).

The mutual support that develops between participants during PR may become one of its most enduring legacies and participants often prefer to continue exercising with their peers, sometimes in a structured environment, without the embarrassment of a public setting (Hogg et al. 2012). This support can be built into self-help groups using Breathe Easy (Appendix B, Links for Patients) or peer outreach when patients are visited by volunteers with lung disease. Social outings together are particularly supportive for people who do not like to be seen in public with their oxygen.

*'To be honest, it wasn't the exercise, it was more the support … just having other people'*
                                            **Witcher et al. 2015**

## OUTCOMES

*The physiological, symptom-reducing, psychosocial and health-economic benefits of pulmonary rehabilitation have been demonstrated convincingly across multiple outcome areas.*
                                            **Vogiatzis et al. 2016**

Evaluation of rehabilitation should be embedded from the start and can include the following:

- number of participants completing the programme
- daily activity, using an exercise diary (Appendix B)
- patient satisfaction
- wellbeing of carers

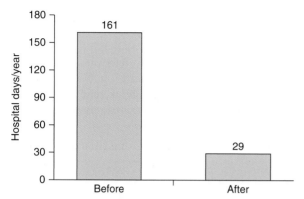

**FIGURE 9.12** Number of days spent in hospital before and after rehabilitation. (From Make 1994.)

- return to hobbies or job
- smoking cessation, normalization of weight
- ↓ general practitioner visits or hospital admissions (Fig. 9.12)

*Specific outcome measures for COPD and other diseases are in Chapter 3. Scales relevant to PR are below.*

For PR and exercise:
- Self-Efficacy Scale (Andenæs et al. 2014), Rating of Perceived Exertion (Ritchie 2012) and activity scales (Williams & Frei 2012), Timed Up & Go test (Albarrati et al. 2016).

For education:
- Lung information needs questionnaire (Cleutjens 2017)
- Inpatient respiratory rehabilitation questionnaire (Pasqua et al. 2012)

For respiratory symptoms:
- Breathlessness, cough and sputum scale (Oliveira & Marques 2016)
- Pulmonary functional status and dyspnea questionnaire (Regueiro et al. 2013).

For anxiety and depression:
- Anxiety inventory for respiratory disease (AIR) scale (Yohannes et al. 2016);
- Hospital anxiety and depression scale (Phan et al. 2016b); a score above 10 for either anxiety or depression should be reported.

For health-related QoL:
- St George's respiratory questionnaire or chronic respiratory questionnaire (McCarthy et al. 2015)
- COPD assessment test, which includes other respiratory diseases (Kon et al. 2013)

For change in behaviour towards exercise:
- obstacles to exercise survey, self-efficacy to exercise scale (Artistico et al. 2013)
- patient activation measure (Roberts et al. 2016b)

For follow-up benefit:
- Nijmegen clinical screening instrument, a short online questionnaire that includes an automated monitoring system (Vercoulen 2012);
- Video clips that demonstrate flexibility, posture and gait.

It is hoped that an abiding legacy of the programme is the friendship and courage that participants give each other. For those labouring under the double burden of disease and ageing, the outcome should be a more optimistic attitude towards a life that can be both active and fulfilling.

*I'm thankful that I have one leg,*
*to limp is no disgrace.*
*Although I can't be number one*
*I still can run the race.*
**Hart, quoted by deLateur 1997**

## CASE STUDY: MR EH

*Identify the problems of this 66-year-old man with COPD from Medellin who was referred as an outpatient after disappointment following rejection for transplantation. Then implement a treatment plan.*

### Background
- Social history: lives with wife, first floor flat with lift
- Drugs: bronchodilators, steroids, diuretics
- History of present complaint: recent admission for exacerbation, discharged with home oxygen, making slow recovery

### Subjective
- Can't do much since leaving hospital
- Able to look after self
- Unable to walk any useful distance
- Don't go out
- Unable to help in house or with shopping
- Poor sleep since hospital
- Not hungry
- Don't use oxygen much
- No phlegm

## Objective

- Leaning forward with hands on knees
- Speaking in short sentences
- Pursed lips breathing

## Questions

1. Analysis?
2. Problems?
3. Goals?
4. Plan?

## CLINICAL REASONING

*Do we need to read further than the title of the following article?*

*'Preoperative pulmonary rehabilitation versus chest physical therapy in patients undergoing lung cancer resection: a pilot randomized controlled trial.'*
**Arch Phys Med Rehabil (2013); 94(1):53–58**

## Response to Case Study

1. Analysis
   - Loss of confidence and exercise tolerance since discharge.
   - Lack of sleep and appetite may relate to depression, possibly triggered by rejection for transplantation and contributing to vicious cycle of inactivity.
2. Problems
   - breathlessness
   - inefficient breathing pattern
   - ↓ exercise tolerance
   - possible depression
   - misuse of oxygen
3. Goals
   - Short term: daily walk to bandstand
   - Medium term: return to preadmission function including steps up to front door
   - Long term: lifelong exercise programme
4. Plan
   - Obtain further information from patient on fluids, nutrition, assessment for oxygen therapy and limitations to exercise tolerance (e.g. anxiety, SOB, deconditioning).
   - Identify cause of poor sleep, discuss possible depression and liaise with multidisciplinary team.

- If oxygen indicated, educate Mr H on its use. Check knowledge of medication. Provide information on PR.
- If patient declines PR, refer to dietician for nutritional advice, educate on SOB and exercise, initiate written daily exercise programme, follow-up in a week to maintain motivation, then monthly, then 6-monthly reviews.

## RESPONSE TO CLINICAL REASONING

Pulmonary rehabilitation and 'chest physical therapy' (chest clearance) are for different problems.

# RECOMMENDED READING

Afolabi, G., Stevens, R., Turner, M., et al., 2013. Development of a pulmonary rehabilitation service for people with COPD. J. Cardiopulm. Rehabil. Prev. 33 (5), 323–327.

Apps, L.D., Mitchell, K.E., Harrison, S.L., et al., 2013. The development and pilot testing of the self-management programme of activity, coping and education for COPD. Int. J. Chron. Obstruct. Pulmon. Dis. 8, 317–327.

Astokorki, A.H.Y., 2017. Transcutaneous electrical nerve stimulation reduces exercise-induced perceived pain and improves endurance exercise performance. Eur. J. Appl. Physiol. 117 (1), 483–492.

Beekman, E., 2013. Course length of 30 metres versus 10 metres has a significant influence on six-minute walk distance in patients with COPD. J. Physiother. 59 (3), 169–176.

Benzo, R.P., Kirsch, J.L., Dulohery, M.M., et al., 2016. Emotional intelligence: a novel outcome associated with wellbeing and self-management in chronic obstructive pulmonary disease. Ann. Am. Thorac. Soc. 13 (1), 10–16.

Bourbeau, J., Lavoie, K.L., Sedeno, M., et al., 2016. Behaviour-change intervention in a multicentre, randomised, placebo-controlled COPD study: methodological considerations and implementation. BMJ Open 6 (4), e010109.

Budde, H., 2016. The need for differentiating between exercise, physical activity, and training. Autoimmun. Rev. 15 (1), 110–111.

Castro, A.A., Porto, E.F., Iamonti, V.C., 2013. Oxygen and ventilatory output during several activities of daily living performed by COPD patients stratified according to disease severity. PLoS ONE 8 (11), e79727.

Dassios, T., 2013. Aerobic exercise and respiratory muscle strength in patients with cystic fibrosis. Respir. Med. 107 (5), 684–690.

Demeyer, H., Burtin, C., Hornikx, M., et al., 2016. The minimal important difference in physical activity in patients with COPD. PLoS ONE 11 (4), e0154587.

Garuti, G., 2013. Pulmonary rehabilitation at home guided by telemonitoring and access to healthcare facilities for respiratory complications in patients with neuromuscular disease. Eur. J. Phys. Rehab. Med. 49 (1), 51–57.

Garvey, C., Bayles, M.P., Hamm, L.F., 2016. Pulmonary rehabilitation exercise prescription in chronic obstructive pulmonary disease: an official statement from the American Association of Cardiovascular and Pulmonary Rehabilitation. J. Cardiopulm. Rehab. Prev. 36 (2), 75–83.

Gillespie, P., O'Shea, E., Casey, D., et al., 2013. The cost-effectiveness of a structured education pulmonary rehabilitation programme for chronic obstructive pulmonary disease in primary care. BMJ Open 3 (11), e003479.

Gupta, S.S., Sawane, M.V., 2012. A comparative study of the effects of yoga and swimming on pulmonary functions in sedentary subjects. Int. J. Yoga 5 (2), 128–133.

Harrison, S.L., 2013. Physical activity monitoring: addressing the difficulties of accurately detecting slow walking speeds. Heart Lung 42 (4), 361–364.

Heerema-Poelman, A., Stuive, I., Wempe, J.B., 2013. Adherence to a maintenance exercise program 1 year after pulmonary rehabilitation. J. Cardiopulm. Rehabil. Prev. 33 (6), 419–426.

Holland, A.E., Wadell, K., Spruit, M.A., 2013. How to adapt the pulmonary rehabilitation programme to patients with chronic respiratory disease other than COPD. Eur. Respir. Rev. 22 (130), 577–586.

Inoue, S., Shibata, Y., Kishi, H., 2017. Decreased left ventricular stroke volume is associated with low-grade exercise tolerance in patients with chronic obstructive pulmonary disease. BMJ Open Respir. Res. 4 (1), e000158.

Jorine, E., 2013. Physical and psychosocial factors associated with physical activity in patients with COPD. Arch. Phys. Med. Rehabil. 94 (12), 2396.e7–2402.e7.

Lan, C.-C., 2013. Benefits of pulmonary rehabilitation in patients with COPD and normal exercise capacity. Respir. Care 58 (9), 1482–1488.

Mador, M.J., Modi, K., 2016. Comparing various exercise tests for assessing the response to pulmonary rehabilitation in patients with COPD. J. Cardiopulm. Rehab. Prev. 36 (2), 132–139.

Markovitz, G.H., Cooper, C.B., 2010. Mechanisms of exercise limitation and pulmonary rehabilitation for patients with pulmonary fibrosis/restrictive lung disease. Chron. Respir. Dis. 7 (1), 47–60.

Moy, M.L., Weston, N.A., Wilson, E.J., et al., 2013. A pilot study of an Internet walking program and pedometer in COPD. Respir. Med. 106 (9), 1342–1350.

O'Neill, B., McDonough, S.M., Wilson, J.J., et al., 2017. Comparing accelerometer, pedometer and a questionnaire for measuring physical activity in bronchiectasis. Respir. Res. 18, 16.

Osthoff, A.R., 2013. Association between peripheral muscle strength and daily physical activity in patients with COPD. J. Cardiopulm. Rehab. Prev. 33 (6), 351–359.

Reid, W.D., Yamabayashi, C., Goodridge, D., et al., 2012. Exercise prescription for hospitalized people with COPD and comorbidities. Int. J. Chron. Obstruct. Pulmon. Dis. 7, 297–320.

Shirreffs, S.M., 2007. Milk as an effective post-exercise rehydration drink. Br. J. Nutr. 98 (1), 173–180.

Spruit, M.A., Singh, S.J., 2013. Maintenance programs after pulmonary rehabilitation. Chest 144 (4), 1091–1093.

Spruit, M.A., Singh, S.J., Garvey, C., et al., 2013. An official ATS/ERS statement: key concepts and advances in pulmonary rehabilitation. Am. J. Respir. Crit. Care Med. 188 (8), e13–e64.

Suler, Y., Dinescu, L.I., 2013. Safety considerations during cardiac and pulmonary rehabilitation program. Phys. Med. Rehabil. Clin. N. Am. 23 (2), 433–440.

Theodorakopoulou, E.P., 2017. Effect of pulmonary rehabilitation on tidal expiratory flow limitation at rest and during exercise in COPD patients. Resp. Physiol. Neurobiol. 238, 47–54.

Wardini, R., Dajczman, E., Yang, N., et al., 2013. Using a virtual game system to innovate pulmonary rehabilitation. Can. Respir. J. 20 (5), 357–361.

Zhang, C., 2013. Development and validation of a COPD self-management scale. Respir. Care 58 (11), 1931–1936.

# 10

# Physiotherapy for People With Cardiovascular Disorders

*Alison Draper, Jo Sharp*

## INTRODUCTION

*It has been estimated that if everyone walked briskly at 3–4 mph on most days, about 30% of deaths from cardiovascular disease would be prevented.*
**WCPT 2009**

Physiotherapists treat problems of movement and function. Cardiovascular (CV) disorders cause symptoms such as chest pain, breathlessness and fatigue, which affect the ability to move and provoke a fear of moving, leading to a spiralling decline in function and quality of life (QoL).

Physiotherapy includes education and exercise. Physical fitness both prevents and treats CV disease, and poor CV fitness is now thought to be the strongest risk factor for these disorders (Lavie et al. 2015).

Education is provided by all team members and can improve function and QoL (Clark et al. 2015), but patients may feel too ill, too well, too tired or too busy to take it all in, and clinicians need to maximize patients' motivation to change the habits of a lifetime (Box 10.1).

Treatment follows the physiotherapy approach of assessing, setting patient-centred goals, following through a plan and assessing outcome.

## PHYSIOTHERAPY FOR PEOPLE WITH HEART FAILURE

*Prescribing physical activity as medicine is desperately needed throughout the health care system.*
**Lavie et al. 2015**

A failing left ventricle leads to pulmonary congestion which increases the work of breathing, especially during exercise (Cross et al. 2012a). Exercise capacity is also limited by fatigue and muscle weakness, augmented by 'heart failure myopathy' (Tzanis et al. 2013). Extra shortness of breath (SOB) is caused by increased ventilatory response to exercise (Witte & Clark 2008).

Patients should be under the care of a specialist team, which leads to improved QoL, reduced hospitalization and extended life (OHTAC 2009).

---

### BOX 10.1    Tips for Improving Adherence

- Ask the patient what they want to know rather than tell them what you think they should know.
- Give the most important information first.
- Be specific: 'Walk for 30 minutes every day' is better than 'Do as much walking as you can'.
- Link self treatment to an event or location ('whenever you make a cup of tea...' is more effective than 'three times a day').
- Tell them what you are going to tell them, then tell them, then tell them what you have told them.
- Write it down or use easy-to-read teaching material.
- Use clear sentences and repeat key information.
- Recruit family members to help with remembering.
- Tailor advice to the individual.
- Ask patients to repeat what they have been told, to check understanding of key points.
- Encourage questions.

---

## Education

*'If I knew I was going to live this long, I would have taken better care of myself'*

**Menezes et al. 2012**

Education is best started with an explanation that the alarming term 'heart failure' simply means that the heart is not pumping as hard as it should and that it is different from a heart attack or cardiac arrest. Advice (Table 10.1) is reinforced by strategies to maintain cognitive functioning and improve independence (Alosco et al. 2013).

Patient-directed goals, along with provision of blood pressure monitors, weight scales, pedometers, DVDs and booklets, can improve autonomy, lower blood pressure and reduce admissions (Shively et al. 2013). Explanation of the benefits and side effects of medication allows patients to make informed decisions. Arthritis is a common comorbidity and patients should be advised that nonsteroidal antiinflammatory drugs can worsen renal function and heart failure (HF) (ESC 2016). If sodium is restricted, patients are advised against low-salt substitutes due to their high potassium content (SIGN 2016). However, there is now doubt about recommending salt restriction (Doukky et al. 2016).

---

### TABLE 10.1    Topics for patient education

| Topic | Patient skills and self care |
|---|---|
| What is heart failure? | • Background, causes and symptoms. |
| How do I manage it? | • Daily weight. |
| | • If dyspnoea or oedema increases or there is sudden weight gain of >2 kg in 3 days, diuretic dose to be increased and/or health team alerted. |
| What do the drugs do? | • Indications, doses, effects and side effects. |
| What about drinking and eating? | • Healthy eating and correct weight. |
| | • Fluid restriction to 1.5–2 L/day with severe heart failure, to relieve symptoms and congestion. |
| | • Restriction of hypotonic fluids if hyponatraemia is a problem. |
| Can I smoke? | • Smoking and illicit drugs to be avoided. |
| How does exercise help? | • Benefits of exercise explained. |
| | • Flexibility to suit the patient. |
| | • Activities of daily living. |
| Can I have sex? | • Normal sexual activity is fine if the condition is stable and undue symptoms are not provoked. |
| Do I need a flu jab? | • Vaccinations against influenza and pneumococcal disease advised. |
| What about how I feel? | • Social support and treatment options for depression and cognitive dysfunction. |
| What's my future? | • End of life choices. |

Adapted from ESC 2016.

Depressed mood impairs concordance. The prevalence of depression is four to five times higher than in the general population, leading to reduced adherence to advice, a more sedentary lifestyle and higher mortality (Adelborg et al. 2016). Patients should be screened using a validated measure such as the Cardiac Depression Scale (ESC 2016) and cognitive therapy may be considered (SIGN 2016). Depression may contribute to erectile dysfunction, which is a risk with HF, especially if patients are taking thiazide diuretics, spironolactone or β-blockers (ESC 2016). Discussion on sleep-disordered breathing is also required because the condition is present in the majority of patients (Cowie 2016).

Motivation to exercise is assisted by explaining that SOB on exercise is not harmful (Witte & Clark 2008). Recognition of acute episodes requires explanation because exacerbations are not usually identified by patients (Reeder et al. 2015). Patients also need to ask for a follow-up appointment within 14 days (McAlister et al. 2016).

## Exercise

The majority of patients experience symptoms during their activities of daily living rather than at rest (Lalande & Johnson 2010). Exercise training has shown the following benefits:

- ↑ functional capacity and QoL (Antonicelli et al. 2016), equivalent to the improvements seen with chronic obstructive pulmonary disease (COPD) (Man et al. 2016);
- ↓ SOB and fatigue (Pineda et al. 2016);
- ↑ peripheral vascular and skeletal muscle function (Lavie et al. 2013);
- ↑ improved mood (ESC 2016);
- protection against the diaphragm dysfunction that is induced by HF (Mangner 2016);
- ↓ hospitalization and mortality by a third (Lavie et al. 2015).

With appropriate testing (Malhotra 2016) and prescription (Box 10.2), improvements in health status occur early and persist over time (Flynn et al. 2009).

Exercise tends to be accompanied by rapid shallow breathing rather than deep breathing because the reduced lung compliance caused by pulmonary oedema means that a deep breath could overstimulate pulmonary stretch receptors and depress heart rate (Fig. 10.1).

Some cardiac rehabilitation programmes exclude patients with a primary diagnosis of HF because these

---

**BOX 10.2 Exercise Prescription for People With Heart Failure**

- Incorporate aerobic and resistance exercise.
- Start with frequent 5–10 min activities for deconditioned or compromised patients.
- For interval exercise: work for 1–6 min and rest for 1–2 min.
- Consider ratios of work:rest at 1:2 or 1:1, sitting:standing at 1:1 or 1:3 and strength:endurance at 1:1 or 2:1.
- Intensity for aerobic exercise: 55%–80% HRR or use RPE.
- Intensity for strength and endurance exercise: 50%–70% of 1RM for lower body, 40%–70% for upper body.
- Include low to moderate intensity large muscle group work e.g. walking, stationary cycling, muscle groups for activities of daily living.
- Emphasize posture and core strength.
- Include breathlessness management and recovery strategies.
- Promote energy conservation and pacing. Exercise heart rates will be approximately 10–20 bpm lower than for individuals without heart failure.

*1RM*, one repetition maximum; *ADL*, Activities of daily living; *bpm*, beats per minute; *HRR*, heart rate reserve; *RPE*, rating of perceived exertion.
Adapted from ACPICR 2015.

---

patients form a different population to those who have been through a sudden event such as myocardial infarct or heart surgery. However, there is progress towards incorporating HF-specific education into these programmes (Keteyian et al. 2014), and beneficial outcomes appear to be consistent (Sagar et al. 2015). Pulmonary rehabilitation programmes are also suitable because people with COPD and HF face similar problems of SOB and slowly progressive disability on a background of multimorbidity, and the conditions often coexist (Man et al. 2016).

Interval training allows higher-intensity training levels, can improve QoL (Chrysohoou 2014) and may reduce arrhythmias (Guiraud et al. 2013), while eccentric muscle exercise suits patients with reduced energetic reserve (Casillas et al. 2016). Dancing carries extra motivation and can bring functional and CV benefits similar to formal exercise training (Kaltsatou et al. 2014). In relation to medical treatment and exercise, some patients profit from added oxygen (Koshy et al.

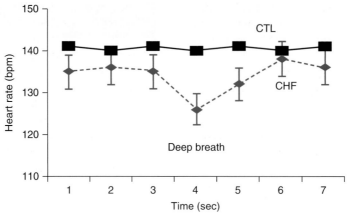

**FIGURE 10.1** Influence of a deep breath on heart rate in patients with chronic heart failure *(CHF)* and controls *(CTL)* during exercise. (From Lalande & Johnson 2010.)

2016), but nitrates can reduce activity levels (Oeser 2016). Patients with implanted devices to restore synchronized contraction between right and left ventricles require specific precautions (Haennel 2012).

> ### PRACTICE TIP
> Warm up and cool down before and after exercise counteract the risks of ischaemia, postexercise hypotension and arrhythmias.

The addition of inspiratory muscle training can add extra QoL, according to a systematic review and meta-analysis (Neto et al. 2016b), possibly because of the association of inspiratory muscle weakness with exercise intolerance and poor nutrition, the latter also requiring attention (Yamada et al. 2016). Functional electrical stimulation of peripheral muscles may improve exercise capacity, QoL and endothelial function (Karavidas 2013).

A home-based programme can reduce mortality and hospitalization (Fergenbaum et al. 2015), with telephone reinforcement for extra benefit (Hoekstra et al. 2013). A cheerful outcome measure named the Worst Symptom Visual Analogue Score is available (AbouEzzeddine et al. 2016).

### Management of Patients With Acute Disease

Breathlessness from pulmonary oedema may be relieved in acutely unwell patients by a hand-held fan (Wong 2013) and upright positioning to displace the fluid downwards, with support of the feet to prevent the inexorable slide down the bed. Poor gas exchange may require continuous positive airway pressure (Mebazaa et al. 2015) which brings the bonus of improved neural control of heart rate in patients who have comorbid COPD (Reis et al. 2010). BiPAP (p. 240) may also be suitable, and more comfortable (Allison & Winters 2016). As soon as the patient is willing, mobilization should follow, after a check for anaemia, which is present in 10%–56% of patients (Piña 2013) but is missed by most cardiologists (Doehner et al. 2013). Rehabilitation maintained after discharge improves survival (Catanzaro et al. 2012).

## PHYSIOTHERAPY FOR PEOPLE WITH CORONARY HEART DISEASE – OVERVIEW

Both aerobic exercise and stress management may each reduce adverse clinical events (Sherwood 2017). Preventive physical activity is recommended to be:
- at least 150 min of moderate intensity aerobic activity or 75 min of vigorous intensity aerobic activity or a mix of moderate and vigorous aerobic activity on two or more days a week;
- muscle-strengthening activities for all major muscle groups (NICE 2016b).

For patients with acute problems related to coronary heart disease, the physiotherapist becomes involved when they are admitted with myocardial infarction or for heart surgery. Once the patient has stabilized, they are best managed through a multidisciplinary cardiac rehabilitation programme (Chapter 11).

## PHYSIOTHERAPY FOR PEOPLE WITH PERIPHERAL ARTERIAL DISEASE

Intermittent claudication (p. 143) limits exercise tolerance and impairs QoL (Fig. 10.2). Goals negotiated with the patient may include increased distance walked or time spent walking, walking to a location which is meaningful to the patient or managing a specific activity.

### Education

For people with peripheral arterial disease (PAD), the aims of education are to modify the risk factors associated with atherosclerosis, explain how exercise helps their condition and advise on foot care. The importance of education is underlined by patients' lack of belief that lifestyle interventions will help, and unrealistic expectations of the outcome of surgery (NICE 2012b).

### Exercise

Exercise can improve walking ability more than stent revascularization (Murphy et al. 2012) as well as enhance QoL and, with follow-up, helps to reduce mortality (ESC 2016). Examples are:

- Ten sets of 2-min walking at a speed corresponding to the onset of claudication pain with a 2-min inter-val between sets, and/or 1 × 10 repetitions of eight resistance exercises plus five 2-min sets of walking, a single session of which can improve blood flow and reduce leg vascular resistance (Lima et al. 2016).
- Three episodes of walking up to 15 min or until claudication becomes intolerable, separated by rest periods long enough for claudication to subside, plus three bouts of resistive calf exercise of up to 5 min or until claudication is intolerable, separated by similar recovery periods; over time this reduces claudication and increases exercise tolerance in a third of patients (Figoni et al. 2016).
- Interval training by walking at varying intensities, from 30 min to 55 min, which can prolong walking times (Collins et al. 2016b).

Exercise prescription is also suggested in Table 10.2.

Treadmill walking is suitable for many patients, but for those who are frail, circulation can be improved by lower limb exercises in sitting (Castro-Sánchez 2013). For patients who cannot tolerate intermittent claudication, effective alternatives include upper limb training (Tompra et al. 2015) and other variations (Lefebvre 2013). The benefits of exercise training are quickly lost if ongoing exercise is not frequent and regular (NICE 2012b). For simple cramps at night, patients may find it helpful to do three 30-s calf stretches during the day,

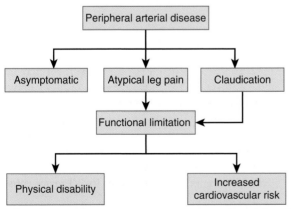

**FIGURE 10.2** Functional consequences of peripheral arterial disease. (From Modified from Hamburg et al. 2011.)

| TABLE 10.2 | **Endurance training for patients with intermittent claudication** |
|---|---|
| Frequency | 3–5 days/week |
| Modality | Walking, e.g. treadmill or free walking. |
| Intensity | Exercise to work rate at which patient experiences onset of claudication. Continue walking until pain score is mild to moderate (3–4 out of 5 points). Stop until pain completely subsides. Resume exercise again at similar intensity. Repeat rest/exercise bouts. Progress to a higher work rate when able to walk for 8-min bouts without needing to stop for leg symptoms. |
| Duration | Total exercise time (including rest periods) should equal 50 min. Continue for at least 6 months. |

From Hamburg & Balady 2011, Lefebvre 2013.

lowering alternate heels from the edge of a step (Daniell & Pentrack 2013).

Exercise testing may reveal evidence of occult coronary heart disease, which should be reported. As exercise tolerance improves, heart disease symptoms may become a limiting factor. Cardiac rehabilitation can be adapted for patients with PAD but patients classified at the most severe level (p. 144, Table 4.5) should not join the exercise sessions.

## CASE STUDY: MR BG

*Identify the problems of this patient awaiting discharge following inguinal hernia repair.*

### Background
- COPD, on bronchodilators
- Smoker

### Nurse report
- Possible chest infection

### Subjective
- Feeling unwell
- Breathless, especially when lying flat
- Coughing up white secretions

### Objective
- Pale
- Apyrexial
- Bilateral basal crackles and wheeze on auscultation
- Swollen ankles
- $SpO_2$ 94%
- Radiology as Fig. 4.3, p. 139

### Questions
1. Analysis?
2. Problems?
3. Goals?
4. Plan?

### CLINICAL REASONING

At the end of a lengthy study, the conclusion was:

*'Postural drainage and chest percussion in patients without sputum production is not indicated.'*
Connors et al. 1980

## Response to Case Study

1. Analysis
   - X-ray suggests pulmonary oedema.
   - Absence of green sputum or pyrexia suggests there is no chest infection.
   - Sudden onset suggests myocardial infarct rather than HF.
   - Need to liaise with medical team for further investigations.

   Note 1: $\beta_2$-agonist bronchodilators may induce tachycardia.

   Note 2: Airway clearance techniques are not effective for pulmonary oedema.

2. Problems
   - Increased work of breathing, due to pulmonary oedema
   - Reduced mobility due to breathlessness

3. Goals
   - Reduce work of breathing
   - Rehabilitate to home environment

4. Plan
   - Check operation notes.
   - Liaise re. medication, including pain relief if required, and diuretics, which will reduce alveolar secretions.
   - Check patient understanding; advise on upright positioning and progressive mobility.
   - Multidisciplinary rehabilitation.

### RESPONSE TO CLINICAL REASONING

Perhaps the time spent trying the clear the chests of 'patients without sputum production' could be directed more usefully, e.g. problem-solving.

## RECOMMENDED READING

Bernocchi, P., Scalvini, S., Galli, T., et al., 2016. A multidisciplinary telehealth program in patients with combined chronic obstructive pulmonary disease and chronic heart failure. Trials 17, 462.

Drozdz, T., Bilo, G., Debicka-Dabrowska, D., et al., 2016. Blood pressure changes in patients with chronic heart failure undergoing slow breathing training. Blood Press. 25 (1), 4–10.

Jaureguizar, K.V., 2016. Effect of high-intensity interval versus continuous exercise training on functional capacity and quality of life in patients with coronary artery disease. J. Cardiopulm. Rehabil. Prev. 36 (2), 96–105.

Lefebvre, K., 2013. A review of exercise protocols for patients with peripheral arterial disease. Topics Geriatr. Rehab. 29 (3), 165–178.

Parmenter, B.J., 2015. Exercise training for management of peripheral arterial disease: a systematic review and meta-analysis. Sports Med. 45 (2), 231–244.

Ponikowski, P., Voors, A.A., Anker, S.D., et al., 2016. ESC Guidelines for the diagnosis and treatment of acute and chronic heart failure. Eur. J. Heart Fail. 18 (8), 891–975.

Rouse, G.W., Albert, N.M., Butler, R.S., et al., 2016. A comparative study of fluid management education before hospital discharge. Heart Lung 45 (1), 21–28.

Sagar, V.A., 2015. Exercise-based rehabilitation for heart failure: systematic review and meta-analysis. Open Heart 2, e000163.

SIGN, 2016. Management of Chronic Heart Failure. Scottish Intercollegiate Guidelines Network, Edinburgh.

Sperling, M.P.R., Simões, R.P., Caruso, F.C.R., et al., 2016. Is heart rate variability a feasible method to determine anaerobic threshold in progressive resistance exercise in coronary artery disease? Braz. J. Phys. Ther. 20 (4), 289–297.

# 11

# Cardiac Rehabilitation

*Alison Draper, Jo Sharp*

## LEARNING OBJECTIVES

*On completion of this chapter the reader should be able to:*
- understand the physiotherapist's role in the management of patients with coronary heart disease;
- outline the importance of patient education in reducing risk and improving adherence;

- describe the principles of exercise therapy for patients with cardiovascular disorders;
- identify a range of outcome measures suitable for this group of patients.

## OUTLINE

## INTRODUCTION

*'Will I have another heart attack? I don't know, but I do know that cardiac rehabilitation has fast-tracked me back to a normal life and given me the knowledge that the chances of another heart attack are greatly reduced'*

**Dalal et al. 2015**

**1RM**: one repetition maximum – maximum load that can be moved once, over a full range of motion without compensatory movements
**HRR**: heart rate reserve – difference between maximum heart rate and resting heart rate, i.e. a measure of fitness, a high maximum heart rate with low resting heart rate representing the highest functional reserve
**Max HR**: available from a stress/exercise test, or calculated as 220 minus age

**MET**: metabolic equivalent – measure of exercise intensity based on oxygen consumption
**RPE**: rating of perceived exertion
**Stress test**: treadmill walking at gradually increasing intensity under electrocardiogram monitoring to identify the heart's response to exercise
$\dot{V}O_2$: oxygen consumption
$\dot{V}O_2max$: maximal rate at which oxygen can be used by an individual during maximal work, i.e. aerobic capacity
$\dot{V}O_2peak$: highest value of $\dot{V}O_2$ attained on a particular exercise test if maximal has not been achieved

Following hospitalization for heart disease or heart surgery, disability rates of 45%–75% have been identified (Dolansky et al. 2011). Cardiac rehabilitation (CR) addresses the causes of this, including exercise intolerance, comorbidities and anxiety. Its aims are to

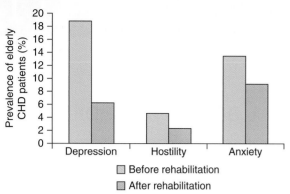

**FIGURE 11.1** Benefits of cardiac rehabilitation in elderly heart disease patients. *CHD,* Coronary heart disease. (From Menezes et al. 2012.)

improve physical health, quality of life (QoL) and self management.

CR involves education, exercise and relaxation, supervised by a multidisciplinary team. Participation rates are low at 20%–50%, due to patient and health system factors (Dalal et al. 2015). Older patients show higher adherence (Azad 2012), and have demonstrated greater improvements in function and QoL (Schopfer & Forman 2016), but older people are underrepresented, possibly because of low expectations and inadequate referrals (Menezes et al. 2012).

Attendance can be maximized by sending phone reminders, arranging parking or volunteer drivers, and considering home-based programmes for lower risk patients (Chen et al. 2016c), including the use of smartphone (Yudi et al. 2016) and other virtual technologies (Brewer et al. 2015). Following myocardial infarction (MI) however, supervision is advised (Coll-Fernández et al. 2016).

Benefits are both social (Fig. 11.1) and physical (Fig. 11.2), including the following:

- physical activity levels consistent with health-related benefits (Ribeiro et al. 2017);
- ↓ hospital admissions (Anderson et al. 2016);
- ↓ readmissions, myocardial reinfarction and anxiety, ↑ QoL, exercise capacity and return to work (ACPICR 2016);
- ↓ mortality and depression, ↑ functional capacity and medication adherence (Servey 2016);
- ↑ $\dot{V}O_2$peak by 14%–31% (Andjic et al. 2016);
- ↓ time in atrial fibrillation for some patients (Malmo et al. 2016);

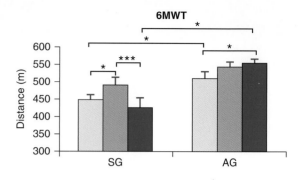

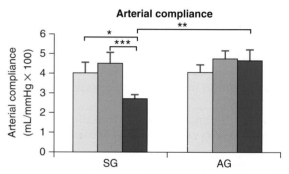

**FIGURE 11.2** Six-minute walk test and arterial compliance at the beginning of cardiac rehabilitation (pale bars), end of the programme (middle) and 18 months afterwards (dark bars). *AG,* Active group; *SG,* sedentary group; $*p < .05$, $**p < .01$, $***p < .001$. (From Freyssin et al. 2011.)

---

**BOX 11.1   Core Components of Cardiac Rehabilitation**

Lifestyle risk management, e.g. smoking cessation
Medical risk management, e.g. cardioprotective therapies
Exercise
Diet
Psychosocial health
Long-term management
Audit and evaluation

Adapted from BACPR 2012.

---

- for people with stable angina: ↓ angina frequency and physical limitation (McGillion et al. 2014);
- for people with severe pulmonary arterial hypertension: improved haemodynamics and ↑ $\dot{V}O_2$peak (Ehlken et al. 2016).

The seven core components are shown in Box 11.1.

## STRUCTURE

CR is divided into phases:

I. Inpatient period.
II. Early postdischarge period.
III. Intermediate postdischarge period, involving multidisciplinary rehabilitation in groups or a home-based individualized programme.
IV. Long-term maintenance.

### Inpatient Period

The patient's physical ability is compromised by the effects of heart disease or surgery, and sometimes by bed rest. Automatic referral to CR is advised (Tiller et al. 2013) and for patients who have had an MI it should begin as soon as possible after admission or at least before discharge (NICE 2013b). Once vital signs are stable, the physiotherapy component is to maintain suitable levels of activity, with exercise intensity governed by heart rate (HR) or rating of perceived exertion (RPE) (Table 11.1).

### Early Postdischarge Period

In this transition stage, patients are advised to build up their activity gradually to around 20–30 min of walking each day, depending on previous fitness levels. Early initiation of moderate intensity aerobic training can reduce cardiovascular risk and increase aerobic capacity, and may be more beneficial than later training (Takagi et al. 2016). When combined with education, both improved exercise tolerance and motivation to attend CR have been demonstrated (Dolansky et al. 2011).

Most postdischarge morbidity and mortality have been attributed to failure to adhere to the new medication regimen (Bernal et al. 2012), which underlines the importance of monitoring and support during this period. Education is usually provided by specialist nurses and involves a combination of home visits, telephone monitoring and clinic appointments.

### Intermediate Postdischarge Period

The structured part of the programme is usually provided to outpatients in supervised groups, starting soon after MI or 4–6 weeks after cardiac surgery (Dalal et al. 2015). Patients need to be screened, including with a stress test to detect ischaemic changes on graded exercise. Patients with a variety of CV disorders can be included (Box 11.2) irrespective of age or clinical status, but a change in condition requires reassessment.

### TABLE 11.1   Rating of perceived exertion

| Rating of perceived exertion | Intensity | Breathing equivalent |
|---|---|---|
| 6 | No exertion | |
| 7 | | Can sing full songs |
| 8 | Extremely light | |
| 9 | Very light | Can sing partial verses |
| 10 | | |
| 11 | Light | Can talk in full sentences |
| 12 | | |
| 13 | Somewhat hard | Can talk in short sentences |
| 14 | | |
| 15 | Hard | Breathing hard |
| 16 | | |
| 17 | Very hard | |
| 18 | | |
| 19 | Extremely hard | |
| 20 | Maximal | |

### BOX 11.2   Patients who benefit from Cardiac Rehabilitation

**Coronary heart disease**
New onset angina or worsening exertional angina
Acute coronary syndrome
Pre- and postrevascularization by angioplasty or coronary artery bypass graft

**Other types of heart surgery**
Pre- and post-heart transplant
Ventricular assist device
Heart valve repair or replacement

**Other heart conditions**
Heart failure and cardiomyopathy
Following implantation of cardiac defibrillator or resynchronization device
Adults with congenital heart disease

**Vascular conditions**
Peripheral arterial disease
Transient ischaemic attack

ACPICR 2016, BACPR 2012, NICE 2013b.

A multidisciplinary team provides one to three sessions a week of education and supervised exercise, with family present if agreeable to the patient.

The team may include:
- cardiologist or specialist general practitioner
- specialist nurse
- physiotherapist
- dietician
- psychologist
- exercise physiologist
- occupational therapist
- clerical administrator

The recommended minimum duration is 8 weeks (NACR 2014). Patients should not be excluded if they choose to attend only specific components, but those who stop attending unexpectedly should be tempted back by phone call, letter or prearranged visit (NICE 2013b).

## Long-Term Maintenance

The final phase is indefinite, the goal being to encourage lifelong adherence to the healthy habits established during earlier phases. Physical activity often drops quickly after the end of the supervised period, and progressively autonomous physical activity has been suggested (Fournier et al. 2016). High intensity interval training is also recommended, with Aamot et al. (2016) finding that it led to the majority of participants meeting the recommended daily level of 30 min moderate physical activity. Meanwhile, the zeal with which occasional participants exercise is a reminder that some need explanations that excessive endurance regimens may not be helpful (Fig. 11.3).

# EDUCATION

Education aims to build confidence and facilitate autonomy. It is useful to establish participants' health perceptions before offering lifestyle advice, and then to use the principles in Box 10.1 and topics from National Institute for Health and Care Excellence (NICE) (2013b), including:
- pathology and symptoms;
- pharmaceutical and surgical options;
- risk factors, including tobacco, alcohol, fast food and inactivity;
- occupational and vocational information, including welfare rights and social support;
- understanding the discharge summary;

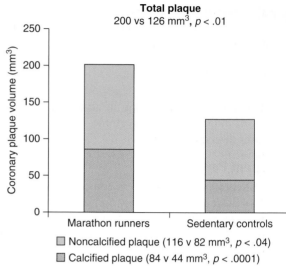

**Total plaque**
200 vs 126 mm$^3$, $p < .01$

FIGURE 11.3 Significantly higher coronary plaque volume in marathon runners compared with control subjects. (From Parto et al. 2016.)

- driving, flying and competitive sport, as required;
- sexual activity, e.g. after recovery from an MI, sexual activity presents no greater risk of triggering a subsequent MI than if the person had never had an MI;
- stress management;
- basic life support;
- living with uncertainty, advance care planning and end-of-life decisions (BACPR 2012).

Discussion on other therapies is also advised because the majority of patients use dietary supplements or complementary therapies (Prasad et al. 2013). Stress management is integral to reducing cardiovascular risk, and treatment options for depression should be included because of the link between depression and physical inactivity (Carney et al. 2016). Depression is most likely in people with heart failure, while anxiety is prominent following MI (Moryś et al. 2016).

# EXERCISE

Exercise training is well-established for lowering BP, improving lipid profiles and reducing morbidity and mortality (Parto et al. 2016), particularly when individualized to each person's needs (Charansonney et al. 2014).

Patients need to build up their exercise tolerance slowly because, although sustained physical training reduces platelet reactivity, acute activity brings an increased risk of atherosclerotic plaque rupturing during and immediately after physical exercise, especially in those who have been sedentary (Kumar et al. 2012).

## Assessment

Participants should bring their antianginal drugs with them for all sessions. Those with diabetes need to bring their glucose tablets. Drinking water must be available throughout, but energy drinks are not recommended because of the risk of adverse cardiac events (Goldfarb 2014).

The 6-min and shuttle walk tests (p. 351–352) relate to $\dot{V}O_2$max, or the 2-min walk test can be used for debilitated patients (Casillas et al. 2013). Patients with implanted cardioverter defibrillators require symptom-limited exercise testing (Flo et al. 2012), but, as always, strategies must be prepared in case of complications. Intensity monitoring uses the measures in Table 11.2.

Assessment identifies any contraindication to exercise training (Box 11.3) and patients are stratified as low, moderate or high risk for exercise prescription and level of supervision.

BP should be taken with the cuff as near heart level as possible. BP and HR are required before each exercise session, as well as during the formal assessment. If HR is irregular or >100 bpm or unusually low for the patient, especially if associated with dizziness, palpitations, chest discomfort, dyspnoea, nausea or sweating, the patient should sit or lie down in a semirecumbent position. If it does not resolve, exercise is contraindicated and the doctor should be called.

The assessment provides an opportunity to offer literature or advice on dietetics, erectile dysfunction or smoking cessation. The benefits of CR are limited for people who continue to smoke (Mlakar 2013).

## Safety

A minimum of two staff members is required at all times, with a staff-to-patient ratio of 1:5 for moderate-risk patients. Warm up and cool down periods of 15 min (or less for lower-functioning patients) are needed for all patients.

Patients on anticoagulation drugs should avoid high impact activity or contact sports in case of bruising or

| TABLE 11.2 | Exercise prescription | | | |
|---|---|---|---|---|
| Requirement | Frequency | Intensity | Time in minutes per day | Type of exercise |
| Cardiovascular fitness | Two to three times per week | Initially 40%–70% $\dot{V}O_2$max, i.e.: <br>• 40%–70% HRR <br>• 11–14 RPE | 20–60 min continuous or interval training (plus 15 min warm up and 10 min cool down) | Large muscle groups worked rhythmically |
| Muscle strength and endurance | Two to three times per week | • Upper body 30%–40% 1RM <br>• Lower body 50%–60% 1RM | Minimum 1–4 sets of 10–15 repetitions | 8–10 different muscle groups |
| Flexibility/ stretching (can be incorporated into cool down) | Two to three times per week when muscles are warm | Hold stretch for 30 s | Repeat stretch two to four times (60 s in total) | Static, ballistic or PNF stretches |
| Deconditioned patient with functional capacity <3 METS | Every day – incorporate into daily routine | Moderate: <br>• Borg RPE 11 <br>• 40% HRR | 5–10 min bouts (gradual increase to accumulated 30 min per day) | Activities to improve function, strength, endurance, posture, balance and coordination e.g. walking, low step-ups, sit to stand, seated activities |

*1RM*, One repetition maximum; *HHR*, heart rate reserve; *METS*, metabolic equivalent; *PNF*, proprioceptive neuromuscular facilitation; *RPE*, rating of perceived exertion; *$\dot{V}O_2$max*, maximum oxygen consumption.
Adapted from ACPICR 2016.

BOX 11.3  **Factors Precluding a Patient From Joining or Continuing the Exercise Component of Cardiac Rehabilitation**

- Unstable angina
- Resting systolic BP >180 mmHg or diastolic BP >110 mmHg
- Exercise-induced hypotension or orthostatic BP drop of >20 mmHg with symptoms
- Critical aortic stenosis (valve area <1 cm$^2$)
- Acute systemic illness or fever
- Uncontrolled atrial or ventricular arrhythmias
- Uncontrolled sinus tachycardia (HR >120 bpm)
- Acute pericarditis or myocarditis
- Uncompensated heart failure
- Third degree atrioventricular block (without pacemaker)
- Thrombophlebitis
- Resting ST segment displacement >2 mm, indicating ischaemia
- Uncontrolled diabetes mellitus
- High or low potassium levels
- Severe rejection following cardiac transplantation
- Severe orthopaedic or arthritic condition for which exercise cannot be adapted without exacerbating the condition

*BP*, Blood pressure; *bpm*, beats per minute; *HR*, heart rate.
Adapted from ACPICR 2016.

bleeding, and those on diuretics should avoid prolonged exercise in hot weather in case of reduced potassium and fluid volume. Patients must not exercise after a large meal or in extremes of heat or cold. For poststernotomy patients, the mode of exercise should not cause a shearing stress on the sternum before union at 8–12 weeks.

Exercise can usually be modified for patients with arthritic conditions, but on days when joint pain is increased by exercise, the patient can take their own decision on whether to continue, with or without analgesia, so long as the pain is not prolonged and they are fully informed about joint protection. They may prefer non-weight-bearing maintenance exercise such as swimming.

A check electrocardiogram (ECG) should be requested if the pulse behaves abnormally, if exercise tolerance declines over two or three sessions, or if a patient feels that their heart is 'not right'. Patients often detect that something is amiss before it becomes obvious. Referral for drug review is required if angina occurs, side effects increase or exercise tolerance is reduced by pulmonary oedema.

If a patient says that they do not feel well or they feel unusually tired, they should sit down and have their BP, HR and respiratory rate taken. If a patient gets angina during exercise, the following steps should be taken:
- the patient sits down and takes their glyceryl trinitrate, one to two sprays or one to two tablets, under their tongue, if prescribed, unless the patient is hypotensive or feels dizzy;
- they wait 5 min for relief of symptoms;
- two further doses may be taken at 5 min intervals;
- if symptoms are relieved, they should rest for a further 5 min, then rejoin the class at a lower intensity; if they wish to leave they must be fully recovered beforehand;
- if symptoms are unrelieved after 15 min of repeated medication, the doctor should be called.

If there is an irregular pulse which takes more than a minute to recover, the patient should lie down. MI is suspected if the pain is more severe than normal or the patient is grey, short of breath and sweaty, in which case assistance is summoned.

When one participant feels unwell and is being cared for, spare staff should attend to the other participants.

## Procedure

A progressive training effect can be achieved by increasing the frequency, intensity and/or duration of exercise (Table 11.2), to include exercise for strength, flexibility, balance and coordination. Examples are:
- walking at 60%–70% of $\dot{V}O_2$peak for 15–30 min (confirmed by a Borg one repetition maximum (RPE) of 11–14);
- resistance exercises at 50% of RPE for 10–15 repetitions;
- aerobic exercise for 30–40 min on the treadmill or exercise bike, plus lower limb resistance training between three and five sets at 50% of 1RM for 10 repetitions (ACPICR 2016).

The magnitude of improvement is related to the duration of training (8–16 weeks, three to five times a week) and intensity (e.g. 11–14 Borg RPE scale for 30 min sessions excluding warm up and cool down).

If HR is used for monitoring (Fig. 11.4), participants take their pulse during exercise to ensure that it is within their prescribed target range, and after the cool down period to check that it has returned to the preexercise

Name .................................. Exercise heart rate zones .................................. 70% ..........

| | Exercise considerations ........................................... ........................................... ........................................... | | | Shuttle outcome Metres ........................................... METS ........................................... Outcome ........................................... | | | | | | | | |
|---|---|---|---|---|---|---|---|---|---|---|---|---|
| | 1 ..../..../.... | | | 2 ..../..../.... | | | 3 ..../..../.... | | | 4 ..../..../.... | | |
| **Exercise** | **Time** | **Pulse** | **Effort** | **Time** | **Pulse** | **Effort** | **Time** | **Pulse** | **Effort** | **Time** | **Pulse** | **Effort** |
| **Walk** | mins | ♡ | effort | mins | ♡ | effort | mins | ♡ | effort | mins | ♡ | effort |
| **Chest press** | Reps | ♡ | effort | Reps | ♡ | effort | Reps | ♡ | effort | Reps | ♡ | effort |
| **Squats** | mins | ♡ | effort | mins | ♡ | effort | mins | ♡ | effort | mins | ♡ | effort |
| **Bicep curls** | Reps | ♡ | effort | Reps | ♡ | effort | Reps | ♡ | effort | Reps | ♡ | effort |
| **Stepper** | mins | ♡ | effort | mins | ♡ | effort | mins | ♡ | effort | mins | ♡ | effort |
| **Upright rows** | Reps | ♡ | effort | Reps | ♡ | effort | Reps | ♡ | effort | Reps | ♡ | effort |
| **Lunges** | mins | ♡ | effort | mins | ♡ | effort | mins | ♡ | effort | mins | ♡ | effort |
| **Triceps** | Reps | ♡ | effort | Reps | ♡ | effort | Reps | ♡ | effort | Reps | ♡ | effort |
| **Sit to stand** | mins | ♡ | effort | mins | ♡ | effort | mins | ♡ | effort | mins | ♡ | effort |
| **Standing rows** | Reps | ♡ | effort | Reps | ♡ | effort | Reps | ♡ | effort | Reps | ♡ | effort |

**FIGURE 11.4** *Effort,* As per Borg rating of perceived exertion scale; *Exercise considerations,* specific needs of the patient; *Exercise heart rate zones,* the two rates between which the most benefit is derived; *METS,* metabolic equivalent, measure of exercise intensity based on oxygen consumption.

rate. Excessively high HR is inadvisable because a short diastole prevents the blood from nourishing cardiac muscle (Böhm & Reil 2013).

β-Blockers and calcium channel blockers dampen the heart's response to exercise, and patients on these drugs should monitor their RPE rather than HR (Scherr 2013). The RPE is explained to patients as the inner feeling of exertion, not leg ache or breathlessness. Self-monitoring encourages long-term exercise maintenance.

## RELAXATION

Relaxation improves haemodynamic variables beyond that promoted by CR alone (Neves et al. 2009), and 5–10 min practice should be slotted into each session so that patients understand how it can be fitted into their daily life. Other techniques that promote relaxation are:
- T'ai Chi, which shows beneficial effects on BP, $\dot{V}O_2$max and QoL (Ng et al. 2012);

- meditation and yoga, which modestly lower BP by altering autonomic balance, and slow deep breathing and other guided breathing techniques, which significantly reduce BP (Brook et al. 2013) so long as hyperventilation is avoided in case of comorbid hyperventilation syndrome;
- massage, which moderately reduces BP (Liao et al. 2016b).

## FOLLOW-UP

Patients have described ongoing support as imperative to help them maintain lifestyle changes and navigate a new way of life (Pryor 2014), e.g. community programmes run by fitness instructors (Adsett et al. 2013) or the use of phone apps (Chow 2016). The recommendations for ongoing exercise are:
- UK: 20–30 min a day to the point of slight breathlessness (NICE 2013b);

- World Health Organization: at least 150 min of moderate intensity exercise or 75 min of vigorous exercise per week (Parto et al. 2016).

Some participants like to work out the physical demands of different activities, found on the Centers for Disease Control and Prevention website.

> '... last week I had worked up in my mind I had to brush my back garden and I had to do that in stages. I did one stage and then came inside and had a drink and then another stage and came in, you know, and just did it that way'
>
> *Tierney et al. (2011)*

## OUTCOMES

The following can be used to evaluate outcomes.

### Exercise Capacity

- Accelerometer (Aamot et al. 2016)
- Six-minute walk test (Bellet et al. 2012)
- Incremental shuttle walk test (Buckley et al. 2016)
- Treadmill or cycle ergometer tests (Lauer 2008)
- Duke activity questionnaire (Fan et al. 2015)

### Quality of Life

- Minnesota Living with Heart Failure questionnaire (Bilbao et al. 2016)
- Behavioural questionnaires, particularly relevant due to the association of, e.g. stress and poor sleep with unhealthy lifestyle choices (Gostoli et al. 2016)
- SF36 and SF12 questionnaires (Mays et al. 2011)
- Heart QoL Questionnaire (Oldridge et al. 2014)
- Hypertension QoL questionnaires (Patil et al. 2016)
- Late Life Function and Disability Instrument for people age >60 years (LaPier et al. 2012)
- MacNew heart disease health-related quality of life questionnaire (Hofer et al. 2012)
- Illness perception questionnaire (Broadbent et al. 2015)

## CASE STUDY: MR TE

*Identify the problems of this patient who has undergone a percutaneous coronary intervention to insert a stent after being admitted following an ST segment elevation MI.*

### Background

- Taxi driver
- Smoker

### Nurse report

- Stable
- No bleeding at puncture site

### Subjective

- Groin tenderness at site of catheter insertion
- Mild chest discomfort
- Tired

### Objective

- ECG sinus rhythm
- HR 85 bpm
- BP 128/95 mmHg
- Peripheral arterial oxygen saturation ($SpO_2$) 97%

### Questions

1. Analysis?
2. Problems?
3. Goals?
4. Plan?

---

**CLINICAL REASONING**

*Cardiac rehabilitation including exercise, group discussion, breath focus, meditation, mindfulness, visualization and cognitive restructuring was found to reduce BP, blood lipids and BMI, and to improve psychological measures and exercise response. The conclusion was that a mind/body CR program reduced medical and psychological risks.*

Casey et al. (2009)

---

### Response to Case Study

1. Analysis
   - Nurse report and objective findings suggest that patient is well enough to mobilize
2. Problems
   - Reduced exercise tolerance due to poor cardiovascular fitness and anxiety
   - Lack of knowledge of self management

3. Goals
   - Prevent postangioplasty complications
   - Restore functional mobility prior to discharge
   - Ensure knowledge of factors which will promote recovery
4. Plan
   - Teach patient to carry out regular exercises until fully mobile
   - Progressive mobilization for up to 20 min, three to four times per day
   - Advice and education re. physical activity and exercise, diet, smoking cessation
   - Referral to CR

### RESPONSE TO CLINICAL REASONING

Multiple components mean that no conclusion can be drawn about any one modality. Lack of a control group means that improvements cannot definitely be attributed to the intervention.

## RECOMMENDED READING

Anderson, L., Taylor, R.S., 2014. Cardiac rehabilitation for people with heart disease: an overview of Cochrane systematic reviews. Cochrane Database Syst. Rev. (2), CD011273.

BACPR, 2012. Standards and Core Components for Cardiovascular Disease Prevention and Rehabilitation (The British Association for Cardiovascular Disease Prevention and Rehabilitation). http://www.cardiacrehabilitation.org.uk/nacr/docs/BACPR_Standards_2012.pdf.

Besnier, F., Labrunée, M., Pathak, A., et al., 2016. Exercise training-induced modification in autonomic nervous system. Ann. Phys. Rehabil. Med. 60 (1), 27–35.

Casillas, J.-M., Gudjoncik, A., Gremeaux, V., et al., 2017. Assessment tools for personalizing training intensity during cardiac rehabilitation. Ann. Physical. Rehab. Med. 60 (1), 43–49.

Chauvet-Gelinier, J.-C., 2017. Stress, anxiety and depression in heart disease patients: a major challenge for cardiac rehabilitation. Ann. Physical. Rehabil. Med. 60 (1), 6–12.

Chou, A.Y., Prakash, R., Rajala, J., et al., 2016. The first dedicated cardiac rehabilitation program for patients with spontaneous coronary artery dissection: description and initial results. Can. J. Cardiol. 32 (4), 554–560.

Clark, R.A., 2015. Alternative models of cardiac rehabilitation: a systematic review. Eur. J. Prev. Cardiol. 22, 35–74.

Emami, Z.A., Sharafkhani, M., Armat, M., et al., 2016. Women's sexual issues after myocardial infarction. Dim. Crit. Care Nurs 35 (4), 195–203.

Filos, D., Triantafyllidis, A., Chouvarda, I., 2016. PATHway: decision support in exercise programmes for cardiac rehabilitation. Stud. Health Technol. Inform. 224, 40–45.

Inder, J.D., Carlson, D.J., Dieberg, G., et al., 2016. Isometric exercise training for blood pressure management: a systematic review and meta-analysis to optimize benefit. Hypertens. Res. 39 (2), 88–94.

Jennings, C.A., 2017. A systematic review of interventions to increase stair use. Am. J. Prev. Med. 52 (1), 106–114.

Kaminsky, L.A., Brubaker, P.H., Guazzi, M., et al., 2016. Assessing physical activity as a core component in cardiac rehabilitation. J. Cardiopulm. Rehabil. Prev. 36 (4), 217–229.

Karagiannis, C., Savva, I., Mamais, M., et al., 2017. Eccentric exercise in ischemic cardiac patients and functional capacity. Ann. Phys. Rehabil. Med. 60 (1), 58–64.

Palau, P., Núñez, E., Domínguez, E., et al., 2016. Physical therapy in heart failure with preserved ejection fraction. Eur. J. Prev. Cardiol. 23 (1), 4–13.

Ribeiro, P.A.B., Normandin, E., Meyer, P., 2017. Comparison of carbohydrate and lipid oxidation during different high-intensity interval exercise in patients with chronic heart failure. Am. J. Phys. Med. Rehabil. 96 (1), 34–44.

Sorensen, L.L., Liang, H.-Y., Pinheiro, A., et al., 2017. Safety profile and utility of treadmill exercise in patients with high-gradient hypertrophic cardiomyopathy. Am. Heart J. 184, 47–54.

White, A., Broder, J., Campo, T.M., 2012. Acute aortic emergencies. Adv. Emerg. Nurs. J. 34 (3), 216–229.

Zapico, A., Fuentes, D., Rojo-Tirado, M.A., et al., 2016. Predicting peak oxygen uptake from the 6-minute walk test in patients with pulmonary hypertension. J. Cardiopulm. Rehabil. Prev. 36 (3), 203–208.

# 12

# Complications

## INTRODUCTION TO SURGERY

Physiotherapists working on a surgical ward need acumen to identify patients who need treatment, and empathy for the individual, because what is routine for the clinician is a unique event for the patient. Patients anticipate surgery with their own mixture of hope and dread.

Open surgery with full-sized incisions (Fig. 12.1) is becoming less common as more organs are accessible to video-assisted keyhole techniques. These minimally invasive procedures involve the insertion of fibreoptic endoscopes through small stab incisions so that the operative field can be viewed by the team on a monitor. Surgery is also possible at the bedside or in the intensive care unit under local anaesthesia.

The need for physiotherapy has increased because of rapid rehabilitation, early discharge and the extra time needed for the sicker and older patients who now undergo surgery. Less physiotherapy is now required to deal with complications related to pain and bed rest.

## CARDIORESPIRATORY COMPLICATIONS

Respiratory complications are the leading cause of prolonged hospital stay, morbidity and mortality (Branson 2013). Chronic obstructive pulmonary disease (COPD) is the main risk factor, others being unplanned surgery (Fig. 12.2) and the factors listed in Box 12.1.

### Atelectasis

Functional residual capacity is reduced by up to 1 L on lying down and a further 0.5 L on induction of anaesthesia (Licker et al. 2007). This predisposes to atelectasis (Fig. 12.3) in dependent lung regions, lasting on average 24 h after laparoscopy and 2 days after major surgery (Duggan & Kavanagh 2005). It becomes problematic in 0%–5% of patients following lower abdominal surgery, 19%–59% after thoracic surgery (Agostini & Singh 2009) and up to 88% after upper abdominal surgery (Dias 2008). Causes of atelectasis are the following:
1. Pain has a direct effect (Narayanan et al. 2016), dull at rest and sharp on movement. After abdominal or

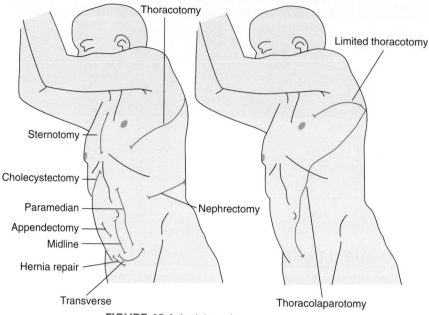

**FIGURE 12.1** Incisions for open surgery.

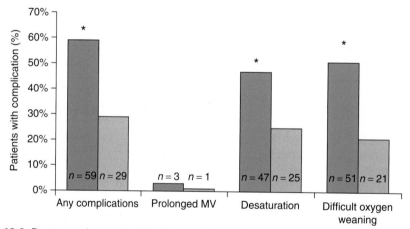

**FIGURE 12.2** Postoperative respiratory complications after nonelective surgery. Intra-operatively (left panel) and postoperatively (right panel). *$p < .05$. *MV*, Mechanical ventilation. (From Chudeau et al. 2016.)

chest surgery, guarding spasm of the trunk muscles and inhibition of breathing brings tidal volume down into the closing volume range (p. 12, Fig. 1.10).

2. Prior to any incision, high oxygen concentration during induction and maintenance of anaesthesia causes absorption atelectasis (p. 151), compression of alveoli depletes surfactant and recumbency causes 15%–20% of the lung to be collapsed basally (Hedenstierna 2010).

3. Immobility and drowsiness obliterate the normal oscillations in tidal volume, which explains why the sedation associated with endoscopic procedures also predisposes to atelectasis (Choe et al. 2016).
4. Abdominal surgery disrupts the diaphragm.
5. Pleural effusion is a common, though usually minor, reaction to perioperative fluid overload.

Atelectasis creates a restrictive defect, reducing lung compliance and depleting surfactant (Davis 2012).

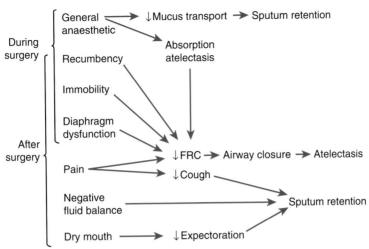

**FIGURE 12.3** Factors relating to physiotherapy. *FRC*, Functional residual capacity.

---

**BOX 12.1   Risks**

Risk Factors for General Postoperative Complications
- Smoking history (Nolan et al. 2017)
- Obesity (Bluth et al. 2016)
- Malnutrition (Weimann et al. 2017)
- Old age (Deyo et al. 2013)
- Steroids (Deyo et al. 2013)
- Emergency surgery (Fujii et al. 2016a)
- Postponed surgery (Kim & Park 2013)

Risk Factors for Postoperative Pulmonary Complications
- Prolonged surgery
- Chronic obstructive pulmonary disease (Craig 2017)
- Surgery close to the diaphragm
- Anaemia
- Pain (Shaffer et al. 2017)
- Congestive heart failure (Craig 2017)
- Obstructive sleep apnoea (Opperer et al. 2016)

---

Greater efforts are needed to inflate poorly compliant collapsed alveoli (see Fig. 1.6) than to prevent this occurring.

**KEY POINT**

Prevention is better than cure, and should begin preoperatively.

## Hypoxaemia

Hypoxaemia (Fig. 12.2) occurs in 37% of patients (Gali et al. 2009), especially in those having abdominal or thoracic surgery (Jaber et al. 2014), and is mainly caused by atelectasis (Martin et al. 2016b). Hypoxaemia can slow wound healing, destabilize the cardiovascular system, impair cognition and cause infection by encouraging bacterial translocation from the gut through its hypoxic lining and into the circulation (Strachan 2001).

When present briefly, hypoxaemia is related to the anaesthetic, and low risk patients only need brief postoperative oxygen therapy. When present for several days it is related to the surgery and postoperative factors, with supplemental oxygen being required for at least 72 h following major surgery (Singh 2011). Night time is particularly precarious, high risk patients being hypoxaemic for two to four nights after surgery (Kehlet & Wilmore 2002) because they are catching up on their oxygen-hungry rapid eye movement (REM) sleep (p. 24), which has been obliterated by sleep disturbance and medication. Patients who have had major surgery, or those with respiratory or cardiovascular disease, should be monitored for nocturnal oxygen desaturation (Fig. 12.4) to prevent premature cessation of oxygen therapy.

In contrast, unnecessary oxygen therapy during surgery can increase lactate levels and cause oxidative stress (Koksal et al. 2016).

## Chest Infection

A slight pyrexia following surgery is a normal reaction to tissue trauma, but fever beyond 48 h suggests infection, often of the wound or lungs. Intubation during surgery overrides upper airway defence mechanisms, and for longer operations the anaesthetic gases dry the

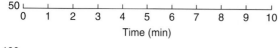

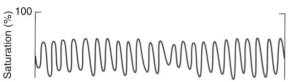

**FIGURE 12.4** Oximetry readings showing damaging episodes of desaturation on the third postoperative night after major surgery. (Adapted from Reeder et al. 2007.)

airway and impair ciliary action. Signs usually emerge some days after surgery, e.g. crackles on auscultation, purulent bronchial secretions, malaise and sometimes rapid breathing. The risk of pneumonia is reduced by a multidisciplinary 'pneumonia bundle' comprising education, incentive spirometry for selected patients, oral care and mobility (Wren et al. 2010).

## Haemodynamic Instability

Atrial fibrillation is a common complication in elderly people and the most frequent problem after cardiovascular surgery. It tends to develop on the second postoperative day and itself predisposes to cardiovascular complications (Omae & Kanmura 2012).

Pre- and postoperative fluid restriction can cause electrolyte disturbance, which may develop into unrecognized hypovolaemia and arrhythmias (Chelazzi 2011). Fluid overload also brings complications (p. 31), which can be life-threatening (Fujii et al. 2016a). The risk is reduced by preemptive 'goal-directed therapy' to monitor and manipulate fluid and drug therapy (Haas 2012). Postural hypotension may be a sign of unrecognized hypovolaemia and is a reminder to avoid sudden position change.

## Ventilatory Instability

Anaesthetic agents depress compensatory responses to hypoxaemia, hypercapnia and airway obstruction (Strachan 2001).

## Obstructive Sleep Apnoea

Obstructive sleep apnoea is common, easily identified, and a predictor of other respiratory complications (Chudeau et al. 2016). Causes are drugs, rebound REM sleep when these are withdrawn (Strachan 2001) or prolonged positioning in supine, when fluid may accumulate in the neck (Lam et al. 2016).

## Thromboembolism

Deep vein thrombosis (DVT) complicates up to a quarter of operations (Dar et al. 2012). Causes are calf compression on the table, immobility, fluid loss, manipulation of blood vessels and the postoperative inflammation and hypercoagulability that can last for a month after surgery (Ulrych et al. 2016). DVT may be clinically silent or cause signs and symptoms. If it breaks free it may lodge in the pulmonary vascular bed, causing pulmonary embolism, reportedly leading to 10% of hospital deaths (Dar et al. 2012). Patients at risk are those who:

- are undergoing lengthy surgery, neurosurgery or surgery that pulls on blood vessels such as knee, hip or pelvic procedures;
- are elderly, immobile, obese, or have malignant, neurological, vascular or blood disorders;
- have a history of DVT.

Prevention and treatment are detailed on p. 145.

## OTHER COMPLICATIONS

Complications are a significant and often long-term predictor of psychosocial problems (Pinto et al. 2016).

**Pain** (p. 297) is one of the main limitations to mobility. **Anxiety** and **stress** predispose to long-term postoperative pain (Reddi 2016) and inhibit healing (Gouin 2012). The majority of patients are fearful of anaesthesia (Ruhaiyem et al. 2016), but anxiety is reduced by giving preoperative information and granting postoperative autonomy. The physiological stress response is modified by preoperative nutritional support and postoperative analgesia (Patel et al. 2012).

Some drugs contribute to the 'big little problem' of **nausea** and **vomiting,** which can be more distressing than pain (Al Jabari & Massad 2016). Risk factors are anxiety, pain, abdominal or breast surgery and inadequate preoperative fluids. Nausea inhibits deep breathing and can lead to dehydration, electrolyte imbalance, wound dehiscence (reopening of the incision) and bleeding (Gan 2006). It can be relieved by:

- hydration and pain relief (Kovac 2013)
- 80% oxygen (Izadi et al. 2016)

- medication such as dexmedetomidine (Song et al. 2016b)
- acupressure (White 2012) or acupuncture (Grube 2009).

**Hypotension** occurs frequently during anaesthesia and is associated with adverse outcomes such as stroke, neurological impairment and myocardial infarction, elderly patients being the least able to tolerate any period of low blood pressure (Wickham et al. 2016).

**Fatigue** is more prolonged than expected by most patients and can be measured by a short questionnaire (Nøstdahl et al. 2016). It is worsened by pain or anaemia (Rubin & Hotopf 2002). Frequent short walks may need to be negotiated postoperatively rather than infrequent long ones.

**Anaemia** increases morbidity and mortality and should be identified and treated before surgery (Muñoz et al. 2016).

**Depression** may occur, especially if surgery affects body image, e.g. head and neck surgery, mastectomy or surgery requiring a colostomy. An understanding ear or referral to a self-help group (App B) may prevent a natural sense of loss degenerating into long-term depression.

**Urine retention, flatulence** or **constipation** impair excursion of the diaphragm. Flatulence can be relieved by gentle bed exercises (Dainese 2004), e.g. pelvic tilting and knee rolling in crook lying.

**Wound infection** is suspected if there is fever, swelling, localized redness or worsening pain. It increases the risk of **dehiscence,** especially if the patient smokes, is malnourished, obese, immunocompromised, diabetic, on long-term steroids or receiving radiotherapy (Havey et al. 2013). Wound, chest or other infection may lead to **sepsis.**

Incessant **hiccups**, due to irritation of the diaphragm, cause sharp pain at the wound site. Suggested remedies are the Valsalva manoeuvre, osteopathic manipulation (Petree 2015), drugs (p. 425), sugar, breath-holding to raise partial pressure of $CO_2$ in arterial blood ($PaCO_2$), pulling on the tongue, pressing on the eyeball, eating peanut butter, rectal massage (Chang & Lu 2012) or prayers to St Jude, the patron saint of lost causes (Howard 1992).

**Cognitive dysfunction** occurs in over half of elderly patients (Smith & Yeow 2016) and in 30%–50% of people after cardiac surgery (Klypa et al. 2016). The incidence is increasing and it is often not noticed until the patient returns home, when it contributes to long-term disability and mortality, but it can be minimized by adequate communication, access to hearing aid or glasses as appropriate, accurate analgesia, day surgery (Steinmetz 2016) and intraoperative monitoring of cerebral oxygenation (Ballard et al. 2012).

Preexisting cognitive dysfunction increases the risk of **delirium**, which occurs in one-third of elderly patients having emergency abdominal surgery, up to 50% of hip fracture patients and in 9%–11% of other surgical patients (Tomlinson 2016). Delirium may precede a chest infection (Killinger 2012), but can be reduced or prevented with early mobilization and nutrition, a familiar clock and calendar, and ensuring a good night's sleep (Rudolph et al. 2011).

Psychogenic **nonepileptic seizures** should not be treated with anticonvulsants (Ramos & Brull 2016) and may relate to hyperventilation syndrome.

**Peripheral nerve injuries** may become apparent 48 h postoperatively, most commonly of the ulnar nerve or brachial plexus. They are caused by compression, stretch ischaemia or direct nerve trauma. Protocols are available for some operations (Blackburn et al. 2016).

Postoperative **haemorrhage**, due to surgical complications or deficient clotting, is suspected if there is:
- obvious bleeding
- rapid filling of drainage bottles
- signs of hypovolaemic shock (p. 549).

**Awareness during anaesthesia** is a feared but rare complication occurring in 1 in 15,000 patients and sometimes leading to posttraumatic stress disorder (Avidan 2013). Risks are day surgery, when anaesthesia is minimized, and trauma surgery (Ghoneim 2000). Brain monitoring is advised (Cascella et al. 2016).

## CASE STUDY: MR MF

*You visit Mr MF at his home after he calls the domiciliary respiratory service feeling 'washed out'.*

### From notes

- 69-year-old musician with COPD, on home oxygen
- No record of assessment for oxygen therapy
- Medication – antibiotics, bronchodilators, steroids – regular drug review, good inhaler technique
- History of recreational drug use

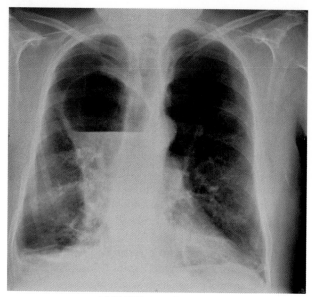

FIGURE 12.5 Mr MF.

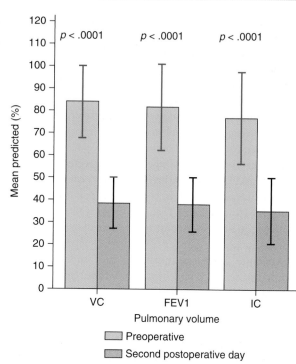

FIGURE 12.6 Lung volumes at percentage of predicted values preoperatively and postoperatively, mean and standard deviation ($n = 107$). $FEV_1$, Forced expiratory volume in 1 s; *IC*, inspiratory capacity; *VC*, vital capacity. (From Urell et al. 2012.)

### Subjective

- Doing little
- Watch TV most of the time
- Occasional sputum, cleared independently
- Nutrition and fluids good
- Using oxygen in the day but not at night

### Objective

- Able to speak in full sentences
- Breathing pattern efficient, respiratory rate normal
- Apyrexial
- Auscultation – Breath sounds (BS) poor generally, ↓ BS right lower lobe (RLL)
- Percussion note hyperresonant right upper zone (RUZ) posteriorly
- Oxygen saturation ($SpO_2$) drops significantly with activity
- Radiology as Fig. 12.5

### Questions

1. Analysis?
2. Problems?
3. Goals?
4. Plan?

### CLINICAL REASONING

Fig. 12.6 shows reduced postoperative lung volumes, as measured by forced respiratory manoeuvres. Would anything else affect postoperative lung volumes when measured in this way?

### Response to Case Study

1. Analysis
   - X-ray shows encapsulated fluid line RUZ, which matches the hyperresonant percussion note. Fluid likely to be in a bulla associated with emphysematous COPD, probably in the lower lobe because the hyperresonant percussion note is in the RUZ posteriorly. Unlikely to be an abscess because of lack of fever. Lost right costophrenic angle, suggesting some RLL atelectasis.
   - ↓ BS RLL confirms atelectasis.
   - Inadequate self management.

2. Problems
- Inappropriate use of oxygen
- Inadequate exercise
- Bulla ? causing problems

3. Goals
- Education on self management
- Oxygen prescription and monitoring
- Exercise programme
- Management of bulla

4. Plan
- Educate on oxygen therapy, monitor $SpO_2$ at rest and exercise, refer to oxygen clinic for day, night and ambulatory oxygen assessment
- Educate on COPD, identification of infection and use of medication
- Discuss pulmonary rehabilitation or progressive home exercise programme, set goals, provide modest exercise tick chart and theraband
- Breathless management, including desensitization, fan and pacing
- Positive expiratory pressure tube and information sheet supplied in case of sputum problems, with a reminder to phone if assistance required
- Discuss bulla with Mr MF and general practitioner, request consultant referral

## RESPONSE TO CLINICAL REASONING

The forced manoeuvres themselves would be painful after surgery and therefore skew the results. Lung volume measurements without effort are available (p. 62).

## RECOMMENDED READING

Andrews, P.L., Sanger, G.J., 2014. Nausea and the quest for the perfect anti-emetic. Eur. J. Pharmacol. 722, 108–121.

Ball, L., Battaglini, D., Pelosi, P., 2016. Postoperative respiratory disorders. Curr. Opin. Crit. Care 22 (4), 379–385.

Moyce, Z., Rodseth, R.N., Biccard, B.M., 2014. The efficacy of peri-operative interventions to decrease postoperative delirium in non-cardiac surgery. Anaesthesia 69 (3), 259–269.

Neto, A.S., Hemmes, S.N., Barbas, C.S., et al., 2016. Association between driving pressure and development of postoperative pulmonary complications in patients undergoing mechanical ventilation for general anaesthesia. Lancet Respir. Med. 4 (4), 272–280.

Radosevich, M.A., Brown, D.R., 2016. Anesthetic management of the adult patient with concomitant cardiac and pulmonary disease. Anesthesiol. Clin. 34 (4), 633–643.

Tsai, A., Schumann, R., 2016. Morbid obesity and perioperative complications. Curr. Opin. Anaesthesiol. 29 (1), 103–108. doi:10.1097/ACO.0000000000000279.

Vutskits, L., Xie, Z., 2016. Lasting impact of general anaesthesia on the brain: mechanisms and relevance. Nat. Rev. Neurosci. 17 (11), 705–717.

Weingarten, T.N., Warner, L.L., Sprung, J., 2016. Timing of postoperative respiratory emergencies. Curr. Opin. Anaesthesiol. 30 (1), 156–162.

Yang, D., Grant, M.C., Stone, A., et al., 2016. A meta-analysis of intraoperative ventilation strategies to prevent pulmonary complications. Ann. Surg. 263 (5), 881–887.

Yang, Y., Xiao, F., Wang, J., et al., 2016. Simultaneous surgery in patients with both cardiac and noncardiac diseases. Patient Prefer. Adherence 10, 1251–1258.

# 13

# Physiotherapy for Surgical Patients

*The single most important pre-operative intervention is to educate patients on manoeuvres to increase lung volumes.*
*Zarmsky 2001*

## PREOPERATIVE PHYSIOTHERAPY

Is physiotherapy necessary before surgery? Occasional patients require assistance with sputum clearance, but advice on activity benefits all patients. Impaired physical capacity is associated with postoperative pulmonary complications (Soares 2013) and preoperative exercise has shown the following benefits:

- ↓ complications after abdominal (Moran et al. 2016), cardiac (Shakouri et al. 2015) and lung surgery (Marseu 2016);
- reduced need for reintubation postoperatively (Piriyapatsom et al. 2016);
- ↓ postoperative sick leave (Angenete et al. 2016).

The benefits of prehabilitation are most marked for patients with the worst pulmonary function and weakest functional capacity (Mujovic et al. 2014). For those unwilling or unable to undertake sufficient systemic exercise, it is claimed that inspiratory muscle training can halve postoperative complications (Mans et al. 2015).

Preoperative assessment of functional capacity helps identify patients who need physiotherapy, but there is significant discrepancy between clinician assessment and patient self-assessment. Although patient-completed surveys are probably at least as reliable as the medical record, patients sometimes overestimate and clinicians sometimes underestimate a patient's functional capacity, and it may be best to ask patients to demonstrate their ability to do a task (Stokes et al. 2016b).

Preoperative education includes advice on postoperative positioning, mobilization and, if necessary, chest clearance, which can reduce postoperative complications, increase $SpO_2$ and improve mobility (Olsén et al. 1997). Information is most important for patients expecting to wake up in the intensive care unit (ICU), where they will feel relieved at the sight of a familiar face. Patients anticipating mechanical ventilation (MV) should be warned of their inability to speak. They need information on the experiences of MV and suction, the fact that they may hear before being able to respond, and reassurance that there will be a nurse watching over them. Visits to the ICU by the patient and family are often helpful, and should be supplemented by written material. Preoperative physiotherapy education, when combined with accurate analgesia, has shown speedier recovery and reduced length of ICU stay (Osseis et al. 2016).

Anxiety increases postoperative pain (Bradshaw et al. 2016). Accurate information relieves anxiety, and anxious patients should be seen early if possible because worry at impending surgery inhibits receptivity. Some patients find it beneficial to have relatives present to help absorb the information. If a patient is not admitted early enough to be seen, preoperative education can take place by phone (Carli et al. 2010) or in the pre-assessment clinic, which should include rehabilitation and discharge planning (Dhesi et al. 2016). At the end of the discussion, it is useful to check patients' understanding. Preoperative anxiety is reflected in higher death rates for people with longer preoperative waiting times for heart surgery (Sobolev et al. 2013).

## PREOPERATIVE TEAMWORK

Multidisciplinary information includes advice for smokers to stop at least 3 weeks previously (Özmen et al. 2016). They are more likely to quit if they hear messages specific to surgery, e.g. that smoking increases wound infections (Tibæk et al. 2016). Some patients also benefit from the opportunity to discuss advance care planning.

The tradition of prolonged preoperative fluid and food restriction is now known to induce metabolic stress, and patients must not fast for longer than 6 h (Abdelhamid et al. 2016), while clear oral fluids up to 2 h before surgery help maintain patient comfort and fluid/electrolyte balance (Gupta & Gan 2016).

The 'Enhanced Recovery' programme incorporates interventions to minimize the stress response to surgery (Fig. 13.1), early mobilization being a key component (Yip et al. 2016). Although some patients express

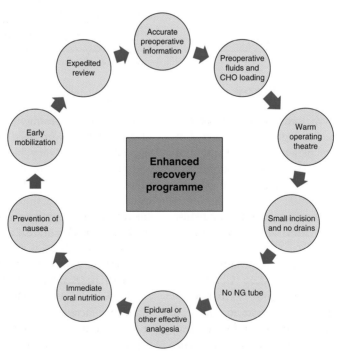

**FIGURE 13.1** Components of the enhanced recovery programme. *CHO*, Carbohydrate; *NG*, nasogastric.

concern at early discharge (Vandrevala et al. 2016), positive outcomes of the programme include:

- ↓ chest infections, ↓ need for analgesia or fluids (Wisely & Barclay 2016);
- ↓ length of stay and readmission (Messenger et al. 2016);
- after thoracic surgery: ↑ patient satisfaction and ↓ costs (Scarci et al. 2016).

Preoperative analgesia reduces acute and chronic postoperative pain by blocking nociceptive signals and central sensitization (Reddi 2016). Preoperative malnutrition occurs in up to two-thirds of patients, increasing infection risk and impairing wound healing (Abdelhamid et al. 2016); nutritional intervention can reduce complications two- to threefold (Leach et al. 2013). A leafy view through a window is not part of the programme but has been found to speed recovery (Ulrich 1984).

'Goal-directed therapy' refers to maximizing oxygen delivery to the tissues by manipulating haemodynamics, especially in avoiding volume depletion or overload (Doyle et al. 2016).

Preoperative physiotherapy for specific operations is covered in Chapter 14.

## PAIN MANAGEMENT

*The heaviest burden of inadequate pain management is borne by the weakest: the elderly, children, people coping with addictions, the mentally ill … patients with cognitive disorders, depression, agitation or dementia.*

**Mędrzycka et al. 2016**

The experience of pain involves both the sensation and the individual's reaction to the sensation, leading to wide variations in patients' perception of pain, as well as unpredictable responses to analgesics (Peiró et al. 2016). However, it is not unusual to hear patients dismissed as having a 'low pain threshold' or being accused of exaggerating (McCaffrey et al. 2005). Unnecessary postoperative pain still occurs in 50%–60% of patients at rest and 14%–15% during mobilization (Geisler et al. 2016). Empathy for another's pain requires activation of the anterior insular and cingulate cortices (Gu et al. 2012) and it is to be hoped that these precious parts of the brain in clinicians are not desensitized by exposure to poor practice in the health system. Other reasons for needless pain are:

- ignorance of the difference between the use and abuse of opioids, some staff thinking that a request for morphine suggests drug dependence (McCaffrey et al. 2005);
- misunderstanding the difference between opioid euphoria and respiratory depression, or an unfounded fear that opioids adversely affect pain assessment (Ranji et al. 2006);
- 'opiophobia', reinforced by British GP Harold Shipman using diamorphine to murder his patients in the 1990s;
- in Western countries, racial and age discrimination, elderly patients having to wait longer for their analgesics and receiving lower doses (Mędrzycka et al. 2016);
- patients' low expectations of pain relief and anxiety about side effects;
- inexperience, staff shortage and poor pain assessment (Moore et al. 2013).

*It seems almost as if many members of the medical profession view 'curing' and 'caring' as mutually exclusive.*

**Lowenstein 2000**

### PRACTICE TIP

Next time you are in the dentist's chair and you see the needle advancing, try to take a deep breath.

### Effects of Pain

*'There are many things that make pain worse, such as the spirit with which it is inflicted. You are indeed acutely vulnerable to the attitude of people surrounding you'*

**Donald 1977**

Pain contributes to the following:

- atelectasis (Fig. 13.2), ↓ ability to deep breathe and cough (Fig. 13.3);
- ↓ cardiorespiratory function, mobility and sleep, ↑ delirium (Reimer-Kent 2003);
- ↑ pulse, immunosuppression and persistent catabolism (ICS 2013);
- ↑ sympathetic tone, inflammatory response, coagulation cascade and oxygen consumption (Piriyapatsom et al. 2013);
- delayed hospital discharge (Wooster et al. 2017);

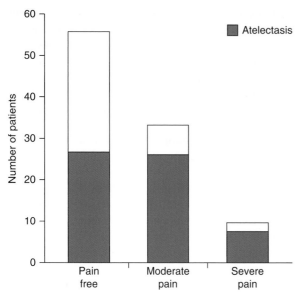

FIGURE 13.2 The effect of pain on atelectasis. (From Embling 1985.)

## Assessment

*With rare exceptions, pain is as the patient describes it.*

*Azzam & Alam 2013*

Pain should be assessed like any other vital sign, including at rest and on movement (Tandon et al. 2016 and Box 13.1). Verbal numerical rating scales are simple and give consistent results, while assessment tools are available for patients with confusional states, intellectual impairment (Macintyre et al. 2010), critical illness (D'Andrea 2016) and with an inability to communicate (Kankkunen 2010). People with learning disabilities may express pain by self-harm, and their carers are best able to interpret behaviours that indicate pain.

People who smoke (Montbriand et al. 2017) or have severe depression (Savitz et al. 2012) are extra sensitive to pain. Elderly people are less likely to report pain and are at particular risk of undertreatment (Mędrzycka et al. 2016) while the majority of patients with dementia have been found to suffer severe postoperative pain (Morrison & Siu 2000).

Objective signs are pallor, sweating, shallow breathing, breath-holding and increased pulse, blood pressure (BP) and respiratory rate (RR), but these indicate severe pain and can also reflect other conditions. Extreme pain causes nausea, vomiting and reduced pulse and BP.

Pain assessment for infants, children and older people are in Chapters 15, 16 and 18.

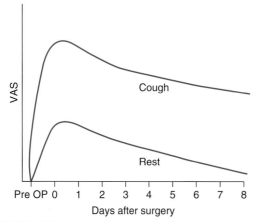

FIGURE 13.3 Postoperative pain with cough *(top)* and at rest *(bottom)* measured by visual analogue scale *(VAS)*. (From Brennan 2011.)

- pneumonia, deep vein thrombosis, infection, delayed healing and the development of chronic pain (Meissner et al. 2016).

Long-term postoperative pain is the second most common reason for referral to a chronic pain clinic (Butrick 2016), the risk being increased by poorly managed acute pain. It develops in half of patients who have a thoracotomy, leg amputation or breast cancer surgery, and 1 in 2.5 after coronary artery bypass surgery (Reddi 2016).

## Handling Patients in Pain

*'The sense of anticipation is honed, to hysteria almost, and one quickly learns to be thoroughly suspicious of the well-meant: "this won't hurt".'*

*Brooks 1990*

There are few rewards greater than relief on the face of a patient whose pain we have eased, and handling and positioning can be as important in relieving acute pain as drugs (Sutcliffe 1993). Some suggestions are in Box 13.2.

For rolling into side-lying position, patients are asked to bend their knees, shift away from the direction in which they are to roll, hold onto the bed rail on the side towards which they are to roll, push with their knees and roll in one piece. They are encouraged to push with their legs more than pull with their arms so that abdominal muscle work is inhibited. After laparotomy, any manoeuvre that entails abdominal muscle work, e.g. eccentric contraction when lying back against the pillows, is eased by facilitating active back extension and reciprocal abdominal relaxation.

During activity, patients need reassurance in words and actions that they will be heard and responded to. 'Tell me if it hurts and I'll stop', is music to their ears. The effect of 'anticipatory anxiety' on the perception of pain (Lin et al. 2013) is a reminder of the need for accurate information in terms the patient understands.

## Medication

*The more patients feel in control of their own pain management, the lower the requirement for analgesia.*

***Starritt 2000***

Pain research is problematic because volunteers know that they can stop the pain at any time, and with animals it is unethical (though sometimes done). However, the following are some of the evidence-based principles of the drug management of pain:

1. Analgesia titrated to the individual's need provides more pain relief for less dosage than time-scheduled prescription (Von Korff et al. 2012).
2. Morphine remains the favourite opioid analgesic, with a half-life of several hours. Side-effects include elimination of spontaneous sighs (Bell 2013), urine retention, pruritus, vomiting, nausea, constipation, risk of falls and, in hypovolaemic patients, hypotension. Fentanyl is a synthetic opioid approximately 100 times more potent than morphine, while alfentanil is an analogue of fentanyl with around one-tenth its potency. The side-effect of respiratory depression is identified by a RR below 8 bpm, and is reversible by the opiate antagonist naloxone. Respiratory depression can also be caused by gabapentin (Cavalcante et al. 2017), although preoperative gabapentin reduces the consumption of postoperative opioids (Arumugam et al. 2012).
3. Multimodal analgesia combines drugs and delivery systems in order to influence different physiological processes, e.g. intraoperative wound irrigation with local anaesthetic, drugs aimed at neuropathic pain, and regional (epidural or nerve block) analgesia (Craig 2017).
4. Drugs are best coordinated by an acute pain team, which also reduces costs and improves care (Kontinen & Hamunen 2016).

The **intravenous** (IV) route works immediately and can be delivered continuously or in boluses. Fentanyl should be injected slowly to reduce the side-effect of coughing (Hung et al. 2010).

**Patient-controlled analgesia** (PCA) delivers a preset dose of drug when the patient presses a button. This encourages mobility, requires less drug to achieve the same pain control, minimizes respiratory depression and can include antinausea medication (Song 2016c). Whether delivered intravenously, orally, transdermally or epidurally, a lock-out interval avoids overdosing, and patients are advised to use the device freely.

The **epidural** route alters spinal processing by delivering drugs to the epidural space by a catheter inserted in the operating theatre and left in situ. Patients should be advised that postoperative epidurals are not the same as those given during childbirth and they will not be numb below the catheter. Administration is by intermittent blockade, continuous infusion or PCA, and it brings a bonus of inhibiting postoperative cognitive dysfunction in elderly people (Wang et al. 2016c).

Advantages of epidurals are improved pain control (Roeb et al. 2016), earlier mobilization, decreased morbidity, mortality and thromboembolic events (Parra et al. 2016) and a halving of pulmonary complications after abdominal, oesophageal, aortic and cardiac surgery (Marseu 2016).

Disadvantages are the risk of nausea, vomiting, hypotension, urinary retention and sometimes partial sensory or motor loss (Kim 2013). High blocks are more associated with hypotension and low blocks with urine retention or motor loss. Respiratory function may be impaired by a block higher than T4. Patients receiving intermittent dosage may need to lie down for 30 min after a top-up to avoid hypotension, but not for too much longer because this allows the drug to move up the epidural space to the brain, causing respiratory depression. Capnography can be used to monitor ventilation.

The **intrathecal** or **spinal** route delivers 'one-shot' drugs to the subarachnoid space below L2, producing profound analgesia without motor, sensory or sympathetic blockade. Complications include spinal headache due to leak of cerebrospinal fluid (CSF) through a punctured dura, leading to loss of the intracranial CSF 'cushion' (Wu et al. 2016b).

The **transdermal** route is useful for local procedures such as taking blood. Anaesthetic cream creates topical anaesthesia when applied to the skin 30–60 min beforehand (Wiles et al. 2010). No child should be submitted to venipuncture, lumbar puncture or, indeed any injection without prior application of their 'magic cream' (Fig. 13.4). Needle-phobic adults also benefit. As well as skin anaesthesia, systemic analgesia can be delivered transdermally, with the result of increased mobility (Oliashirazi et al. 2016) and less pain and side effects than IV morphine by PCA (Glaun et al. 2016).

The **transmucosal** route uses 'fentanyl lollipops', or the nasal route, or tablets under the top lip for rapid analgesia (Yang et al. 2016d), mucous membranes imposing less of a barrier than skin, as cocaine users have discovered.

The **intramuscular** route is rarely used because it is relatively ineffective, especially if given 'p.r.n.' (otherwise known as 'pain relief never').

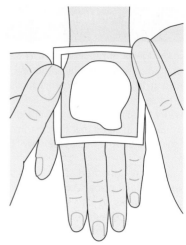

**FIGURE 13.4**  Local anaesthetic skin patch using 'EMLA' (eutectic mixture of local anaesthetics) cream.

The physiotherapist may take more direct action by using transcutaneous nerve stimulation (TENS) (Silva 2012), acupuncture (Taghavi 2013) or acupressure (Chung et al. 2014). The latter is also sometimes used to reduce the pain of venipuncture (Hosseinabadi et al. 2016).

*Freedom from pain should be a basic human right.*
***Liebeskind & Melzack 1987***

## POSTOPERATIVE PHYSIOTHERAPY

Is physiotherapy necessary after surgery? Research has shown positive outcomes when delivered accurately (Agostini & Singh 2009, Souza et al. 2013) but not when provided routinely (Fernandes et al. 2016). Techniques to expand the lungs, in particular, can halve pulmonary complications (Marseu 2016). Most patients gain from physiotherapy input to the team management of positioning and mobility, but those with the risk factors in Box 12.1 (p. 289) are most likely to need direct intervention. Risks are higher in patients who have problems with cognition, gait, balance, nutrition or function (Hulzebos 2016), and atelectasis is a particular risk in obese patients (Fig. 13.5). Risk scoring models help to identify patients needing physiotherapy (Anderson et al. 2010, Bruton et al. 2009).

Physiotherapy is based on techniques to increase lung volume and clear secretions (Chapters 6 and 8).

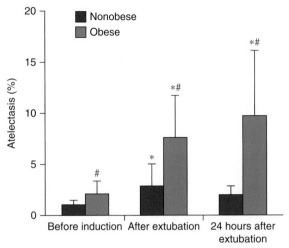

**FIGURE 13.5** Percentage of atelectasis between morbidly obese and nonobese patients before and after surgery. (From Eichenberger et al. 2002.)

Specific modifications are discussed below, with variations for different operations in the next chapter.

## Mobility

Both immobility and surgery invoke the inflammatory cascade (Havey et al. 2013) and early mobilization improves outcomes (Leeden et al. 2016), including restored lung volume, improved $SpO_2$, easier chest clearance (Stiller et al. 2004), shortened hospital stay and improved functional mobility at discharge (Schaller et al. 2016). If surgically and medically acceptable, this should be on the first postoperative day. Patients can have targets such as walking along increasing lengths of a coloured line painted along the corridor. IV equipment that is plugged into the mains can usually be temporarily unplugged, so long as the battery is functioning. For patients with a urinary catheter, leg bags are more dignified than loose catheter bags.

Posture correction is incorporated as soon as discomfort has eased. Safety aspects are on p. 182, with specific precautions for epidurals below:

- check local protocol to identify if two staff members are required for mobilization;

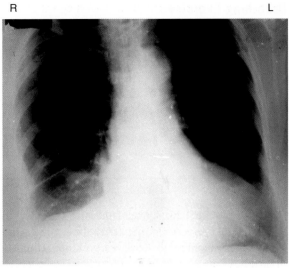

**FIGURE 13.6** Upward shift of the right hemidiaphragm suggests lower lobe collapse, and loss of the right heart border indicates some middle lobe involvement. Opacity of the left lower zone could be breast shadow, especially as it is not possible to compare it to the right, but clinical assessment revealed bronchial breathing, indicating consolidation. *L*, Left; *R*, right.

- check lower limb strength to ensure that there is no motor block;
- check BP to ensure that there is no sympathetic block.

## Positioning

If pain, surgical procedure or instability delay mobilization, the emphasis should be on accurate and comfortable positioning, as upright as possible, or side-lying. Sitting shows better gas exchange than supine (Duggan & Kavanagh 2005) and, in half the research surveyed by Nielsen (2003), side-lying was preferable to supine. Regular position change, including alternate side-lying, helps prevent atelectasis. If side-lying pulls on the incision, the position is modified, or the patient can hold a pillow against the wound.

Clinical and radiological assessment assists in decisions about positioning. Fig. 13.6 suggests that the patient should lie primarily on the left so that the collapsed lobe (R) is uppermost, but also to spend time on the right side to avoid the consolidation (L) developing into collapse.

## Breathing Exercises

Breathing exercises have not been indicated routinely for uncomplicated surgery since Stiller et al.'s seminal work in 1994, but if mobilization is delayed, positioning limited, or atelectasis develops, deep breathing may be beneficial (Duggan & Kavanagh 2005). Following high risk procedures such as oesophagectomy or upper abdominal surgery, regular prophylactic deep breathing is advisable, though this suggestion comes from physiological reasoning and auscultatory outcomes rather than research. For these patients, the 10 deep breaths an hour advised by Bartlett et al. in 1973 still make physiological sense today.

Pain must first be minimized, then deep breathing is done in a position that achieves a balance between comfort and optimal ventilation, usually a well-forward side-lying position. For patients who cannot achieve this, upright sitting is the next option, but this tends to compress the lower chest and is unlikely to inflate dependent lung regions. Patients who are able to stand and lean against a wall can take relaxed deep breaths while upright (p. 181).

Incentive spirometry has been called 'the number one best tool for preventing postoperative complications' (Zarmsky 2001). Even so, it is only required for patients who need the incentive to achieve the quality or quantity of breaths required.

Accumulated secretions are usually cleared without assistance postoperatively as mucociliary transport regains its momentum, but if sputum retention occurs, breathing techniques (p. 205) can be effective if pain does not dampen the huff. Coughing, percussion, vibrations and unnecessary forced expiration are not used routinely because they may cause pain and muscle splinting. If coughing is required, patients may prefer to remain in side-lying, but if they are willing, sitting over the edge of the bed is mechanically efficient and allows maximum support (Fig. 13.7). Pressing on the incision

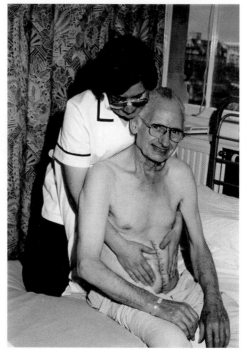

**FIGURE 13.7** Manual support for postoperative coughing after laparotomy. For thoracotomy, the physiotherapist can sit beside the patient on the opposite side to the wound in order to support the wound while providing counterpressure to the patient's body. Gentle firm pressure is directed at holding the wound edges together. (This is an historic picture: the physiotherapist would now kneel on a plastic apron and use gloves.)

with a pillow is less effective than sensitive and accurately timed manual support, but when patients are on their own, they may find a cough belt (Fig. 13.8), pillow or towel.

If patients are too weak, fatigued or drowsy to cooperate, mechanical aids may be useful, such as continuous positive airway pressure for hypoxaemia (Chung et al. 2016c), intermittent positive pressure breathing for reduced lung volume or sputum clearance, and noninvasive ventilation for excess work of breathing or low oxygenation (Jaber et al. 2016).

**PRACTICE TIP**

Practice Fig. 13.7 in pairs, the 'patient' giving feedback on the timing and pressure of the manual support.

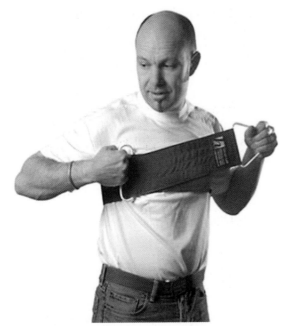

**FIGURE 13.8** The 'Cough lok' is designed for chest surgery but is also useful for abdominal surgery. It may be purchased from www.hawksley.co.uk, or a similarly functioning device might be homemade.

## Prevention of Deep Vein Thrombosis (DVT)

There is no evidence that postoperative leg exercises have any place in the prevention of DVT, and clinical reasoning suggests that near-continuous ankle exercises would be required both during and after surgery. Also, although it is good to get out of bed, there is no evidence that this is preventive, especially as most cases become apparent after discharge (Dahl 2012). This does not apply to other situations such as long-haul flights.

If a patient develops a DVT, this should not confine them to bed. A systematic review suggests that they should get up, mobilize and, if ready for discharge, go home (Anderson et al. 2009) so long as they are on anticoagulant drugs (pp. 145–146).

### Discharge and Outcomes

*We may experience them as recovered at discharge, but many patients say that they do not understand where their strength has gone.*

*Allvin et al. 2008*

Assessment for discharge from physiotherapy can be facilitated by a scoring tool using mobility, breath sounds, secretion clearance, $SpO_2$ and RR (Brooks et al. 2002). Discharge advice is to encourage progressive paced activity suited to the individual's lifestyle, along with regular rest because fatigue becomes troublesome mainly after participants have returned to regular activities (Allvin et al. 2008). For patients who have been doing breathing exercises, a reminder to stop prevents conscientious patients continuing indefinitely. Liaison with the community team may be required for patients who are able to do stairs in the safe hospital environment but do not have the confidence to do so at home. Wireless monitoring of mobility may be available (Cook 2013).

Bowyer & Royse (2016) provide a variety of outcome measures and state that:

- outcomes should incorporate physical function, emotional after-effects, pain and cognition;
- subjective assessment may be limited by impaired postoperative insight or cognition, but this does not make it subordinate to objective measures;
- recovery from surgery is best viewed as a process.

Physiotherapy outcomes may need to be based on an endpoint at discharge, but liaison with community teams will provide more useful information.

## CASE STUDY: MR MW

*A 71-year-old male with a history of COPD is admitted with empyema and a bronchopleural fistula.*

### Social history

- Lives alone
- Exercise tolerance 30 steps
- History of asbestos exposure; no information in notes on possible after-effects

### Subjective

- Breathless for 2 weeks
- Feeling less ill since antibiotics
- Weak
- Can't get to toilet

### Objective

- X-ray as Fig. 13.9
- Pyrexial
- pH 7.46, $PaCO_2$ 4.9, $PaO_2$ 7.9, $HCO_3^-$ 26, BE 2.6

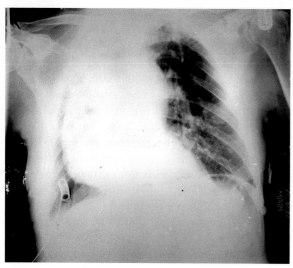

**FIGURE 13.9** Mr MW.

- No oxygen therapy
- Tending to breath-hold
- Tending to rush

## Questions

1. What else does the X-ray show?
2. Analysis?
3. Problems?
4. Goals?
5. Treatment plan?

### CLINICAL REASONING

Would you read further than the title of this article?

*'Lung function can be increased significantly when incentive spirometry and specific inspiratory muscle training are used before and after operation.'*
*J Thorac Cardio Surg* (1997), 113, 552–557

## Response to Case Study

1. X-ray
   - Lack of lung markings in RLZ indicates a pneumothorax
   - Chest drain in RLZ
   - White shadow represents the empyema: unlike a pleural effusion, there is no fluid line because the pleural fluid of an empyema is thick
2. Analysis
   - Breathlessness → pH at high end of normal, $PaCO_2$ at low end of normal

- COPD ± empyema → hypoxaemia
- Lack of oxygen therapy possibly relates to Mr MW being on a surgical ward, where there may be anxiety about oxygen and COPD

3. Problems
   - Hypoxaemia
   - Breathlessness
   - Weakness } Inability to reach toilet
   - Tendency to rush
4. Goals
   - Accurate oxygen therapy
   - Patient to reach toilet independently by end of first day
   - Rehabilitate to home circumstances
5. Plan
   - Teamwork:
     - discuss oxygen therapy, provide oxygen guidelines (BTS 2017) (tactfully, e.g. by asking for advice), ensure that prescription and monitoring are instigated, request local anaesthetic for blood gases (BTS 2017)
     - discuss investigations on possible asbestosis or mesothelioma, go back through previous X-rays and lung function tests
   - After initiation of oxygen therapy, mobilize to toilet, with oximetry
   - Suggest day clothes
   - Pacing
   - Graduated exercise programme
   - Liaise with community care

### RESPONSE TO CLINICAL REASONING

- The techniques described are for different problems: incentive spirometry is to increase lung volume, and inspiratory muscle training is to reduce the work of breathing.
- There is a double whammy of variables: which of these modalities is the effective one, and is it before or after surgery that they are effective?
- And that old chestnut – if lung function is measured with tests of forced exhalation, this does not control for postoperative pain.

## RECOMMENDED READING

Carli, F., 2017. Promoting a culture of prehabilitation for the surgical cancer patient. Acta. Oncol. 56 (2), 128–133.

Castro, M.A., Dedivitis, R.A., Salge, J.M., et al., 2016. Validation of methodology for assessment of pulmonary function in patients who undergo total laryngectomy. Head Neck 38 (Suppl. 1), E2030–E2034.

Chou, R., Gordon, D.B., de Leon-Casasola, O.A., et al., 2016. Management of postoperative pain: a clinical practice guideline. J. Pain 17 (2), 131–157.

Filbet, M., Larkin, P., Chabloz, C., et al., 2017. Barriers to venipuncture-induced pain prevention in cancer patients: a qualitative study. BMC Palliat. Care 16, 5.

Hariharan, S., 2016. Do patient psychological factors influence postoperative pain? Pain Manag. 6 (6), 511–513.

Hijazi, Y., Gondal, U., Aziz, O., 2017. A systematic review of prehabilitation programs in abdominal cancer surgery. Int. J. Surg. 39, 156–162.

Keller, D.S., 2017. Impact of long-acting local anesthesia on clinical and financial outcomes in laparoscopic colorectal surgery. Am. J. Surg. 214 (1), 53–58.

Ledowski, T., Averhoff, L., Tiong, W.S., et al., 2014. Analgesia Nociception Index (ANI) to predict intraoperative haemodynamic changes: results of a pilot investigation. Acta Anaesthesiol. Scand. 58 (1), 74–79.

Moran, J., Wilson, F., Guinan, E., et al., 2016. Role of cardiopulmonary exercise testing as a risk-assessment method in patients undergoing intra-abdominal surgery. Br. J. Anaesth. 116 (2), 177–191.

Onerup, A., Angenete, E., Bock, D., et al., 2017. The effect of pre- and post-operative physical activity on recovery after colorectal cancer surgery (PHYSSURG-C): study protocol for a randomised controlled trial. Trials. 18, 212.

Ongley, D., Hayward, A., Allan, C., 2014. Severe respiratory depression associated with perioperative opioid-sparing gabapentin use. Anaesth. Intensive. Care 42 (1), 136–137.

Rana, M.V., Desai, R., Tran, L., et al., 2016. Perioperative pain control in the ambulatory setting. Curr. Pain Headache Rep. 20 (3), 18.

Shunsuke, T., Kenji, M., Moeka, F., et al., 2017. Deep breathing improves end-tidal carbon dioxide monitoring of an oxygen nasal cannula-based capnometry device in subjects extubated after abdominal surgery. Respir. Care 62 (1), 86–91.

Smith, C.S., Guyton, K., Pariser, J.J., et al., 2017. Surgeon–patient communication during awake procedures. Am. J. Surg. 213 (6), 996–1002.

Van Boekel, R.L., 2016. Comparison of epidural or regional analgesia and patient-controlled analgesia. Clin. J. Pain 32 (8), 681–688.

Wildgaard, K., 2014. The post-thoracotomy pain syndrome: epidemiological, psychophysical and social consequences. Acta Anaesthesiol. Scand. 58, 129.

# 14

# Modifications for Different Types of Surgery

## LEARNING OBJECTIVES

*On completion of this chapter the reader should be able to:*
- understand different forms of surgery;
- adapt physiotherapy to the needs of patients on thoracic, cardiac, transplant, head/neck and general surgical wards;
- discuss the management of a patient with a tracheostomy.

## OUTLINE

## ABDOMINAL SURGERY

*The effect of an upper abdominal incision seems to strike at the root of normal respiration.*

***Bevan 1964***

Abdominal surgery impinges less on respiration now that most abdominal organs are amenable to the laparoscope, leading to lower morbidity and mortality than open laparotomy (Bulus et al. 2013). However, procedures such as laparoscopic cholecystectomy take longer than open laparotomy and entail tilting the patient head-down and pumping $CO_2$ into the peritoneum. This impairs diaphragmatic function, and residual $CO_2$ can refer pain to the right shoulder, although the pain can be minimized by two recruitment manoeuvres before extubation (Khanna et al. 2013).

## Complications

Pulmonary complications remain the most significant cause of morbidity following open upper abdominal surgery (Branson 2013). In addition, to those previously described, the following may occur:
1. Pain tends to be taken less seriously than after chest surgery, even though pain after laparotomy is often worse on movement because most activity requires abdominal muscle contraction. Patient-controlled analgesia is mandatory (Niiyama et al. 2016).
2. Abdominal distension and guarding spasm require attention to positioning in order to reduce pressure on the diaphragm. The position chosen best follows patient comfort, auscultation and oximetry.
3. Paralytic ileus is a normal postoperative delay to gut motility. It becomes problematic if prolonged beyond

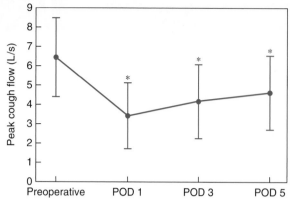

**FIGURE 14.1** Perioperative peak cough flow. *, $P < .001$ compared with previous measurements; *POD*, postoperative day. (From Colucci et al. 2015.)

the usual 1–2 days, causing nausea and exacerbating diaphragm dysfunction. Management is by early mobilization, nonopioid pain relief, timely oral feeding and chewing gum (Terzioglu et al. 2013).

4. Cough strength is halved on postoperative day one and only gradually recovers (Fig. 14.1).

5. Fatigue is a particular problem with abdominal surgery (Havey et al. 2013), but responds well to a balanced exercise programme (Wiskemann et al. 2016).

6. Malnourishment may occur because of:
   - preexisting gut pathology;
   - preoperative fasting;
   - the catabolic effects of surgery;
   - intestinal handling that affects the delicate mucosal lining;
   - postoperative nausea and precarious appetite;
   - unfamiliar hospital food.

### Oxygen, Fluids and Nutrition

Hyperoxaemia during and after surgery can reduce infection rates (Schietroma et al. 2016) and improve anastomotic integrity in gastric and colorectal surgery (BTS 2017), but long-term heart problems have been linked to excessive $FiO_2$ perioperatively (Fonnes et al. 2016). The physiotherapist's job, as always, is to ensure that oxygen is both prescribed and monitored.

Patients should be encouraged to drink clear liquids up to 2 h before induction of anaesthesia, and the postoperative goal is to eat and drink without IV fluids (Gupta et al. 2016). Preoperative oral carbohydrates

are thought to speed recovery (Awad et al. 2013), and early postoperative enteral nutrition reduces postoperative complications, with most patients eating normally in the immediate postoperative period, regardless of traditional markers of gut function (Kirchhoff et al. 2010). Other options are:

- a **gastrostomy** tube to deliver food directly into the stomach via a percutaneous endoscopic gastrostomy (PEG) tube through the abdominal wall;
- a **jejunostomy** tube placed percutaneously directly into the jejunum.

Local anaesthesia during surgery speeds the recovery of bowel function and brings an agreeable advantage of inhibiting cancer dissemination (Votta-Velis 2013).

### Physiotherapy

Patients having lower abdominal surgery require no more than a reminder about mobility and posture, unless they fall into a high-risk category. For others, benefit has been found with:

- mobilization (Silva et al. 2013, Choi et al. 2013);
- positioning, deep breathing and mobilization (Olsén 2000);
- deep breathing and abdominal breathing, which can improve $SpO_2$ (Manzano et al. 2008);
- incentive spirometry, which may improve pulmonary function and exercise tolerance (Kumar et al. 2016);
- for high-risk patients, prophylactic postoperative continuous positive airway pressure (CPAP), which reduces the incidence of pneumonia and atelectasis, so long as high pressures are avoided (Singh et al. 2016).

Mobilization may not be accompanied by increased abdominal excursion in the early stages because of diaphragmatic inhibition (Zafiropoulos et al. 2004), but when started early, it can reduce pulmonary complications and fatigue, promote return of gut function and bring earlier discharge (Havey et al. 2013). Wound dehiscence (p. 291) is more likely with vertical than transverse incisions (Havey et al. 2013), and abdominal belts are sometimes used (Czyżewski et al. 2016).

Suggestions for specific operations are below.

An **abdominal aortic aneurysm** (p. 144) may require open or endovascular repair, following which there is a risk of cardiovascular instability and limitations on mobility. For elective surgery, supervised preoperative exercise can reduce postoperative complications

(Barakat et al. 2016) Epidural analgesia provides better pain relief, quicker extubation and reduced cardiorespiratory complications than systemic drugs (Guay & Kopp 2016).

**Bariatric surgery** by gastric bypass, sleeve gastrectomy or gastric band can reduce obesity-related mortality by 30% (Neff 2013). Preoperative recommendations include an exercise programme (Floody et al. 2015) and early smoking cessation because smoking poses a greater risk than weight (Morgan 2016). Preoperative and/or postoperative noninvasive ventilation may reduce complications (Carron et al. 2016), but postoperative hypoxaemia is common (Edmark et al. 2016) and nearly one-third of patients are rehospitalized (Gribsholt 2016). Patients with a 'buffalo back' may develop brachial plexus injuries during surgery if elevated arm boards are not used.

Aftercare includes a structured exercise programme (Thibault et al. 2016), which can be facilitated by intraoperative peritoneal analgesia (Ruiz-Tovar et al. 2016). After-effects of surgery include osteoporotic fractures (Rousseau et al. 2016), a high incidence of substance misuse if the cause of an eating disorder has not been addressed (Conason 2013) and long-term deterioration in mental health, with higher than expected suicide rates (Canetti et al. 2016).

## LUNG SURGERY

### Procedures

An open posterolateral thoracotomy (see Fig. 12.1) involves an incision below the scapula, dividing latissimus dorsi and retracting or resecting one or more ribs, leading to restricted shoulder and chest wall movement. Keyhole video-assisted thoracic surgery (VATS) can be used to reduce complications for pulmonary (Fig. 14.2), pleural, cardiac or oesophageal procedures (Falcoz et al. 2016), especially with the use of epidural anaesthesia (Guo et al. 2016a).

To remove a cancerous tumour from a lobe (Fig. 14.3), **lobectomy** may be curative if mediastinal lymph nodes are not involved. The vacated space is accommodated by expansion of the rest of the lung and some reorganization of moveable structures. A **segmentectomy** or smaller **wedge resection** are sublobar resections which may be adequate for early-stage peripheral lesions.

A **bilobectomy** removes two lobes, and a **sleeve resection** removes the T-junction of a bronchus with its lobe.

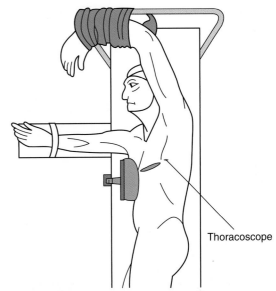

**FIGURE 14.2** Patient in position for minimal-access lung surgery. The shoulder joint ligaments are vulnerable to overstretch. (Redrawn from Benetti et al. 1996.)

Sleeve resection is commonly followed by atelectasis and sputum retention due to oedema around the anastomosis and ciliary damage from nerve involvement.

A complete lung is removed by **pneumonectomy**, sometimes accompanied by chest wall resection if the tumour has spread. Stretch of the remaining lung stimulates some growth (Filipovic et al. 2013), but most of the vacated space fills with air, blood and fibrin (Fig. 14.4), the quantity of which is regulated by one of the following:

- a chest drain, which is kept clamped except when drainage is required;
- a small thoracic catheter;
- needle aspiration.

A chest drain allows recognition of haemorrhage and, if sutures break down, prevents a pneumothorax. It must never be attached to suction, nor clamped or unclamped except by instruction of the surgeon. Too much drainage of the vacated space pulls the remaining lung into the space, risking a pneumothorax on the good side, and too little drainage leads to the bronchial stump becoming soggy.

If all goes well, the air is absorbed over 4–6 weeks. In the ensuing months, the space shrinks by upward shift of the hemidiaphragm, lateral shift of the mediastinum

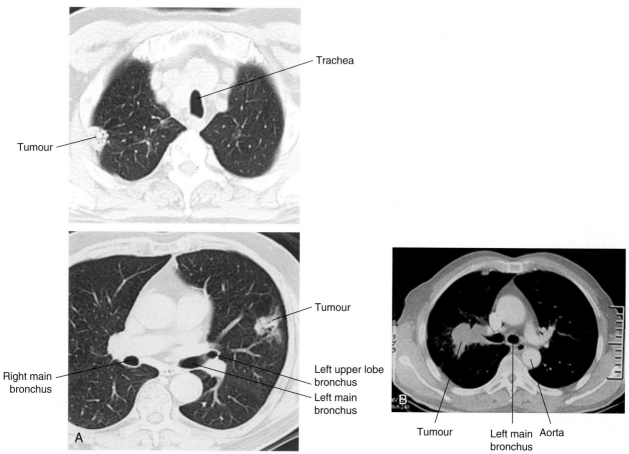

**FIGURE 14.3** (A) Scan of two peripheral lung tumours (A from Hsu et al. 2016b). (B) Central tumour in right upper lobe, requiring sleeve resection. (B from Ma & Liu 2016.)

and crowding of the ribs (Fig. 14.5). The remaining lung expands, undergoes some remodelling, and its perfusion doubles (Dane et al. 2013).

Positive pressure techniques such as manual hyperinflation are contraindicated immediately after lung resection because of potential damage to the anastomosis or stump, and risk of a pneumothorax.

In patients with hyperinflation due to emphysema, **lung volume reduction** is achieved by either surgically removing an area of nonfunctioning lung, or inserting one-way endobronchial valves to block inspiratory flow to a lobar bronchus. These reduce residual volume, relieve hyperinflation and improve exercise capacity (Faisal et al. 2016b). The diaphragm returns to a functional dome shape, which, in one patient, increased exercise tolerance from dyspnoea at rest to walking a

kilometre (Saxena et al. 2013). A giant bulla can be removed by **bullectomy**.

**Thoracoplasty** is a historic procedure involving rib resection so that part of the chest wall collapses and obliterates underlying tuberculosis-infected lung, thus suffocating the tubercle bacillus. The procedure may make a comeback if drug-resistant tuberculosis overwhelms the pharmacological industry, and is still an option for chronic empyema (Botianu 2012). The space is sometimes filled with ping pong balls to prevent chest wall deformity (Fig. 14.6).

**Lung transplantation** is on p. 322.

## Complications

Risk factors for developing complications are weak quadriceps (Irie et al. 2016), smoking and chronic

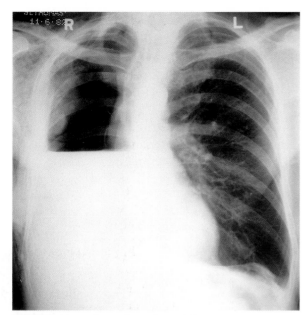

FIGURE 14.4 One day after right pneumonectomy showing a horizontal fluid line below an empty air space without lung markings. The trachea is shifted towards the vacated space. Compared to a pleural effusion, the fluid line shows no meniscus because it is not tracking up the pleura as the visceral pleura is now in the bin. The speckled appearance just visible in the soft tissue outside the right ribcage is subcutaneous emphysema.

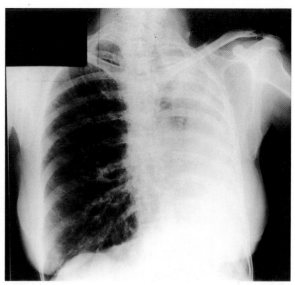

FIGURE 14.5 Some months after left pneumonectomy in a female patient, showing the vacated space now opaque. The deviated trachea is clearly visible against the opacity, healed rib and stitches.

obstructive pulmonary disease (COPD), but not necessarily old age (Lugg et al. 2016).

Atelectasis is common, usually on the operated side, but both sides are vulnerable (Fig. 14.7A). Diaphragm dysfunction occurs if the phrenic nerve is damaged (see Fig. 14.7A–B). During pneumonectomy, some surgeons deliberately cut the phrenic nerve to shrink the residual space.

An air leak is escape of air from the lung into the pleura, then out through a chest drain, as demonstrated by bubbling through the underwater seal drainage bottle. The chest drain must not be removed until bubbling stops.

Escape of air into subcutaneous tissue may occur, causing subcutaneous emphysema. This is rarely of more than cosmetic significance, and resolution usually occurs naturally, though this can be hastened by 100% oxygen (Lin et al. 2015) or subcutaneous drainage with compressive massage (Funakoshi et al. 2016). If secretions are a problem, the active cycle of breathing

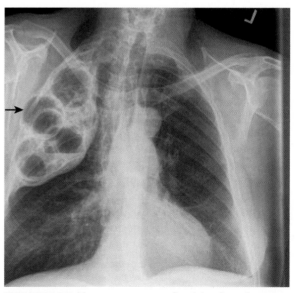

FIGURE 14.6 X-ray some years after 'plombage' surgery for TB, with some ping-pong balls filling with fluid. (From Galen 2016.)

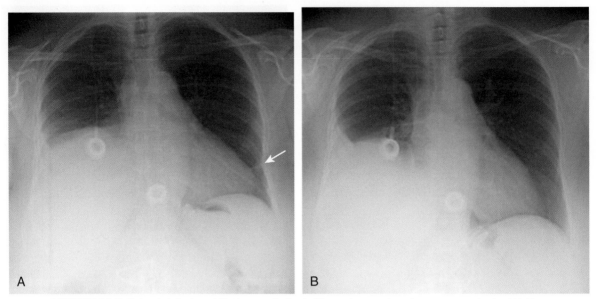

**FIGURE 14.7** Raised right hemidiaphragm in both films shows phrenic nerve paralysis. (A) Five days after right lower lobectomy, showing a band of atelectasis *(arrow)* on the left. (B) Atelectasis resolved after physiotherapy. Note also a pronounced rise in the right hemidiaphragm due to phrenic nerve paralysis. (Reproduced from Bommart et al. 2016.)

technique (ACBT) and/or autogenic drainage (AD) are preferable to coughing. If subcutaneous emphysema causes the face to swell and eyes to close, relatives can be shown how to massage the eyelids to allow temporary vision.

**Recurrent laryngeal nerve damage** may occur after left pneumonectomy or upper lobectomy, impairing speech and cough (Gelpke et al. 2010).

**Bronchopleural fistula** is a breach between the lung and pleura, which has the same effect as a pneumothorax and is often accompanied by empyema. It is usually delayed and is most likely to occur with mechanical ventilation, being suspected if there is a spiking temperature, X-ray evidence of a decreasing fluid level after pneumonectomy, or expectoration of bloody-brown secretions. Spread of infected material is minimized by the patient sitting up or lying with the fistula side downwards. Large fistulae need a chest drain or sealing via bronchoscopy or surgery (Fuso et al. 2016). Positive pressure physiotherapy techniques are contraindicated.

**Shoulder pain**, caused by positioning during surgery or pleural irritation, is experienced by the majority of patients, with 8% continuing to experience pain a year later (Blichfeldt et al. 2017).

**Long-term pain** (Fig. 14.8) after 1–3 years is present in 33% of patients after thoracotomy and 25% after VATS. It relates to preoperative pain, surgical technique including nerve damage and rib retraction, and inadequate postoperative analgesia (Kampe et al. 2016). Neurofeedback-based relaxation shows promise (Gorini et al. 2015).

## Physiotherapy

Physiotherapists may be involved in assessing suitability for surgery by exercise tests (Benattia et al. 2016). Patients at risk of sputum retention can be predicted by a history of COPD or absence of regional analgesia (Bonde et al. 2002).

If postoperative pain hinders treatment, a nerve block can be requested (Saby et al. 2016). Postoperative complications are reduced by early mobilization, deep breathing with or without incentive spirometry, chest clearance if required and progressive shoulder and thoracic mobility exercises (Rodriguez-Larrad et al. 2016). Kinesiology taping may help if pain is a problem (Imperatori et al. 2016).

For cancer patients, preoperative exercise has led to decreased postoperative complications and shorter

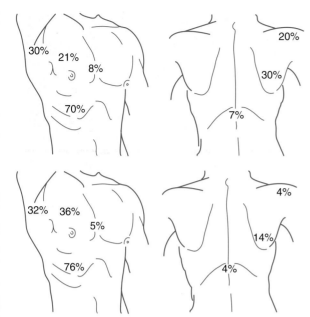

**FIGURE 14.8** Distribution of long-term pain (top) and sensory changes (bottom) after thoracotomy and VATS. (From Wildgaard et al. 2014.)

length of stay, while postoperative exercise training can improve quality of life (QoL), exercise tolerance (Ni et al. 2017) and fatigability (Hoffman et al. 2016a). Baddeley (2016) suggests that postoperative patients walk for increasing distances four times a day at Borg level 3–4 (p. 251, Fig. 9.2). Interdisciplinary education further improves quality of life (QoL) (Raz et al. 2016).

Noninvasive ventilation may be needed, sometimes prophylactically (Chiumello 2012). High-flow nasal oxygen provides some positive pressure and can shorten hospital stay (Ansari et al. 2015). Concerns have been raised about using positive pressure if there is bubbling through the chest drain, although CPAP has been investigated and found not to prolong an air leak (Nery et al. 2012).

Portable oxygen on exercise is required if $SpO_2$ falls below 90% on air at rest, and blood pressure (BP) monitoring is needed if there is an epidural (Yeung et al. 2016). High-intensity endurance and strength training is well tolerated and improves fitness and QoL (Edvardsen et al. 2015), and 2 weeks of inspiratory muscle training has improved oxygenation in high-risk cancer patients (Brocki et al. 2016). Shoulder exercises begin once pain allows and after liaison with the surgeon.

Points to note in relation to pneumonectomy are the following:

1. Patients should not lie on the *nonoperated* side, to prevent fluid spilling onto the stump. Some surgeons require this to be life-long.
2. After radical pneumonectomy, which entails entering the pericardium, patients should not lie on *either* side in case of cardiac herniation (Gadhinglajkar et al. 2010).
3. If sputum clearance is necessary, ACBT/AD is preferred to coughing, to avoid pressure on the stump.
4. There should be no head-down tip and, for some patients, no lying flat.
5. Pharyngeal suction, if necessary, should be shallow, as with any surgery involving the airway.

Chest wall resection or reconstruction requires liaison with the surgeon if muscle flaps or plastic surgery are involved.

Fast track surgery means that patients may be sent home before complications develop, and a system of symptom monitoring with automatic email alerts has proved beneficial (Cleeland et al. 2011). Postoperative pulmonary rehabilitation is recommended (Sterzi 2013), followed by home-based exercise (Hoffman et al. 2014), with a final check on shoulder range of movement and posture.

## PLEURAL SURGERY

The commonest indication for pleural surgery is recurrent, bilateral or persistent pneumothorax, caused by a breach in either layer of the pleura. Other indications are problematic pleural effusion or bronchopleural fistula. Pleural surgery leaves a long-term mild restrictive defect.

**Pleurodesis** introduces irritant chemicals, tetracycline, fibrin glue or laser pulses into the pleura via thoracoscopy, setting up a sterile and brutally painful inflammation, leading to fibrosis and adherence of the two layers of the pleura. Kindly surgeons instill local anaesthetic into the pleura before closure. The procedure relies on an inflammatory response and should not be followed by antiinflammatory analgesia (Suárez et al. 2013). Chest drains facilitate lung and chest wall apposition, but hypoxaemia can be a problem (Lui et al. 2016).

**Pleurectomy** strips off the parietal pleura so that a raw surface is left at the chest wall, to which the visceral pleura adheres.

Empyema is normally managed by chest tube drainage, but if it is large or loculated, thoracoscopic surgery may be required, entailing debridement or, if infection is not contained, **decortication**, which involves peeling off the restrictive fibrosed visceral pleura and releasing the trapped lung. The parietal pleura is spared unless long-standing empyema and deformity mean that it will impair lung expansion. Surgical patients are debilitated from extended infection and require graded exercise.

## CHEST DRAINS

Simple wound drains are adequate to remove blood from the affected site after most forms of surgery, but if the pleura has been cut, large-bore, underwater-seal drains are usually required to restore negative pleural pressure. The proximal end is inside the pleura, with one end-hole to drain fluid and air, and several small side-eyes to prevent catheter occlusion. The last side-eye can be identified radiologically by an interruption in its radiopaque line. The distal end, outside the patient, drains into a collection chamber. The airtight system becomes an extension of the patient's pleura and allows air and blood to escape from the pleural space while preventing re-entry, thus allowing the lung to re-expand.

These pleural chest drains may be used after lobectomy, pneumothorax, pleural effusion, haemothorax or empyema. One is traditionally placed in the apex to remove air and the other in the base to remove blood, but both air and blood will usually find the drains, especially when suction is applied. Pleural drains may also be required if the pleura has been cut during oesophageal, kidney or upper abdominal surgery, either by mistake or of necessity. Pain is reduced by applying lignocaine jelly to the drains before insertion (Kang et al. 2014), 8-hourly intrapleural local anaesthesia thereafter (BTS 2003), or using only one drain, which appears to be as effective as two (Dawson 2010).

Nonpleural chest drains may be used after:
- pneumonectomy, when they are placed in the space vacated by the lung to drain blood and debris and prevent excessive displacement of the mediastinum;
- heart surgery (although some cardiac surgeons find that simple wound drains are sufficient), when one drain is usually placed inside the pericardium to prevent cardiac tamponade, and one outside the pericardium to drain blood from the mediastinum.

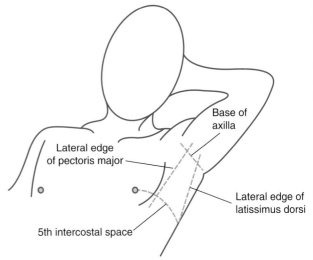

**FIGURE 14.9** Safe zone for insertion of chest drain.

### Procedure

All tissues down to the pleura are infiltrated with local anaesthetic (BTS 2010b), and after this has taken effect, the drains are inserted above a rib, where there are fewest nerves and blood vessels, and within the 'safe triangle' (Fig. 14.9).

### Mechanism

Chest drain units incorporate one to three bottles or chambers: one for drainage, one to act as a water seal, and a suction-control chamber, sometimes as separate bottles but usually as one system (Fig. 14.10):

1. The collection/drainage chamber collects expelled fluid and debris.
2. The water-seal chamber measures negative pressure in the chest, determines the degree of air leak and acts as a one-way valve so that air and fluid escape from the negative pressure inside the chest but cannot return.
3. The suction-control chamber regulates the amount of negative pressure that sucks fluid and/or air from the chest.

Fluid from the pleura enters the drainage chamber and cannot return so long as the system is below the level of the patient's chest. Air from the pleura enters the drainage chamber and then the water-seal chamber, where it bubbles through the water, which acts as a seal to prevent its return.

Drainage depends on gravity or suction. Gravity drainage occurs when the exit tube is open to the

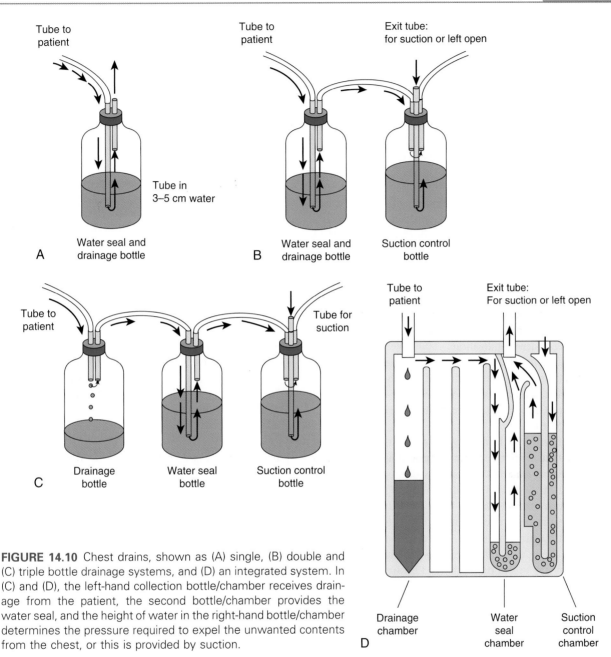

**FIGURE 14.10** Chest drains, shown as (A) single, (B) double and (C) triple bottle drainage systems, and (D) an integrated system. In (C) and (D), the left-hand collection bottle/chamber receives drainage from the patient, the second bottle/chamber provides the water seal, and the height of water in the right-hand bottle/chamber determines the pressure required to expel the unwanted contents from the chest, or this is provided by suction.

atmosphere. This allows the water level in the tubing of the water-seal chamber to swing, reflecting the change in pleural pressure with breathing. It rises by 5–10 cm on inhalation and falls on exhalation, but goes the opposite way if the patient is on positive pressure ventilation. If a suction system is not in place, the exit tube must be open to allow free drainage.

An air leak is present if air is bubbling through the water, having passed from the lung and through the visceral pleura at each breath. The hole in the visceral pleura should seal in time. If there is any change in air leak after treatment, this should be reported. Persistent air leaks can be sealed by insertion of endobronchial valves.

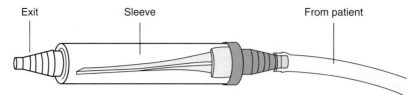

**FIGURE 14.11** Heimlich flutter valve. When negative pressure is created in the chest by the patient breathing in, the sleeve closes to prevent air being sucked into the pleura. When air escapes from the pleura, the sleeve opens to allow it to escape.

Exit    Sleeve    From patient

If the negative pressure of the patient's breathing is inadequate to reinflate the lung, e.g. if there is excess fluid drainage or large air leak, suction is applied at a pressure that should not normally exceed −8 cm $H_2O$, (George 2016) or sufficient to produce slow, consistent bubbling without turbulence in the water column (Bar-El et al. 2001). Suction pressure is provided from a dedicated pump or from wall suction via an adaptor to avoid too high a pressure. Some patients can have their systems on suction at night and on water seal during the day, allowing easier mobilization.

Patients with an uncomplicated pleural effusion, haemothorax or pneumothorax usually only require one bottle, which acts as both drainage and water-seal chamber. Chest drain protocols are described by French et al. (2016).

Alternatives to the underwater seal system are a digital device that provides continuous portable suction while maintaining negative pleural pressure regardless of the volume of air leak (Pompili et al. 2017) and a flutter valve such as the Heimlich (Fig. 14.11), which releases air on expiration but collapses shut by the negative pressure on inspiration. It does not require a bottle system and is cheap, safe, effective unless suction is required, and can stay in situ on discharge (Tavare et al. 2016).

## Management

Patients on suction must be nursed on a specialist ward (BTS 2003), but they take responsibility for some of the care of their drains, e.g. avoiding dependent loops in the tubing where drainage can collect, and keeping the system below chest level so that fluid cannot be siphoned back into the patient. They are advised that movement is good for encouraging drainage, as is turning towards the side of the drain, and occasionally coughing.

Clamping should be avoided unless there is accidental disconnection of a junction in the system, or when lifting the bottle temporarily above the patient's chest.

**BOX 14.1  Tips on Managing Chest Drains**

- Before treatment, the location of the clamps should be identified in case of need.
- Junctions in the tubing should not be taped, otherwise disconnection might be missed.
- Bottles should be kept upright and not raised above chest level.
- Drainage is assisted by deep breathing and exercise, with care taken to avoid disconnection.
- When handling patients, the tubing should be held in alignment along the patient's chest to minimize discomfort.
- The bottles and tubing should be kept exposed throughout treatment, to avoid accidental knocking or kinking.
- The system should be observed before and after treatment to check for any change in drainage, air leak or swing in water level. Extra drainage is expected after treatment, but excessive loss suggests haemorrhage and should be reported.

If there is an air leak, clamping is forbidden, otherwise a tension pneumothorax (p. 510) could be created. The principles of safe handling of chest drains are in Box 14.1.

If there is no pressure swing in the water seal chamber of a pleural drain, either the system is on suction, which overrides the swing to some degree, or the tube is blocked. If the lung has successfully re-expanded, the pleural end of the tube has been occluded and the swing is reduced.

Chest drains are removed by nursing staff once drainage is no more than 300 mL/day (Yao et al. 2016), there is no air leak and the lung has fully expanded. A more accurate estimate of the timing for removal is by a wi-fi-based digital system (Cho et al. 2016b). Removal has been described as 'the most distressing and intensely painful experience of all' (Fox et al. 1999), and neither opioids nor Entonox alone are adequate (Bruce et al. 2006, Akrofi et al. 2005). Additions include local anaesthesia, EMLA cream (Rosen et al. 2000) as well as systemic analgesia and/or techniques that avoid tightening the purse-string suture (Kim & Cho 2017). A spontaneously breathing patient is asked to perform a Valsalva manoeuvre during removal to prevent air being drawn into the chest.

Physiotherapy incorporates exercise, posture correction, shoulder mobility and, for some patients, respiratory care. When self-mobilizing, patients can carry the drain(s) in a bucket.

## Complications

If a patient with a clamped drain becomes breathless or develops subcutaneous emphysema, the drain should be unclamped and the doctor informed.

If any junction in the system becomes disconnected, the tubing nearest the patient is clamped, both the disconnected ends are cleaned and reconnected, the tubing unclamped, the patient asked to cough a few times to force out any air that has been sucked into the chest, and the incident reported and documented.

If the tubing becomes disconnected from the patient, the following steps should be taken:

1. Ask the patient to exhale and, at the same time, press a hand against the wound at end-exhalation, preferably using a dressing or glove but speed taking precedence over sterility.
2. Ask the patient to breathe normally.
3. Summon assistance.
4. If air is heard leaking from the site, or the drain was previously bubbling, the hand should be removed periodically (with the patient breathing out) to allow air to escape and to prevent a tension pneumothorax.
5. Explain to the patient that the drain will probably need to be reinserted and the pressures will then regain their equilibrium.
6. Observe breathing rate and chest symmetry.
7. Give oxygen if $SpO_2$ drops.

## HEART SURGERY

*'[Waiting for surgery] is like driving a car with no brakes. When I get the pain, all I can think about are those five blocked arteries'*

***Fitzsimons 2003***

Most forms of heart surgery improve QoL (Westerdahl et al. 2016). Coronary artery bypass grafting (CABG) is the commonest, using a native blood vessel to connect the aorta to the coronary artery. It is usually performed if there are recurrent symptoms after percutaneous coronary intervention (p. 141) because of progressive atherosclerosis. Some of the 20% of patients who do not achieve improved QoL are thought to suffer long-term cognitive defects or traumatic memories from their intensive care experience (Schelling et al. 2003).

## Procedures

Open surgery involves sternotomy (see Fig. 12.1), division of the aponeurosis of pectoralis major, retraction of the sternum and instigation of cardiopulmonary bypass (CPB) to allow surgery on a quiescent heart in a bloodless field. CPB involves the heart being stopped, the aorta cross-clamped to separate outflow of the heart from the systemic circulation, the circulating blood removed from the right atrium, filtered and oxygenated outside the body, then pumped back into the ascending aorta. Neither heart nor lungs are functioning during this period, and the lungs are partially collapsed. The pericardial sac is often filled with chilled saline to reduce tissue oxygen demand and the flow required for bypass.

Off-pump techniques avoid cardiopulmonary bypass and use an 'octopus' to stabilize the beating heart. This reduces the inflammatory response, but the same multimodal analgesia is required (Sondekoppam et al. 2014).

Minimally invasive surgery reduces pain, cardiorespiratory complications, sternal instability and hospital stay, with early return to normal activity (Malik et al. 2016).

To replace the diseased coronary arteries, the saphenous vein, radial artery and/or internal mammary artery (IMA) are used (Fig. 14.12). IMA grafts last longer (Ennker 2012) but the artery is harvested from the chest wall, usually puncturing the pleura (Ghavidel et al. 2013), and can cause shoulder pain and greater impairment of lung function than saphenous vein grafts.

## Complications

Enhanced recovery principles (p. 296) reduce morbidity (Fleming et al. 2016). The education component is relevant preoperatively because waiting for cardiac surgery evokes a greater stress response than with other types of surgery (Rosiek et al. 2016).

For patients spending time on mechanical ventilation postoperatively, **ventilator-associated pneumonia** is the major independent risk factor for hospital mortality (Tamayo et al. 2012).

Postoperative **cardiovascular instability**, although minimized by control of pain, fluids and oxygenation, may contraindicate turning or other forms of physiotherapy. Atrial fibrillation is the commonest problem (Perrier et al. 2017), increasing the risk of stroke, cerebral

dysfunction and respiratory complications (Phan et al. 2016c). Venous thromboembolism occurs in a quarter of patients (Viana et al. 2017).

**Atelectasis** is ubiquitous (Westerdahl & Tenling 2014) but generally resolves in a few days (Khan et al. 2009a). Causes are compression from the heart (Neves et al. 2013), the lung deflation that accompanies bypass or trauma/cold injury to the phrenic nerve. This can be treated with a preextubation recruitment manoeuvre (Claxton et al. 2003). Manual hyperinflation has the same effect, though only temporarily (Fig. 14.13), and not to be done routinely (Paulus et al. 2011).

Atelectasis can cause **hypoxaemia** (Parida 2016). Following bypass, the shunt is typically 25% (Kotani et al. 2000), reducing to an average 15% after 48 h (Rasmussen et al. 2006). Compromised **oxygen delivery** is indicated by $ScvO_2$ (p. 472) below 70%, indicating a poor prognosis (Méndez 2017).

Hypoxaemia and/or hypotension contribute to **acute kidney injury**, which complicates recovery in up to 30% of patients. This impairs function of the brain, lungs and gut, and increases risk of death fivefold (O'Neal et al. 2016).

**Anaemia** should be corrected preoperatively because as many as 30% of patients have surgery when anaemic, which doubles the risk of acute kidney injury (Murphy 2015), impairs mobility and increases morbidity and mortality (Padmanabhan et al. 2016).

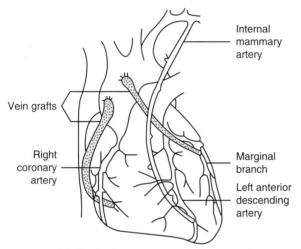

**FIGURE 14.12** Grafts to the heart. (From Adam & Osborne 2005.)

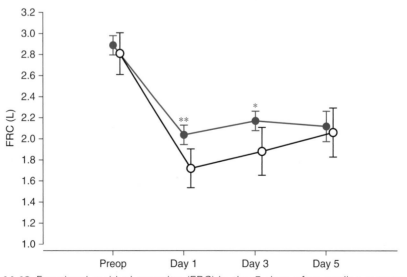

**FIGURE 14.13** Functional residual capacity *(FRC)* in the 5 days after cardiac surgery. Closed symbols represent 6-hourly manual hyperinflation until extubation, and open symbols represent the control group. *, $P < .04$; **, $P < .002$; *Preop,* preoperative. (From Paulus et al. 2011.)

**Brain** complications range from delirium in 20%–30% of patients, cognitive and functional decline (Li et al. 2015a), stroke in a few patients and silent ischaemic lesions in as many as two-thirds (Školoudík et al. 2016). Causes are sedation (Mayr et al. 2016), CPB, sleep deprivation, acid–base imbalance and anxiety (Bruce et al. 2013). Effects may be temporary, as represented by Bill Clinton's strange speeches after his bypass surgery (Johnson 2016) or permanent (Rasmussen et al. 2016). Monitoring brain perfusion reduces the risk (Mohandas et al. 2013).

**Pain** contributes to atelectasis. Wound pain may be compounded by musculoskeletal pain if the sternum and ribs have been retracted, for which TENS may be beneficial (Lima et al. 2011). Pain is greatest during coughing, and one study found it to be less during incentive spirometry than deep breathing (Milgrom et al. 2004), possibly due to the distraction of using a device. Chronic pain continues in 3.8% of patients (Gjeilo et al. 2016).

Cardiogenic **pulmonary oedema** may be caused by over-eager fluid replacement or the effect of cardio-pulmonary bypass on capillary permeability. The risk of developing **acute respiratory distress syndrome** is reduced by ventilator manipulations and avoidance of fluid overload (Hoegl et al. 2016). **Pleural effusion** can result from fluid disturbance, IMA harvesting, diaphragm dysfunction or surgical technique (Özülkü & Aygün 2015).

**Peripheral nerve injuries**, especially with diabetes, can be caused by the position of the body or limbs on the table, chest wall retraction or vein canulation (Gavazzi et al. 2016).

**Haemorrhage** is a particularly dangerous complication after surgery if blood is trapped in the pericardium, causing **tamponade** (p. 509).

**Anxiety** has been linked to pain, whereas **depression** relates to major adverse cardiac events (Poole et al. 2016), or reduced attendance at cardiac rehabilitation and increased risk of the return of angina (Tully 2012). **Fatigue** indicates the need for graded exercise and discharge advice tailored to the individual.

**Sternal complications** have been linked to smoking, obesity, diabetes, intense coughing (Adams et al. 2016) and IMA grafting (Fig. 14.14). If the sternum is heard or felt to click on movement, a cough belt (see Fig. 13.8) or towel is needed to stabilize the chest wall during deep breathing and coughing. Sternal instability in the first 2

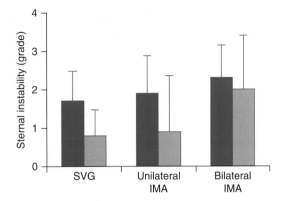

**FIGURE 14.14** Sternal instability, as indicated by grade of movement on palpation, after saphenous vein grafting *(SVG)* and internal mammary artery *(IMA)* grafting. (From Al-Ansary et al. 2000.)

**TABLE 14.1 Post-CABG symptoms reported at 3, 6 and 12 weeks**

| Symptom | 3 weeks (%) | 6 weeks (%) | 12 weeks (%) |
|---|---|---|---|
| Fatigue | 52.2 | 30.2 | 27.5 |
| Sleep problems | 38.6 | 25.7 | 19.4 |
| Poor appetite | 33.6 | 13.3 | 2.7 |
| Depression | 16.8 | 7.6 | 8.6 |
| Constipation | 15.9 | 2.5 | 0.4 |
| Neuromuscular problems | 6.0 | 3.9 | 2.2 |
| Nausea | 2.6 | 1.7 | 0.4 |

From Schulz et al. 2011.

weeks is usually associated with infection. After 6 weeks it becomes nonunion, which is suspected if the X-ray shows broken sutures or a gradually widening lucent line at the sternotomy site. Unilateral arm movement, or any upper limb movement that increases sternal pain, should be avoided.

Long-term symptoms are outlined in Table 14.1.

## Physiotherapy

The following postoperative benefits of preoperative physiotherapy have been identified:

1. Exercise may reduce atelectasis and pneumonia (Hulzebos et al. 2012).

2. For high-risk patients, incentive spirometry, deep breathing and mobilization reduce the incidence of atelectasis (Yánez-Brage et al. 2009).
3. Preoperative and postoperative cardiac rehabilitation leads to fewer complications and shorter hospital stay (Herdy et al. 2008).
4. Preoperative and postoperative inspiratory muscle training may reduce respiratory complications and shorten length of stay (Neto et al. 2016c).

Postoperatively, BP should be observed before, during and after treatment. Diastolic pressure is more significant than systolic pressure because coronary artery perfusion is highest during diastole. The operation notes indicate the limits within which BP should be maintained.

A proportion of patients appear euphoric on the first day, possibly as a reaction to their survival, but then sink into depression. When identified, these patients should be encouraged to take things gently on the first day to help avoid mood swings that interfere with rehabilitation.

Some surgeons request that the patient not be turned immediately after CABG, to avoid a shearing stress on the sternum, and with IMA graft to protect the graft. If side-lying is acceptable to patient and surgeon, the upper arm should rest on a pillow to maintain symmetry and prevent strain on the sternum.

For spontaneously breathing patients, deep breathing exercises are not required routinely (Brasher et al. 2003) so long as the patient is able to mobilize. Urell et al. (2011) claim that 30 deep breaths an hour improve oxygenation, but these were against positive pressure so it is not known which variable was beneficial. If deep breathing is indicated, this can be encouraged with incentive spirometry, which may improve blood gases (Yazdannik et al. 2016). Deep breathing or incentive spirometry is usually more effective with manual support of the wound on inspiration to improve comfort and allow greater excursion. Airway clearance is sometimes required.

Sitting out and walking should begin on day one if possible, early mobility helping to prevent complications, improve functional capacity and reduce length of stay (Santos et al. 2017). Assessment for musculoskeletal problems and neurological damage is required (El-Ansary et al. 2000b), and frequent musculoskeletal problems require liaison with theatre staff.

Shoulder elevation should normally be limited to 90 degrees for 24 h after sternotomy, especially after IMA grafting, and should be performed bilaterally to protect the sternum. Exercise and functional activities should keep the arms within an imaginary tube (Fig. 14.15), using Fig. 14.16 as a teaching aid (Adams et al. 2016). If patients have to use their arms to stand up, they should be used bilaterally, and if a walking aid is required, weight-bearing must use the upper limbs equally.

Epidural analgesia speeds up mobilization (El-Morsy 2012). Precautions to mobilization are:

- unstable BP;
- complete heart block reliant on external cardiac pacing;
- atrial fibrillation with compromised cardiovascular stability;
- heart failure requiring inotropic drugs;
- intravenous vasodilator drugs;
- pulmonary artery catheter in situ;
- new myocardial infarct or symptomatic angina;
- neurological event.

Before discharge, it is useful to check the breathing pattern and posture to make sure that there are no lingering signs of tension, which could become a habit. Patients need to understand the distinction between incisional pain and angina, receive written information and advice on rest/exercise balance. Before and after discharge, early cardiac rehabilitation can reduce complications, improve cardiac function and reduce length of stay, beginning with exercise at <13 on the 6–20 rate of perceived exertion (p. 279), e.g.:

- Walking three–four times a day from postoperative day 1, with gradually increasing distances.
- Intermittent bouts of exercise lasting 3–5 min with rest periods (ACPICR 2016).

CABG is effective in reducing angina, but atherosclerosis continues (Burazor & Susak 2016). Patients are well advised to cultivate a lifestyle that retards the disease process in the grafted vessels, including regular exercise, which continues to improve QoL 5–6 years after surgery (Diane 2007).

## TRANSPLANTATION

*'Each new day is welcomed with open arms come sun, rain or snow. Gone are the excuses for putting off activities until the weather is better or the time more opportune'*

**Marsh (post-transplant patient) 1986**

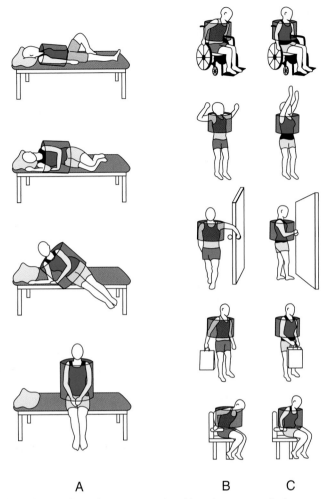

**FIGURE 14.15** Teaching tool to demonstrate load-bearing upper limb movements after sternotomy. 'B' movements should be avoided. (From Adams et al. 2016.)

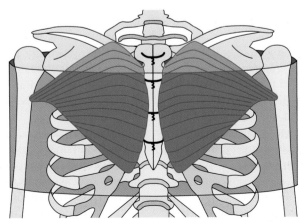

**FIGURE 14.16** Illustration to teach patients about their sternotomy, the attachments of pectoralis major and the imaginary tube forming the basis of a 'Keep Your Move in the Tube' approach. (From Adams et al. 2016.)

Receiving a transplanted heart, lung or both sometimes causes profound change in a patient's attitude to life. Postoperative feelings of resurrection are not unusual, but the patient's mood may swing between euphoria and depression (Xu et al. 2012b), sometimes complicated by conflicting emotions including 'recipient guilt' and being in possession of part of someone else. However, for many who survive the waiting list, operation and complications, each day is precious and life is usually sweet.

The indication for transplantation is end-stage organ failure and the capacity for rehabilitation. Examples are:

- heart transplant for cardiomyopathy;
- double lung or heart–lung transplant for cystic fibrosis (CF);
- single lung transplant for noninfective lung disorders such as pulmonary fibrosis or occasionally COPD.

Preoperatively, smokers must have quit for 6 months, and family members are also exhorted to stop. Nutrition should be optimized and steroids minimized (Mahida et al. 2012).

The operations are no longer technically awesome, and now that immunosuppressive therapy is better able to prevent organ rejection, the main limiting factor is lack of donor organs. Delays can sometimes be bridged by left ventricular assist devices for heart transplant and extracorporeal membrane oxygenation (ECMO) for lung transplant.

## Procedures

Cardiopulmonary bypass is used for heart and occasionally double lung transplant.

For single lung transplant, a thoracotomy incision is required. For double lung transplant, a massive transsternal bilateral thoracotomy (clamshell incision) allows sequential single lung transplant.

To retain collateral circulation with lung transplant, both heart and lung may be transplanted, with the recipient's healthy heart donated to a second recipient. To maximize the donor pool, living related donation allows a lower lobe to be given, for example, by both parents and used as two full lungs by the recipient. This brings the added benefit of elective surgery, well-tested donors and well-perfused donor organs.

## Complications

All transplants are complicated by the side effects of lifelong drugs to inhibit organ rejection, bringing risks of infection, malignancy and muscle weakness (Dudley 2012). Uchiyama et al. (2012) claim that listening to Mozart helps prolong graft survival.

## Heart

Complications include emotional repercussions specific to heart transplant (Conway et al. 2013). Acute rejection is suspected if there are temperature or ECG changes, confirmed by biopsy. Chronic rejection accelerates atherosclerosis of the transplanted arteries and is identified by annual angiography or biopsy (Strecker et al. 2013). The only treatment for chronic heart rejection is retransplantation. The 5-year mortality is 27% for recipients below age 60, 30% for those aged 60–69 and 30.8% at ages >70 years old (Cooper et al. 2016).

## Lung

The lung is the only organ in contact with the atmosphere and has evolved a strong protective immunity to anything foreign. This mechanism is compromised by transplantation, and the risk of infection is increased by immunosuppression, dysphagia, lymphatic interruption and hilar stripping during surgery (Glanville 2013). Infection is the leading cause of death in the first year (Dickson et al. 2016).

Denervation of the lung contributes to mucociliary transport being reduced to <15% of normal (Caster et al. 2011) and may lower the patient's awareness of the presence of secretions, which people with CF have developed to a fine art. Excess secretions continue to be produced from the native airway of CF patients above the anastomosis. A short-term hindrance to secretion clearance is oedema around the anastomosis. Long-term effects include a 50% incidence of gastroesophageal reflux (Davis et al. 2010). Denervation is often long term but the bronchial arteries and lymphatic system are thought to regenerate in some weeks (Oh 2009). Bilateral lung transplantation results in complete denervation, which may impair the hypercapnic respiratory drive and exercise capacity (Scherer et al. 2016).

Pulmonary oedema can be caused by initial loss of lymphatic drainage or the ischaemic insult of surgery followed by reactive reperfusion. This 'reperfusion pulmonary oedema' peaks 8–12 h postoperatively, causing hypoxia and reduced lung compliance. Treatment with fluid restriction and diuretics may cause thick airway secretions and a dry mouth.

Prolonged air leak may occur, especially if the new lobe or lung does not fit snugly into the chest, and empyema can develop.

Acute or chronic rejection may occur from a few days to several years postoperatively. $FEV_1$ should improve by as much as 70% in the first 6 months and then plateau (Mulhall 2016), but a subsequent reduction of 10%–15% is a warning of possible rejection. Suspicions are confirmed if there are fever, breathlessness, hypoxaemia and fine crackles on auscultation. Radiological signs are similar for both rejection and opportunistic infection, and gentle bronchoscopy is needed to distinguish the two. Treatment of rejection is by steroids. Exercise training should be temporarily ceased or modified.

Obliterative bronchiolitis may follow repeated episodes of rejection, creating a combined obstructive and restrictive defect. The small airways become obstructed by inflammation and then obliterated by granulation tissue, which then fibroses. It can extend into alveoli and develop into pneumonia or 'BOOP' (p. 117). Retransplantation may be required, but carries high mortality.

One year survival after lung transplant is 80% and median survival 5.5 years, non-adherence to immunosuppressive drugs being a factor (Castleberry et al. 2017).

## Physiotherapy

*Pulmonary rehabilitation in the pretransplant phase is a crucial component for positive functional outcomes.*

**Hatt et al. 2017**

Preoperative physiotherapy takes place at the assessment clinic because there is no time once a donor has been found. Assessment includes exercise capacity, muscle function, mobility and activities of daily living (Wickerson et al. 2016). An individual exercise programme is needed because many patients are debilitated, and deconditioning predicts poor postoperative outcomes and worse survival (Walsh et al. 2016). Patients with tenuous pulmonary reserve can still improve their exercise tolerance (Thrush & Skrzat 2016), and even housebound people with pulmonary fibrosis can improve their physical activity levels and respiratory symptoms (Polastri et al. 2016). With pulmonary hypertension, precautions include avoidance of hypoxemia, chest pain, dizziness, presyncope, nausea and visual changes, and training at Borg score 2–3 or slight to moderate intensity (Wickerson et al. 2016). High-intensity aerobic and resistance training and Valsalva manoeuvres are to be avoided.

The wait for an organ is a feat of endurance, during which patients feel in limbo. Active preoperative care needs to be integrated with palliative care because many patients will not reach the front of the queue (Colman et al. 2013). Physical activity can also be maintained for people on mechanical ventilation or ambulatory ECMO (Wickerson et al. 2016).

Postoperative treatment is similar to that after other forms of chest surgery, with extra attention to prevention of infection, plus the specific considerations in Hatt et al. (2017), Wickerson et al. (2016) and as discussed below.

Following lung transplant, secretions below the anastomosis do not elicit a cough reflex so continuous humidification and sometimes other techniques may be needed at first, but long-term chest clearance is not usually required. If manual hyperinflation or other positive pressure technique is needed, the operation notes should be checked for the pressure to which the anastomosis has been tested, and pressures during physiotherapy kept well below this. Suction, if needed, should not allow the catheter to reach the anastomosis, which in ventilated patients is just below the end of the endotracheal tube. Rehabilitation is outlined in Table 14.2.

Transplanted hearts are denervated so that the transmission of angina is impaired, the pulse is not a reliable monitoring tool and there is a delayed heart rate response to exercise, requiring ample warm-up and cool-down periods. After 6–12 months of exercise, responses may become near-normal, although the intensity and duration of exercise will be limited.

Ongoing exercise training brings sustained gains in QoL (Wickerson et al. 2016), with awareness that patients are at risk of secondary osteoporosis because of anti-rejection drugs (Tabarelli et al. 2016).

Attention is focused on the recipient, but the donor's relatives are vulnerable at this time. The wife of one donor, herself a health professional, described her concern about staff 'not being nice to him' (Fulbrook et al. 1999). Respiratory physiotherapy may be requested to maintain oxygenation to the organ, and even if the donor is brain-dead, he or she must be cared for as any moribund patient, especially as physical responses to painful stimuli have been identified (Wu 2013). Conversation with relatives must avoid terminology such as

## TABLE 14.2   Overview of lung transplant rehabilitation

| Pre-transplant | Early post-transplant | 1–6 months post-transplant | Long-term |
| --- | --- | --- | --- |
| **Outpatient**<br>Aerobic, resistance and flexibility<br>Oxygen titration to support activity, as required | Early mobility on ICU or ward<br>Progression to independent function: transfers, walking, self-care, stairs<br>Exercise training<br>Oxygen titration to support activity, as required | **Uncomplicated course**<br>Exercise training | **Exercise training**<br>Home or community<br>Education on long-term exercise, barriers and motivators, relapse planning, restarting after illness<br>Return to leisure activities and sports |
| **Inpatient, on ward or ICU**<br>Exercise as tolerated<br>± oxygen | | **Complicated course**<br>Progression to independent function<br>Referral to inpatient rehabilitation if required<br>Exercise training ± oxygen | Transplant games and charity events |

Adapted from Wickerson et al. 2016.

'harvesting' the organs, or comments on the importance of maintaining vital signs.

## REPAIR OF AORTIC COARCTATION

Coarctation of the aorta is a congenital localized narrowing of the vessel. It may not be picked up until routine imaging shows an abnormal aorta or inferior notches on ribs 3–8. Surgery is advisable before hypertension wreaks damage in later life. Repair is by resection of the narrowed segment and insertion of a graft or stent.

The following precautions are needed postoperatively to avoid a sudden rise in BP that might strain the anastomosis:

1. The head-down tip should be avoided. Some surgeons prefer the patient not to lie flat.
2. Mobilization should be slow and fatigue avoided. Extra care is needed when patients are beginning to feel well enough to exert themselves.
3. Vigorous exercise should be discouraged for several months.

After this, benefit is gained from regular exercise but myocardial reserve remains below normal (Chen et al. 2016d). Patients remain at risk of exercise-induced hypertension, and cardiopulmonary exercise testing helps guide clinical decision making (Buys et al. 2013).

## OESOPHAGECTOMY

*Patients who do not recover physical function, pain and fatigue scores within 6 months … are at significant increased risk of shorter survival.*

**Lococo et al. 2012**

The above is a reminder of the importance of rehabilitation for this debilitated group of patients. Risk factors for oesophageal cancer are, for the squamous cell variety, tobacco, alcohol and searingly hot drinks, and for adenocarcinoma, Barrett's oesophagus (p. 126) or drugs that relax the lower oesophageal sphincter such as anticholinergics (Lagergren 2000).

Open oesophagectomy is a harrowing operation, with access by thoracolaparotomy, thoracotomy and laparotomy, or thoracotomy with a neck incision. This brings the highest rate of respiratory complications of any operation, although these are reduced by perioperative rehabilitation (Oikawa et al. 2016). More usual is minimally invasive surgery, which entails various combinations of thoracoscopy and laparoscopy and requires a period of one lung ventilation and sometimes the prone position to improve oxygenation (Otsubo et al. 2016). Endoscopic resection is feasible in early-stage disease (Knabe et al. 2016).

Pain is substantial even after keyhole surgery, and regional analgesia such as a paravertebral block is essential (Rucklidge et al. 2010). Other complications include:

- significant atelectasis because the stomach is pulled up into the chest and anastomosed to the oesophageal stump;
- recurrent laryngeal nerve injury;
- atrial fibrillation;
- pleural effusion;
- aspiration pneumonia, a risk that is reduced by a swallowing evaluation prior to starting oral feeds (Berry et al. 2010);
- chronic pain in approximately half of patients, reinforcing the importance of acute pain management (Olsén et al. 2009);
- anastomotic leak, empyema (Fig. 14.17) or abscess.

A third of complications occur after discharge, and 5-year survival is just 15%–40% (Chen et al. 2016e).

Preoperatively, a balanced exercise regimen is advised, especially as sarcopaenia increases respiratory complications (Makiura et al. 2016).

Postoperative precautions are:

- avoid the head-down tilt in case reflux of gastric contents damages the anastomosis (some surgeons prefer patients to maintain head elevation);
- avoid neck movements that might stretch the anastomosis;
- with a high resection and after extubation, avoid deep suction because the catheter might accidentally enter the oesophagus;
- positive pressure techniques should first be discussed with the surgeon due to possible stomach insufflation or damage to the anastomosis (Pedoto 2012).

Preston et al. (2013) suggest the following regimen:

- evening of surgery: sit up in bed, optimize fluid status;
- day 1: walk two–three times a day as far as the patient is able, instigate jejunal tube feeding;
- day 2: walk three–four times a day;
- day 3: walk four times a day;
- follow-on: progressive rehabilitation and intensive dietetic input.

Pneumonia is reduced by immediate postoperative oral nutrition (Weijs et al. 2016), but sputum retention is common and a request for early minitracheostomy is advisable in high-risk patients.

Soon after discharge, a multidisciplinary pulmonary rehabilitation programme leads to improved QoL and long-term outcome (Lococo et al. 2012). Ongoing nutritional support is required.

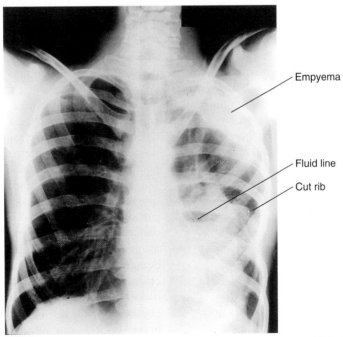

Empyema

Fluid line

Cut rib

**FIGURE 14.17** Opacity in the left upper zone represents an empyema which developed after oesophagectomy in this 17-year-old. A rib was cut for the thoracotomy, and the colon, containing fluid, was transplanted in place of the oesophagus.

# BREAST SURGERY

Breast cancer is the most common cancer in women, accounting for nearly 1 in 3 cancers (Wisotzky et al. 2017). Any surgery to the breast is distressing, and this distress affects postoperative outcomes (Montgomery et al. 2010), so preoperative care should provide individualized information.

For women who require a full mastectomy, immediate breast reconstruction is usually feasible. Postoperative complications include shoulder stiffness and pain, and muscle weakness, especially after axillary node dissection. The risk of developing neuropathic postmastectomy pain, characterized by burning and stabbing sensations, may be reduced by the anaesthetist creating a paravertebral block, which also reduces nausea (Bansal et al. 2012).

Patients require advice on preoperative activity because this speeds physical recovery (Nilsson et al. 2016). Postoperatively, early rehabilitation improves shoulder mobility, reduces pain and improves QoL (Testa et al. 2014), and ongoing exercise further increases shoulder movement and reduces breast and chest wall pain (Wong 2012), with extra benefit when balance and posture are emphasized (Winters-Stone 2011). Motivation to continue an individually tailored exercise programme is advised (Appendix B) because ongoing physical inactivity contributes to worsening health status (Vardar et al. 2015) and over half of patients experience chronic pain (Bruce et al. 2016).

Immediate or delayed lymphoedema requires manual lymphatic drainage, compression garments, exercise and skin care (Melam et al. 2016). A stiff shoulder may not become evident for some weeks, so prevention and follow up are advised (Campbell 2012), as well as attention to the opposite shoulder, which shows above-average morbidity (Adriaenssens et al. 2012).

# HEAD AND NECK SURGERY

*Patients are often faced with physical disfigurement and altered abilities to breathe, speak, smell, taste, chew or swallow, while simultaneously enduring pain and fatigue.*

**Eades et al. 2013**

Distressing effects of head and neck surgery include mucous discharge, limited ability to express feelings, difficulties with breathing and nose-blowing, dysphagia, dental problems, sense disturbance, disfigurement, depression, difficulties with eating and drinking, and a proclivity towards alcohol and nicotine dependence (Simcock & Simo 2016).

Types of surgery include **selective** neck dissection to excise a tumour, and **radical** neck dissection to also remove malignant lymph nodes. **Transoral laser microsurgery** reaches the tumour through the mouth, with improved cosmetic outcomes, and may be used if the cancer has not spread to the lymph nodes in the neck (Fink et al. 2016). **Reconstructive surgery** may be required if speech, swallowing or appearance are affected

## Head and Neck Cancers

The incidence of oropharyngeal cancer is increasing, the main causes being tobacco and alcohol (Perdomo et al. 2016). Cancer of the larynx is most common in Western countries (Sheahan 2014). It can be identified early by voice changes, and 70% of patients are cured (Chen et al. 2010). The larynx is preserved when possible, but if it is lost, voice restoration may be possible surgically. Either way, 'voice rehabilitation' is required (Ouyoung et al. 2016), along with swallowing and mouth-opening exercises for those receiving radiotherapy (NICE 2016c).

## Complications

Postoperative complications include shoulder pain and limited neck movement, which can become long-term (Guru et al. 2012), and difficult or painful swallowing, which may lead to dehydration, a 75% incidence of malnutrition (Abdelhamid et al. 2016) and a 50% incidence of aspiration (Jung et al. 2011). Positions that minimize aspiration can be identified by fluoroscopy, and exercises for dysphagia are detailed by Pauloski (2008). Respiratory complications develop in 10%–15% of patients, including atelectasis, pneumonia and respiratory failure (Genç et al. 2008).

Hospital stay is shortened by an enhanced recovery programme specific to head and neck surgery, including patient diaries, nutritional optimization, avoiding tracheostomy when possible and specific management protocols (Coyle et al. 2016). Tracheostomy can sometimes be avoided by 'debulking' the tumour, followed by chemotherapy and/or radiotherapy (NICE 2016c). Intensive dietary advice and oral nutritional supplements are required, because most patients continue to lose weight in the year following surgery (Vlooswijk et al. 2016).

For disfiguring surgery, a mirror should be given to patients only with prior explanation, and they should not be alone for their first view. Relatives also need preparation before their first visit. Women may have extra difficulty adapting if their voice has become low-pitched.

## Physiotherapy

Postoperatively, hourly deep breathing with an end-inspiratory hold may improve oxygenation (Genç et al. 2008) and patients need posture correction, with advice to avoid traction to the brachial plexus. If grafts allow, an exercise regimen begins with gentle range of motion, along with advice on supporting the shoulder and arm. Neck dissection requires progressive resistance training to regain shoulder function (NICE 2016c). A comprehensive exercise programme begins at 10–14 days, after liaising with the surgical team to ensure that there is no risk of delayed wound healing, fistula formation or carotid blowout (Guru et al. 2012).

Surgery or radiotherapy may lead to spinal accessory nerve dysfunction, requiring attention to trapezius strengthening and functional scapula movements (McGarvey et al. 2013a), with the compensatory role of rhomboid and serratus anterior accessory muscles being considered (McGarvey et al. 2013b). If the sternomastoid muscle has been excised, the patient's head will need support postoperatively during activity. Connecting tubes must also be supported. Patients need to keep the head up to minimize oedema for the first few days. Liberal mouthwashes are required, even for patients with excess salivation. Suction of the mouth should be with low pressures.

With a tracheostomy, ACBT/AD can still be performed. An incentive spirometer can be attached with a connector. Inhaled medication can be delivered by metered-dose inhaler, paediatric face mask and small volume spacer (Nandapalan 2000).

After discharge, multidisciplinary rehabilitation helps prevent social isolation and empower patients to improve their QoL (Eades et al. 2013).

## TRACHEOSTOMY

> **Stoma**: surgical opening from the inside to the outside of the body
> **Tracheostomy**: opening into the trachea
> **Tracheotomy**: surgical creation of an opening into the trachea

Breathing through a tracheostomy bypasses the nose, pharynx and larynx. The cough is weakened, and filtering and humidification functions are lost.

A tracheostomy is formed for the following reasons:
- during and after surgery, if the airway needs protection from aspiration or swelling;
- permanently after laryngectomy;
- to provide airway access for patients on ventilators or after facial trauma.

Full surgical tracheostomy is done in theatre, but percutaneous dilatational tracheotomy causes less inflammation and can be done under local anaesthesia at the bedside.

Fig. 14.18A shows the location of a tracheostomy with its tube, and 14.18B shows a permanent stoma following laryngectomy.

### Tracheostomy Tubes

For the first few days after surgery, there is an inflated cuff encircling the tube within the trachea to minimize aspiration (Fig. 14.19A).

For nonlaryngectomy patients, the cuff is deflated as soon as there is a cough reflex and swallowing is adequate. If the tube is to be removed, it will then be plugged, with the cuff deflated so that the patient can breathe, for lengthening periods until the plug can be left in situ for 4 h without distress. If oxygen is required when the tube is plugged, it needs to be delivered by face mask and not tracheostomy mask.

For laryngectomy patients, the cuffed tube is removed after about 48 h, when haemorrhage is no longer a risk, and replaced with an uncuffed tube (Fig. 14.19B). An uncuffed and hypoallergenic silver tube (Fig. 14.19C) is used for people needing a permanent tracheostomy.

Most tubes have an inner cannula (Fig. 14.19D), which increases the work of breathing (Henderson 2017) but helps prevent blockage and trauma from repeated tube changes. It is left in place for suction, but needs to be removed and cleaned regularly.

For people without a laryngectomy but requiring long-term tracheostomy, speech is possible with a fenestrated tube (Fig. 14.19E). This has inner and outer cannulae and matching windows (fenestrations) on their posterior curves. With the cuff deflated and stoma occluded by a plug or gloved finger on expiration, the patient can speak because the breath is directed out through the holes and up through the larynx. An unfenestrated inner

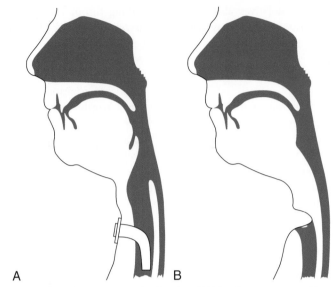

**FIGURE 14.18** (A) Tracheostomy tube in situ. (B) Tracheostomy and laryngectomy.

cannula is used for suction and when eating or drinking. Fenestrated tubes should not be used with mechanical ventilation.

A tracheostomy button (Fig. 14.19F) acts as a stent to maintain the patency of a mature stoma. It is usually kept closed and does not extend into the tracheal lumen, so if frequent suction is required it should be replaced with a tracheostomy tube to protect the back of the trachea. It is used for neurological patients who may need repeated tracheostomies, or as a step to decannulation, or during rehabilitation.

Minitracheostomies are used for suction rather than to facilitate breathing and are discussed on p. 220.

## Complications

*'We can never make the sounds of crying, shouting or laughter'*

*Ulbricht 1986*

Unavoidable complications of a tracheostomy tube are the following:

• communication difficulty;
• impaired cough because there is no closed glottis behind which pressure can build up;
• impaired swallow because of reduced muscle coordination, disturbed pressure gradients, compression of the oesophagus and anchoring of the larynx so that

swallowing feels like there is a lump in the throat, especially with an inflated cuff;
• loss of taste and smell.

Other complications are below:

1. Occlusion, which is most likely by a mucous plug.
2. Haemorrhage due to tracheal erosion into an artery. This may be obvious, or indicated by pulsation of the tracheostomy tube synchronously with the pulse. If suspected, the airway should be suctioned and cuff inflated. This will temporarily limit aspiration of blood into the lungs until medical attention arrives and bronchoscopy instigated.
3. Displacement, which can occur especially if there is uncontrolled coughing, loose tracheal ties or excessive movement of the tube in the immediate postoperative period.
4. Subcutaneous emphysema, and sometimes other forms of barotrauma (Fig. 14.20).
5. Aspiration, often without symptoms but is sometimes accompanied by an unstable breathing pattern (Martin-Harris 2012). Secretions can trickle past an inflated cuff, but aspiration is more common with the cuff deflated. A deflated cuff may be necessary during eating, but patients with neurological disorders must be assessed by a speech language therapist before cuff deflation, which should be preceded by suction above the cuff, i.e. via the mouth.

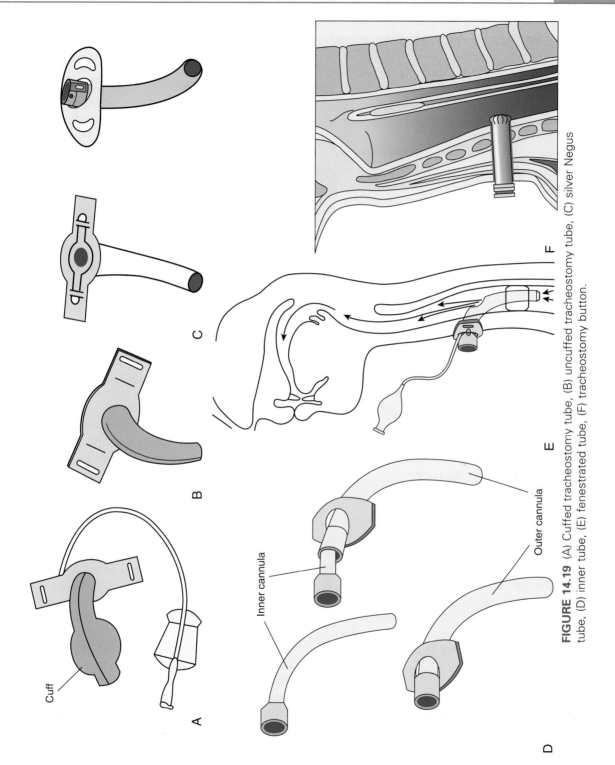

**FIGURE 14.19** (A) Cuffed tracheostomy tube, (B) uncuffed tracheostomy tube, (C) silver Negus tube, (D) inner tube, (E) fenestrated tube, (F) tracheostomy button.

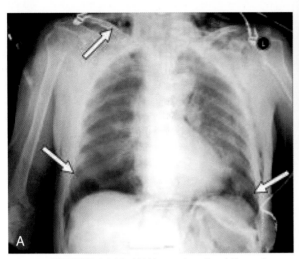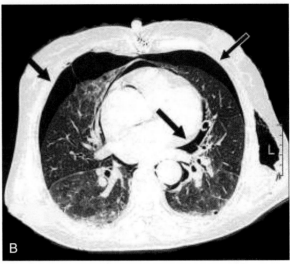

**FIGURE 14.20** (A) X-ray showing bilateral pneumothoraces, pneumomediastinum, pneumoperitoneum and subcutaneous emphysema. (B) Scan showing pneumothorax and pneumomediastinum. (From Kim & Kim 2012.)

6. Dysphagia, nausea and vomiting which are experienced if pressure is exerted on the posterior wall of the trachea and oesophagus by the wrong sized tube.
7. Weight loss that is due to dysphagia, reduced appetite or impaired taste and smell.
8. Infection, which occurs partly because the oropharynx is teeming with bacteria and partly because poor suction technique is widespread.
9. Tracheoesophageal fistula, which is suspected if suctioned secretions contain food or drink.
10. Damage to the trachea, which increases by pull on the tube if connected to a ventilator, or by mishandling.
11. Late-onset stricture following damage to the trachea, which is due to granulation tissue as eroded areas heal.
12. Stenosis, which may be indicated by cough, difficulty clearing secretions and breathlessness, occurring weeks, months or years after decannulation (Crooks et al. 2012). Laser treatment or surgery may be required.

## Management

> **KEY POINT**
>
> The greatest fear of tracheostomy patients during their early postoperative days is an inability to summon help, and a bell must always be within reach.

Patients should be under the care of a multidisciplinary tracheostomy team (Mah et al. 2017). Their bed must be in sight of the nurses' station and not in a side room. Sterile gloves should be worn for all contact with the tracheostomy site, and the patient should support the neck plate when coughing or sneezing. Questions to the patient are best framed for a 'yes' or 'no' answer, and time is needed for lip-reading and deciphering written requests.

It takes about a week after tracheostomy for fascia and muscle to fuse and form a tract from the skin to the trachea, during which time tracheal dilators are on hand in case the tube becomes dislodged. The tape securing the tube around the neck is best secured with Velcro and should be loose enough to fit one or two fingers between the tape and neck, depending on local protocol.

Two spare tracheostomy tubes must be at the bedside, one the same size and one a size smaller in case a tube change is needed urgently. Also required is an obturator, a solid insert that assists insertion of a new tracheostomy tube but which must be removed immediately after tube change so that the patient can breathe. Tracheostomy tubes should only be changed by a specifically trained nurse, physiotherapist or doctor.

With long-term tracheostomy, patients are taught to huff out their secretions, but a suction unit at home is required, with instructions to the patient and their carers on its use, and how to deal with a blocked tube (see the following section).

If hydrotherapy is undertaken, two staff are needed in the water, plus sufficient staff at the pool side for an emergency exit from the water, including one staff member proficient in tracheostomy tube change. Also required are suction, oxygen and a tracheostomy change kit. The patient needs a Swedish nose, and assistance to keep their shoulders above the water level and away from splashing patients.

## Humidification

A heat–moisture exchanger (HME) is inadequate in the acute stage, especially if oxygen is added (Chikata et al. 2013), and continuous hot water humidification is needed for the first 48 h, connected to a T-piece or tracheostomy mask. An HME can be used when mobilizing (Foreman et al. 2016). A permanent tracheostomy leads to acclimatization of the airway lining by metaplasia from respiratory to squamous epithelium. Patients will then need to maintain adequate fluid intake, and are supplied with a Swedish nose, or a bib to hang over the stoma (Fig. 14.21), which also filters out large particles. Humidification is restarted if infection occurs, and people with chronic lung disease may need a nebulizer at home to use with saline if secretions become thick.

If suction of the mouth is needed, low pressures are advised. Tracheal suction, if required, should be with the inner tube in situ. Premarked catheters should be used and deep suction avoided unless essential because of the risk of epithelial damage (Lee et al. 2016f). Patients should be assisted with mobilizing secretions, with secretions huffed out when possible.

## Communication

The majority of patients having a laryngectomy can regain communication with speech therapy, preferably begun preoperatively (Gordon 2011). Examples are:

- an electrolarynx held at the neck that produces Dalek-like speech as the user mouths the words;
- oesophageal speech, in which the patient learns to compress air into the oesophagus and release it, creating a more normal sound than the electrolarynx;
- a valve inserted into a surgical tracheo-oesophageal puncture through which patients can learn to generate another form of oesophageal speech;
- laryngeal transplants;
- text messaging or iPod touch, with which patients become expert.

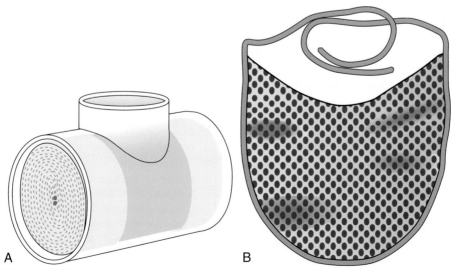

**FIGURE 14.21** (A) Swedish nose heat moisture exchanger to fit over the tracheostomy tube, and (B) bib to tie round the neck and hang over the stoma.

Speaking valves such as the Passy-Muir or Blom (Leder et al. 2013) can be used with patients who have not had a laryngectomy, including those on a ventilator. Practical points when using the Passy-Muir valve are to:

- monitor humidification and $FiO_2$;
- before connecting the valve, suction the airway, then suction above the cuff, then let the cuff down slowly, with another suction catheter prepared in case of need;
- if the patient finds it hard to breathe, or they are unable to speak or they begin to sound wheezy, remove the valve and identify the cause of the problem;
- ensure that the valve is removed for sleep to avoid impaired gas exchange due to extra dead space, and ask the patient to take precautions against falling asleep with the valve in situ;
- increase tolerance gradually to allow accommodation to the extra dead space.

## Nutrition

The speech language therapist assesses for swallowing with cuff inflation and deflation. When eating, the patient sits up if possible, flexes the neck slightly and then the cuff is deflated if safe to do so. Sips of sterile water are initially given, and if tolerated without coughing, desaturation, fatigue or signs of aspiration, then thickened fluids may be introduced, followed by a soft diet. The patient should stay sitting upright for 20 min after eating.

## Inner tube change

Local policy varies about frequency of change. A suggested procedure is to:

- explain the procedure, preoxygenate and suction if required;
- ask the patient to slightly extend the head;
- support the neck plate with one gloved hand;
- unlock or unclip the inner cannula with the other gloved hand, then remove the inner tube outwards and downwards, while stabilizing the tracheostomy tube;
- insert a new inner cannula and ensure that it is locked or clipped into place;
- discard the old inner cannula, or clean with sterile water or normal saline and foam sponges, then leave to air dry.

## Blocked Tracheostomy Tube

Half of airway-related deaths are attributable to complications such as occlusion or displacement, and information on the nature of the stoma and who to contact in an emergency should be clearly displayed (Darr et al. 2016). If a tracheostomy tube becomes blocked with thick secretions, blood or a foreign body, as shown by difficulty breathing or respiratory arrest, the steps in Box 14.2 should be taken (ICS 2008). The crash team should have arrived before this is completed, but the steps may be needed in quick succession.

Once the patient is stabilized, a new tracheostomy tube can be reinserted by a suitably experienced member

---

**BOX 14.2  Management of a Blocked Tracheostomy Tube**

1. Press the crash button and call for help.
2. Explain to the patient what is happening while encouraging them to cough.
3. If this is not sufficient, remove the inner cannula.
4. If this is not sufficient, suction the airway.
5. If this is not sufficient, deflate the cuff.
6. If this is not sufficient, move the patient's head in case this relieves the obstruction.
7. If the patient is breathing, apply oxygen to the tracheostomy, or to the nose and mouth if the natural airway is patent (and there is no inflated cuff), or to both, which may require oxygen from the crash trolley as well as the wall/cylinder.
8. If the patient is not breathing, ventilate by attaching the resuscitation bag to the tracheostomy tube, or by blowing down the stoma, using a paediatric face-mask or laryngeal mask airway if available, while occluding the nose and mouth (or use a resuscitation bag and mask to the nose and mouth if patent, while occluding the stoma).
9. If this is inadequate, remove the tracheostomy tube:
   - cut the securing tape or undo the Velcro;
   - insert a suction catheter to allow oxygen administration;
   - slide out the tube over the catheter, using tracheal dilators to maintain patency of the stoma;
   - continue ventilation, keeping tracheal dilators in situ, by either encouraging the patient to breathe spontaneously, or blowing down the stoma;
   - if the airway is still blocked, suction with a Yankauer or other large-bore suction catheter.

of the team, or a nasopharyngeal tube can be temporarily used.

## Discharge

Patients with permanent tracheostomies should receive a full checklist of emergency supplies and the following information:

- how to remove a blocked tube and replace it in an emergency;
- sterile suction procedure;
- protecting the stoma from water and dust;
- the importance of winter flu vaccination, and avoiding people with chest infections;
- instructions for carers on mouth-to-stoma resuscitation;
- a contact number in case of problems;
- information on support groups.

Decannulation of a tracheostomy tube is described on p. 457.

## CASE STUDY: MR LS[a]

*Identify the problems of this 74-year-old man 2 days after a left upper lobectomy for small cell carcinoma.*

### Subjective

- Pain on coughing
- Bringing up thick green phlegm
- Unable to sleep

### Objective

- Notes: pseudomonas chest infection;
- Charts: intermittent intramuscular analgesia, pyrexia, $SpO_2$ 94%, no target saturation documented;
- Patient slumped in bed, on 40% dry oxygen;
- Rapid, shallow breathing pattern;
- Auscultation: ↓ BS LLL, coarse crackles;
- AP film shows two fluid-filled cavities in the left upper zone (Fig. 14.22A), which the lateral film shows to be in the LUL (Fig. 14.22B). Scan at tracheal level identifies the largest cavity (Fig. 14.22C). Radiology report states that these may relate to an abscess, empyema or bronchopleural fistula.

[a]*BS*, Breath sounds; *LLL*, left lower lobe; *LUL*, left upper lobe; *PA*, postero-anterior.

### Questions

1. Analysis?
2. Patient's problems?
3. Precaution?
4. Plan?

**CLINICAL REASONING**

Comment on the following:

*A trial concluded that 'the routine use of respiratory physiotherapy after abdominal surgery does not seem to be justified'.*
  *The key words excluded 'positioning' and 'exercise'.*
  *Methods: 'trials were included if they investigated prophylactic respiratory physiotherapy'.*
                    *Chest (2006):130:1887–1899*

### Response to Case Study

1. Analysis

```
┌─ Inadequate analgesia
├→ Pain
├→ Loss of lung volume
├→ Potential sputum retention
├→ Poor sleep ──────────┐
└→ Potential poor motivation ←
```

↓ BS over LLL and raised left hemidiaphragm indicates atelectasis (the lower lobe would expand to fill much of the space from the lobectomy, i.e. these signs are not just attributable to removal of the upper lobe).

2. Problems
   - Pain
   - Poor sleep
   - ↓ Lung volume LLL → poor gas exchange
   - Potential sputum retention → poor gas exchange

3. Precaution
   - Avoid right side-lying position to prevent infected fluid spreading from abscess or bronchopleural fistula.

4. Plan
   - Liaise with team to optimize analgesia, instigate pain chart and documentation of target $SpO_2$ and its monitoring;

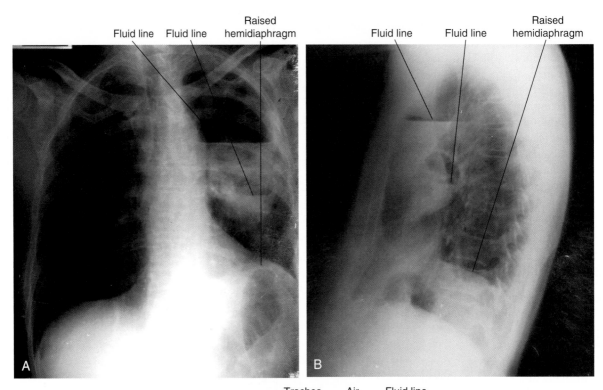

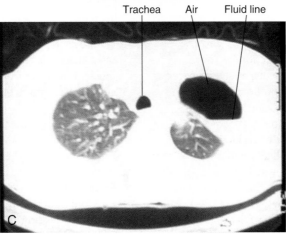

**FIGURE 14.22** Mr LS.

- Identify cause of poor sleep, e.g. pain/anxiety/noise, then remedy with the team;
- Humidify oxygen;
- Identify goals with patient, then initiate, according to patient preference:
  - controlled mobilization;
  - sitting out in chair;
  - deep breathing, end-inspiratory hold, incentive spirometry;
  - ACBT or positive pressure device or both, to clear secretions;
  - when drip is down, monitor fluid balance;
  - progressive exercise programme to include shoulder range of motion, posture and exercise tolerance, using tick chart and involving family.

## RESPONSE TO CLINICAL REASONING

The authors appear to be confusing 'prophylactic' with 'routine'.

Positioning and exercise are techniques that might be used prophylactically after surgery (and selectively, not routinely).

# RECOMMENDED READING

Amri, R., Bordeianou, L.G., Sylla, P., et al., 2014. Obesity, outcomes and quality of care: body mass index increases the risk of wound-related complications in colon cancer surgery. Am. J. Surg. 207 (1), 17–23.

Brand, L.R., 2013. The effect of hand massage on preoperative anxiety in ambulatory surgery patients. AORN J. 97 (6), 708–717.

Brocki, B.C., Andreasen, J., Nielsen, L.R., et al., 2013. Short and long-term effects of supervised versus unsupervised exercise training on health-related quality of life and functional outcomes following lung cancer surgery. Lung Cancer 83 (1), 102–108.

D'Agostino, R.S., Jacobs, J.P., Badhwar, V., et al., 2017. The Society of Thoracic Surgeons adult cardiac surgery database. Ann. Thorac. Surg. 103 (1), 18–24.

Damian, D., Esquenazi, J., Duvvuri, U., et al., 2016. Incidence, outcome, and risk factors for postoperative pulmonary complications in head and neck cancer surgery patients with free flap reconstructions. J. Clin. Anesth. 28, 12–18.

Guo, Y., Sun, L., Li, L., et al., 2016. Impact of multicomponent, nonpharmacologic interventions on perioperative cortisol and melatonin levels and postoperative delirium in elderly oral cancer patients. Arch. Gerontol. Geriatr. 62, 112–117.

Hansen, D., Roijakkers, R., Jacvkmaert, L., 2017. Compromised cardiopulmonary exercise capacity in patients early after endoscopic atraumatic coronary artery bypass graft: implications for rehabilitation. Am. J. Phys. Med. Rehabil. 96 (2), 84–92.

Havey, R., Herriman, E., O'Brien, D., 2013. Guarding the gut: early mobility after abdominal surgery. Crit. Care Nurs. Q. 36 (1), 63–72.

Ibañez, J., Riera, M., Amezaga, R., et al., 2016. Long-term mortality after pneumonia in cardiac surgery patients. J. Intensive. Care Med. 31 (1), 34–40.

Lugg, S.T., Agostini, P.J., Tikka, T., et al., 2016. Long-term impact of developing a postoperative pulmonary complication after lung surgery. Thorax 71 (2), 171–176.

Morris, L.L., Afifi, M.S., 2010. Tracheostomies: The Complete Guide. Springer, New York.

Peres, A.C.A.M., 2017. Body posture after mastectomy. Phys. Res. Intern. 22 (1), e1642.

Perry, A., Lee, S.H., Cotton, S., et al., 2016. Therapeutic exercises for affecting post-treatment swallowing in people treated for advanced-stage head and neck cancers. Cochrane Database Syst. Rev. (8), CD011112.

Pryor, L.N., Baldwin, C.E., Ward, E.C., et al., 2016. Tracheostomy tube type and inner cannula selection impact pressure and resistance to air flow. Respir. Care 61 (5), 607–661.

Pryor, L.N., Ward, E.C., Cornwell, P.L., et al., 2016. Clinical indicators associated with successful tracheostomy cuff deflation. Aust. Crit. Care 29 (3), 132–137.

Satoh, Y., 2016. Management of chest drainage tubes after lung surgery. Gen. Thorac. Cardiovasc. Surg. 64 (6), 305–308.

Schenker, Y., 2016. An enhanced role for palliative care in the multidisciplinary approach to high-risk head and neck cancer. Cancer 122 (3), 340–343.

Vandrevala, T., Senior, V., Spring, L., et al., 2016. 'Am I really ready to go home?': a qualitative study of patients' experience of early discharge following an enhanced recovery programme for liver resection surgery. Support. Care Cancer 24 (8), 3447–3454.

# 15

# Infants

*Kath Ronchetti, Paul Ritson, Alexandra Hough*

## LEARNING OBJECTIVES

*On completion of this chapter the reader should be able to:*
- describe the anatomical and physiological differences between adults and infants;
- discuss the common medical and surgical conditions of infants;
- understand the principles of care for infants on a neonatal intensive care unit;
- identify the main physiotherapy problems in relation to neonatal conditions, and describe their management.

## OUTLINE

## INTRODUCTION

Central to a baby's universe is his or her mother. Separation at birth is felt by both mother and baby (Nagasawa et al. 2012) and for the infant this can lead to possible neural dysfunction in later life (Wieck et al. 2013). Babies need to hear and feel their mother, and parents should be involved in their care and comfort. Handling by health staff can destabilize preterm infants, but stroking and gentle handling may be beneficial (Harrison 1996) whereas handling by the mother can reduce stress and oxygen consumption (Ludington 1990).

Premature infants are those born before 37 weeks' gestation. Neonates are preterm or term infants up to 28 days after birth. Infants are children under 1 year old.

## How the Neonatal Cardiorespiratory System Works

Infants are not small adults. Their different cardiorespiratory systems (Table 15.1) mean that changes are more abrupt.

### Prematurity

> *The emergence of the baby into the outside world is perhaps the most cataclysmic event of his or her life*
> **West (2016) p.176**

The birth of an infant at <32 weeks' gestation is a medical emergency (McCormick & Litt 2017). The preterm infant is in effect a displaced foetus, experiencing heightened responses to external stimuli (Honda

**TABLE 15.1   Cardiorespiratory differences between infants and adults**

| Difference | Effect | Clinical implications |
|---|---|---|
| Ribs more horizontal. Chest has greater AP diameter (Fig. 15.1). | No bucket handle motion. Diaphragm at a mechanical disadvantage. | Less able to increase $V_T$ therefore need to ↑ RR in response to heavy workload. |
| Thoracic cage more compliant due to ribs being more cartilaginous. Underdeveloped intercostal muscles. | Less thoracic cage stability. Breathing predominantly diaphragmatic. FRC sometimes below closing volume. | Recession of the thoracic cage in response to heavy workload until age 2. In side-lying, dependant lung is more difficult to expand. Expiratory vibrations can ↓ FRC, but manual techniques are better transmitted to lungs. |
| Less diaphragmatic fibres are of the fatigue-resistant slow-twitch variety (25% in neonates, 50% at 8 months old). | More prone to fatigue. | Limited reserve. Prompt intervention required if fatigue becomes evident. |
| Narrow airways. | Increased airflow resistance. | Airflow obstruction with small amount of secretions or inflammation. |
| Immature respiratory control. | RR varies widely and is more responsive to disease and emotion. | Irregular breathing and episodes of apnoea. |
| Fewer and smaller alveoli: neonatal lungs possess only 25% of their alveolar potential, with rapid increase in first 2 years of life. | Reduced area for gas exchange. | Hypoxaemia can develop quickly. Hypoxaemia may cause ↓ cardiac output. |
| Immature cilia. More mucus glands. | Less effective mucociliary transport. | ↑ risk of retained secretions, airway collapse and infection. |
| Lack of collateral channels: pores of Kohn develop age 1–2, channels of Lambert and channels of Martin from 6 years. | Less ability for air to bypass an area of collapse. | Tendency to retention of secretions and atelectasis. |
| Soft tracheal cartilage. | Reduced support of airway. | Prone to tracheal occlusion. |
| Predominately nasal breathers, mouth normally reserved for ingestion, exploration and communication. Relatively large tonsils, adenoids and tongue. | Vulnerable if upper airway obstruction. | Nasal secretions or NG tube can increase WOB. Unable to feed if nasally congested. |
| BP regulation is unrefined. | | BP and cardiac output more sensitive to stimuli. |
| Underdeveloped sympathetic nervous system. | Hypoxaemia tends to cause bradycardia rather than tachycardia. | Stressors such as handling can lead to apnoeic episodes and bradycardia. |

*AP,* anteroposterior; *BP,* blood pressure; *bpm,* beats per minute; *FRC,* functional residual capacity; *NG,* nasogastric; *RR,* respiratory rate; $V_T$, tidal volume; *WOB,* work of breathing. (Adapted from Jauncey-Cooke et al. 2015, Gao & Raj 2010, Minowa et al. 2016.)

2013) and being more in need of skin-to-skin contact (Buil et al. 2016). The respiratory system expects to provide only intermittent stretch to stimulate structural development of the lung, not deliver oxygenation, so 'apnoea of prematurity' occurs intermittently until term gestation (Di Fiore et al. 2013).

Prematurity leaves the infant with limited defence mechanisms and sometimes without the basic capacity for temperature control. They are at risk of long-term cognitive and neurobehavioral problems (Hauglann et al. 2015), which has led some units to monitor cerebral oxygen saturation (Baik et al. 2015). Prematurity

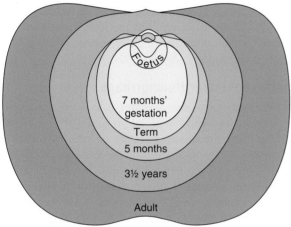

FIGURE 15.1 Changes in anteroposterior chest configuration with age. (From Wilkins et al. 2010.)

also predisposes to bone disease (Arani et al. 2015), reduced exercise capacity, respiratory disease (Lowe et al. 2016) and hypertension (Fig. 15.2), which may last into adulthood (Tikanmäki et al. 2016). Surfactant is not produced until 35 weeks' gestation.

## Care of the Family

*Feeling her minute pink fingers holding so hard to mine, I was hit sideways and bowled over by the purest, tenderest, most passionately committed love I have ever felt…*

*Every time I touched her, she relaxed and the monitors showed it, her heart rate settled, her limbs were calmer, her eyes searched less frantically about…*

*I had never held her to me and I ached to do so, she seemed so alone in there amongst all the wires and drips and tubes and monitors.*

**Hill 1989**

Parents need to be involved in all aspects of care in order to reduce the helplessness that is one of the greatest stresses for parents (Matricardi et al. 2013) and to help avoid the 'medicalization of parenting'. Parental presence during invasive procedures is recommended and, with support, during resuscitation, if acceptable to the parent (Curley et al. 2013). Parents require confidence in their own competence and credit for being the experts on their children. Diary writing has been found helpful

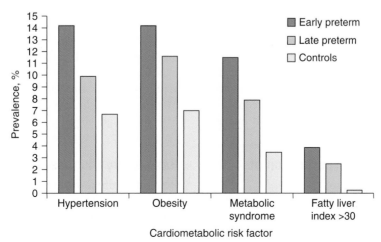

FIGURE 15.2 Increased likelihood of developing cardiometabolic disorders in people born prematurely. (From Sipola et al. 2015.)

(Kadivar et al. 2016) as well as unrestricted visiting, including grandparents and siblings. Siblings require involvement because they may feel a variety of responses including jealousy, anxiety, isolation and guilt. If their brother or sister is disabled, they are likely to suffer bullying at school, as are preterm-born children (Wolke et al. 2015).

## MEDICAL CONDITIONS

### Meconium Aspiration Syndrome

Infants who suffer distress in utero or asphyxia during labour or Caesarean section (Swarnam et al. 2012) may pass meconium (faecal material) before birth, then gasp and suck it into their mouth. Meconium aspiration occurs when this material is inhaled into the lungs, leading to 5%–10% developing meconium aspiration syndrome (Chettri et al. 2015), manifesting as alveolar inflammation, surfactant depletion and epithelial injury. Hypoxaemia, poor lung compliance and sometimes pneumothorax ensue. Airflow obstruction causes gas trapping if incomplete, and atelectasis if complete.

Surfactant replacement and supplemental oxygen are required, and a nonvigorous infant may need continuous positive airway pressure (CPAP). Nearly half require mechanical ventilation (MV), sometimes with high pressures to ventilate the stiff lungs, leading to a 15%–30% incidence of barotrauma and 5%–12% mortality (Nangia et al. 2016). High-frequency ventilation, inhaled surfactant or extracorporeal membrane oxygenation (ECMO) may allow the lungs to recover with less risk of barotrauma.

If caught early, physiotherapy may clear the fresh meconium by intensive postural drainage, percussion, vibrations, saline instillation and suction as required. This is continued until secretions are free from the dark colour of meconium. Suction alone produces mixed results, different studies showing that this reduces the need for bag and mask ventilation, or that it increases the need for MV (Nangia et al. 2016).

### Persistent Pulmonary Hypertension of the Newborn

In utero, a high pulmonary vascular resistance shunts blood away from the lungs and through the ductus arteriosus. After birth, the pulmonary circulation dilates within a few breaths, enabling oxygen to enter the bloodstream so that the placental circulation becomes redundant, pulmonary vascular resistance reduces fivefold and pulmonary blood flow increases threefold (Hughes 2016). If the pulmonary circulation does not dilate, the pressure in the lungs remains high and the ductus arteriosus stays open, shunting blood away from the lungs and through the patent foramen ovale, leading to profound hypoxaemia.

Risk factors are infection, prematurity, and maternal diabetes, obesity or advanced age (Steurer et al. 2017). Signs are cyanosis, tachypnoea, respiratory distress, hypoxaemia and tachycardia, and diagnosis is by echocardiography and oximetry. Medical management is with sildenafil or selective pulmonary vasodilators, steroids, inhaled nitric oxide (iNO), surfactant and/or ECMO. Oxygen is given, but the high shunt limits its benefit. Complications include pneumothorax and acute kidney injury (Nakwan 2016).

### Intraventricular Haemorrhage

Prematurity may cause bleeding into the cerebral ventricles due to swings in blood pressure (BP) or arterial blood gases. Precipitating factors are pain (Mainous & Looney 2011), intubation without sedation (Wren 1989), repeated intubation attempts (Sauer et al. 2016), early cord clamping (Katheria et al. 2016), extreme prematurity (Durães et al. 2016) and MV (Aly et al. 2012). Physiotherapy is contraindicated, including suction unless essential.

### Pulmonary Haemorrhage

Pulmonary haemorrhage is an acute, often catastrophic event in which bleeding may involve more than a third of the lungs, sometimes spreading to other areas (Zahr et al. 2012). Causes are prematurity, birth asphyxia, bleeding disorders, toxaemia of pregnancy, breech birth, hypothermia, respiratory distress syndrome or interventions such as surfactant administration or ECMO. Management includes immediate suction, oxygen and MV with high airway pressures to inhibit the bleed. Physiotherapy is contraindicated.

### Respiratory Distress Syndrome

Respiratory distress syndrome (RDS) is the commonest cause of death in the preterm infant (Smart & Princivalle 2012). Lack of surfactant leads to patchy atelectasis, stiff lungs and increased work of breathing (WOB). Alveoli inflate with difficulty and collapse between respiratory efforts. Signs of respiratory distress develop in the first hours of life. Reduced breath sounds are heard on auscultation, along with faint crepitations. The X-ray shows hyperinflation, mottling and air bronchograms. Respiratory distress may persist for 24–48 h, followed by improvement over several days as surfactant is produced, or protracted disease.

Prevention is by prophylactic instillation of artificial surfactant on delivery of preterm babies, administered in different positions to ensure even distribution (Rojas-Reyes et al. 2012).

Management is by regulation of temperature, fluid and nutrition, and respiratory support with humidified high-flow oxygen (Lavizzari et al. 2016), CPAP, noninvasive ventilation, low-pressure MV (Kallio et al. 2016), and sometimes ECMO or iNO. Both oxygen and MV come with their own complications:

- oxidative stress (an imbalance between oxidative reactive species and antioxidant defences) predisposes to chronic lung disease of prematurity (Ozsurekci 2016);
- high-pressure ventilation in surfactant-deficient alveoli can lead to atelectrauma, and high tidal volumes can cause barotrauma.

Physiotherapy is limited to advice on positioning in the early stages. Prone improves oxygenation (Di Fiore et al. 2013) and periods in alternate side-lying assist secretion mobilization and postural orientation, with the head of the incubator raised to minimize reflux. Intubation irritates the airways and may stimulate excess secretions, which need to be cleared in the recovery phase when the infant is stable, usually with suction and occasionally with manual techniques. Monitoring should be continuous, especially in prone. Manual hyperinflation is contraindicated because of the risk of gas trapping and air leaks, but if high-frequency ventilation is used, individualized oxygenation-guided lung recruitment through the ventilator can stabilize lung volume, with a low risk of air leaks (De Jaegere et al. 2016).

Late-gestation RDS is associated with birth asphyxia and encephalopathy rather than surfactant deficiency (Mehrabadi et al. 2016).

## Chronic Lung Disease (CLD) of Prematurity

With prematurity comes the risk of a continuum of lung injury, progressing from RDS, sometimes pulmonary interstitial emphysema (p. 447) and then CLD, also known as bronchopulmonary dysplasia. The process is exacerbated if the infant has required high volume MV.

Inflammation is the basis of CLD, interfering with surfactant production and leading to scarring, disordered lung growth, stiff lungs and pulmonary hypertension, which strains the right ventricle (Xie et al. 2016). Signs are persistent respiratory distress and high oxygen requirements. X-ray changes vary from 'grey' lungs to widespread cystic areas or hyperinflation (Dassios et al. 2016).

Treatment is by minimally invasive surfactant instillation (Rigo et al. 2016), steroids, targeted $SpO_2$, caffeine, vitamin A, optimum nutrition and if necessary lung protective ventilation. An unstable breathing pattern may indicate the need to increase $FiO_2$ (Coste et al. 2015) but oxygen therapy must be finely tuned.

The damaged lungs are prone to recurrent infection and atelectasis, for which physiotherapy is often indicated. Depending on presentation and age, this may entail alternate side-lying with the head elevated, manual techniques and suction. Manual hyperinflation may be required if atelectasis is present in an intubated baby without air leak. Treatment should be modified or discontinued if the child becomes wheezy or develops pulmonary hypertension.

After long hospitalization, parents need comprehensive preparation for discharge so that they build up confidence and do not feel that they have 'borrowed' their baby to take home. Domiciliary oxygen or noninvasive ventilation may be needed, and sometimes advice on physiotherapy. Adult survivors continue to experience respiratory symptoms and low exercise tolerance (Caskey et al. 2016).

## Bronchiolitis

Acute viral bronchiolitis is the most common disorder in infants under age 2, with respiratory syncytial virus being the main culprit (Allen 2016). Infection depletes the mucous layer water content, damages epithelial architecture and impairs mucociliary clearance. Sputum retention and mucosal oedema lead to airway obstruction and hyperinflation. Signs are excess oral secretions, wheeze, fine crackles, nasal congestion and breathlessness. Air trapping may prevent sternal recession, unlike croup or pneumonia.

Treatment is by maintenance of the head-up position, environmental temperature regulation, hydration, assisted feeding and minimal handling. Medication is not indicated (NICE 2016d). Hospital admission is required if there is:

- grunting (exhaling through a closed glottis to generate intrinsic PEEP, equivalent to pursed lip breathing in adults);
- chest recessions and cyanosis;
- RR >50/min or below normal;
- apnoea for more than 10 s;
- exhaustion (sleepiness, irritability or floppiness);
- feeding at less than $\frac{1}{2}$ to $\frac{3}{4}$ of normal, or no wet nappy for 12 h (NICE 2016d).

Oxygen therapy can be fine-tuned by using lung ultrasound (Basile et al. 2015), with some positive pressure provided via humidified high-flow nasal cannulae, or CPAP if required (Turnham et al. 2017). Noninvasive or invasive ventilation may be needed, but can be minimized by good fluid balance (Ferlini et al. 2016).

Nebulized saline is usually beneficial, using either normal saline half-hourly for mild disease (Anil et al. 2010) or 3% hypertonic saline to reduce airway oedema (Khanal et al. 2015). Nasal irrigation with saline may improve $SpO_2$ but not wheeze or RR (Schreiber et al. 2016a). Physiotherapy with manual techniques is not recommended in the acute stage because of the risk of desaturation, wheeze or vomiting (Roqué et al. 2016). If sputum retention is a problem, and the infant has been stabilized, an experienced physiotherapist can sometimes coax the secretions to mobilize using modified postural drainage, manual techniques, assisted autogenic drainage manual hyperinflation and saline instillation. For spontaneously breathing infants, nasal suction may be required to maintain patent nostrils, but deep suctioning is inadvisable (Ralston et al. 2014).

The acute illness normally subsides in a week, with recovery over 2–3 weeks, but over 50% of infants experience recurrent cough and wheeze (Midulla et al. 2012).

**Bronchiolitis obliterans** is a particularly severe form of the disease in which inflammation partially obliterates the small airways, causing ventilation inhomogeneity and gas trapping (Gur et al. 2016) and leading to long-term obstructive airway disease (Colom et al. 2015).

## Tracheobronchomalacia

Repeated upper airway infections or prolonged intubation can lead to softened airway cartilages, causing a cough, harsh wheeze, chest recession and sputum, especially with increased workloads such as crying, feeding, pain or discomfort. Often the first sign is inability to wean from MV. The condition is resistant to steroids and inhaled bronchodilators, and diagnosis by CT scan

obviates the need for bronchoscopy (Chetambath 2016). Protracted ventilatory support and tracheostomy may be needed until the infant grows and the cartilaginous rings become more rigid.

If physiotherapy is required, positive pressure in the airway must be maintained to minimize airway collapse, unless a stent has been inserted. This is provided if the infant is receiving MV, but spontaneously-breathing infants benefit from an age-appropriate positive expiratory device (PEP) device.

## Spinal Muscular Atrophy

This autosomal recessive neuromuscular disease is characterized by degeneration of alpha motor neurons in the spinal cord, resulting in progressive weakness, predominately in the proximal limb muscles. The most severe and common form presents within months of birth, the infant showing profound hypotonia, little or no antigravity movements, no head control and no independent sitting. Inspiratory muscle weakness leads to paradoxical breathing, diminished lung and chest wall development, hypoventilation and areas of atelectasis. Expiratory muscle weakness results in poor cough and inadequate airway clearance (Gormley 2014). Involvement of the bulbar motor neurons leads to poor swallow. The combination leads to respiratory infections, which, if untreated, are the prime cause of mortality. Respiratory support includes noninvasive ventilation and assisted cough, and some neuroprotection might be created by prudent exercise (Chali et al. 2016).

## Gastro-Oesophageal Reflux

Gastro-oesophageal reflux (GOR) is common, sometimes causing severe hypoxaemia and bradycardia with feeding (Minowa et al. 2016).

## SURGICAL CONDITIONS

The commonest major postoperative complications in newborns are haemodynamic compromise, multisystem failure and respiratory failure requiring mechanical ventilation (Michelet et al. 2016).

## Congenital Heart Disease (CHD)

CHD is the most common birth defect, usually identified by routine oximetry (Saxena et al. 2015). Classification is according to whether the baby is blue or not (Table 15.2), cyanosis indicating that 30%–40% of the

## TABLE 15.2   Noncyanotic and cyanotic congenital heart disease

| Acyanotic defects | Cyanotic defects |
| --- | --- |
| Ventricular septal defect | Tetralogy of Fallot |
| Atrial septal defect | Transposition of the great arteries |
| Patent ductus arteriosus | Tricuspid atresia |
| Aortic stenosis | Total anomalous pulmonary venous drainage |
| Pulmonary stenosis | Truncus arteriosus (may be acyanotic) |
| Coarctation of the aorta | Pulmonary atresia with VSD |
| Atrioventricular septal defect | Pulmonary atresia with intact ventricular septum |
| Aorto-pulmonary window | Hypoplastic left-sided heart syndrome |
| Partial anomalous pulmonary venous drainage | Ebstein anomaly of the tricuspid valve |

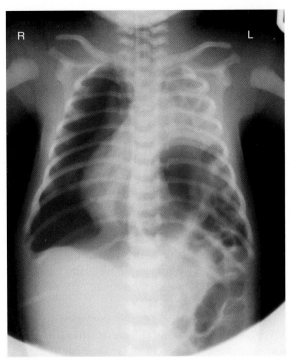

**FIGURE 15.3** Left congenital diaphragmatic hernia, showing bowel gas in left hemithorax, plus right tension pneumothorax.

blood supply is shunted from the right to left side of the heart without passing through the lungs. Other features are compression atelectasis from an enlarged heart (Healy et al. 2012), pulmonary oedema and, later, atherosclerosis (Lui et al. 2017), obesity (Lerman 2017) and exercise intolerance (Ginde et al. 2013). Over 90% of patients survive to adulthood (Zomer 2013), but cerebral oxygen saturation is low in the days after birth (Mebius et al. 2016), and persistent cognitive deficits are observed in more than half the survivors (Birca et al. 2016).

Defects require immediate repair, sometimes in utero (Pedra et al. 2014). Staged surgery may be needed throughout life. Complications of repair include:

- damage to the recurrent laryngeal nerve, leading to a weak cough, hoarse voice, difficulty weaning from MV and vocal cord palsy;
- damage to the phrenic nerve, causing unilateral diaphragmatic palsy, which may require further surgery to make tucks in the diaphragm;
- hypoxia, especially in the first postoperative hours (Andrés et al. 2015).

Physiotherapy precautions are the following:

1. The target saturation should be ascertained before treatment, as specified in the notes. Supplemental oxygen can upset the balance between pulmonary and systemic blood flow (AARC 2002b).
2. Robust analgesia is required, e.g. neuraxial drugs added to local anaesthesia (Walker 2012).
3. Newly diagnosed infants with transposition of the arteries are on a drug called dinoprostone (Prostin) to maintain a patent ductus arteriosus. The antagonist to this drug is oxygen, so medical staff should be consulted before $FiO_2$ is increased as this may cause the duct to close.
4. Infants can desaturate spectacularly and without warning if they become stressed.

## Congenital Diaphragmatic Hernia

If the diaphragm fails to fuse properly during foetal development, the abdominal contents herniate up into the thorax (Fig. 15.3), inhibiting lung development and leading to pulmonary hypertension and lung hypoplasia. Antenatal diagnosis by ultrasound improves the likelihood of safe delivery and timely surgery, but respiratory insufficiency may be lethal (Burgos et al. 2017). Physiotherapy depends on cardiovascular stability.

## Necrotizing Enterocolitis

This condition is characterized by bowel necrosis and multisystem failure, sometimes precipitated by exposure to antibiotics (Shimamura 2016). Early detection is via biomarkers (Ng et al. 2015) but it typically becomes evident in the second to third week of life, with abdominal distension, bloody stools and air in the bowel wall. Prevention is aided by breastfeeding and probiotics (Müller et al. 2016). Supportive care is by bowel rest with parenteral nutrition, gastric decompression and control of fluids, electrolytes and BP, and continuous morphine because of extreme pain associated with the condition (Meesters et al. 2016).

If the abdomen is sufficiently distended to require MV, physiotherapy consists of assessment to ascertain if respiratory care is needed, and involvement in the team management of positioning, usually avoiding prone and supine. Bowel perforation requires resection of the dead bowel and/or formation of a colostomy.

## Oesophageal Atresia With Tracheo-Oesophageal Fistula

Discontinuation or atresia of the oesophagus is usually combined with a connection or fistula between the oesophagus and trachea, the most common being oesophageal atresia with a distal fistula (Fig. 15.4). Aspiration of oral feeds leads to rattly breathing and inability to tolerate feeds, attempts leading to choking episodes or cyanosis. Surgery is required. Preoperative chest clearance is not needed if the rattly breathing only relates to the upper airway.

Postoperative physiotherapy is indicated if there is secondary lung disease due to repeated aspiration. Airway clearance may include manual techniques in modified postural drainage positions, assisted autogenic drainage, PEP devices and activity.

## NEONATAL INTENSIVE CARE

*The quiet epidemic of extreme prematurity rolls on. Left in the wake are infants and children with diminished function, particularly in the brain and lung.*

***Truog 2015***

The neonatal intensive care unit (NICU) provides the technology and skill to care for sick infants or those born prematurely. It is not an ideal environment for the baby, with its bright lights, noise that can be 10 times above recommended levels (Marik 2013), frequent disturbance and resistant bacteria (Akturk et al. 2016). The infant's neurological system is vulnerable to injury, sensory bombardment and the deprivation of normal stimuli or maternal skin contact (Symington & Pinelli 2009). Bonding between child and mother is hindered by the barrier of the incubator and the mother's fear of touching equipment. Premature NICU 'graduates' show a 6% incidence of major neurodisability (Sujatha 2016), and follow-up clinics are advised (Ralser et al. 2012).

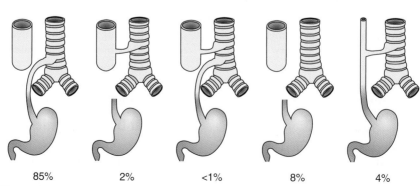

85%    2%    <1%    8%    4%

**FIGURE 15.4** Percentage incidence of variations in oesophageal atresia with tracheo-oesophageal fistula. (From Smith 2014.)

## Stress Management

The brain undergoes a dramatic sequence of maturation in the third trimester of pregnancy and the first months of postnatal life. Untimely exposure to some environmental influences, especially in preterm infants, can affect brain function throughout life (Arichi et al. 2012).

> **KEY POINT**
>
> A stressed parent means a stressed baby

Parents benefit from help to cuddle their child when attached to awesome equipment, and advice on stroking, which reduces stress and improves sleep (Parashar et al. 2016), and massage, which can improve growth in preterm infants, alleviate motor problems and enhance immune function (Matricardi et al. 2013).

Skin-to-skin and chest-to-chest contact ('kangaroo care') with a parent (Fig. 15.5) shows improvements in pain, $SpO_2$ (Boundy et al. 2016), survival, neurodevelopment, as well as long-term social and behavioural benefits over 20 years (Charpak et al. 2017). Benefit is greatest when started straight after birth and maintained for as much time as possible (Blomqvist et al. 2013). Being close to the mother brings the added advantage for the infant of being close to her familiar heartbeat, smell and voice (Welch 2012). Marx & Nagy (2015) found that the foetus responds to her voice and touch in the 21st to 33rd week of gestation.

### Noise and light

> *The NICU environment … should be as close as possible to that of the intra-uterine environment.*
> **Rakhetla 2016**

The auditory, visual and central nervous systems are the last to mature, and for premature babies these stages occur in the incubator. Cerebral plasticity and cognitive development are intimately linked to early sensory experience (Lejeune et al. 2016), but noise and light are consistently above recommended levels in the NICU (Capó 2016). Noise, especially from alarms, provoking a painlike stress response, leading to disrupted sensory learning, BP, sleep, neurological development, breathing (Lejeune et al. 2016 and Fig. 15.6), and even DNA damage (Ceylan et al. 2016). Simple remedies are ear muffs, soft-close bins, dimmed lights when not needed, avoidance of equipment on top of the incubator and quiet conversation.

### Sleep

Babies require 16 h of sleep per day, evenly distributed in 2–4 h periods (Primhak & Kingshott 2012). Maintenance of this pattern promotes brain development

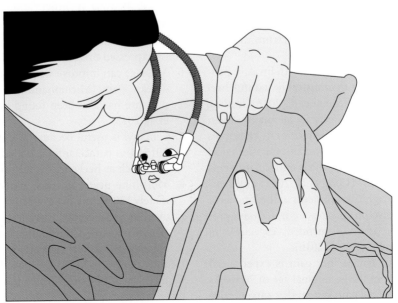

**FIGURE 15.5** Kangaroo care, a baby's ideal ecological niche.

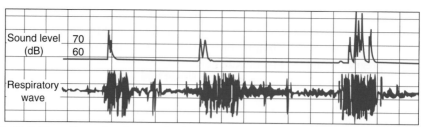

**FIGURE 15.6** The effect of noise on the breathing pattern of a premature infant. (From Long et al. 1980.)

(Tarullo et al. 2012). This is aided by an 'I am sleeping till … pm' sign above the cot.

## Pain

*Painful procedures in the NICU are common, undertreated and lead to adverse consequences.*

**Hall 2012**

Newborns are more sensitive to pain than children or adults, and preterm infants even more so (Courtois et al. 2016). The physiological effects of neonatal pain are:
- ↑ BP, respiratory rate (RR), heart rate (HR) and intracranial pressure;
- ↓ $SpO_2$, vagal tone, peripheral and cerebral blood flow;
- ↓ immune function (Hatfield & Umberger 2015);
- with crying: respiratory inhibition and sometimes hypoxaemia (Minowa 2016);
- sustained changes in central neural function (Courtois et al. 2016);
- in preterm infants, apnoea of prematurity (Karen et al. 2013) and possibly autism spectrum disorder (Lee et al. 2016h).

Preterm infants can be subjected to 10–16 invasive procedures per day, including demonstrably painful heel pricks and venepunctures (Bellieni et al. 2015), leading to the risk of detrimental effects in all major organ systems (Cong et al. 2012). Behavioural responses diminish when acute pain abates, but physiological responses may continue, risking intraventricular haemorrhage in the short term (Cong et al. 2012) and neurological, social and cognitive problems in the long term (Honda 2013). Invasive procedures are not always preceded by analgesia, as recommended, especially in parental absence (Courtois et al. 2016).

Some staff do not realize that pain is experienced from before birth. From the gestational age of 20 weeks the foetus has a functional pain system that can perceive

tissue injury (Lundeberg 2015). Even after birth, knowledge has often not been translated into practice (Harrison et al. 2015b), and the physiotherapist can check that a stepwise approach to analgesia is used (Fig. 15.7), and contribute some practical suggestions:
1. Validated pain scores should be used routinely (Milesi et al. 2010), e.g. the premature infant pain profile (Bellieni et al. 2015). Preterm infants display different pain behaviours to term babies and need assessment at a cortical level (Holsti et al. 2012).
2. One blood sample should be used for multiple measurements, or a central line placed to avoid frequent puncture. Anaesthetic ('EMLA') cream should be used before all skin punctures (Kucukoglu et al. 2015).
3. Heel sticks are more painful than venepuncture (Shrestha 2012) but less painful with an automatic lancet (Hwang 2015).
4. Kangaroo care reduces pain-induced hypoxaemia (Choudhary et al. 2015).
5. Minor pain can be eased by sucrose, pacifier sucking, radiant warmth and breastfeeding (Gray et al. 2015) or expressed breast milk (Rosali et al. 2015).
6. Massage can improve weight and height gain as well as ease pain (Mirmohammadali et al. 2015). Acupressure has also been found beneficial (Abbasoğlu et al. 2015).
7. Fentanyl is useful because it is short acting (Pacifici 2015), but paracetamol is not advised for procedural pain such as heel sticks (Ohlsson & Shah 2016).
8. Morphine needs to reach blood levels of approximately 120 ng/mL to be effective in neonates, whereas overdose effects start once levels exceed 300 ng/mL (Pacifici 2016). Continuous morphine infusion is inadequate for heel sticks (Courtois et al. 2016).

Healthy newborns are also exposed to pain if the birth requires vacuum extraction or forceps, and if blood is taken for screening tests (Ohlsson & Shah 2016). If an

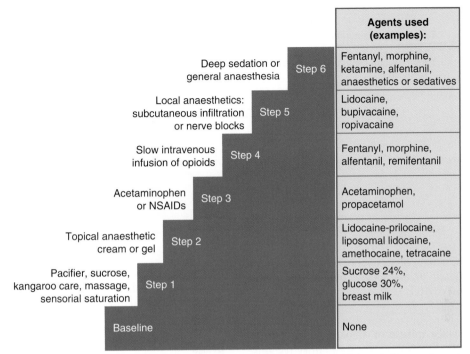

| | | Agents used (examples): |
|---|---|---|
| Deep sedation or general anaesthesia | Step 6 | Fentanyl, morphine, ketamine, alfentanil, anaesthetics or sedatives |
| Local anaesthetics: subcutaneous infiltration or nerve blocks | Step 5 | Lidocaine, bupivacaine, ropivacaine |
| Slow intravenous infusion of opioids | Step 4 | Fentanyl, morphine, alfentanil, remifentanil |
| Acetaminophen or NSAIDs | Step 3 | Acetaminophen, propacetamol |
| Topical anaesthetic cream or gel | Step 2 | Lidocaine-prilocaine, liposomal lidocaine, amethocaine, tetracaine |
| Pacifier, sucrose, kangaroo care, massage, sensorial saturation | Step 1 | Sucrose 24%, glucose 30%, breast milk |
| Baseline | | None |

**FIGURE 15.7** Stepwise approach to pain relief. *NSAIDs,* Nonsteroidal antiinflammatory drugs. (From Hall 2012.)

umbilical artery blood sample is needed, it should be withdrawn slowly to protect the brain from hypoxia (Schulz et al. 2003).

## Support Systems
### Humidification and temperature regulation
The more immature the baby, the less efficient is heat conservation because of minimal subcutaneous fat, fragile skin, inability to sweat or shiver and a large surface area in relation to body mass. Heated humidification is required immediately for intubated infants (Chidekel et al. 2012), and for spontaneously breathing preterm infants (Meyer et al. 2015). Heat–moisture exchangers are inadequate because they increase the work of breathing and do not prevent loss of body heat. During physiotherapy, the head, in particular, must be protected from heat loss.

### Oxygen therapy
Antioxidant systems to counteract toxic oxygen free radicals do not develop until late in the third trimester (Walsh et al. 2009), and the developing brain, kidneys, lungs and eyes of premature infants may be damaged by high or fluctuating oxygen administration (Wang 2015). These can disrupt the development of the delicate retinal capillaries, leading to a form of blindness called retinopathy of prematurity. Fine-tuning is required because the $SpO_2$ response to $FiO_2$ adjustments varies widely (Fathabadi et al. 2016), whereas oxygen restriction (Fig. 15.8) may increase mortality (Manja et al. 2015), especially in extremely preterm infants, whose oxygen saturation must not drop below 90% (Stenson et al. 2013). Interestingly, the eyes of the earliest premature babies were not damaged because the first American NICU was run by a businessman who was not willing to buy oxygen.

As with adults, intermittent hypoxaemia is particularly harmful, occurring more often with a low-oxygen target saturation range and contributing to neurodisability and eye damage (Di Fiore et al. 2012). Control of inspired oxygen is aided by closed-loop (Claure & Bancalari 2015) or automated systems (Kaam 2015, Waitz et al. 2015). Reference values on nocturnal $SpO_2$ for term infants are provided by Terrill et al. (2015).

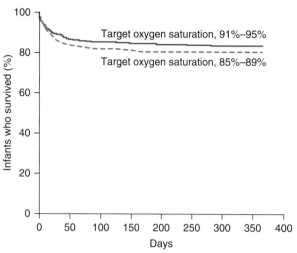

**FIGURE 15.8** Estimate of survival to hospital discharge or 1 year of life with different levels of inspired oxygen. (From SUPPORT 2010.)

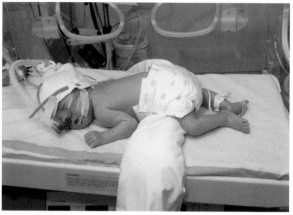

**FIGURE 15.9** CPAP with nasal prongs.

Maternal substance misuse or smoking during pregnancy is associated with impaired ventilatory response to hypoxia in her offspring (Ali et al. 2017).

The mode of administration also requires fine-tuning. Infants do not tolerate oxygen masks, and supplemental oxygen is usually by soft-pronged nasal cannulae or a humidified Perspex head box. Disadvantages of the box include a variable $FiO_2$, the need for a minimum 7 L/min flow to prevent accumulation of $CO_2$, bacterial contamination and harmful noise levels (Walsh et al. 2009). High-flow nasal cannulae bring the advantage of mini-CPAP levels of positive pressure, with similar WOB and oxygen saturation (Shetty et al. 2016) but, although they are more comfortable, the pressure is too much for some preterm infants, who may experience decreased oral feeding and increased eye damage (Hoffman et al. 2016b).

### Nutrition

Term babies can coordinate breathing and sucking, but this is compromised in preterm infants, who may aspirate or desaturate while feeding (Sakalidis et al. 2012). Breastfeeding minimizes the risk, but if this is not possible, a bottle nipple is available that feels like a normal breast and vents to air when the child sucks (Jenik et al. 2012). Otherwise the $FiO_2$ can be increased during feeds.

Infants who become breathless with oral feeds are usually fed by nasogastric tube, sometimes via a pump to reduce intermittent loads on the diaphragm. Severely compromised babies require intravenous feeds, which should be initiated early to minimize complications (Maas et al. 2015).

### Drugs

Most drugs given to neonates are unlicensed (Coppini et al. 2016) because research is limited in this age group. Standardized doses for discrete weight categories have been recommended (Robinson et al. 2014) but medication is affected by prolonged gastric emptying time, a high body surface area-to-weight ratio and the influence of developmental changes on the pharmacokinetics and pharmacodynamics of drugs (Matalová et al. 2016).

Analgesia is usually required before physiotherapy, but infant and monitors should be observed for postanalgesia respiratory depression, which can happen suddenly.

Drugs can be delivered direct to the lung by inhalation (Steinhorn 2012) or instillation (Jeng et al. 2012).

### Continuous positive airway pressure (CPAP)

The low FRC of infants requires them to avoid exhaling too far, using eccentric diaphragmatic activity and glottic closure during exhalation. CPAP fulfils the latter function when the baby is unable to do so, raising FRC either conventionally with nasal prongs (Fig. 15.9) or with a bubble system (Fig. 15.10). Risks are pneumothorax (Hishikawa et al. 2015) skin breakdown around the nose with nasal CPAP or, for infants with cardiovascular compromise, impaired cardiac output (Beker et al. 2015).

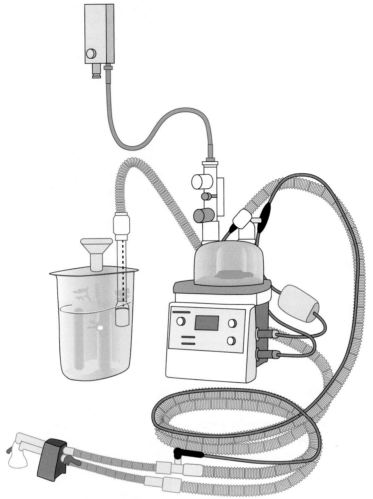

**FIGURE 15.10** Bubble CPAP. Pressure is generated at 3–10 cm $H_2O$, controlled by the amount of water in the CPAP generator (From Fisher & Paykel).

### Noninvasive ventilation

If neither oxygen nor CPAP are able to maintain oxygenation, or if ventilatory failure supervenes, assisted ventilation is needed. Noninvasive mask ventilation is preferred to MV, and may offer some advantages over CPAP because inspiratory and expiratory pressures can be titrated separately (Cummings & Polin 2016).

### Mechanical ventilation

Intubation without anaesthesia is almost always fatal in injured adults (Lockey 2001) and babies should be anaesthetized for the procedure (Barois & Tourneux 2013) to help prevent the complications of hypoxaemia,

bradycardia, hypertension and intracranial hypertension (Maheshwari et al. 2016).

Accidental intubation of the right main bronchus and beyond the right upper bronchus leads to right upper lobe collapse more often than with adults. The subglottic area is the narrowest part of the airway and young children tend to move their heads more than adults, so to protect the mucous membranes, a nasal endotracheal tube (ETT) is used which either has no cuff or, if ventilation is compromised by the leak, a high-volume low-pressure microcuff. Elaborate fixation systems help prevent such a heavy contraption becoming disconnected from such a tiny nose.

Complications are similar to those in adults, but the compliant rib cage and low lung collagen afford little protection against overdistension and barotrauma is more likely:

1. Pulmonary interstitial emphysema (PIE) is identified radiologically as lucent streaks radiating from the hila, representing air in the interstitium (Fig. 15.11). Unlike air bronchograms, the streaks do not branch or taper. Extension to the periphery can lead to pneumothorax. Lung ultrasound and CT scans help confirm the diagnosis.

2. Pneumomediastinum presents as a halo of air adjacent to the heart borders (Fig. 15.11B).

3. Pneumothorax is suspected if there is rapid deterioration without obvious cause. Chest drainage in a female infant requires careful placement to avoid long-term breast damage (Rainer & Gardetto 2003). Ventilator-induced lung injury is more likely in the immature lung, but can be reduced by high-frequency ventilation (González et al. 2016). For conventional ventilation, pressure control is used in order to avoid high peak airway pressures and to allow flow to increase automatically to compensate for the leak if there is no cuff.

MV requires continuous analgesic infusion to maintain synchrony with the ventilator, improve oxygenation and stabilize BP (Ancora et al. 2012). The stress response is reduced if the ventilator is set so that the infant can trigger his or her own breaths (Brown & DiBlasi 2011).

Transitioning between levels of respiratory support may be assisted by oximetry histograms (Mascoll et al. 2016) or cerebral oxygen saturation (Pichler et al. 2016).

## PHYSIOTHERAPY

### Consent

Consent should be obtained from a parent or legal guardian (Table 15.3), but if this is unavailable, treatment may be given if it is deemed in the patient's interest.

### Assessment

The main role of the physiotherapist is to judge if intervention is required. Treatment itself may be carried out by the physiotherapist, neonatal nurse or in part by the parent. The approach is to assess, identify problems, and balance up the benefits and risks of treatment. Scrutiny of the notes is complemented by reports from nursing and medical staff, preferably with parental presence

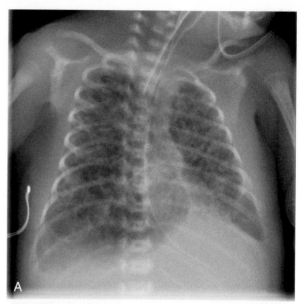

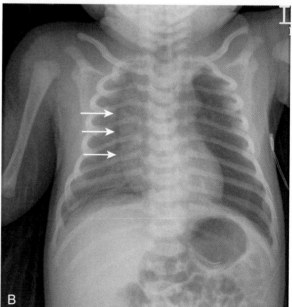

**FIGURE 15.11** (A) Intubated infant of 5 weeks' gestation, showing the multiple cysts of PIE, with hyperinflation and downward displacement of the right lung. (B) Pneumomediastinum, the arrows indicating the air outlining the right heart border. (From Greenough 2012.)

| TABLE 15.3 | Parental responsibility in the UK |
|---|---|
| Child's mother | Responsible unless the child is adopted, placed for adoption or under a placement order. |
| Child's father | Responsible if married to the mother or has legal responsibility by:<br>• joint birth registration with the mother<br>• parental responsibility agreement with the mother<br>• parental responsibility order made by the court. |
| Social services/court | Responsible if parental responsibility is removed. May be temporary or permanent. |

From BMA 2010.

| TABLE 15.4 | Normal values for infants | |
|---|---|---|
| | Premature infant | Infant |
| RR | 40–60 | 30–40 |
| SpO$_2$ | 92%–95% | 93%–98% |
| PaO$_2$ | 8–10.6 kPa | 10–13 kPa |
| | (60–80 mmHg) | (75–100 mmHg) |
| PaCO$_2$ | 5–6 kPa | 5–6 kPa |
| | (37–45 mmHg) | (37–45 mmHg) |
| HR | 120–200 | 100–150 |
| BP | 50/25–60/30 | 70/40–80/50 |

BP, Blood pressure; HR, heart rate; RR, respiratory rate. From APLS 2011.

(Abdel-Latif et al. 2015) plus identification of the acceptable limits for SpO$_2$ and other vital signs.

## History

Medical and birth history provide the first indications of precautions to be taken, for example:

1. Neurological insults such as intraventricular haemorrhage or encephalopathy may show as altered tone, abnormal postures, aspiration or difficulty clearing secretions. The head-down position is banned in these infants, and any other respiratory treatment avoided unless essential because of the risk of raising intracranial pressure. Physiotherapy should also be avoided if there are uncontrolled seizures.

2. Cardiorespiratory instability indicates the need for minimum intervention. Neonates are prone to bradycardia and desaturation with suction and handling. Physiotherapy, if required, may be preceded by analgesia, sedation and preoxygenation, with closed-circuit suction and minimum saline instillation recommended.

3. Deranged clotting increases the risk of internal bleeding, and manual techniques should be minimized.

## Subjective

Examples of information from the parent or nurse include the following:

- handling responses: e.g. desaturations or bradycardia are present;
- feeding regimen: physiotherapy assessment can take place at any time but treatment should normally be given at least an hour after a feed to avoid vomiting;
- secretions: colour, consistency, ability to cough are noted;
- pain: signs may include withdrawal, increased extensor tone, irritability, inconsolable crying or clenched fists, but it should not reach this extreme, and assessment is aided with pain scales, e.g. Fig. 15.12.

## Objective

Much reliance is placed on objective information because of the limitations of clinical and subjective assessment. Throughout assessment and treatment, speaking softly is soothing for the infant and reassuring for parents.

The chart identifies trends in vital signs (Table 15.4) and response to handling, as well as ventilator parameters, fluid balance and oxygenation related to FiO$_2$. Preterm infants have a left-shifted dissociation curve because of foetal haemoglobin, and desaturation may reflect a lower PaO$_2$ than with adults. The chart also documents response to medication, weight gain or loss, mode and frequency of feeds, response to suction, results of the last suction, and whether the baby has rested since the last intervention.

Observations from the end of the cot include:

- consciousness, irritability and muscle tone;
- stridor, wheeze, grunting, tracheal tube leak or the coarse crackles of upper airway secretions heard at the mouth;
- pallor, flushing or cyanosis, the latter being a late sign of deterioration;

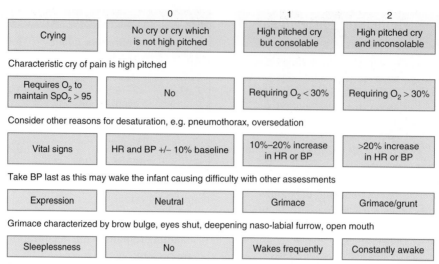

| | 0 | 1 | 2 |
|---|---|---|---|
| Crying | No cry or cry which is not high pitched | High pitched cry but consolable | High pitched cry and inconsolable |

Characteristic cry of pain is high pitched

| | 0 | 1 | 2 |
|---|---|---|---|
| Requires O₂ to maintain SpO₂ > 95 | No | Requiring O₂ < 30% | Requiring O₂ > 30% |

Consider other reasons for desaturation, e.g. pneumothorax, oversedation

| | 0 | 1 | 2 |
|---|---|---|---|
| Vital signs | HR and BP +/– 10% baseline | 10%–20% increase in HR or BP | >20% increase in HR or BP |

Take BP last as this may wake the infant causing difficulty with other assessments

| | 0 | 1 | 2 |
|---|---|---|---|
| Expression | Neutral | Grimace | Grimace/grunt |

Grimace characterized by brow bulge, eyes shut, deepening naso-labial furrow, open mouth

| | 0 | 1 | 2 |
|---|---|---|---|
| Sleeplessness | No | Wakes frequently | Constantly awake |

Based on infant's state during the hour preceding assessment

**FIGURE 15.12** Pain scale for babies from 32 weeks' gestation. (From Krechel & Bildner 2007.)

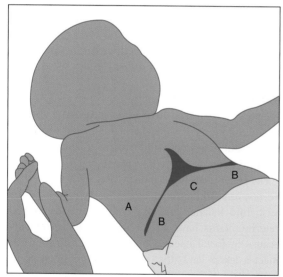

**FIGURE 15.13** Recessions indicating respiratory distress. *A,* Intercostal; *B,* subcostal; *C,* substernal. (From Wilkins et al. 2010.)

- breathing pattern;
- observation of the unclothed chest for expansion, atelectasis often being suspected because of the compliant rib cage;
- respiratory distress, e.g. Fig. 15.13, Table 15.5.

**TABLE 15.5    Signs of cardiorespiratory distress**

| Mild | Moderate | Severe |
|---|---|---|
| ↑ RR | Chest recessions | ↓ RR or apnoea |
| ↑ HR | Tracheal tug | Cyanosis |
| Reduced activity / irritability | Paradoxical breathing | Head bobbing (unfixed accessory muscle contraction) |
| | Nasal flaring | ↓ HR |
| | Grunting | Pallor, mottling of skin |
| | Inability to feed | Exhaustion |

*HR,* Heart rate; *RR,* respiratory rate.

Physical assessment must avoid noise, sudden movement or cold hands. Auscultation, with a warmed stethoscope, identifies atelectasis or secretions. Sounds are often referred through such a diminutive chest: upper lobe collapse can sometimes only be detected posteriorly. It may be difficult to identify the location of crackles and it is best to first listen to the upper airways. The high RR also makes it difficult to identify where they come in the respiratory cycle. In ventilated infants, the slight hiss of the intentional air leak can be heard by ear or stethoscope.

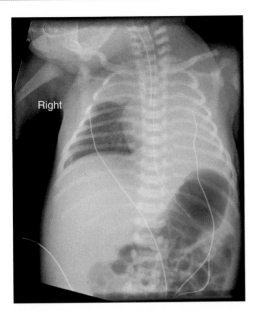

FIGURE 15.14 Right upper lobe and left lung collapse following right endobronchial intubation.

Atelectasis or consolidation show on X-ray, the middle and upper lobes being especially inclined to collapse. A large thymus may look similar to right upper lobe consolidation, and atelectasis of the left lower lobe may be missed on a portable X-ray if it is hidden by the heart. Air bronchograms projected against the heart shadow may not be significant but are pathological when seen peripherally. Overenthusiastic intubation may lead to the tube passing into the right main bronchus and past the right upper bronchus, leading to collapse of the right upper lobe and left lung (Fig. 15.14).

Lung ultrasound reduces exposure to ionizing radiation and contrasts aerated lung with an interstitial or alveolar pattern more easily than in adults because there is less fat and muscle (Yousef 2016), e.g. a pneumothorax is easier to identify (Cattarossi et al. 2016).

## Monitoring

Noninvasive monitoring is available for arterial blood gases (Chatterjee et al. 2015). For $SpO_2$, the oximeter probe site must be changed every 4 hours to prevent pressure sores. Conscious level can be assessed with bispectral monitoring (Sammartino et al. 2010).

## Indications for Treatment

Physiotherapy is indicated if there is evidence of atelectasis, or excess secretions that cannot be cleared by humidification and the nurse's use of manual hyperinflation, saline instillation and suction. Increased work of breathing (WOB) may be responsive to physiotherapy unless it is due to a pathological process. Poor gas exchange is responsive to physiotherapy if it relates to increased secretion load. Treatment may also be indicated after extubation if airway irritation has created secretions that the infant does not cough and swallow spontaneously.

## Contraindications

Physiotherapy must be avoided if the infant is hypothermic, has suffered a pulmonary haemorrhage, or received surfactant treatment in the last 6 h. Other contraindications are cardiovascular instability (unless this is due to hypoxia caused by a problem amenable to physiotherapy), or fresh blood-stained secretions (unless there is significant mucous plugging).

Manual hyperinflation is contraindicated if there is PIE or other barotrauma, and any physiotherapy is contraindicated in infants with an undrained pneumothorax.

Manual techniques are contraindicated if there is osteopaenia, due to the risk of rib fractures.

Any intervention should also be avoided within 24–48 h of an intraventricular haemorrhage to prevent further bleeding, or with infants under 1500 g in the first 2–4 days of life due to the risk of intraventricular haemorrhage (Price & Ronan 2014).

## Precautions

Added to the precautions identified from the history are the following:

• Treatment should only take place after the infant has been stabilized medically. Observation and monitoring are required more frequently during treatment than with adults. Large swings in BP, in particular, risk causing brain injury (Marlow 2014).

- Hand washing and universal precautions are required even more strictly than with adults because of the immature defence mechanisms of infants. Staff with any infection should not enter the NICU.
- If treatment is necessary within an hour of feeding, the gastric contents can be aspirated by syringe through the nasogastric tube and replaced afterwards. If the infant is receiving phototherapy for jaundice, it can be suspended temporarily for treatment.
- Desaturation episodes may be precipitated by suction or caused by secretions, breath holding, pulmonary hypertension or upper airway obstruction. The infant's head falling into flexion can obstruct the airway and may cause stridor. Following extubation, subglottic oedema may develop immediately or over 24 h.

After treatment, the cot sides must be raised or incubator ports closed.

---

**PRACTICE TIP**

Physiotherapy sessions should be structured into the daily plan so that infants can receive prolonged rest and adequate sleep

---

## Methods to Increase Lung Volume
### Positioning

The cardiorespiratory system is not happy to remain in the same position for prolonged periods, and infants should have their position changed as regularly as their condition and response to handling allows. Raising the head of the incubator lessens the risk of GOR (Button et al. 2005) and in spontaneously breathing infants, reduces the load on the diaphragm. Side-lying allows greater diaphragmatic excursion than supine, with trunk and limbs supported in a flexed position to optimize neurodevelopment. If there is a pneumothorax or unilateral PIE, side-lying with the affected lung dependent may assist absorption of the gas (Miller et al. 2015), with close monitoring of $SpO_2$.

In preterm infants, the prone position (see Fig. 15.9) stabilizes HR and RR (Ghorbani et al. 2013), and increases $SpO_2$ (Eghbalian 2014), but spontaneously breathing infants must be monitored because of the risk of sudden infant death syndrome (Pease et al. 2016). Extended time in prone may lead to a flattened frog position because of hypotonia, which can be avoided by raising the pelvis on a roll (Guidetti et al. 2017).

The effects of repositioning should be closely monitored, especially in preterm infants. For ventilated babies, traction on the ETT must be avoided, and the leak around the ETT reassessed in the new position.

### Hyperinflation

For the ventilated infant who has not responded to positioning, hyperinflation can be used to increase lung volume. A device such as the Neopuff (Fig. 15.15) provides hyperinflation at a preset flow, peak inspiratory pressure and PEEP, thus reducing the risk of barotrauma and derecruitment. If this is not available, manual hyperinflation (MH) is used. Specialist training is required for this, particularly with younger infants, because of the risk of barotrauma (Morrow et al. 2008). Precautions to MH are similar to adults, with three additions:

- hyperinflation conditions such as meconium aspiration and bronchiolitis;
- extreme prematurity due to the risk of pneumothorax;
- infants whose RR is over 40/min because it is difficult to achieve an effective hyperinflation at such a high rate, although extra sedation and muscle relaxants may be helpful.

A 500 mL reservoir bag is used for infants and children under two years old. These bags have an open tail which is squeezed between finger and thumb to regulate the pressure more sensitively than a valve (Fig. 15.16). The following technique is suggested:

1. A manometer should be incorporated into the circuit, plus a pop-off valve that opens above $40\pm5$ cmH$_2$O (Oliveira et al. 2011), which is especially important because pressure varies with flow (Oliveira et al. 2013b).
2. Each hyperinflation should be interposed with 2–3 tidal breaths.
3. The chest should rise just slightly more than during MV.
4. Some positive pressure should be maintained at the end of expiration to maintain PEEP and prevent derecruitment.
5. The monitors must be kept under observation, any significant drop in BP indicating a need to return the infant to MV and advise nursing or medical staff.

## Methods to Reduce the Work of Breathing

Excess WOB can be for respiratory, neurological or postural reasons. An unstable breathing pattern may be caused by excess WOB but also by pain or stress. Once

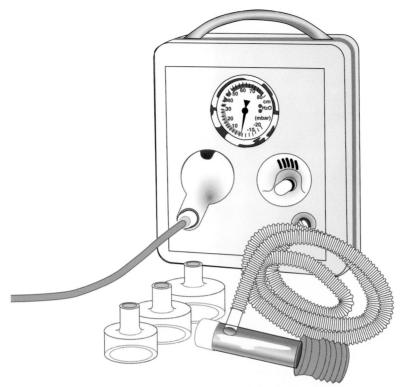

**FIGURE 15.15** Neopuff infant T-piece resuscitator (From Fisher & Paykel).

distress has been minimized, repositioning may reduce the WOB. Noninvasive ventilation for infants who become exhausted, hypercapnic and acidotic can be used in the youngest age groups so long as apnoeas and technical problems are overcome (Abadesso 2012).

## Methods to Clear Secretions
### Assisted autogenic drainage
In order to reach the lung volume at which secretions have been identified, gentle pressure is applied during each inspiration. This gradually restricts the inspiratory level so that the infant exhales slightly more than the previous breathing cycle. By altering the pressure, airflow is manipulated at different lung volumes, thus mobilizing secretions until a spontaneous cough is achieved. In an able older infant this can also be combined with bouncing gently on a gym ball in order to increase expiratory airflow (Ginderdeuren et al. 2016).

### Postural drainage
Preterm infants, or term infants who tolerate handling poorly, should have their position changed minimally. Other babies can be posturally drained in alternate side-lying or prone on a parent's lap, avoiding the head-down position.

### Percussion and vibrations
Manual techniques can be soothing as well as effective. Vibrations with the finger tips are applied on every second or third exhalation. Percussion can be performed with a soft-rimmed face mask or a 'palm cup' (Fig. 15.17) directly on the skin, taking care to stay within the surface markings of the little lungs.

Precautions are similar to adults, with the following additions:
1. The head must be supported throughout because of the risk of causing a form of brain damage similar to 'shaken baby syndrome' (Hassam & Williams 2003).

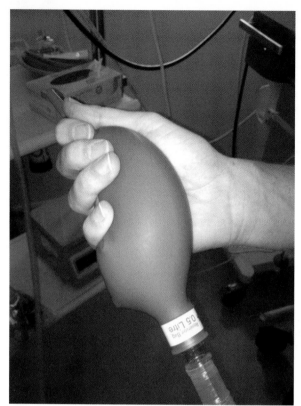

FIGURE 15.16 Hand position for manual hyperinflation (From Paul Ritson).

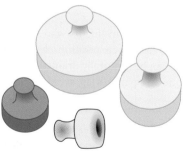

FIGURE 15.17 Palm cups made for percussion on babies and young children (From Henleys).

2. Manual techniques should be avoided in premature infants or others at risk of rickets (Nehra et al. 2013).
3. Strong chest vibrations may increase airflow resistance (Schechter 2007).
4. Monitoring must be maintained throughout because responses can be unpredictable.

## Mechanical insufflation–exsufflation

Assisted cough (p. 217) in infants requires extra attention to insufflation in order to reverse any collapse of small airways caused by exsufflation.

## Suction

For **nonintubated infants**, positioning and manual techniques may mobilize secretions so that they are swallowed. If not, or there is a poor swallow, suction may be necessary, but with minimal distress because this is associated with the physiological responses that accompany other painful interventions (Ivars et al. 2012) and crying increases transpulmonary pressure swings and the risk of lung damage (Walsh et al. 2011). Nasopharyngeal airways should not be used in infants routinely because the narrow airway lumen increases WOB. Oral airways should not be used unless the infant is unconscious or does not have airway protective mechanisms. The precautions and techniques described in Chapter 7 are modified by the following:

For nasal suction:

1. Have the baby side-lying, wrapped up comfortably but firmly, and if possible with a second person supporting the infant behaviourally (Cone et al. 2013).
2. For preterm infants, pre-oxygenate by no more than 10% above baseline (Walsh et al. 2011).
3. Set the vacuum pressure to 8–10 kPa (60–80 mmHg) (GOSH 2013).
4. Use a catheter that is no more than half the diameter of the smallest nostril, usually size 5–6 FG.
5. Measure the depth of suction from the tip of the nose to the tragus of the ear, and then to the base of the neck (Fig. 15.18). If the child has a significant kyphoscoliosis, depth is measured on both sides of the head, added up and divided by two (Alder Hey 2009).
6. Using a small amount of water-soluble jelly or the child's nasal secretions as a lubricant on the catheter tip, insert it gently into the nose to the measured depth, but no further than the point at which a cough is stimulated.
7. Withdraw while applying suction.
8. Suction the nostril on the other side.
9. Observe monitors throughout.
10. Reassess, repeat only if necessary.
11. Invite the parent to cuddle the baby.

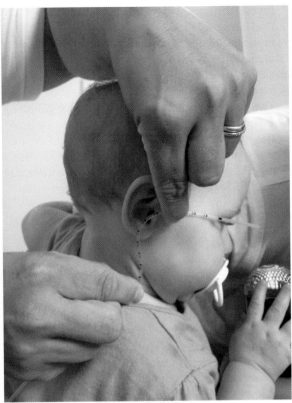

**FIGURE 15.18** Measurement for nasopharyngeal suction in an infant.

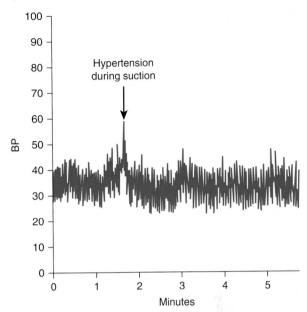

**FIGURE 15.19** Hypertension in an infant during suction. *BP*, Blood pressure. (From McIntosh 1989.)

For oral suction, as points 1–3, then:

- Gently insert a clean catheter or Yankauer down either side of the mouth following the gum line.
- Take the catheter or Yankauer as far as the back of the tongue and mouth (deeper if necessary and if tolerated).
- Avoid stimulating gagging or vomiting.
- Only apply suction when it is in place and on withdrawal.

Then continue with points 9–11, as outlined previously.

Long-term use of oral suction should be avoided if possible because it can lead to oral aversion and problems with feeding.

For **ventilated infants**, secretions may be present even if not heard on auscultation or felt on palpation. Liaison with the nurse is helpful, but for babies without hypersecretory disease, suctioning every 6–12 h is adequate if no indication for more frequent suction is apparent (Walsh et al. 2011).

Complications include hypoxaemia, bradycardia, tachycardia, atelectasis, infection, arrhythmias (Cone et al. 2013) and abrupt peaks in BP (Fig. 15.19). Open suction risks more hypoxaemia than a closed system (Cardoso et al. 2015). Suction should be avoided if there is low cardiac output or shock (pallor or cyanosis, sweating or decreased peripheral temperature).

Modifications to the technique described on p. 219 are the following:

1. Extra sedation is required to blunt the stress response, so long as the infant is not at risk of hypotension.
2. To reduce the stress of the procedure, a parent can hold the infant in a flexed position (Axelin et al. 2015).
3. Preoxygenation is by increasing ventilator $FiO_2$ to 10%–20% above baseline (Walsh et al. 2011), or by using MH, with monitoring by oximetry.
4. The catheter should not advance more than 1 cm beyond the end of the ETT. Its length can be checked against the length of an equivalent-sized ETT, which is usually taped to the outside of the incubator for emergencies, or a graduated catheter can be used (Ritson 2000).

5. The catheter size is calculated by doubling the ETT size, e.g. a size 4 requires a size 8 catheter (Walsh 2011).
6. For postoperative infants, ensure that someone supports the wound.
7. Ensure that monitors can be observed throughout.
8. After disconnection from the ventilator (for open suction), the catheter is inserted to the premeasured depth. If resistance is felt, it is withdrawn 0.5 cm before suction is applied. Suction should be kept to within 5 s if possible, or a maximum 10 s.
9. In a weak or paralysed infant, vibrations or a manually assisted cough can be applied during suction.
10. After reconnection to the ventilator, the mouth and nostrils usually need suction.
11. Increased $FiO_2$ may be required, which is automatic on ventilators with a suction mode. If values do not return to the target $SpO_2$, or the infant is unsettled, further suction may be indicated.

If the infant does not respond as expected, or does not settle, liaison with nursing or medical staff is required. The nurse will know if bradycardia caused by stress might be reversed by physical input such as gently rubbing the sternum.

If sputum retention continues despite efficient humidification and the previous technique, saline instillation may be required, preferably with a low-sodium solution to reduce infection risk (Walsh et al. 2011). Suggested boluses are 0.5 mL for preterm infants and 1–3 mL for term babies, but this varies with the stability and tolerance of the infant (Ridling et al. 2003).

## Nonbronchoscopic bronchoalveolar lavage (NBBAL)

For persistent atelectasis caused by mucous plugging, NBBAL has been found effective in 84% of ventilated infants who have not responded to conventional physiotherapy (Morrow et al. 2006), and can also be used to obtain samples for diagnosis.

Precautions are:
- haemodynamic instability
- pulmonary haemorrhage
- pulmonary oedema
- pulmonary hypertension
- raised intracranial pressure
- congestive heart failure
- coagulopathy
- surfactant therapy
- prematurity, or small for gestational age
- inadequate sedation
- bronchospasm (Morrow et al. 2006, ERS 2002)

Complications include hypoxaemia or cardiovascular instability, which may require escalation of respiratory of haemodynamic support.

The following equipment is required, for collecting two samples:
- two sputum traps
- two syringes, two white syringe adaptors
- two NBBAL suction catheters of appropriate size for ETT
- two Y connectors
- catheter mount, heat–moisture exchanger, MHI circuit
- 0.9% saline
- sterile towel
- gloves, apron, visor
- suction catheters

A suggested procedure is below:
- Assess cardiorespiratory stability.
- Ensure adequate sedation and analgesia, plus paralysing agent in order to suppress cough if lower airway sample is required.
- Prime catheters with saline and attach the syringes to the catheters (Fig. 15.20A). Use 1 mL/kg for each sample up to 10 mL maximum.
- Position infant, depending on which lobe is being targeted or whether samples are required for unilateral or diffuse lung pathology.
- Preoxygenate by manual inflation.
- If collecting samples, connect the sputum trap as in Fig. 15.20B.
- Don a sterile glove, remove the catheter (with syringe connected) from its packet and introduce it via the catheter mount, while continuing to manually inflate, until resistance is felt (Fig. 15.20C).
- Stop manual inflation, instil saline, give 1–2 breaths and if collecting samples connect sputum trap to the catheter, apply suction (Fig. 15.20D), give expiratory vibrations if necessary.
- After collection, resume manual inflation.
- Reassess; if the infant is stable and if another sample is required, repeat the process.
- To finish, perform suction with or without manual techniques to clear remaining secretions.
- Observe closely; the infant may need increased $FiO_2$ and/or ventilation.

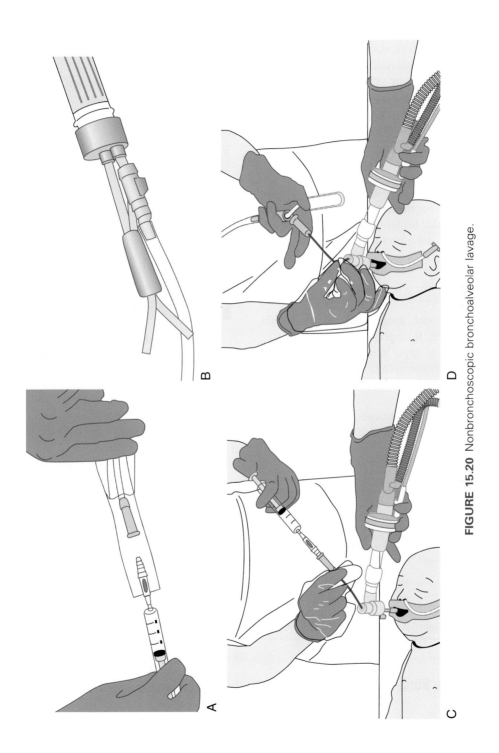

**FIGURE 15.20** Nonbronchoscopic bronchoalveolar lavage.

## Exercise and Rehabilitation

Passive movements are normally unnecessary, but for very low birth-weight babies, daily gentle exercise can improve weight and bone mineralization (Moyer-Mileur 2000). Monitors should be observed throughout. Referral to specialist colleagues is required for infants needing developmental input, including rehabilitation for ventilator-dependent infants with chronic respiratory insufficiency (Dumas et al. 2013).

## CASE STUDY: HOLLY

*Holly is a 1-week-old neonate, born at 38 weeks' gestation, after which she aspirated her feed. She was sedated, intubated and ventilated, using pressure support ventilation with FiO$_2$ of 0.75, and showing the following:*

- SpO$_2$ 94%;
- pH 7.23, PaO$_2$ 9.3 kPa (70 mmHg), PaCO$_2$ 10.2 kPa (77 mmHg), HCO$_3^-$ 22;
- auscultation: ↓ breath sounds left side and right upper zone, crackles throughout;
- X-ray shows bilateral upper lobe collapse (Fig. 15.21);
- suction → thick creamy secretions.

### Questions

1. Analyse the arterial blood gases?
2. Analysis?
3. Problems?
4. Goal?
5. Plan?

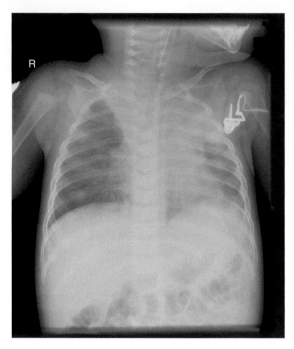

**FIGURE 15.21** Holly.

---

### CLINICAL REASONING

Consider the following:

*Unless it can be shown that the fetus has a conscious appreciation of pain ... the responses to noxious stimulation must still essentially be reflex.*
**Do fetuses feel pain?** *BMJ* (1996), 313, 795–799

---

## Response to Case Study

1. Blood gases:
   Uncompensated respiratory acidosis, borderline oxygenation with high FiO$_2$

2. Analysis:
   X-ray and secretions suggest mucous plugging
3. Problems:
   Loss of volume in both upper lobes and retained secretions
4. Goal:
   Reinflate upper lobes and clear secretions
5. Plan:
   1. Care with positioning throughout because of the high ETT seen on the X-ray, meaning that it could become dislodged
   2. Instil saline to right lung, monitor
   3. Turn to left side-lying
   4. MH, vibrations and suction, monitor
   5. Reassess
   6. Instil saline to left lung, monitor
   7. Turn to right side-lying
   8. MH, vibrations and suction, monitor
   9. Reassess
   10. Plan for improvement
   11. Plan for deterioration.

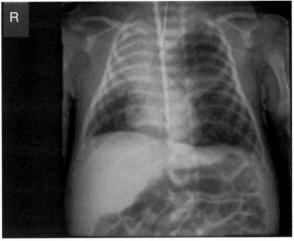

**FIGURE 15.22** Jack.

## CASE STUDY: JACK[a]

*Jack is 6 weeks old (corrected gestational age 36/40) and has bronchiolitis. He is sedated, intubated and ventilated using pressure control ventilation. He is on morphine, IV fluids, nasogastric feeds.*

FiO$_2$ and ventilatory requirements have increased, and nursing staff are unable to clear his chest, although some thick yellow secretions have been suctioned.

### Observations

- HR 140, BP 85/64, temperature 38°C
- Hb 9.0, WCC 18, CRP 150, platelets 400 (normal values: Hb 8–15, WCC 4–12, CRP <10 mg/L, platelets 100–800)
- FiO$_2$ 80, PEEP 8, peak inspiratory pressure 28, RR 45, back up RR set at 35
- SpO$_2$ 86%, end-tidal CO$_2$ 8.0
- ABGs: pH 7.3, PaCO$_2$ 8.5, PaO$_2$ 7.0, HCO$_3^-$ 23, BE 1
- Reduced chest wall movement on the right
- Patient well sedated

### Auscultation

- Breath sounds ↓ on the right, scattered crackles throughout
  Palpable secretions centrally.

### Questions

1. Analysis?
2. Problems?
3. Plan?

---

[a]*ABGs*, arterial blood gases; *BE*, base excess; *CRP*, C-reactive protein; *Hb*, haemoglobin; *HCO$_3^-$*, bicarbonate; *WCC*, white cell count

### Response to Case Study

1. Analysis
   - X-ray (Fig. 15.22) suggests right upper lobe collapse: mediastinum shifted towards the opacity.
   - Hypoxaemia probably caused by sputum plugging.
   - Respiratory acidosis may be secondary to lung protective ventilation, but high ventilator pressures reflect ↓ lung compliance due to bronchiolitis.
   - High oxygen requirements due to bronchiolitis and sputum retention.
   - Increased WCC and CRP indicate infective and inflammatory processes, respectively.
2. Problems
   - Reduced volume RUL
   - Sputum retention
3. Plan
   - Position right side-lying
   - Instil saline
   - Manual hyperinflation
   - Position left side-lying
   - Manual hyperinflation, percussion, vibrations, suction
   - Reassess and repeat if necessary
   - Advise nursing staff on positioning

# RECOMMENDED READING

Allegaert, K., van den Anker, J.N., 2016. Neonatal pain management: still in search of the Holy Grail. Int. J. Clin. Pharmacol. Therapeut. 54 (7), 514–523.

Bailes, S.A., Firestone, K.S., Dunn, D.K., et al., 2016. Evaluating the effect of flow and interface type on pressures delivered with bubble CPAP in a simulated model. Respir. Care 61 (3), 333–339.

Barbosa, V.M., 2013. Teamwork in the neonatal intensive care unit. Phys. Occup. Ther. Pediatr. 33 (1), 5–26.

Borenstein-Levin, L., Synnes, A., Grunau, R.E., et al., 2017. Narcotics and sedative use in preterm neonates. J. Pediatr. 180, 92.e1–98.e1.

Brady, A., Smith, P., 2015. A competence framework and evidence based practice guidance for the physiotherapist working in the neonatal intensive care and special care unit in the United Kingdom. Association of Paediatric Chartered Physiotherapists Neonatal Committee. Available from: http://apcp.csp.org.uk/publications/competence-framework -evidence-based-practice-guidance-physiotherapist-working -neo.

Cerritelli, F., 2013. Effect of osteopathic manipulative treatment on length of stay in a population of preterm infants. BMC Pediatr. 13, 65.

CFN, 2016. Committee on Fetus and Newborn. Prevention and management of procedural pain in the neonate: an update. Pediatrics 137 (2), e20154271. doi:10.1542/ peds.2015-4271.

Doreswamy, S.M., Chakkarapani, A.A., Murthy, P., 2015. Saturation oxygen pressure index for assessment of pulmonary disease in neonates on non-invasive ventilation. Indian Pediatr. 52 (1), 74–75.

Duman, N., Tüzün, F., Sever, A.H., et al., 2016. Nasal intermittent positive pressure ventilation with or without very early surfactant therapy for the primary treatment of respiratory distress syndrome. J. Matern. Fetal Neonatal Med. 29 (2), 252–257.

Eichenwald, E.C., 2016. Apnea of prematurity. Pediatrics 137 (1).

Fathabadi, S.O., Gale, T.J., Lim, K., et al., 2016. Characterisation of the oxygenation response to inspired oxygen adjustments in preterm infants. Neonatology 109 (1), 37–43.

Fotiou, C., Vlastarakos, P.V., Bakoula, C., et al., 2016. Parental stress management using relaxation techniques in a neonatal intensive care unit. Int. Crit. Care Nurs 32, 20–28.

Frawley, G., 2017. Special considerations in the premature and ex-premature infant. Anaesth. Int. Care. 18 (2), 79–83.

Gencpinar, P., Duman, M., 2016. Importance of back blow maneuvers in a 6 month old patient with sudden upper airway obstruction. Turk. J. Emerg. Med. 15 (4), 177–178.

Gilmour, D., Davies, M.W., Herbert, A.R., 2017. Adequacy of palliative care in a single tertiary neonatal unit. J. Paediatr. Child Health 53 (2), 136–144.

Glanzmann, C., Frey, B., Vonbach, P., et al., 2016. Drugs as risk factors of acute kidney injury in critically ill children. Pediatr. Nephrol. 31 (1), 145–151.

Gold, J.I., Nelson, L.P., 2012. Palliative care in a neonatal intensive care unit. J. Crit. Care 27 (1), 95–96.

Goldstein, R.D., Trachtenberg, F.L., Sens, M.A., et al., 2016. Overall postneonatal mortality and rates of SIDS. Pediatrics 137 (1), 1–10.

Gupta, P., 2014. Caring for a teen with congenital heart disease. Pediatr. Clin. North Am. 61 (1), 207–228.

Hansmann, G., Apitz, C., Abdul-Khaliq, H., et al., 2016. Expert consensus statement on the diagnosis and treatment of paediatric pulmonary hypertension. Heart 102 (Suppl. 2), ii86–ii100.

Harris, J., 2016. Clinical recommendations for pain, sedation, withdrawal and delirium assessment in critically ill infants and children. Int. Care Med. 42, 972–986.

Iyer, N.P., Mhanna, M.J., 2016. Association between high-flow nasal cannula and end-expiratory esophageal pressures in premature infants. Respir. Care 61 (3), 285–290.

Kemper, A.R., Prosser, L.A., Wade, K.C., et al., 2016. A comparison of strategies for retinopathy of prematurity detection. Pediatrics 137 (1), 1–10. doi:10.1542/ peds.2015-2256.

Kherani, T., Sayal, A., Al-Saleh, S., et al., 2016. A comparison of invasive and noninvasive ventilation in children less than 1 year of age. Pediatr. Pulmonol. 51 (2), 189–195.

Lanza, F.C., Wandalsen, G., Dela Bianca, A.C., et al., 2011. Prolonged slow expiration technique in infants: effects on tidal volume, peak expiratory flow, and expiratory reserve volume. Respir. Care 56 (12), 1930–1935.

Liu, J., Cao, H.Y., Wang, X.L., et al., 2016. The significance and the necessity of routinely performing lung ultrasound in the neonatal intensive care units. J. Matern. Fetal Neonatal Med. 29 (24), 4025–4030.

Livshitz, I., 2015. Preventative strategies in the management of ROP. Open J. Pediatr 5 (2), 121–127.

Lorch, S.A., 2017. Determining the optimal neonatal care for preterm infants in the era of personalized medicine. Pediatrics 139 (1), e20162442.

Lum, S., Bountziouka, V., Wade, A., et al., 2016. New reference ranges for interpreting forced expiratory manoeuvres in infants and implications for clinical interpretation. Thorax 71 (3), 276–283.

Martinez, F.D., 2017. Bending the twig does the tree incline: lung function after lower respiratory tract illness in infancy. Am. J. Respir. Crit. Care Med. 195 (2), 154–155.

Mikalsen, I.B., Davis, P., Øymar, K., et al., 2016. High flow nasal cannula in children. Scand. J. Trauma. Resuscit. Emerg. Med. 24, 93.

Morley, S.L., 2016. Non-invasive ventilation in paediatric critical care. Paediatr. Respir. Rev. 20, 24–31.

Neumann, R.P., 2014. The neonatal lung – physiology and ventilation. Paediatr. Anaesth. 24 (1), 10–21.

NICE Guideline, 2015. Bronchiolitis in children: diagnosis and management [NG9].

NICE Guideline, 2016. End of life care for infants, children and young people with life-limiting conditions [NG61].

Oei, J.L., Saugstad, O.D., Lui, K., et al., 2017. Targeted oxygen in the resuscitation of preterm infants, a randomized clinical trial. Pediatrics 139 (1), e20161452.

Pal, S., Curley, A., Stanworth, S.J., 2015. Interpretation of clotting tests in the neonate. Arch. Dis. Child. Fetal Neonatal Ed. 100, F270–F274.

Polglase, G.R., Dawson, J.A., Kluckow, M., et al., 2015. Ventilation onset prior to umbilical cord clamping (physiological-based cord clamping) improves systemic and cerebral oxygenation in preterm lambs. PLoS ONE 10 (2), e0117504.

Riviere, D., McKinlay, C.J.D., Bloomfield, F.H., 2017. Adaptation for life after birth: a review of neonatal physiology. Anaesth. Int. Care. 18 (2), 59–67.

Rocha, G.M., Flor-DE-Lima, F.S., Guimaraes, H.A., 2016. Persistent grunting respirations after birth. Minerva Pediatr. PMID: 27607482.

Sadeghi, N., Hasanpour, M., Heidarzadeh, M., et al., 2016. Information and communication needs of parents in infant end-of-life. Iranian Red. Crescent Med. J. 18 (6), e25665.

Schilleman, K., van der Pot, C.J., Hooper, S.B., et al., 2013. Evaluating manual inflations and breathing during mask ventilation in preterm infants at birth. J. Pediatr. 162 (3), 457–463.

Stijn, E.V., Sacreas, A., Vo, R., et al., 2016. Advances in understanding bronchiolitis obliterans after lung transplantation. Chest 150 (1), 219–225.

Sun, R., Liu, M., Lu, L., et al., 2015. Congenital heart disease: causes, diagnosis, symptoms, and treatments. Cell Biochem. Biophys. 72 (3), 857–860.

Sury, M., 2014. Brain monitoring in children. Anesthesiol. Clin. 32 (1), 115–132.

Vento, M., 2017. Oxygen supplementation in neonatal resuscitation. An. Pediatr. 86 (1), 1–3.

Vesoulis, Z.A., Lust, C.E., Liao, S.M., et al., 2016. Early hyperoxia burden detected by cerebral near-infrared spectroscopy is superior to pulse oximetry for prediction of severe retinopathy of prematurity. J. Perinatol. 36 (11), 966–971.

Vutskits, L., 2014. Cerebral blood flow in the neonate. Paediatr. Anaesth. 24 (1), 22–29.

Walker, S.M., 2014. Neonatal pain. Pediatr. Anesth. 24, 39–48.

Williams, G., 2017. Acute pain management in the neonate. Anaesth. Int. Care. 18 (2), 84–89.

Witt, N., Coynor, S., Edwards, C., et al., 2016. A guide to pain assessment and management in the neonate. Curr. Emerg. Hosp. Med. Rep. 4, 1–10.

Zareen, Z., Hawkes, C.P., Krickan, E.R., et al., 2013. In vitro comparison of neonatal suction catheters using simulated 'pea soup' meconium. Arch. Dis. Child. Fetal Neonatal Ed. 98 (3), F241–F243.

# 16

# Children

*Kath Ronchetti, Paul Ritson, Alexandra Hough*

## LEARNING OBJECTIVES

*On completion of this chapter the reader should be able to:*
- describe the anatomical and physiological differences between adults and children;
- discuss the common medical and surgical conditions of children;
- understand the principles of care for children on a paediatric intensive care unit;
- identify the main physiotherapy problems and describe their management;
- develop an insight into palliative care for children.

## OUTLINE

## INTRODUCTION

*We should look at the care of children with a child's eyes, in a child's manner.*

**Collins 1999**

Adult patients can say to themselves: 'I understand that I'm not in hospital for the rest of my life and that the nasty things they are doing to me are for my own good'. Young children do not have these resources of reasoning and may be overwhelmed by bewilderment, uncertainty about the behaviour expected of them and sometimes feelings that they are abandoned or being punished.

Despite progress in humanizing children's experience in hospital, long-term emotional disturbance still occurs. Children need to be listened to, believed and given some control over what is done to them. Teenagers in particular need autonomy because they often feel that they have outgrown the paternalistic environment of a paediatric unit. It is not surprising that children in hospital can exhibit different behaviours than those that are normal for them.

Children appreciate having the same physiotherapist throughout their stay. They need their own toys and belongings, and all but the sickest are best dressed in their day clothes.

A child is defined as aged from 1 year to adolescence. Adolescence is between 10 and 19 years.

### Differences Between Children and Adults

Following on from the differences with infants (p. 338) are the following:
1. By 2 years old, the bucket handle action of the ribs has developed and the rib cage and lungs become equally compliant. By 3 years old, when more time is

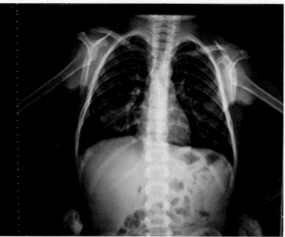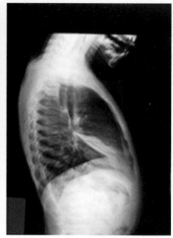

**FIGURE 16.1** Atelectasis of middle lobe in a 5-year-old child. (From Soyer et al. 2016.)

spent upright, the ribs are oblique rather than horizontal.

2. Collateral ventilation continually develops until approximately 8 years of age.

3. Young children's lungs are more prone to atelectasis due to smaller and more collapsible airways, a compliant chest wall and inefficient collateral ventilation, the middle lobe being particularly vulnerable because of its long narrow bronchus (Fig. 16.1).

4. Children are physically resilient, with bones and wounds healing quickly, but emotionally they are only resilient if they have a background of emotional security and have been encouraged to express what they are thinking and feeling.

From age 3, children should be involved in treatment planning with health staff and their parents. Over age 10 they are considered adults anatomically and physiologically, but they are not psychologically or emotionally mature for many years. At any age they may show an exaggeration of the behaviour patterns that they normally use to cope with stress, and social maturation may be delayed by potentiation of the sick role from professionals and families.

The transition from paediatric to adult care needs to be strategically managed. For inpatients, the provision of an adolescent unit means that teenagers do not have to sit in a ward full of toys or be surrounded by elderly patients with advanced pathology. Teenagers also appreciate having some control over which visitors they receive.

# CARDIORESPIRATORY CONDITIONS

Modifications from Chapters 3 and 4 are described below.

## Cystic Fibrosis

For chest clearance, regular physical exercise slows the decline in airflow obstruction (Almajed & Lands 2012), and trampoline or cycle exercise can increase sputum clearance and $SpO_2$ (Kriemler et al. 2016). When combined with forced expiratory manoeuvres, these may be an acceptable substitute for the active cycle of breathing (ACBT) in children with mild disease (Reix et al. 2012). Children should normally avoid head-down postural drainage because of the likelihood of reflux.

For adolescents, Withers (2012) makes the following observations:

1. From their early teens, patients should have some private time with their clinician.

2. Problems such as delayed puberty are visible and distressing at this age.

3. The full significance of a life-limiting condition emerges, and screening for depression should be routine.

4. The need for independence is hampered by ongoing dependence on the health system, and some dependence on their family may continue if employment is limited.

For children and adolescents, adherence is improved by providing a wide choice of patient-friendly chest clearance techniques, and ensuring strong relationships with care teams and structured routines (Sawicki et al. 2015).

Irons et al. (2013) identify singing as an enjoyable extra; they also recommend the children and youth version of the International Classification of Functioning, Disability and Health (ICF) as an outcome measure. Smoking parents need to be advised that passive smoking can stunt growth and facilitate infection (Kopp et al. 2015).

## Asthma

*Cough as a symptom of asthma has been so drummed into us that there is a real danger that every cough of any duration is treated as asthma.*

**Bush 2002**

The incidence of childhood asthma is increasing, the suspected culprits being lack of breastfeeding, fast food, obesity (Ding et al. 2015) and traffic pollution (Federico et al. 2016). The disease is also overdiagnosed, one study finding that only 16% of children identified as having asthma received a confirmation lung function test, as recommended, leading to unnecessary treatment and impairing quality of life (Looijmans et al. 2016). Children are often given steroids for self-limiting viral-induced wheezing or for 'exercise-induced asthma', which is actually deconditioning (Rubin 2015a). Only a third of children with recurrent wheeze develop asthma (Malka 2016).

However, those who have multitrigger wheezing (e.g. from exercise, viruses and allergens) plus a family history of atopy are likely to develop asthma (Hull et al. 2015). Severe disease has detrimental effects on the cardiovascular system through arterial stiffness (Steinmann et al. 2015).

Impaired clearance of inhaled allergens may play a role in airway inflammation, and assistance with mucociliary clearance may aid children with allergic asthma (Fritzsching et al. 2017). Exacerbations may be prevented by avoiding allergens and possibly drinks such as Coca Cola (Bush 2002). Over half of children with asthma have allergies, in comparison to adult-onset asthma which is less likely to be atopic (Rubin 2015). Immunotherapy is effective in some children (Tosca et al. 2014), and all children should be routinely screened for sleep-disordered breathing (Li et al. 2015b).

Most children outgrow their asthma, and it is thought to be more than coincidence that this is the time that they outgrow their fears (Gillespie 1989). Education has shown rapid and beneficial effects (Julian et al. 2015), for example:

- colourful diaries and stickers, available from asthma organizations or manufacturers;
- inhaler practice, preferably in front of a group to improve confidence at school;
- for children aged over 6 years practice in electronic monitoring of peak flow (BTS 2012b);
- healthy eating, including fresh fruit (Varraso 2012);
- hard and enjoyable physical activity because many children with asthma are deconditioned and associate exercise with anxiety;
- cough control because of an above-average incidence of incontinence (Soyer 2013);
- a personalized management plan, e.g. Fig. 16.2 and, when possible, involvement of a school-based clinic.

The early use of inhaled steroids does not affect the natural history of asthma nor prevent lung function decline, and may impair lung development (Rubin 2015a), bone density and adult height (Sutter & Stein 2016). Some parents prefer nedocromil (pp. 83 and 85), which inhibits histamine release but is an unfashionable drug, partly because its patent is out of time; it is effective in 70% of children (Korhonen et al. 1999), is safer than inhaled steroids and is useful for mild to moderate asthma (Sridhar & McKean 2006). Montelukast also provides some control while sparing steroids (Dilek et al. 2016). Nevertheless, steroids are required if asthma is persistent (Vichyanond et al. 2012) or acute (Redman & Powell 2013). For those aged 5 or older with a severe exacerbation, this should be within an hour of presentation (NICE 2013a). Questionnaires help identify if the goals of asthma management are reached (Bergen et al. 2015).

For acute episodes, the perception of breathlessness may be blunted, as with adults (Douros et al. 2015), which, along with some parents' tendency to underestimate the gravity of their child's asthma, could delay the family seeking medical assistance (Mitselou et al. 2016). Up to three bronchodilator nebulizers can be used in a row, which takes roughly an hour. Then:

- if there is no improvement, they will need intravenous drugs;
- if there is improvement, they can be reassessed in an hour, after which another nebulizer can be given if required; hourly assessment will then indicate if further nebulizers are needed; once this is down to 4 h, inhalers are indicated.

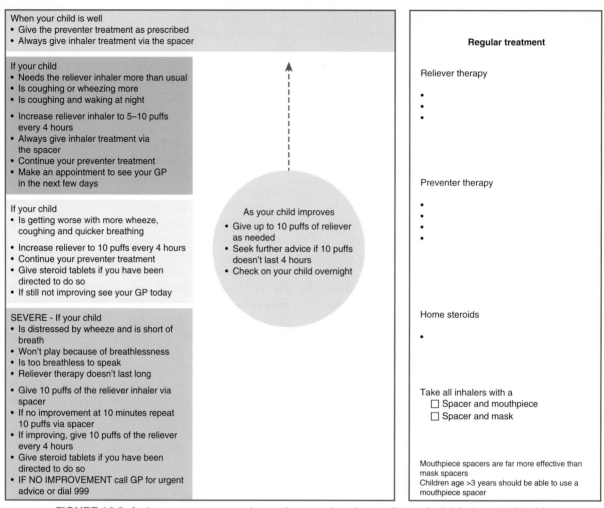

When your child is well
• Give the preventer treatment as prescribed
• Always give inhaler treatment via the spacer

If your child
• Needs the reliever inhaler more than usual
• Is coughing or wheezing more
• Is coughing and waking at night

• Increase reliever inhaler to 5–10 puffs
  every 4 hours
• Always give inhaler treatment via
  the spacer
• Continue your preventer treatment
• Make an appointment to see your GP
  in the next few days

If your child
• Is getting worse with more wheeze,
  coughing and quicker breathing

• Increase reliever to 10 puffs every 4 hours
• Continue your preventer treatment
• Give steroid tablets if you have been
  directed to do so
• If still not improving see your GP today

SEVERE - If your child
• Is distressed by wheeze and is short of
  breath
• Won't play because of breathlessness
• Is too breathless to speak
• Reliever therapy doesn't last long

• Give 10 puffs of the reliever inhaler via
  spacer
• If no improvement at 10 minutes repeat
  10 puffs via spacer
• If improving, give 10 puffs of the reliever
  every 4 hours
• Give steroid tablets if you have been
  directed to do so
• IF NO IMPROVEMENT call GP for urgent
  advice or dial 999

As your child improves
• Give up to 10 puffs of reliever
  as needed
• Seek further advice if 10 puffs
  doesn't last 4 hours
• Check on your child overnight

**Regular treatment**

Reliever therapy
•
•
•

Preventer therapy
•
•
•
•

Home steroids
•

Take all inhalers with a
☐ Spacer and mouthpiece
☐ Spacer and mask

Mouthpiece spacers are far more effective than
mask spacers
Children age >3 years should be able to use a
mouthpiece spacer

**FIGURE 16.2** Asthma management plan, to be completed according to individual need. (Noah's Ark Children's Hospital for Wales.)

Treatment may include continuous positive airway pressure (CPAP) to assist bronchodilation as well as oxygenation (Gomes 2013), and middle lobe collapse will need attention to reduce the risk of recurrent inflammation (Soyer et al. 2016). Manual deflation of a hyperinflated chest may be required (Masuda et al. 2014). Fatalities, although very rare in children, have shown a link with obesity and low income (Rubin & Pohanka 2012).

## Chest Infections

The risk of chest infections is decreased by breastfeeding (Ghimire 2012), increased by prematurity (Drysdale 2011) and doubled by passive smoking (Sconce 2013).

Young children react more severely to respiratory infections than adults because of their narrow airways. Those with neurological impairment or primary airways disease such as cystic fibrosis are more susceptible to lower respiratory tract infections, e.g. acute bronchitis or pneumonia, which themselves are usually preceded by upper respiratory tract infection such as the common cold, tonsillitis or epiglottitis. Physiotherapy is usually indicated for those who are unable to independently clear their secretions.

### Croup

Croup (laryngotracheobronchitis) is acute obstructive inflammation of the upper airway, usually caused by a

| TABLE 16.1 | Upper airway obstruction | |
| --- | --- | --- |
| | **Croup** | **Epiglottitis** |
| Age | 6 months to 3 years | 2 to 6 years |
| Aetiology | Viral | Bacterial |
| Onset | Days | Hours |
| Temperature | <38.5°C | >38.5°C |
| Cough | Barking | Minimal |
| Stridor | Only if severe | Yes |
| Voice | Hoarse | Weak |
| Can drink? | Yes | No |
| Child active? | Yes | No |

viral infection. It occurs mainly from ages 6 months to 6 years, with children born prematurely being most at risk. Clinical features include a harsh barking cough, hoarseness, painful breathing and sometimes stridor, which is a rasping sound on inspiration indicating upper airway obstruction. Croup is usually benign and self-limiting, requiring just encouragement of fluids. Severe disease with stridor requires hospitalization, steroids, sometimes nebulized adrenaline (Eghbali et al. 2016) and occasionally intubation.

### Epiglottitis

Epiglottitis is a less common but more vicious form of upper airway obstruction, caused by fulminant infection of the soft tissues around the entrance to the larynx. Tachypnoea is evident, along with a severe sore throat so that swallowing saliva is difficult and drooling occurs. The child usually sits bolt upright or in a tripod position with neck extended and arms providing support for the accessory muscles. Prompt antibiotics and steroids are required.

With both croup and epiglottitis, physiotherapy is contraindicated in the acute phase because of the risk of increasing obstruction, but if the airway is protected with an endotracheal tube (ETT) and sputum retention is evident, chest clearance may be indicated. Table 16.1 identifies the differences between the two conditions.

### Pneumonia

Viral infection is the most common cause of pneumonia in young children (Wagner 2016) and the clinical course is more acute than in adults. The child presents with tachypnoea, fever, cough, wheeze and chest pain. Complications include empyema, as suggested by absent breath sounds and a dull percussion note, and sometimes abscess or bronchopleural fistula.

Physiotherapy may include positioning and CPAP (Chisti et al. 2015). Secretion clearance is sometimes needed in the later stages if the child is unable to clear airway debris. The presence of a chest drain indicates the need for posture correction and shoulder exercises.

### Pertussis (whooping cough)

Whooping cough is a highly infectious lower respiratory tract bacterial infection, spread by aerosol droplets from coughing or sneezing. A recent resurgence has been attributed to adolescents and adults missing their booster immunization (Zlamy 2016). For children admitted to the paediatric intensive care unit (PICU), mortality is 4.8% (Straney et al. 2016).

Signs are coughing spasms that terminate in a 'whoop' as air is gasped into the lungs, accompanied in younger children by vomiting and apnoea. The disease can be lengthy (hence the nickname '100-day cough') and coughing severe, occasionally causing complications such as barotrauma, rib fracture (Rocha et al. 2015) or bronchiectasis in later life. Physiotherapy is only required if there is sputum retention, and treatment must avoid any stimulus that irritates the sensitive airways and sets off more coughing.

## Paediatric Acute Respiratory Distress Syndrome (ARDS)

The following recommendations emerged from a consensus conference to identify differences in the management of paediatric and adult ARDS (Jouvet et al. 2015):

- $SpO_2$ should be maintained at 92%–97%;
- if plateau airway pressures with conventional mechanical ventilation exceed 28 cmH$_2$O, high-frequency oscillatory ventilation with recruitment manoeuvres may be substituted;
- suction, with saline instillation if required, should avoid derecruitment if possible, usually by using closed-circuit systems;
- prone positioning can be considered for children with the severest form of the condition;
- physical, neurocognitive, emotional, family, and social function should be evaluated within 3 months of discharge.

## Inhaled Foreign Body

Children are notorious for inserting unseemly objects into their nose and mouth, from where they may find their way into the airway. Physiotherapy is contra-indicated until removal, and only then if airway clearance is required. Without treatment, airway damage can lead to chronic respiratory disease (Martin 2016). Details are described on p. 99.

## Hypertension

Systemic hypertension in children has traditionally been secondary to kidney disease, coarctation of the aorta or medications, but the 'explosion of childhood obesity' has uncovered primary hypertension, which occurs in more than 20% of obese children (Patel & Walker 2016). Older children may present with symptoms related to end organ abnormalities involving the heart, eye and brain, and prompt recognition is needed to prevent further damage (Anyaegbu 2014).

## Conduction Disorders

Supraventricular tachycardia is the most common symptomatic tachyarrhythmia in childhood, manifest as palpitations, shortness of breath and dizziness, or in neonates as pallor, lethargy or respiratory distress. Treatment includes carotid sinus massage, drugs, cardioversion or handstands (Hare & Ramlakhan 2015).

## Hyperventilation Syndrome

Hyperventilation syndrome is commonly missed and may incorporate vocal cord dysfunction, fear of suffocation, throat clearing or habit cough (Grüber et al. 2012). It occurs in about 18% of children, or 55% of those with asthma (Gridina et al. 2013). Treatment is similar to adults (Chapter 17).

## CONDITIONS WITH CARDIORESPIRATORY COMPLICATIONS

### Gastro-oesophageal Reflux Disease

Episodes of gastro-oesophageal reflux (GOR) are common in infancy and childhood. This usually resolves spontaneously and is not considered pathological unless frequent enough to cause gastrointestinal or respiratory symptoms (Puntis 2015). It is thought to occur in up to 80% of asthmatic children (Hamdan et al. 2016), and sometimes leads to bronchiectasis (Zaid et al. 2010). Signs include regurgitation or vomiting after meals, failure to gain weight, unwillingness to eat, eating small amounts, choking, and wheezing after food. Management is by feeding little and often with thickened feeds.

There is limited evidence for the benefit of antacids (Berman 2015), and safety concerns have been raised when these are used in infants (Slaughter et al. 2016).

Physiotherapy must be avoided after eating. If postural drainage is required, opinions are conflicted. Some observers have described the head-down tilt as safe (Doumit et al. 2015) but others have claimed the opposite (Schechter 2007). Clinical reasoning suggests that in the absence of convincing evidence, head-down postural drainage is inadvisable unless essential, and certainly should be avoided if symptoms are present. Prone and left side-lying give some protection (Ewer et al. 1999). However, children vary in the position at which reflux occurs, and symptoms should be monitored closely.

## Neuromuscular Conditions

Respiratory illness is the leading cause of hospitalization and death in children with severe neurological compromise. Immobility and oromotor dysfunction are particular risks (Blackmore et al. 2016). Neurological disease may also bring respiratory muscle insufficiency, low lung volumes, impaired cough, swallowing dysfunction, GOR, chronic aspiration or sleep-disordered breathing (BTS 2012c).

In children and adolescents, peak cough flow (PCF) below 270 L/min indicates the need for mechanical cough assistance (BTS 2012c), and vital capacity (VC) dropping below 1.1 L or PCF <160 L/min denotes a risk of chest infection serious enough to require hospital admission (Bush 2007). 'Whistle mouth pressures' provide child-friendly measurements of expiratory muscle strength (Aloui et al. 2016). Cough augmentation may also be required at home (Moran et al. 2015), which, as with neonates, should end with an insufflation breath to restore lung volume. Families require information on the earliest signs of chest infection and a personalized management programme.

Success in respiratory management has led to cardio-myopathies emerging as a cause of mortality, but limited physical activity means that symptoms may not emerge until cardiac involvement is advanced. Cardiopulmonary exercise testing supports early referral to cardiology if required and may assist safe exercise prescription (Case & Hartzell 2015). An example of a child's information sheet is shown in Fig. 16.3.

Children with **cerebral palsy** who are non-ambulant or have oromotor dysfunction may need daily airway

## NaME *Date of Birth/Hospital number*
### Ventilation information sheet

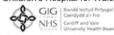

Children's Hospital for Wales

GIG | Bwrdd Iechyd Prifysgol
CYMRU | Caerdydd a'r Fro
NHS | Cardiff and Vale
WALES | University Health Board

*respiratory nurse & physiotel number*
*paediatric respiratory consultant*

## Background information

### Spinal muscular atrophy type 2
........... has SMA2. He is very weak and from a respiratory perspective needs ventilation overnight. This is delivered through mask ventilation. He has difficulties with secretion clearance because of his weakness and has a chest physiotherapy regimen twice a day which incorporates the cough assist machine. He has had spinal surgery and requires regular rod extension procedures.

### When ............ is well
When ............. is well his respiratory health is good. Ventilation at night helps prevent secretion retention in the lungs.
### Physiotherapy
.............has chest physiotherapy twice a day. He has percussion, Mechanical cough assist and mother also knows how to do manual assisted cough via thoracic compression.

**VENTILATOR SETTINGS**
### Pressure control 20/8 I.T 1.0, RR 20

**PHYSIOTHERAPY PROGRAMME**
### COUGH ASSIST +20/–40
- 6 breaths in/exsuff- programme 1 } ×3
- 4 breaths in to finish

## Managing a chest exacerbation

With 24 hour mask ventilation and physiotherapy using the cough assist, it should be possible to prevent intubation and PICU admission. Please contact the paediatric respiratory service at the Children's Hospital for Wales for advice.

- Ventilator pressures may need to be increased during exacerbations
- NIV should be maintained 24 hours/day until ............. is in air and has minimal secretions.
- He should be placed on a humidified circuit
- Use cough assist in programme 3 as and when required but at least twice a day with increase exsufflation of –45 cm $H_2O$
- When............. is in air and has minimal secretions, weaning should be achieved by incrementally increasing time off the ventilator each day. This is best achieved by having 2 short periods off the ventilator, one in the morning and one in the afternoon with a rest on the ventilator in between.
- Weaning to four hours off ventilation twice a day may take 7–10 days

## Equipment

................is ventilated using a ***B&D Nippy junior+ ventilator*** and a ***Respironics Wisp Mask***
He has a ***Respironics E70 Cough Assist*** machine and *Laerdal* suction machine
He has oxygen saturation monitoring to help guide physiotherapy-Saturations to be ≥95%

All equipment is serviced by UHW Clinical Engineering:

Last updated 16/10/2015

**FIGURE 16.3** Ventilation instruction sheet for a child with spinal muscular atrophy. (Noah's Ark Children's Hospital for Wales.)

clearance and a safe feeding regimen to safeguard the lungs. Techniques and positions must be carefully chosen, e.g. side-lying and supported sitting, because abnormal muscle tone and postural deformities may cause breath-holding and spasms. Side-lying and supported sitting may be most effective for reducing respiratory rate (RR) and effort, whereas supine is often least tolerated (Littleton et al. 2011).

For children with **spinal muscular atrophy** or **Duchenne muscular dystrophy**, regular assessment of pulmonary function when awake and asleep enables early recognition of deterioration and the instigation of non-invasive ventilation (NIV) when required, along with humidification (BTS 2012c). Respiratory failure is the primary cause of death, and NIV has improved both quality and longevity of life (Katz et al. 2013). Respiratory function may be enhanced by positioning, the most comfortable often being upright or high side-lying. Twice daily lung volume recruitment (p. 112) can attenuate the decline in VC and maintain assisted PCF (Katz et al. 2016b).

### Trauma

Trauma is the main cause of childhood morbidity and mortality worldwide (Ivashkov 2012). Survivors show surprisingly high rates of posttraumatic stress disorder, at 69% in the short term (Herbert 2005) and 27% in the long term (Holbrook et al. 2005). Parental distress is a contributing factor, underlying the importance of care for the family. Children may mistake flashbacks for reality and keep their feelings to themselves so as not to upset their parents.

Burns can be sustained from steam vaporizers used to humidify room air, especially for toddlers (Lonie et al. 2016) and from steam inhalers (Al Himdani et al. 2016). Severe burns can lead to hypermetabolism for at least 2 years after injury, during which time an exercise programme is beneficial (Porter et al. 2016).

The causes of chest trauma are in Table 16.2, the main immediate complication being hypoxia and the main late complication empyema (Okonta 2015), the predisposing factors for which are in Table 16.3.

## SURGERY

*Untreated anxiety and pain have significant implications for children's short- and long-term recovery.*
**Fortier & Kain 2015**

### Preoperative Care

Parents have not always explained an operation to the child, and, without explanation, the boundary between reality and fantasy may be blurred, e.g. being 'put to sleep' can have fearful connotations if this has happened to a family pet. Children have been known to mistake a bone marrow test for a 'bow-and-arrow test' and a dye injection for a 'die injection'. Both preoperative anxiety and youth increase the intensity of postoperative pain (Pagé 2012).

**TABLE 16.2   Aetiology of chest injury**

| Cause | Percentage |
|---|---|
| Fall | 41.9 |
| Road traffic accident | 32.2 |
| Stab injury | 12.9 |
| Gunshot injury | 9.7 |
| Child abuse | 3.2 |

From Okonta 2015.

**TABLE 16.3   Injuries associated with chest trauma**

| Cause | No of patients | Pneumothorax | Haemothorax | Pneumohaemothorax | Contusion | Rib fracture |
|---|---|---|---|---|---|---|
| Fall | 13 | – | 7 | 1 | 9 | 3 |
| Road traffic accident | 10 | 2 | 3 | – | 8 | 2 |
| Stab injury | 4 | 1 | 1 | – | – | – |
| Gunshot injury | 3 | 1 | 3 | 1 | 1 | – |
| Child abuse | 1 | 4 | 1 | – | – | – |

From Okonta 2015.

Explanations can be helped by pictures, visits, discussion with children who have had the same operation and rehearsal of procedures such as trying the anaesthetic mask (Fortier 2011). Physical sensations and their reasons should be explained, and a play specialist enrolled when possible. Truth is essential, otherwise cooperation is lost. For cardiac patients, preoperative advice on breathing and mobility can lead to more rapid recovery (Carmini et al. 2000). Parents require highly detailed explanations.

Children must not be excessively starved, and should be allowed free fluids until the moment they are called for surgery (Ragg 2015).

At induction of anaesthesia, parental presence reduces postoperative agitation (Zand et al. 2011). Children are more accepting of the face mask if their choice of flavoured lip balm is smeared inside before induction (Walpole 2003).

## Postoperative Care

Postextubation laryngospasm is a greater risk in children than in adults, and is three times higher in infants than in older children, with stridor being a risk if the endotracheal tube has been tight (Pawar 2012). Other problems may be tachycardia, caused by pain, anxiety or fluid deficit, or bradycardia, caused by hypoxia or medication. Oxygen saturation must not be allowed to drop below 93%.

To improve cooperation with physiotherapy, multimodal analgesia should be used that does not compromise mobilization (Visoiu 2015), e.g. combined regional and systemic analgesia (Murphy et al. 2016). Medication may also be needed to prevent vomiting, which is more common in children than adults (Bassanezi 2013).

Children like to be touched as little as possible after surgery. Manual techniques to the chest are usually counterproductive and are not effective in preventing atelectasis (Schechter 2007). However, if required, other forms of chest clearance, with adequate analgesia and including mobility, can reduce complications (Felcar et al. 2008). If coughing is necessary, children prefer to splint the incision themselves by leaning forward with their arms crossed and using a clean teddy bear or rolled up towel.

Following lung surgery, positive expiratory pressure can assist sputum clearance, and mobilization can improve lung expansion (Kaminsk 2013). Following cardiac surgery, multidisciplinary management has been emphasized by Bacha & Kalfa (2014), the goal being to 'treat more while hurting less'.

## PAEDIATRIC INTENSIVE CARE UNIT (PICU)

The PICU is a high stress environment. Sensory overload and sleep disturbance can lead to delirium in children (Schieveld et al. 2015). Restraints should not be used unless the child is in danger, e.g. by pulling out lines and tubes, and sedation requires specific paediatric protocols (Altamimi et al. 2015). The physiotherapist should be watchful after the sedative propofol, which can cause tachycardia in young children (Dewhirst et al. 2013), or dexmedetomidine, which can cause bradycardia and hypotension (Kim et al. 2014).

### Pain Management

*Pain management represents one of children's largest unmet needs.*

***Thompson 2013***

Children at most risk of inadequate pain assessment and treatment are those who are preverbal, neurologically compromised or cognitively impaired (Schreiber et al. 2016b), especially if they have been subject to prior pain experiences in the neonatal intensive care unit, which can sensitize pain pathways and damage central nervous system development (Walker 2014). Guidelines are often not adhered to (Ozawa & Yokoo 2013), and the consequences could bring prosecution if applied to animals.

The causes of poor pain management in children include the following:

1. Children's subjective complaints may not be taken seriously.
2. Distinguishing pain from agitation is challenging in young children, and some do not express pain in terms that are easily understood by adults. Absence of crying does not necessarily mean absence of pain.
3. Inexperienced doctors may underprescribe analgesia due to fear of side effects. They can be reassured that adequate analgesia is safe in the youngest children (Elkomy et al. 2016) and, from age 3 months, ventilatory depression from morphine or fentanyl is no greater than that seen in adults with similar plasma concentrations (Ivashkov 2012). However, meticulous prescription is required (Elkomy et al. 2016).

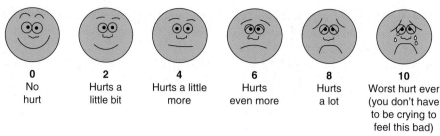

FIGURE 16.4 Faces pain scale. (Wong–Baker Faces Foundation.)

4. Children may not report pain if they anticipate the dreaded needle, and pain scores are often not used (Lord et al. 2016b).
5. Children are easily held down by force (see Clinical Reasoning, p. 385).

Parents' opinions must be actively sought because they tend to assume that everything to minimize pain is done routinely. Older children can be asked directly about their pain, which gives an indication of any associated fear. Children over age 3 can use colour intensity scores, charts with body outlines or face scales (Fig. 16.4). Those aged over 7 can use an adult visual analogue scale, and most children benefit from a combination of self-report and at least one other measure. Assessment tools are also available for prelingual and nonverbal children (Voepel-Lewis 2002, Sikka et al. 2015).

Physiological measures such as changes in RR, heart rate, blood pressure (BP) and $SpO_2$ are not specific to pain, not sustained with continued pain and only occur with extreme pain, as evident by a trebling of serum cortisol levels (Paix & Peterson 2012). Apparent sleeping after a painful procedure may be 'dissociative shock' rather than an indication that all is well.

Multimodal analgesia includes patient-controlled analgesia (Rai 2013), opioids (Arenas et al. 2017), neuroaxial blockade (Lundblad 2016), nitrous oxide (Entonox) (Kurien et al. 2016), or distraction with virtual reality games (Das et al. 2005), medical clowning (Meiri et al. 2016) and iPads (Shahid et al. 2015).

Ineffective pain management has been found with procedural pain such as needle sticks (Pickup & Pagdin, 2001). Local anaesthetic cream is required (Schreiber et al. 2013) or novel options such as a cooling vibration device (Schreiber et al. 2016b). The child must have a measure of control over the process (Brown et al. 2012).

## Oxygen Therapy

Hypoxaemia correlates strongly with mortality in children (Stevenson et al. 2015) and oxygen should be prescribed for a target $SpO_2$, normally >92%. For children with pulmonary hypertension, chronic lung disease of prematurity or cyanotic heart disease, individual target saturations must be determined. Although rare in children, $CO_2$ narcosis can occur with high oxygen concentrations in those with severe lung disease or neuromuscular weakness. Table 16.4 summarizes the oxygen delivery systems used in paediatrics.

Venturi masks are preferred to low-flow systems in hypoxaemic children with a high RR (Uygur et al. 2016). High-flow nasal cannulae are also used as an intermediate level of support between conventional oxygen therapy and noninvasive ventilation, but with occasional complications of barotrauma and abdominal distension. The pressure cannot be controlled, as with CPAP, but depends on flow, diameter of the cannula and whether the child is mouth breathing (Mikalsen et al. 2016). 'Wafting' oxygen provides noncontact oxygen for children unhappy with conventional delivery devices, the highest concentrations being achieved with oxygen tubing 5–15 cm in front of the face, or either tubing or a paediatric nonrebreather mask 5–10 cm below the face at 10–15 L/min flow (Blake et al. 2014).

Home oxygen may be needed for children with obliterative bronchiolitis, using assessment by oximetry rather than arterial blood sampling (BTS 2009).

## Respiratory Drugs

For ventilated children with proven airflow obstruction, aerosolized salbutamol can increase functional residual capacity and assist lung recruitment (Ramsi et al. 2015). For nonventilated children, whether in or outside the

### TABLE 16.4  Paediatric oxygen devices

| Device | Indications | Advantages | Limitations |
|---|---|---|---|
| **Headbox**<br>Humidified and warmed, $FiO_2$ 0.24–0.60 | Infants with acute respiratory disease | Well tolerated in infants | $CO_2$ build up <7 L/min, difficult access |
| **Nasal cannulae**<br>Max flow 2 L/min, variable $FiO_2$ | Minimal oxygen requirement, weaning off from acute episode, long-term oxygen | Easy talking and eating, well tolerated, no rebreathing | $FiO_2$ variable: affected by flow setting, RR and $V_T$, mucosal drying and nasal irritation |
| **Simple facemask**<br>5–15 L/min, $FiO_2$ affected by flow setting and RR | Patients who do not require exact $FiO_2$ | Useful in children who are mouth breathers, have nasal irritation, can also be used as wafting $O_2$ if not tolerated | Minimal delivery of 5 L/min to avoid rebreathing $CO_2$, $FiO_2$ variable |
| **Nonrebreathe mask**<br>6–15 L/min, $FiO_2$ 0.60–1.00 | Often used in emergencies | Delivers high $FiO_2$ | Minimal flow 6 L/min to avoid rebreathing $CO_2$, oxygen delivery affected by mask fit and leak, drying of mucosa and secretions |
| **Humidified facemask**<br>$FiO_2$ 0.28–0.98 delivered at variable flow rates | For children with acute respiratory disease or thick secretions | Controlled $FiO_2$, aids expectoration of secretions | Noisy |

*FiO$_2$*, Fraction of inspired oxygen; *RR*, respiratory rate; *V$_T$*, tidal volume.
From the Noah's Ark Children's Hospital for Wales Cardiff Paediatric Oxygen Working Group (2011).

PICU, inhalers should suit a child's lack of coordination, short inspiratory time, reduced ability to breath-hold and low inspiratory flow rate. The following are suitable but must be reviewed regularly (BTS 2011):

1. Some large-volume spacers need to be tipped downwards towards the child during inhalation to allow the valve to open.
2. From birth to age 5, a metered-dose inhaler (MDI) and spacer are preferred. A face mask is required until the child can use a spacer mouthpiece. If a mask is frightening, it can be used to gently stroke the child's cheek beforehand, or demonstrated on a teddy. Crying means that most of the aerosol does not reach the lower airways (Amirav & Newhouse 2012).
3. Children aged 3 years or older can use a dry powder inhaler or inhaler with spacer.
4. A child aged 10 years and upwards can manage an MDI independently.

In countries where spacers are not available, a 500-mL plastic bottle can be substituted.

Nebulizers are less effective than with adults due to a child's rapid and variable RR, low tidal volumes and high resistance from narrow airways. Infants and toddlers tend to show better results when nasal breathing and older children when mouth breathing (DiBlasi 2015). Practical suggestions are the following:

- Masks should be as tight-fitting as is acceptable to the child (Fig. 16.5) until the child is old enough to use a mouthpiece.

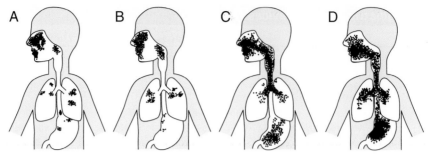

**FIGURE 16.5** Inhaled drug deposition. (A) Metered-dose inhaler (MDI) with spacer through loosely fitted face mask. (B) Nebulizer with loosely fitted face mask. (C) MDI with tightly fitted face mask. (D) Nebulizer with tightly fitted face mask. (Adapted from DiBlasi 2015.)

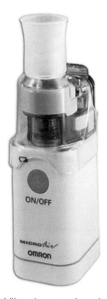

**FIGURE 16.6** Vibrating mesh nebulizer (Omron).

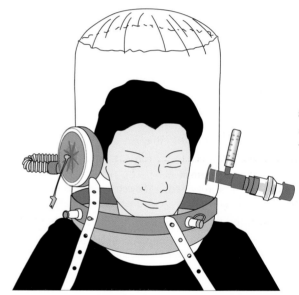

**FIGURE 16.7** Hood.

- Nebulizers should be placed before the Y-piece to the ventilator (Berlinski 2015) or within a nasal high-flow circuit (Réminiac et al. 2017).
- Nebulizers can be tried on a doll first, or used with children when they are asleep, under supervision.
- For children requiring several nebulizers a day, e.g. those with cystic fibrosis, vibrating mesh nebulizers are portable, silent and quick (Fig. 16.6).

## Continuous Positive Airway Pressure and Noninvasive Ventilation

For spontaneously breathing children, continuous positive airway pressure (CPAP) or noninvasive ventilation (NIV) can be used if adequate oxygenation or ventilation cannot otherwise be maintained (Platt 2014). Administration can be by face mask, nasal prongs or a hood (Fig. 16.7).

In the absence of chronic lung pathology, a starting pressure of 5 cmH$_2$O is used for CPAP, then gradually increased until grunting stops or oxygenation is optimum, so long as the child does not start to exhale forcefully, indicating excess work of breathing. Pressures above 10 cmH$_2$O bring a risk of gastric distension and diaphragmatic splinting, so if the child has a nasogastric tube, it should be left on free drainage to enable escape of trapped gas. Accurate monitoring of pressure, using a separate manometer, is required to minimize the risk of pneumothorax.

For NIV, inspiratory pressures of 8–12 cmH$_2$O are set initially, then gradually adjusted to a level that overcomes excess work of breathing, as observed by a stable breathing pattern. Expiratory pressures start at 3–5 cmH$_2$O and are adjusted to achieve upper airway patency at end-expiration, as reflected by improved SpO$_2$ and normalised PaCO$_2$. Children going home with a long-term portable ventilator will need:

- a well-fitting comfortable interface
- an oximeter
- family training from a specialist team (ATS 2016)

---

**KEY POINT**

Children at risk of vomiting should not use a hood or full face mask without a nasogastric tube, in case of aspiration.

---

## Mechanical Ventilation

Intubation and mechanical ventilation (MV) can cause haemodynamic compromise in children (Jones 2012), and inotropic support (p. 459) may be needed to stabilize BP. This acts as a warning that if physiotherapy is indicated, the response to each intervention should be monitored before proceeding to the next step.

'VAP bundles' (p. 440) help prevent ventilator-associated pneumonia (Hill 2016). Lung protective strategies limit ventilator-induced lung injury, but the lung recruitment manoeuvres that sometime accompany this, for example increased duration and pressure at end-inspiration, may cause alveolar overdistension in these vulnerable lungs (Jauncey-Cooke et al. 2015). Examples are the neurally adjusted ventilatory assist mode (Kallio et al. 2015), or high-frequency oscillation (Morgan et al. 2016).

Intubation means that the child cannot grunt when in respiratory distress, and loss of positive end-expiratory pressure (PEEP) may cause derecruitment and hypoxia, so if manual hyperinflation is indicated, PEEP should be maintained (Boriosi et al. 2012).

Falling tidal volumes may be due to bronchospasm or retained secretions. Excess secretions or agitation both increase the risk of unplanned extubations, which are more common in children than adults, and are usually followed by reintubation, both events bringing their own risks (Tripathi et al. 2015).

## Extubation

A spontaneous breathing trial, with pressure support to compensate for the loss of PEEP, can predict successful extubation (Gaffari et al. 2015). Upper airway obstruction is the commonest cause of extubation failure, and children who have been ventilated for several days, or have a risk of postextubation stridor (e.g. Down syndrome or cerebral palsy) may need steroids beforehand to minimize airway swelling. Stridor can be managed by heated humidified oxygen, nebulized adrenaline or sometimes heliox (Martinón-Torres 2012). Children with neurological disorders and an ineffective cough need a clear protocol for extubation including secretion clearance, cough augmentation and NIV (BTS 2012c, Appendix B).

---

**KEY POINT**

Nasopharyngeal suction should be avoided in the presence of stridor because of the risk of obstruction. If suction is essential, a doctor experienced in intubating children must be on hand.

---

## Tracheostomy

Early tracheostomy is advised if lengthy MV is anticipated (Holloway et al. 2015). Differences from adult tubes are the following:

- Fenestrated tubes are not used for small children due to the risks of obstruction with granulation tissue.
- Inner tubes are impractical because of the size of the tracheostomy tube.
- Cleaning the tube requires its complete removal and replacement.
- Uncuffed tubes are used unless excessive leak around the tube prevents adequate ventilation.
- The stoma path is a curve rather than an opening straight to the back of the neck.
- The short neck may pose problems for access and cause discomfort. Some tubes have longer and more flexible connectors to accommodate this (Fig. 16.8)

To assist communication, an uncuffed tube can be occluded with a gloved hand on expiration if the child is attempting to talk, laugh or cry. This must only be

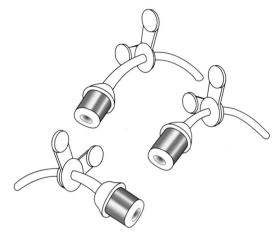

**FIGURE 16.8** Silicone tracheostomy tubes (Smiths Medical).

done if there is sufficient leak to allow air to move past the vocal cords so the child can breathe out. Occlusion must be brief and explained to the child beforehand. Toddlers learn to drop their chin to occlude the tube when wanting to talk. For intubated children who are preverbal, delayed communication can be prevented by speech–language therapy (Jiang & Morrison 2003).

Decannulation is usually preceded by downsizing to a tube that is small enough to let the child breathe around the tube but wide enough to allow suction if required. The smaller the child, the more likely are problems related to airway resistance created by a smaller tube, unexpected anatomical problems or a mucous plug. Close monitoring is required, particularly at night.

The families of children going home with a tracheostomy need training in suction, feeding, bathing, tracheostomy care and resuscitation. Unlike adults, children requiring an ongoing tracheostomy need humidification rather than a heat–moisture exchanger (McNamara et al. 2014).

## PHYSIOTHERAPY

*You need to obtain as much information as you can before touching the child.*

**Isaacs 2015**

Parents should be welcomed during assessment and treatment. If this causes the child to express anxiety more noisily than when unaccompanied, this is healthier than withdrawal. Children must not be discouraged from crying, nor told to be brave, although they can be awarded a brave sticker afterwards. If they are 'difficult', it is usually because they are frightened.

Clear, quiet and honest explanations to the child and family are required, including details such as the experience of disconnection from the 'breathing machine', the beeping of alarms and how manual techniques will feel. Demonstrations can be given on a teddy or doll. Hand puppets can give instructions in funny voices, sometimes hiding under clothes. The puppet can fall down with a squeal of joy if good breaths are done, or sulk if not so good. If the child's favourite toy, TV programme, food or game is documented, these can be used to engage their interest. Story-telling enables the child to look forward to the rest of the story in the next session. Babies can be given rattles and toys to watch during treatment.

Children must be reassured that the procedure can be stopped, sometimes temporarily, at any time (Lundeberg 2015). Reluctance can often be overcome by cajoling, distraction, joking, enlisting the help of a parent/play specialist or giving the child a choice, e.g. whether to keep the TV on or off, to have incentive spirometry or a walk outside, or have parents present or not.

### Consent

Children should not simply be deemed competent if they agree and incompetent if they disagree. Those aged over 16 are able to consent to treatment unless they lack capacity (p. 437). A child under 16 may consent to treatment if he or she fully comprehend what is involved. If he or she refuses treatment, it can be overridden by an adult who has parental responsibility (Lynch 2010).

Emergency treatment can be given without consent if this is required to prevent serious deterioration. Treatment may be provided in the absence of a guardian if that treatment is deemed in the patient's best interests, so long as this is not used as an excuse to avoid seeking consent.

### Assessment

Assessment of a child can be on a parent's lap, with a description of what is being examined and why. Wound drains and intravenous lines can inhibit children from moving and they should be reassured that these will be supported throughout. If the child is nil-by-mouth,

## TABLE 16.5  Normal values for children

| Parameter | Values |
|---|---|
| RR | 16–30 |
| SpO$_2$ | 93%–98% |
| PaO$_2$ | 10–13.2 kPa (75–100 mmHg) |
| PaCO$_2$ | 5–6 kPa (35–45 mmHg) |
| HR | 60–100 beats/min |
| BP | 90/55–110/65 |

*BP*, Blood pressure; *HR*, heart rate; *PaCO$_2$*, partial pressure of CO$_2$ in arterial blood; *PaO$_2$*, partial pressure of oxygen in arterial blood; *RR*, respiratory rate; *SpO$_2$*, peripheral oxygen saturation. From APLS 2011.

## BOX 16.1  Questions to Ask a Child[a]

1. What do you think asthma is?
2. How did you learn that you had asthma?
3. What do you think can be done to help it go away?
4. How do you feel when you have an attack?
5. Why do you think you got asthma?
6. How do you feel about asthma?

[a]Can be modified for other conditions (Gillespie 1989).

he or she can be distressed and not understand why drinking is not allowed. The notes and charts indicate any variation in normal values (Table 16.5).

### Subjective

Both the parent and child's views are required, including, for chronic conditions, how these are managed at home. Asking the child to draw a picture may indicate the effect of the illness on them. Some suggested questions are in Box 16.1.

A cough may be caused by foreign body aspiration, GOR, hyperventilation syndrome, passive smoking or, in preschool-aged children, bacterial bronchitis that may presage bronchiectasis (Kantar 2016). It can disrupt sleep and schooling, and disturb family members. Management is by identifying the cause, and cough facilitation (p. 216) or suppression (Appendix B). Medication is largely ineffective (Shields et al. 2008).

Fatigue may manifest as a change in sleep–wake times, continuous lack of interest, or concentration difficulties. Breathlessness can be measured with picture scales (Tulloch et al. 2012).

## BOX 16.2  Signs of Respiratory Distress

- Unstable RR or apnoea, unstable HR, tracheal tug, nasal flare or grunting
- Apical breathing pattern
- Paradoxical breathing (abdominal paradox in younger children, neck and shoulder accessory muscles in older children)
- Increased accessory muscle use ± tripod position
- Lethargy

*HR*, Heart rate; *RR*, respiratory rate.

### Objective

#### KEY POINT

Children in respiratory distress assume a position that promotes airway patency and they should be allowed to maintain this position, especially if stridor is present.

Objective signs of respiratory distress are in Box 16.2. Signs of deteriorating gas exchange include pallor, sweating, restlessness, agitation, glazed eyes or, in ventilated children, fighting the ventilator. Cyanosis or reduced consciousness indicates severe hypoxaemia. For hypoxia, capillary refill time of 3 s or more after moderate pressure for 5 s is considered abnormal (Fleming et al. 2015). Before auscultation, children can be given the opportunity to see and feel the stethoscope, and use it to listen to themselves or a parent. Identification of catheters, tubes and drains on X-ray is illustrated by Concepcion et al. (2016), as shown in Figs 16.9 and 16.10. Reference curves for exercise tests are available for children (Saraff et al. 2015).

### Precautions

- The assessment, in particular questioning the nurse and parents, indicates if the child is unstable and should be touched minimally.
- All forms of physiotherapy except education, and sometimes positioning, are contraindicated if there is an undrained pneumothorax or airway compromise not caused by secretions.
- Most forms of physiotherapy should be avoided if there are blood-stained secretions or cardiac instability.
- Desaturation episodes may be caused by secretions, breath holding, distress or suction.

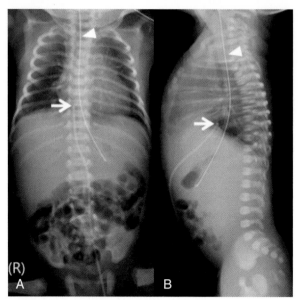

**FIGURE 16.9** A boy born at 33-weeks' gestation demonstrating an umbilical venous catheter coursing antero-superiorly with its tip *(arrows)* at the junction of the inferior vena cava and right atrium. A feeding tube is also in place *(arrowheads)*. (From Concepcion et al. 2016.)

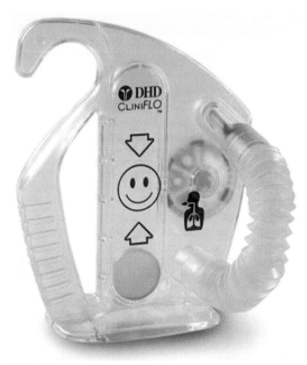

**FIGURE 16.11** Incentive spirometer (Courtesy Smiths Medical).

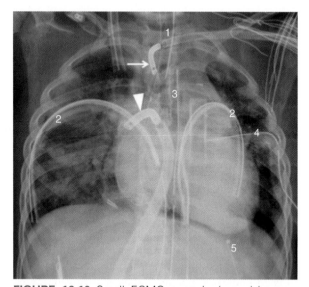

**FIGURE 16.10** Small ECMO cannula *(arrow)* is seen with its tip near the aortic arch, while the tip of the bigger cannula *(arrowhead)* is at the superior vena cava. Endotracheal *(1)*, Blake *(2)*, mediastinal *(3)*, left-sided chest *(4)* and feeding *(5)* tubes are also seen. A pneumopericardium is seen inferior to the heart. (From Concepcion et al. 2016.)

- Reassessment is necessary throughout treatment because deterioration can occur rapidly.

## Methods to Increase Lung Volume

Modifications of the techniques described on pp. 181 and 354 are discussed below.

**Positioning** is fundamental to both respiratory and developmental physiotherapy. For respiratory care, alternate high side-lying and supported upright sitting are usually effective and well tolerated. Oximetry guides positioning for gas exchange.

**Breathing exercises** can be done by children aged more than 2 years if taught imaginatively, and a paediatric incentive spirometer can be motivating (Fig. 16.11). The use of blowing games utilizes the deep breath that is taken before blowing out, e.g. paper mobiles, bubble-blowing, blowing a tissue or, better still, messy paint-blowing. Abdominal breathing can be taught by putting a toy on the abdomen 'like a boat on the sea'. Crying upsets the flow rate without increasing lung volume (Fig. 16.12) and should be avoided, particularly in children with stridor.

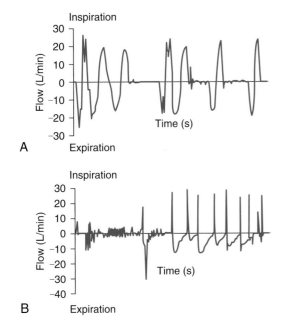

**FIGURE 16.12** Breathing patterns of (A) a 2-year-old child at rest and (B) a 20-month-old child while crying (left half) and sobbing (right half). (From Nikander 1997.)

| TABLE 16.6   Size of manual hyperinflation bag | | |
|---|---|---|
| **Weight of child (kg)** | **Size of bag (L)** | **Flow rate required (L/min)** |
| 0–20 | 0.5 (open ended) | 6 |
| 20–40 | 1 | 6–10 |
| >40 | 2 | 10–15 |

For intubated children, **manual hyperinflation** uses a bag to suit the weight of the child (Table 16.6). The following technique is suggested:

1. A manometer should be incorporated into the circuit to avoid high pressures.
2. If inhaled nitric oxide is being delivered, this should be included in the circuit in order to prevent swings in pulmonary artery pressure.
3. Ensure adequate sedation and prepare the child for a different breathing pattern and cold air.
4. For the 0.5 L open-ended bag, pressure and PEEP are controlled by the user squeezing the open tail (p. 354).
5. Each hyperinflation should be interposed with 2–3 tidal breaths

6. The chest should rise just slightly more than during MV.
7. Some positive pressure should be maintained at the end of expiration to maintain PEEP and prevent derecruitment.
8. The monitors must be kept under observation, any significant drop in BP indicating a need to return the infant to MV and advise nursing or medical staff.
9. If vibrations are added to the expiratory phase, they should be timed accurately: too early can cause high inspiratory pressures and too late renders the technique ineffective (Shannon et al. 2010).

**Ventilator hyperinflation**, or lung recruitment, for example inspiratory holds at 30–40 cmH$_2$O, can also improve lung volume and gas exchange, but not all studies document the complications of this technique, e.g. overdistension in nondependent lung regions, so positioning is key. Using the lower inflection point of the pressure–volume curve as a target is inadvisable because ventilators with this facility do not distinguish between hyperinflation and recruitment, and provide no information on the distribution of ventilation (Jauncey-Cooke et al. 2015).

Added to the usual precautions (p. 492) are to avoid pressures above 45 cmH$_2$O and PEEP over 30 cmH$_2$O because they can cause barotrauma or damage to the alveolar–capillary membrane sufficient to cause translocation of inflammatory cytokines into the circulation (Halbertsma 2010).

## Methods to Reduce the Work of Breathing

Breathlessness may be caused by increased work of breathing, deconditioning, anxiety, metabolic acidosis or decreased power due to muscle weakness or structural abnormalities. As with adults, it can be relieved by positioning, a fan or noninvasive ventilation.

## Methods to Clear Secretions

Children have more viscous secretions and relatively more mucus-secreting glands than adults. They benefit from airway clearance according to their condition (Table 16.7) and techniques can be disguised in a range of blowing games and activities. Once they are old enough to produce adequate expiratory flow and mouth control, they become more independent with positive expiratory pressure (PEP) devices.

To aid motivation, airway clearance techniques are best chosen by the child when possible.

| TABLE 16.7 | Evidence of benefit from airway clearance with some conditions | | |
|---|---|---|---|
| **Proven benefit** | **Probable benefit** | **Possible benefit** | **Minimal or no benefit/ counterproductive** |
| Cystic fibrosis | Neuromuscular disease Atelectasis in mechanically ventilated children | Prevention of post-extubation atelectasis in neonates | Acute asthma Bronchiolitis Respiratory distress syndrome Respiratory failure without atelectasis or secretions |

From Schechter 2007.

## Mucociliary clearance

**Postural drainage** can be enjoyable over a bean bag, or wedges and frames can be used for the longer term, with the usual precautions in case of GOR (p. 370). For infants, who spend much time in supine, the sitting position helps drain the apical segments of the upper lobes, with particular attention to the right upper lobe. **Manual techniques** are modified according to the child's age and comfort, and have been shown to improve flow bias, lung compliance, tidal volume and oxygenation, so long as patients are accurately selected (Hawkins & Jones 2015). **Rebound therapy** on a trampoline is enjoyed by older children.

The **active cycle of breathing** and **autogenic drainage** can be done by children from age 3–4, but they may not be able to put the components together consistently until aged 6–7. Huffing can be facilitated by misting up a mirror, using a peak flow mouthpiece to blow cotton wool or ping pong balls, or using the story of the big bad wolf who 'huffed and puffed and blew the house down'. For younger children, the physiotherapist can apply passive autogenic drainage.

**Positive expiratory pressure** can be delivered via a mask (Fig. 16.13A) or the ever-popular 'bubble PEP' (Fig. 16.13B), in which the child blows out through tubing or a straw into a bottle of soapy coloured water. For children who are nil-by-mouth, care is required to avoid them drinking the water.

## Cough

Coughing can be encouraged by laughter and rewarded by earning a star on a cough score sheet. Children are encouraged to expectorate more than saliva by looking for 'froggies' in their spit. Cough augmentation may be required for children with neuromuscular conditions.

If a sputum specimen is needed, children under age 4 can rarely expectorate. A **cough swab** may be successful, in which the child coughs and secretions are collected from the back of the throat by a swab, then sent to microbiology in a sterile container. If a specimen of **nasopharyngeal aspirate** is requested in order to obtain epithelial cells for diagnostic purposes, nasal suction should be performed into the postnasal space, to a depth that has been measured from nose to ear (Fig. 16.14). However, contamination by oral flora limits success. **Nasal swabs** are as sensitive as nasopharyngeal aspirate for the detection of major respiratory viruses except respiratory syncytial virus (Blaschke et al. 2011).

## Suction

### PRACTICE TIP

Nasopharyngeal suction is unnecessary if the child is coughing effectively, even if secretions are swallowed.

Suction that is followed by manual hyperinflation (MHI) tends to increase lung volume and compliance, but the opposite occurs without MHI (Hawkins & Jones 2015).

Variations from the procedure on p. 219 are the following:

- If regular suction is anticipated in an older child, a nasopharyngeal airway can be inserted to minimize trauma.
- Depth of insertion of the suction catheter is measured from the tip of the nose to the tragus of the ear and then to the base of the neck, with the head facing forwards (Fig. 16.15). If the child has a significant kyphoscoliosis, the depth is measured on both sides of the head, then the measurements added up and divided by two.

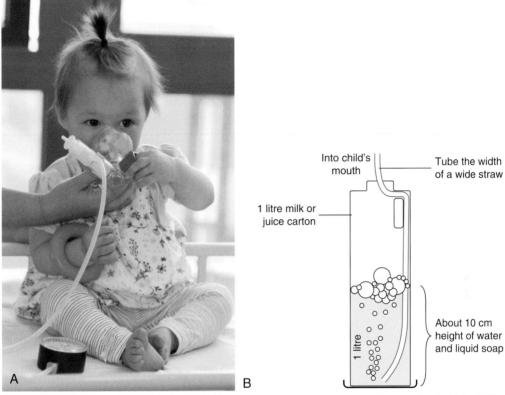

Into child's mouth

Tube the width of a wide straw

1 litre milk or juice carton

About 10 cm height of water and liquid soap

1 litre

A

B

FIGURE 16.13 (A) Child using a PEP mask (Children's Hospital for Wales). (B) Bubble PEP, particularly enjoyable if water sprays over the physiotherapist.

- There is little research on the pressure at which damage occurs, but limits of 13.3–16 kPa (100–120 mmHg) have been advised (AARC 2004).
- For intubated children, closed suction systems are usually preferred because they minimize derecruitment associated with disconnection from the ventilator, but open suction allows greater control of the negative pressure (Jauncey-Cooke et al. 2015), so discussion with the team is advisable.

If the rare complication of laryngospasm occurs in a nonintubated child, after summoning assistance, firm digital pressure should be directed inward at the notch bounded by the mastoid process posteriorly, the mandibular condyle anteriorly, and the base of the skull superiorly, identified just medially and slightly superior to the earlobe, while simultaneously performing a jaw thrust (Abelson 2015).

Saline instilled before suction may be beneficial (O'Leary 2017) so long as it does not cause haemodynamic instability, bronchospasm or hypoxaemia (Owen et al. 2016). Accurate NBBAL (p. 358) can be used to reverse atelectasis caused by mucous plugging.

## Exercise and Rehabilitation

Physical activity may open up the lung or assist airway clearance (Dwyer et al. 2011), with the added benefit of improving vascular health (Daniels 2015b) and cognitive performance (Chen 2015). Games can become increasingly energetic as the child progresses, building up to wheelbarrow races. Paediatric rehabilitation programs for asthma and cystic fibrosis may reduce symptoms and enhance self-management (Jung 2012).

In the PICU, the physiotherapist may be the first person to identify critical care weakness, which is

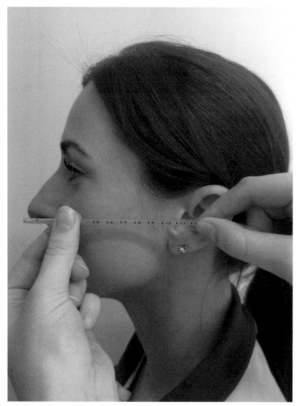

**FIGURE 16.14** Measurement for nasopharyngeal aspirate (Paul Ritson).

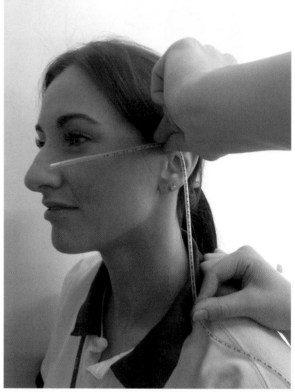

**FIGURE 16.15** Measurement for nasopharyngeal suction (Paul Ritson).

associated with some treatments and invasive procedures but is often missed (Field-Ridley et al. 2016).

Early mobilization contributes to a reduction in the after-effects of a stay in the PICU such as weakness and cognitive impairment (Hopkins et al. 2015). After discharge, children may also experience depression, altered relationships (Rennick 2015), an 80% risk of sleep disturbance and a 34% incidence of posttraumatic stress symptoms (Als et al. 2015).

A physiotherapy discharge planning tool has been developed (Ellerton et al. 2011), and the need for ongoing rehabilitation is emphasized by increased post-PICU survival (Hawkins & Jones 2015).

## Transition

Active referral to adult services is required for teenagers with asthma (Srivastava 2012) and cardiac disease (Moceri et al. 2015) to avoid them disappearing into a void. Communication and education aids the transition

so that young adults feel in control of their own health needs, and some paediatric services offer to escort them to their first adult appointment to ease anxieties and ensure a thorough handover.

## PALLIATIVE CARE

*It is every dying child's right to be helped to 'live while dying'.*

*Wellings 2001*

Children have a right to grieve. They have the capacity to do so, and begin to develop an understanding of death from 2 to 3 years old (Slaughter & Griffiths 2007). They may be prevented from grieving because of a natural desire by others to protect them from suffering. Children understand more than they can articulate and it is thought that they usually know that they are going to die (Tamburro et al. 2011). Evasion can leave them with a sense of bewilderment, betrayal and fantasies that are more frightening than reality.

Communication with dying children should be based on honesty. If death is compared to sleep, for example, they may develop an unhealthy fear of bedtime. Many children are able to take decisions about whether to have active or supportive therapy (Tamburro et al. 2011). As well as experiencing their own responses to dying, children have the burden of their parents' grief. Parents, grandparents, brothers and sisters may carry the added burden of being avoided by friends.

Tools are available to assess the needs of parents (Meert et al. 2012), whose main concern usually is to minimize suffering. The most prevalent symptoms at the end of life are pain and breathlessness, but over a quarter of children are not given opioids or sedatives, more so in the case of black children (Derrington 2015), despite strong opioids achieving pain control without serious complications (Urtubia et al. 2016). The family benefit from timely palliation of symptoms, continuity of personnel, the opportunity to bathe and hold their child, clear explanations and written summaries of options before making any decisions, including the timing of withdrawal of life support if necessary.

Physiotherapy focuses on symptom control. Children can use the hydrotherapy pool with oxygen cannulae, tracheostomies and ventilators, with appropriate safeguards. Withdrawal of PICU support sometimes enables the child to transfer to a hospice (Gupta & Harrop 2013), with the physiotherapist maintaining continuity of care when possible.

Comprehensive family support before and after the death helps reduce the high incidence of distress, divorce and sibling neglect that may ensue. Siblings often recognize their parents' grief and may themselves suffer survivor guilt, parental overprotection, or the effect of idealization of the deceased child (Miller et al. 2015). They may worry about their own vulnerability, feel confused by a mixture of what they have been told, overheard, observed or imagined, and may experience the functional loss of their parents. They should not be told 'Susie is going away on a long trip' euphemisms or they may wait for her return. They need information, open family communication, active involvement in the dying child's care and sometimes contact with others in a similar situation.

The family needs respect for the child's body, and sometimes locks of hair, attendance of staff at the funeral and follow-up phone calls (Brooten et al. 2013). It is unhelpful to tell parents that they will get over their child's death and it is rarely true. Parents can sometimes find ease in reflecting that it may have been better to have loved and lost a child than not to have had the child at all.

## CASE STUDY: MARK

*Four-year-old Mark has cerebral palsy. He was admitted with a severe chest infection, then developed respiratory failure and was ventilated for 2 days. Now extubated, he has suddenly dropped his $SpO_2$ and shows the following signs:*

- RR 40, $FiO_2$ 0.6, $SpO_2$ 88%
- ABGs: pH 7.10, $PaCO_2$ 13.2 kPa (100 mmHg), $PaO_2$ 7.9 kPa (60 mmHg) $HCO_3^-$ 29
- Auscultation: ↓ BS and crackles on the left
- ↓ expansion left chest
- See-saw breathing pattern
- Secretions thick and yellow

### Questions

1. Analyse the ABGs
2. Analyse the CXR (Fig. 16.16)
3. Overall analysis?
4. Problems?
5. Goal?
6. Plan?

> ### CLINICAL REASONING
>
> *'…these patients vigorously object to having an arterial puncture done even if they are relatively sick. Because of this, more than one person is usually required to obtain the sample'*
> Deming 1995, p. 213

### Response to Case Study

1. ABGs
   - Severe partially compensated respiratory acidosis. Poor oxygenation with high $FiO_2$

---

*ABGs*, Arterial blood gases; *BS*, breath sounds; *CXR*, chest X-ray; *RR*, respiratory rate.
*CPAP*, Continuous positive airway pressure; *NIV*, noninvasive ventilation.

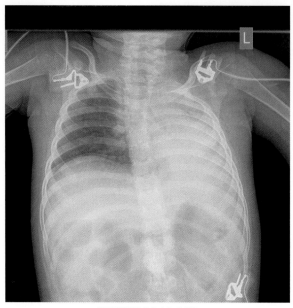

**FIGURE 16.16** MK.

2. CXR
   • Left lung collapse with mediastinal shift to left
3. Analysis
   • Acute left lung collapse, probably due to mucous plugging
   • Poor respiratory function, borderline for CPAP/NIV or intubation and ventilation
4. Problems
   • Loss of volume left lung
   • Retained secretions
5. Goal
   • Left lung reinflated within two treatments
6. Plan
   • Preoxygenate patient, monitor
   • Administer nebulized saline or hypertonic saline
   • Position patient onto right side-lying, monitor
   • Percussion and vibrations, monitor
   • Cough stimulation
   • If unsuccessful, consider cough augmentation with in–exsufflator
   • If unsuccessful, consider nasopharyngeal suction, monitor
   • Reassess
   • Plan for improvement
   • Plan for deterioration, including the need for mechanical assistance

## RESPONSE TO CLINICAL REASONING

This demonstrates the low priority given to children's pain by some medical textbooks and shows little awareness of the ethical, legal and humane implications of forcibly holding down a child in order to impose a painful procedure.

## CASE STUDY: HANNAH

*Hannah is a 10-year-old gastrostomy-fed cerebral palsy patient and has been admitted with increased work of breathing, excess secretions and low oxygen levels. Her parents have been performing her normal regimen of percussion, vibrations and suction at home. Hannah has a poor swallow reflex and rarely coughs spontaneously. She deteriorated after retching at home. The gastroenterology team suspect a failed fundoplication.*

On examination:
• awake and distressed, increased tone demonstrating an extensor pattern;
• tracheal tug and sternal recession;
• audible inspiratory stertor and crackles;
• RR 25, HR 160, temperature 35.7°C;
• $SpO_2$ 97% on 10 L via rebreathe mask; 85% on air;
• awaiting blood gases and X-ray;
• inspiratory stertor and crackles transmitted throughout chest;
• breath sounds ↓ on the right;
• secretions palpable throughout;
• increased tone with handling;
• susceptible to breath-holding.

**Questions**
1. Analysis?
2. Problems?
3. Plan?

**Response to Case Study**
1. Analysis
   • Retained secretions in the right lung, causing high oxygen requirements and increased work of breathing.

---

*Fundoplication*: Surgical strengthening of the lower oesophageal sphincter to stop acid reflux, *HR,* heart rate; *RR,* respiratory rate; *Stertor,* low-pitched snoring or snuffly sound caused by airflow obstruction above the larynx.

- Cause – probable aspiration from gastric reflux due to failing fundoplication. Poor swallow so unable to protect airway from aspiration. Right sided changes and normal temperature also support this.

2. Problems
   - Sputum retention
   - Poor gas exchange
   - ↑ work of breathing
   - ↑ tone and distress

3. Plan
   - Gain consent from parents
   - Changed to humidified oxygen
   - Liaise with parents about effective secretion clearance
   - Liaise with parents about managing Hannah's distress. Sedatives discussed, including possible effect on respiratory drive and cough reflex. Decision to communicate with Hannah and use sensitive handling.
   - Positioned sitting up and left side-lying
   - Percussions and expiratory vibrations → slight increase in tone
   - Assisted autogenic drainage → no increase in tone, therefore continued
   - Suction
   - Sputum sample sent to microbiology and virology
   - Consider nebulized hypertonic saline
   - Liaise with domiciliary physiotherapist

## RECOMMENDED READING

Allen, K.A., 2016. Pathophysiology and treatment of severe traumatic brain injuries in children. J. Neurosci. Nurs. 48 (1), 15–27.

Alzouebi, M., Roberts, I., 2005. Paediatric chest radiographs. Student. Br. Med. J. 13, 309–352.

Amedro, P., Picot, M.C., Moniotte, S., et al., 2016. Correlation between cardio-pulmonary exercise test variables and health-related quality of life among children with congenital heart diseases. Int. J. Cardiol. 203, 1052–1060.

Andrzejowski, P., Carroll, W., 2016. Salbutamol in paediatrics: pharmacology, prescribing and controversies. Arch. Dis. Child Educ. Pract. Ed. 101 (4), 194–197.

Anon, 2015. Assessing dehydration. Arch. Dis. Child. 100 (10), 1005.

Aynsley-Green, A., 2015. Improving the care of children and young people in the UK: 20 years on. Arch. Dis. Child. 100 (1), 4–7.

Backeljauw, B., Holland, S.K., Altaye, M., et al., 2015. Cognition and brain structure following early childhood surgery with anesthesia. Pediatrics 136 (1), e1–e12.

Banasiak, N.C., 2016. Understanding the relationship between asthma and sleep in the pediatric population. J. Pediatr. Health Care 30 (6), 546–550.

Barkman, C., 2013. Clowning as a supportive measure in paediatrics. BMC Pediatr. 13, 166.

Baudin, F., Bourgoin, P., Brossier, D., et al., 2016. Noninvasive estimation of arterial $CO_2$ from end-tidal $CO_2$ in mechanically ventilated children. Pediatr. Crit. Care Med. 17 (12), 1117–1123.

Berlinski, A., 2013. Nebulized albuterol delivery in a model of spontaneously breathing children with tracheostomy. Respir. Care 58 (12), 2076–2086.

Bianchi, C., Baiardi, P., 2008. Cough peak flows: standard values for children and adolescents. Am. J. Phys. Med. Rehabil. 87, 461–467.

Bilan, N., 2015. Validity of $SpO_2$/$FiO_2$ ratio in detection of acute lung injury and acute respiratory distress syndrome. Int. J. Pediatr. 3 (1.2), 429–434.

Bilan, N., Barzegar, M., Habibi, P., 2015. Predictive factors of respiratory failure in children with Guillain-Barre Syndrome. Int. J. Pediatr. 3 (1.2), 33–37.

Blackmore, A.M., Bear, N., Blair, E., et al., 2016. Prevalence of symptoms associated with respiratory illness in children and young people with cerebral palsy. Dev. Med. Child Neurol. 58 (7), 780–781.

Bokov, P., Mahut, B., Flaud, P., et al., 2016. Wheezing recognition algorithm using recordings of respiratory sounds at the mouth in a pediatric population. Comput. Biol. Med. 70, 40–50.

Bontant, T., Matrot, B., Abdoul, H., et al., 2015. Assessing fluid balance in critically ill pediatric patients. Eur. J. Pediatr. 174 (1), 133–137.

Carnevale, F.A., Gaudreault, J., 2013. The experience of critically ill children. Dynamics 24 (1), 19–27.

Chang, A.B., Oppenheimer, J.J., Weinberger, M., et al., 2016. Use of management pathways or algorithms in children with chronic cough. Chest 149 (1), 106–119.

Chikata, Y., Sumida, C., Oto, J., 2012. Humidification performance of heat and moisture exchangers for pediatric use. Crit. Care Res. Pract. 2012, 439267.

Choi, J.Y., Rha, D., Park, E.S., 2016. Change in pulmonary function after incentive spirometer exercise in children with spastic cerebral palsy. Yonsei. Medical. J. 57 (3), 769–775.

Conti, G., Piastra, M., 2016. Mechanical ventilation for children. Curr. Opin. Crit. Care 22 (1), 60–66.

Craig, F., Henderson, E.M., Bluebond, M., 2015. Management of respiratory symptoms in paediatric palliative care. Curr. Opin. Supp. Palliat. Care 9 (3), 217–226.

Davidson, J.E., Aslakson, R.A., Long, A.C., et al., 2017. Guidelines for family-centered care in the neonatal, pediatric, and adult ICU. Crit. Care Med. 45 (1), 103–128.

Davies, F.C.W., 2013. A patient survey for emergency care designed by children, for children. Arch. Dis. Child. 98 (4), 247.

De Weerd, W., van Tol, D., Albers, M., et al., 2015. Suffering in children: opinions from parents and health-care professionals. Eur. J. Pediatr. 174 (5), 589–595.

Dumas, H.M., 2013. Cardiorespiratory response during physical therapist intervention for infants and young children with chronic respiratory insufficiency. Pediatr. Phys. Ther. 25 (2), 178–185.

Eisenbrown, K., Nimmer, M., Ellison, A.M., et al., 2016. Which febrile children with sickle cell disease need a chest x-ray? Acad. Emerg. Med. 23 (11), 1248–1256.

Feiten, T. dos S., Flores, J.S., Farias, B.L., 2016. Respiratory therapy: a problem among children and adolescents with cystic fibrosis. J. Brasileiro Pneumologia 42 (1), 29–34.

Fuijkschot, J., Vernhout, B., Lemson, J., et al., 2015. Validation of a paediatric early warning score. Eur. J. Pediatr. 174 (1), 15–21.

Gencpinar, P., Duman, M., 2015. Importance of back blow maneuvers in a 6 month old patient with sudden upper airway obstruction. Turkish. J. Emerg. Med. 15 (4), 177–178.

Guilliams, K., Wainwright, M.S., 2016. Pathophysiology and management of moderate and severe traumatic brain injury in children. J. Child Neurol. 31 (1), 35–45.

Hauer, J.M., 2015. Treating dyspnea with morphine sulfate in nonverbal children with neurological impairment. Pediatr. Pulmonol. 50 (4), E9–E12.

Hawkins, E., Jones, A., 2015. What is the role of the physiotherapist in paediatric intensive care units? Physiotherapy 101 (4), 303–309.

Hoo, Z.H., Daniels, T., Wildman, M.J., 2015. Airway clearance techniques used by people with cystic fibrosis in the UK. Physiotherapy 101 (4), 340–348.

Hoppe, J.E., Towler, E., Wagner, B.D., et al., 2015. Sputum induction improves detection of pathogens in children with cystic fibrosis. Pediatr. Pulmonol. 50 (7), 638–646.

Horridge, K.A., 2015. Advance care planning: practicalities, legalities, complexities and controversies. Arch. Dis. Child. 100 (4), 380–385.

Ivy, D., 2016. Pulmonary hypertension in children. Cardiol. Clin. 34 (3), 451–472.

Kaiser, S.V., Bakel, L.A., Okumura, M.J., et al., 2015. Risk factors for prolonged length of stay or complications during pediatric respiratory hospitalizations. Hosp. Pediatr. 5 (9), 461–473.

Knollman, P.D., Baroody, F.M., 2015. Pediatric tracheotomy decannulation. Curr. Opin. Otolaryngol. Head Neck Surg. 23 (6), 485–490.

Leigh, M.W., Ferkol, T.W., Davis, S.D., et al., 2016. Clinical features and associated likelihood of primary ciliary dyskinesia in children and adolescents. Ann. Am. Thorac. Soc. 13 (8), 1305–1313.

Lilley, A., Turner, L., 2016. Assessing the benefits of having a specialist paediatric pharmacist and physiotherapist in the community to improve childhood asthma outcomes. Arch. Dis. Child. 101 (9), e2.

Mhanna, M.J., 2016. Ventilator-associated events in neonates and children: a single definition for a heterogeneous population. Crit. Care Med. 44 (1), 233–234.

Ming, X., Patel, R., Kang, V., et al., 2016. Respiratory and autonomic dysfunction in children with autism spectrum disorders. Brain Dev. 38 (2), 225–232.

Mosier, M.J., Peter, T., Gamelli, R.L., 2016. Need for mechanical ventilation in pediatric scald burns. J. Burn Care Res. 37 (1), e1–e6.

Nanda, M.K., LeMasters, G.K., Levin, L., et al., 2016. Allergic diseases and internalizing behaviors in early childhood. Pediatrics 137 (1), 1–10.

NICE Guideline, 2016. End of life care for infants, children and young people with life-limiting conditions [NG61].

NICE Guideline, 2016. Transition from children's to adults' services for young people using health or social care services [NG43].

O'Leary, F., Hayen, A., Lockie, F., et al., 2015. Defining normal ranges and centiles for heart and respiratory rates in infants and children. Arch. Dis. Child. 100 (8), 733–737.

Packel, L., Sood, M., Gormley, M., et al., 2013. A pilot study exploring the role of physical therapists and transition in care of pediatric patients with cystic fibrosis to the adult setting. Cardiopulm. Phys. Ther. J. 24 (1), 24–30.

Parslow, R.C., 2015. Defining normal heart and respiratory rates in children. Arch. Dis. Child. 100 (8), 719–720.

Prabhakaran, P., Sasser, W.C., Kalra, Y., et al., 2016. Ventilator graphics. Minerva Pediatr. 68 (6), 456–469.

Richards, A.M., 2016. Pediatric respiratory emergencies. Emerg. Med. Clin. North Am. 34 (1), 77–96.

Rizza, A., Bignami, E., Belletti, A., et al., 2016. Vasoactive drugs and hemodynamic monitoring in pediatric cardiac intensive care: an Italian survey. World J. Pediatr. Congenit. Heart Surg. 7 (1), 25–31.

Rodríguez-Rey, R., Alonso-Tapia, J., 2016. Development of a screening measure of stress for parents of children hospitalised in a paediatric intensive care unit. Aust. Crit. Care 29 (3), 151–157.

Sauthier, M., Rose, L., 2017. Pediatric prolonged mechanical ventilation: considerations for definitional criteria. Respir. Care 62 (1), 49–53.

Shein, S.L., Speicher, R.H., Filho, J.O.P., et al., 2016. Contemporary treatment of children with critical and near-fatal asthma. Rev. Bras. Ter. Intensiva. 28 (2), 167–179.

Smallwood, C.D., Walsh, B.K., Bechard, L.J., et al., 2015. Carbon dioxide elimination and oxygen consumption in mechanically ventilated children. Respir. Care 60 (5), 718–723.

Sng, Q.W., He, H.G., Wang, W., et al., 2017. A meta-synthesis of children's experiences of postoperative pain management. Worldviews Evid. Based Nurs. 14 (1), 46–54.

Tabata, H., Hirayama, M., Enseki, M., et al., 2016. A novel method for detecting airway narrowing using breath sound spectrum analysis in children. Respir. Invest. 54 (1), 20–28.

Tovar, J.A., Vazquez, J.J., 2013. Management of chest trauma in children. Paediatr. Respir. Rev. 14 (2), 86–91.

Tschauner, S., Marterer, R., Gübitz, M., et al., 2016. European Guidelines for AP/PA chest X-rays. Eur. Radiol. 26 (2), 495–505.

Ullman, A., Long, D., Horn, D., et al., 2013. The kids safe checklist for pediatric intensive care units. Am. J. Crit. Care 22 (1), 61–69.

Vece, T.J., Young, L.R., 2016. Update on diffuse lung disease in children. Chest 149 (3), 836–845.

Vendrusculo, F.M., 2016. Inspiratory muscle strength and endurance in children and adolescents with cystic fibrosis. Respir. Care 61 (2), 184–191.

Verd, S., Garcia, M., 2015. Acid-base equilibrium in premature infants. Eur. J. Pediatr. 174 (1), 55.

Walter, J.K., 2013. How to have effective advanced care planning discussions with adolescents and young adults with cancer. JAMA Pediatr. 167 (5), 489–490.

Wang, L.A., 2016. Advances in pediatric pharmacology, therapeutics, and toxicology. Adv. Pediatr. 63 (1), 227–254.

Watts, R., Vyas, H., 2013. An overview of respiratory problems in children with Down's syndrome. Arch. Dis. Child. 98 (10), 812–817.

Werkman, M.S., Hulzebos, E.H., Helders, P.J., et al., 2014. Estimating peak oxygen uptake in adolescents with cystic fibrosis. Arch. Dis. Child. 99 (1), 21–25.

White, C.C., 2013. Bronchodilator delivery during simulated pediatric noninvasive ventilation. Respir. Care 58 (9), 1459–1466.

# Hyperventilation Syndrome

*On completion of this chapter the reader should be able to:*
- appreciate the relationships between the origin, triggers, pathophysiology and consequences of hyperventilation syndrome;
- recognize the symptoms and ensure that all team members are aware of the disorder and its presentation;
- plan a flexible management regimen related to the patient's needs;
- ensure that the patient is able to maintain improvement;
- evaluate the outcomes of treatment.

## OUTLINE

## INTRODUCTION

*Respiration is situated strategically at the interface of mind and body.*

**Wilhelm et al. 2001**

Hyperventilation is breathing in excess of metabolic needs. Acute hyperventilation is an adaptive response preparing for fight or flight. Chronic hyperventilation may be linked to stress, disorders associated with shortness of breath, or both. It appears to affect up to 10% of the population to some degree, or 30% if they also have asthma (Depiazzi & Everard 2016). It is associated with some alarming symptoms, often intermittently, which deplete the body's stress-coping mechanisms.

Chronic hyperventilation may also be termed 'dysfunctional breathing', an umbrella term describing abnormal patterns of breathing (Fig. 17.1). More specific is the term hyperventilation syndrome (HVS). Attempts to understand the condition have led to other labels such as irritable heart, autonomic imbalance, cardiovascular neurosis, effort syndrome, neurocirculatory asthenia, soldiers' heart, factor X syndrome and, as a last resort, fat file syndrome. Links with cardiology and warfare relate to its symptomatology and association with stress via the amygdala and hypothalamus (Ramirez 2014). The condition was first identified during the American Civil War and again in the 20th century World Wars (Depiazzi & Everard 2016), when many thousands of young soldiers were invalided out with 'heart disease'. Symptoms that mimic heart disease led to both Florence Nightingale and Charles Darwin being diagnosed with cardiac problems at an early age, but both lived long lives and their ill health has since been ascribed to HVS (Timmons & Ley 1994).

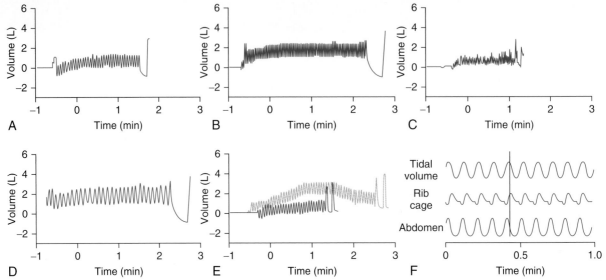

**FIGURE 17.1** Tidal breathing at rest, followed by maximal expiration then inspiration: (A) a healthy volunteer; (B) HVS, showing tidal breathing closer to inspiratory capacity than normal; (C) erratic breathing; (D) thoracic dominant breathing, with large volume breaths and minimal inspiratory reserve capacity; (E) forced expiratory pattern before (pale) and after (dark) exercise, showing minimal expiratory reserve volume; (F) thoracoabdominal asynchrony. (From Boulding et al. 2016.)

Widespread failure to diagnose the syndrome was considered a 'disgrace' nearly 30 years ago (Paulley 1990), and continues today. Reasons are:

- cursory coverage in medical texts;
- physiological adaptation so that not all patients are conspicuously breathless;
- nonspecific and variable symptoms;
- lack of an unequivocal diagnostic test.

HVS occupies the boundary between body and mind, a 'no-man's land' in Western medicine. If it is not identified, patients trek from clinic to clinic, accruing ever fatter case files, being labelled as neurotic and submitting to invasive investigations and sometimes years of debilitating medication. Without treatment, the condition persists or worsens in 75% of people, through intertwining vicious circles (Fig. 17.2).

Children with HVS, are less likely to be diagnosed than adults, but they have shown dramatic improvements after four sessions of physiotherapy (Depiazzi & Everard 2016), and Enzer et al. (1967) found that 86% were misdiagnosed with epilepsy or panic disorder. At any age, acute hyperventilation can provoke seizures (Kang 2015).

HVS is eminently treatable and symptoms can be abolished in 75% of patients (Timmons & Ley 1994). Relaxation and breathing retraining appear to be more effective than psychological methods or drugs (Kraft 1984). Sedatives such as diazepam are inadvisable (Munemoto et al. 2013).

## CAUSES, TRIGGERS AND EFFECTS

*The thread of the breath is woven throughout the tapestry of a person's life experience.*

***Harris 1996***

Certain religious sects and individuals deliberately hyperventilate in order to reach trancelike states of consciousness. Some of these effects are similar to the symptoms of HVS, but they do not incorporate the anxiety and loss of control that accompany unintentional and chronic hyperventilation. The overlap

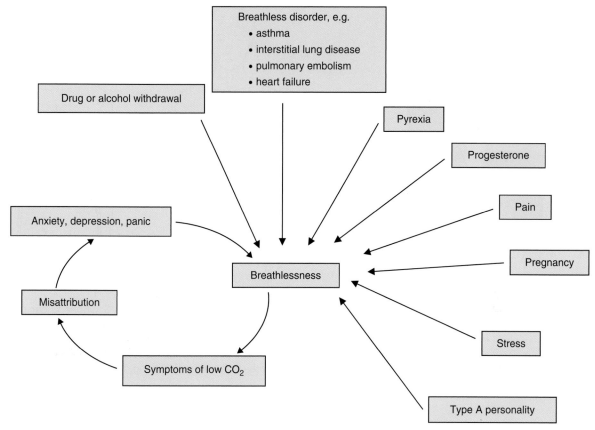

**FIGURE 17.2** Interrelation of some of the factors which cause and exacerbate hyperventilation syndrome.

between cause, effect, pathophysiology and clinical features reinforces the difficulty in identifying HVS, even though physiologically the syndrome is simply an abnormality of respiratory control (Chenuel 2008).

A person's respiratory drive varies twofold to fourfold under normal circumstances, but this can be modulated by life events (Strohl et al. 1998). HVS may originate from bereavement, a traumatic birth (Brennan 2011), adverse life experiences (Bakal 2013) especially if crying out is prevented, or incidents around fear and breathing, e.g. a ducking in the school swimming pool or a forcefully applied anaesthetic mask. The outcome is a hyperventilatory respiratory drive (Jack et al. 2004). Breathing occupies a central role in translating psychological changes into somatic symptoms (Gilbert 1999a), and body memory is thought to be held particularly in the breathing pattern (Harris 1996).

Other causes are chronic or acute pain; dental anxiety, emergence from anaesthesia (Tomioka et al. 2015); drugs such as salicylates, adrenaline or nicotine (Kitterer

et al. 2015); and hypermobility affecting thoracic joints (Innocenti & Troup 2008).

Whether or not an original cause is identified, there is usually a trigger, often stress-related, that the patient may identify as setting off an acute episode. This may be as simple as prolonged conversation, or a recognized stressor such as viral illness, surgery (Moon et al. 2011) or a difficult work environment (Fig. 17.3).

The trigger sets off an overly sensitive 'suffocation alarm', which may have become sensitized by the original cause. This can lead to disproportionate dyspnoea, fear of asphyxia and panic symptoms. One patient described how she constantly listened for her next breath and did not like travelling in cars because she could not hear it (Paulley 1990).

$PaCO_2$ tends to be kept low by chronic hyperventilation in order to avoid triggering the alarm (Meuret et al. 2012), but hyperventilation-induced alkalosis can itself increase serum lactate and set off a panic attack (Ridder et al. 2010).

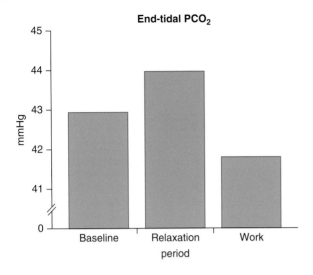

End-tidal PCO$_2$

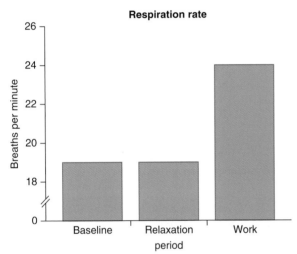

Respiration rate

FIGURE 17.3 Effect of relaxation and work stress on respiratory rate and CO$_2$ levels. (From Schleifer et al. 2002.)

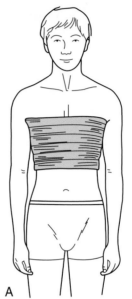
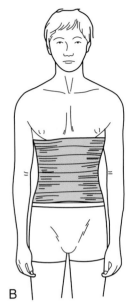

FIGURE 17.4 (A) Patient with HVS whose chest pain was abolished after 2 days of chest strapping to facilitate abdominal breathing. (B) Person without HVS who had chest pain created by strapping the abdomen to enforce upper chest breathing. (From Gilbert 1999c.)

Cause and effect then become interchangeable. The question that continues to tease researchers is whether hyperventilation or anxiety comes first, but in practice they augment each other. Either way, the syndrome is associated with:

- conditions such as chronic fatigue syndrome (Ocon 2013), hypertension, sleep disorder, Raynaud disease, migraine, agoraphobia and vocal cord dysfunction, the latter mimicking or coexisting with asthma and being set off by autonomic imbalance (Ayres 2002) related to stress (Barker & Everard 2015);
- conditions that cause overbreathing and may reprogramme the respiratory centres, e.g. heart failure, pain, interstitial lung disease, long-term low-grade fever, or acidosis caused by liver cirrhosis (Passino et al. 2012);
- spinal and pelvic instability (Chaitow 2007), poor balance (David et al. 2012) and upper limb musculoskeletal disorders related to job stress (Schleifer et al. 2002);
- the premenstrual week because progesterone is a respiratory stimulant (Moon et al. 2011);
- chemical sensitivities, food allergy, irritable bowel syndrome (Kanaan et al. 2007) or high caffeine intake (Wemmie 2011);
- emotional exhaustion, physical tiredness, cognitive difficulties involving memory and concentration (Ristiniemi et al. 2014), fear, suppressed anger, depression, orgasm or laughter;
- occupations that entail deep breathing or prolonged speaking such as teaching, call centre work, playing sports, singing or using a wind instrument (Widmer et al. 1997);
- restrictive clothes around the abdomen (Fig. 17.4), leading in Victorian times to corseted women

collapsing with the 'vapours', and a century later the alternative name 'designer jeans syndrome';
- in children, family discord or anxiety, sometimes leading to fainting in school assembly or 'mass psychogenic illness' (Jones et al. 2000).

There is overlap between hyperventilation, panic attacks and agoraphobia (Wemmie 2011), the latter being found in 60% of people with HVS, whereas HVS has been found in 60% of people with agoraphobia (Garssen 1983). The combination responds to breathing retraining (Meuret et al. 2012).

Although hyperventilation is a recognized stress response, it is not known why some people respond to stress with chronic hyperventilation whereas others develop different somatic symptom disorders. Somatization has been considered one of medicine's blind spots and is thought to be the body's way of expressing distress via autonomic dysregulation without conscious appreciation (Dreher 1996).

Personality plays a part because people who respond to stress in this way tend to suppress their emotions and are often conscientious, sensitive, high-achieving and perfectionist (Barker & Everard 2015). It is these qualities, along with the high motivation that accompanies their relief at finding constructive help, which makes people with HVS a delight to treat.

## PATHOPHYSIOLOGY

*Body and mind can live in two different worlds…*
*this odd mismatch can create a morass of symptoms*
*and no end of distress.*

**Gilbert 1999a**

Overbreathing washes out the body's $CO_2$ stores, leading to high and sometimes unstable pH in blood and cerebrospinal fluid. Alkalosis leads to:
- ↓ hydrogen ions in intracellular fluid, shifting extracellular potassium into the cells to maintain the balance of intracellular ions → hypokalaemia → ECG disturbance;
- ↓ calcium ions in plasma → excitable sensory and motor neurons → muscle twitching, cramps, tetany and convulsions (Parasa et al. 2014);
- ↓ cerebral blood flow (Pearson 2007), leading to headaches (Moon et al. 2011);
- vasoconstriction of other blood vessels (Fig. 17.5C) causing widespread symptoms;

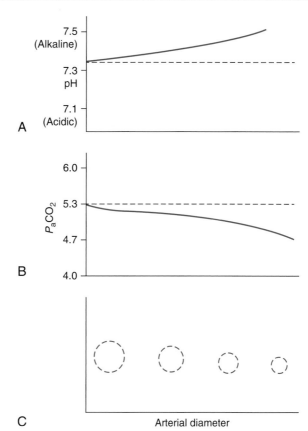

**FIGURE 17.5** Hyperventilation causing (A) respiratory alkalosis, (B) hypocapnia, (C) vasoconstriction. (From Gilbert 1999.)

- oxygen dissociation curve shifted to the left → less oxygen released to the tissues, which reinforces the cerebral hypoxia caused by unstable blood vessels;
- ↓ phosphate levels → fatigue, disorientation, paraesthesia and muscle cramps (Widmer et al. 1997);
- ↓ magnesium → further muscle spasm, fatigue, headache and ECG upset.

An increased drive to breathe resets the respiratory centres in order to maintain normal pH, obliging the patient to continue low-grade hyperventilation despite a persistently low $PaCO_2$.

Stress may also cause the diaphragm to become hypertonic, flattened and relatively immobile (Barker & Everard 2015). The diaphragm acts as a roof to the abdominal cavity and attaches to the spinal musculature, playing a key role in trunk stabilization. When the system is under stress, breathing dominates at the expense of voice and postural control (Depiazzi & Everard 2016).

# CLINICAL FEATURES

*Breathing is the very essence of life. When this function is under threat it is impossible not to feel frightened.*
**Syrett & Taylor 2003**

Once pH reaches 7.5, symptoms emerge in some people, and at 7.6 they are universal (Gilbert 1999a). When compensation has returned pH to normal, albeit with some instability, a low $PaCO_2$ may be maintained with occasional deep breaths or sighs, which can be imperceptible subjectively (Moynihan 2001) and only noticeable by an attentive clinician. Patients whose minute volume is not labile and has stabilized at a higher level may not complain of dyspnoea. Further signs and symptoms are described below.

1. Cerebral vasoconstriction can cause nausea, dizziness, blackouts, fainting (David 2003), fear of falling (Clague 2000), visual disturbance and sometimes a dissociated state of unreality that feels like the person is floating outside the body. Humphriss et al. (2004) found that 23% of patients with vestibular problems were found to have HVS.

2. Chest pain is due to coronary vasoconstriction, hypocapnia and/or musculoskeletal imbalance (Barker & Everard 2015), the latter being caused by dysfunctional postures or overuse and tension in the accessory muscles (CliftonSmith & Rowley 2011). Up to 90% of noncardiac chest pain is thought to be associated with HVS (DeGuire et al. 1992) but a misdiagnosis of heart disease may occur (Kannivelu 2013). Unlike heart pathology, the ST segment of the ECG may be depressed and the T wave flattened (Moon et al. 2011), while other changes may disappear with exercise (Missri & Alexander 1978).

3. Chronic pain sometimes may be a cause or trigger (Kvåle et al. 2002), but one of the effects of neuronal excitability on large nerve fibres is to dampen pain. Hyperventilation is sometimes used as a coping strategy for pain, and HVS can be a legacy of torture (Hough 1992) or a component of posttraumatic stress disorder (Depiazzi & Everard 2016).

4. A wheeze is often reported due to adduction of the vocal cords on inspiration (Groot 2011). Despite being inspiratory, misdiagnosis of asthma is common, which may lead to escalating medication without relief of symptoms (Barker & Everard 2015).

Symptoms are ten times more common in subjects with asthma than in those without (D'Alba et al. 2015).

Thomas et al. (2001) found that a third of women and a fifth of men diagnosed with asthma have HVS, and so-called 'steroid-resistant asthma' may in fact be HVS (Thomas 2003). HVS is also relatively common in asymptomatic asthmatics (Barker & Everard 2015).

Alkalosis and paraesthesia may lead to further misdiagnoses, one study finding that 86% of patients referred with carpal tunnel syndrome have HVS (Aslam et al. 2012).

The dyspnoea of HVS is distinctive. It is disproportionate, fluctuating, poorly correlated with exercise, greater with inspiration than expiration and exacerbated with crowds, conversation and some social situations. It is sometimes described as air hunger, heaviness on the chest or a smothering feeling. Negative trials of nitroglycerin or bronchodilators help to eliminate a diagnosis of heart disease or asthma, and a normal peak flow reading when breathless can be reassuring.

Exercise may relieve symptoms due to extra metabolism catching up with the breathing, but sometimes loss of fine tuning means that breathing may not adjust to activity and symptoms may worsen or become chaotic (Fig. 17.6). Fatigue is a common symptom, but some patients choose to work out because it provides the opportunity to take deep breaths. However, activities that heighten arousal without an accompanying increase in activity, e.g. driving, can worsen symptoms.

Breathing usually stabilizes at night when it is driven by the metabolic system (Slutsky & Phillipson 1994), but patients with unstable blood sugar, e.g. after a late carbohydrate-laden meal, sometimes complain of feeling toxic on waking, when their blood sugar has plummeted.

Signs and symptoms are summarized in Table 17.1 and described in the next section.

---

**SCENARIO**

A young woman was referred in some distress following bilateral carpal tunnel release.

Surgery had been performed due to tingling and numbness in both hands, but these symptoms were related to undiagnosed HVS and her paraesthesia was unrelieved. Postoperatively she developed reflex sympathetic dystrophy and the resulting hyperaesthesia led her to cool her hands by blowing on them. This exacerbated her HVS.

Paraesthesia and other HVS symptoms resolved after physiotherapy but her reflex sympathetic dystrophy remained.

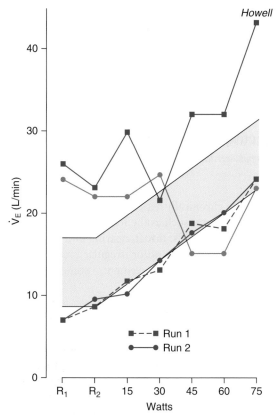

**FIGURE 17.6** Ventilatory response to graded exercise in a patient with HVS before (top 2 lines) and 2 weeks after (bottom 2 lines) education on the disorder. The shaded area represents the range in normal subjects. (From Howell 1997.)

## ASSESSMENT

*Accurate assessment and diagnosis can prevent excessive use of drug therapy.*
**_Depiazzi & Everard 2016_**

People with HVS may have received a selection of diagnoses varying from peripheral neuropathy or neurosis to myocardial infarction or multiple sclerosis. Some have been dismissed as malingerers or told that it is all in their mind. Others have been told that it is 'only hyperventilation', somehow disqualifying further consideration. The first priority therefore is to ensure that patients feel welcome and know that their problem is taken seriously. They need space, time, privacy and an attentive ear.

| System | Manifestation |
|---|---|
| Neurological and vascular | Tingling or numbness of extremities or around mouth |
| | Cold extremities |
| | Tremor or tetany, especially in extremities |
| | Chest, shoulder or arm pain |
| | Headache, dizziness, migraine, blurred vision |
| | Weakness |
| | Poor memory and concentration |
| | Hypersensitivity to lights and sounds |
| | Palpitations |
| | Faintness or a spaced out feeling |
| Emotional | Depersonalized feelings of unreality |
| | Depression |
| | Suppression of emotion |
| | Anxiety ± heightened vigilance |
| | Panic attacks ± fear of going mad or dying |
| | Phobias (especially claustrophobia and agoraphobia) |
| | Mood swings |
| Gastrointestinal | Gastroesophageal reflux |
| | Difficulty swallowing |
| | Dry mouth |
| | Nausea |
| | Indigestion |
| | Flatus and belching |
| | Irritable bowel |
| | Food intolerance |
| Musculoskeletal | Tense and/or fatigued neck and shoulder muscles |
| | Tense posture |
| | Myalgia, stiffness, cramps |
| | Weakness |
| General | Air hunger |
| | Fatigue |
| | Insomnia |
| | Hypoglycaemia |
| | Blurred body image |

TABLE 17.1 Clinical features associated with hyperventilation syndrome

The case notes should be scrutinized for conditions that cause breathlessness and for comorbid or alternative diagnoses, such as the following:
- Low haemoglobin means that breathing retraining can exacerbate the dyspnoea of anaemia.

- If patients are on β-blockers, these can either exacerbate HVS by causing bronchospasm, or ameliorate autonomic symptoms and help break the vicious cycle of sympathetic stimulation and hyperventilation.
- β$_2$-Agonists given for asthma can provoke palpitations and agitation.
- If patients are being weaned off sedatives, relaxation will be difficult unless treatment coincides with the peak effect of the drug.

> **KEY POINT**
>
> Whether the patient has been medically screened or not, an open mind must be maintained because some symptoms may indicate serious disease.

## Subjective

*'Feelings of flying apart, absolute terror, falling down through the world, spinning through the universe…'*

**Patient quoted by Bradley 2012**

Feelings vary from anxiety to a dread of impending madness or dying (Timmons & Ley 1994). There may be a fear of flying, of being trapped in a lift or feeling unable to escape from a crowded supermarket. Patients may complain of an inability to take a satisfying breath, or may in fact be unaware of any breathing abnormality. If symptoms worsen while they are on a waiting list, this may be because a common response to a diagnosis of a breathing disorder is to practice deep breathing exercises. While on the waiting list, patients with a wheeze can also be asked to record it on their mobile phone to help confirm or exclude asthma.

It is useful to identify factors that precede symptoms and patients' interpretation of them. They are often puzzled as to why symptoms affecting so many parts of the body can be caused by a breathing disorder, and may not report 'irrelevant' symptoms. Specific questions about symptoms that are likely to be caused by HVS help elicit these, and also facilitate acceptance of the diagnosis.

Questions on lifestyle may reveal a hyperactive trait and a pattern of rushing to meet deadlines. Many patients are high achievers, and a majority tend to perform tasks quickly, impatiently, often several simultaneously and with a tendency to think ahead, whereas only 20% of normal subjects show these characteristics

(van Dixhoorn 1986). Other common factors are a general sensitivity and hyperresponsiveness (Garssen 1980), as shown in the patient's breathing, emotions, and sometimes allergy to food or medication.

Patients should say all they want at this stage because it reduces their need to talk during treatment, which upsets their breathing pattern.

## Objective

*Hyperventilation is the great mimic.*

**Lum 1981**

People who chronically hyperventilate may have a labile breathing pattern, such as the following:

- sighs, yawns, sniffs, throat-clearing or a dry cough;
- shallow, fast, apical and/or irregular breaths;
- excessive thoracic movement, sometimes with abdominal paradox;
- breath-holding;
- breath-stacking, as if the patient dare not let the air out;
- prolonged inspiration and curtailed expiration, as if the patient wants to hold onto their precious air.

The breathing required to maintain hypocapnia is less than that required to induce it, and resting $CO_2$ levels may be halved with only a 10% increase in minute ventilation (Gardner 2004).

Other signs are a stiff posture and gait, lack of coordination between talking and breathing, accentuated increase in ventilation when moving from supine to standing (Malmberg et al. 2000), rapid speech as if the patient is trying to cram several sentences into one, excessive hand movements or other indication of tension, and strategies to sneak in more air such as chest heaving before speaking. Belching may be caused by air swallowing, and cold hands by vasoconstriction. If chest wall tenderness is present, palpation can reassure patients that it is not cardiac pain. Patients are further reassured if thoracic mobilizations ameliorate this tenderness (Innocenti & Troup 2008).

## Questionnaires

Suspicions of HVS are raised when there is an unusual mix of clinical features, which include some of the above. The Nijmegen questionnaire (Table 17.2) is then used, which demonstrates a sensitivity of up to 91% and specificity up to 95% (Groot 2011). The normal score is 5–11 out of 64, but for those with HVS it is usually

| TABLE 17.2 Nijmegen questionnaire[a] | 0 | 1 | 2 | 3 | 4 |
|---|---|---|---|---|---|
| Chest pain | ☐ | ☐ | ☐ | ☐ | ☐ |
| Feeling tense | ☐ | ☐ | ☐ | ☐ | ☐ |
| Blurred vision | ☐ | ☐ | ☐ | ☐ | ☐ |
| Dizzy spells | ☐ | ☐ | ☐ | ☐ | ☐ |
| Feeling confused | ☐ | ☐ | ☐ | ☐ | ☐ |
| Faster or deeper breathing | ☐ | ☐ | ☐ | ☐ | ☐ |
| Short of breath | ☐ | ☐ | ☐ | ☐ | ☐ |
| Tight feelings in chest | ☐ | ☐ | ☐ | ☐ | ☐ |
| Bloated feeling in stomach | ☐ | ☐ | ☐ | ☐ | ☐ |
| Tingling fingers | ☐ | ☐ | ☐ | ☐ | ☐ |
| Unable to breathe deeply | ☐ | ☐ | ☐ | ☐ | ☐ |
| Stiff fingers or arms | ☐ | ☐ | ☐ | ☐ | ☐ |
| Tight feelings around mouth | ☐ | ☐ | ☐ | ☐ | ☐ |
| Cold hands or feet | ☐ | ☐ | ☐ | ☐ | ☐ |
| Palpitations | ☐ | ☐ | ☐ | ☐ | ☐ |
| Feelings of anxiety | ☐ | ☐ | ☐ | ☐ | ☐ |

[a]Tick the relevant box and add up the score.

above 23 (Courtney et al. 2011b). It is not validated for children, but specificity can be improved by combining it with symptom-limited exercise testing, and other questionnaires may be helpful, e.g. the Self Evaluation of Breathing Questionnaire, or using manual assessment of respiratory motion (Boulding et al. 2016).

## Tests

The following are not validated but may aid acceptance of the diagnosis.

1. A short breath-hold time is suggestive of HVS. People with normal control of their breathing can often hold their breath for 60 s at end-inspiration, whereas those with HVS may only manage 20 s (Courtney et al. 2011).

2. People with HVS have an exaggerated increase in ventilation when changing from supine to standing (Stewart et al. 2006).

3. A provocation test entails the patient taking 20 consecutive deep breaths, or breathing rapidly for 3 min (Warburton & Jack 2006). This may bring on familiar symptoms in people with HVS, not just the dizziness that is a normal response to acute hyperventilation. If capnography is available, the $CO_2$ takes longer than normal to return to baseline (Fig. 17.7). The provocation test can be distressing for patients, but may reassure them of the validity of their symptoms and

show that they have some control, but it is not reliable (Groot 2011). Vasospasm may be caused by the test and a crash trolley should be on hand. Cerebral vascular disease, epilepsy, sickle cell disease (Brashear 1983) and coronary heart disease are contraindications.

4. A low $PaCO_2$ is not itself diagnostic because the syndrome is intermittent, but HVS is suspected if resting $CO_2$ is low or erratic, if a low $CO_2$ is sustained during an exercise test (Warburton & Jack 2006), or voluntary overbreathing reduces it to <4 kPa (30 cmH$_2$O). Capnography may also be used to provide feedback for patients and outcome measures for physiotherapists (p. 466).

> **KEY POINT**
>
> I ask my patients when they do their Christmas shopping.
> If it's August, I'm pretty sure they've got HVS.

## EDUCATION

*Many patients who have been treated with ever increasing medication improve significantly when the condition is explained to them.*

**Depiazzi & Everard 2016**

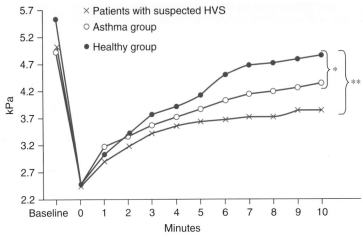

**FIGURE 17.7** Capnography measurement of end-tidal $CO_2$ measured at baseline and for 15 min after provocation.*, $P < .05$; **, $P < .01$. (From Ringsberg & Åkerlind 1999.)

The main sustaining factor with hyperventilation is misattribution of symptoms to a sinister cause (Singh 2001) and education therefore comes first. If a waiting list precludes prompt treatment, education can begin in advance. Sending a handout (Appendix B) or information about a patient-friendly book such as that by Bradley (2012) will do much of the physiotherapist's work, and a Nijmegen questionnaire to be filled out in advance saves time and may give the patient some 'aha' moments as they identify familiar symptoms.

At the first appointment, expectations are checked and goals agreed, e.g. in the short term to cope with panic attacks, and in the long term to integrate a normal breathing pattern into everyday life, as identified by elimination of symptoms. The mechanism of HVS can be explained using the vicious cycle on the handout, and this information itself normally reduces anxiety. Patients are reassured that HVS does not cause harm, nor does it indicate physical damage. It is a response to stress or other trigger, not a psychiatric illness. When patients understand that their symptoms stem from chemical changes in the blood, they sometimes feel exonerated from the stigma of not having had their complaints validated by a 'proper' diagnosis.

The following advice may be helpful:
1. Physiotherapy will not eliminate the original cause nor remove precipitating factors, but triggers should be identifiable.

2. Commitment is required, in the early stages when learning to control the breathing, and later when incorporating practice into everyday life.
3. It is useful, and sometimes essential, to integrate a small but fundamental shift in attitude and lifestyle that allows time for relaxation and reflection.
4. A nice deep breath does not help relaxation.
5. Relearning a new lower level of breathing involves experiencing the discomfort of air hunger, but after practice the respiratory centres become retuned to registering and regulating a more normal breathing pattern.

To anticipate the feelings experienced with breathing retraining, 'bad breathlessness' can be explained as the patient's familiar and distressing sensation of uncontrolled air hunger, whereas 'good breathlessness' is a similar physical feeling but without distress because this can now be consciously initiated and controlled as part of the treatment. Although 'good', this breathlessness is not comfortable, and patients appreciate acknowledgment of this.

Patients are advised that physical symptoms may occasionally become worse during or after the first session. This may be due to a paradoxical but transient increase in minute ventilation if the respiratory centres interpret the effects of the breathing re-education as a threat of smothering.

Education enables patients to step out of their vicious cycle and begin to take control of their breathing.

Fig. 17.6 shows the ventilatory response to graded exercise before and after gaining insight into the nature of the condition.

## BREATHING RETRAINING

Voluntary control can be exerted over the pattern and rate of respiration, and breathing retraining is recognized as a first line treatment for adults (Barker & Everard 2015). According to psychoanalyst Wilhelm Reich, changing a person's breathing pattern is tantamount to emotional surgery (Gilbert 1999b), which may relate to the blocking of emotions by tension in chest wall and postural muscles (Kvåle et al. 2002). The environment of a physiotherapy department is unlikely to excavate the depth of emotion that emanates from the analyst's couch, but feelings may surface, and if this brings tears, a proffered box of tissues lets patients know that this is acceptable.

A quiet room is required with an open window or fan. The patient is positioned in any relaxed position, e.g. half lying with a pillow under the knees and head supported.

### Awareness of Breathing

Patients learn the feel of their breathing, using some (but not all) of the following:

1. Rest one hand on your upper chest and one on your abdomen to distinguish chest and abdominal breathing.
2. Experiment with slight alterations in the depth and rate of breathing, to distinguish the two.
3. Try alternate nose and mouth breathing to feel the difference.
4. Feel the passage of the breath as it passes through your nose, down your windpipe and into your lungs, then visualize the air gently returning along the same route.
5. Feel cool air on the in-breath and warm air on the out-breath.
6. To help keep the throat relaxed, imagine breathing in gently through your eyes (Brennan 2011).
7. Try a pause between the out-breath and the in-breath.
8. Check for tension in the rest of your body.

The patient will need to be observed closely throughout to ensure that minute volume does not creep up.

### Nose Breathing

*Man should no more breathe through his mouth than take food through his nose.*

**Clifton-Smith 2004**

A habit of breathing in and out through the nose should be established during the session, after explanation, with ongoing role modelling from the physiotherapist. This may be combined with localized relaxation by the patient keeping their jaw loose and lips together. Reminders may be needed throughout the session.

---

**PRACTICE TIP**

Patients can use their screen time to remind themselves to nose breathe.

---

### Relaxation

Breathing cannot be reeducated in a tense person, and most patients need to learn relaxation (p. 263). Some people find that the thought of being 'obliged' to relax causes tension itself and may prefer to do their relaxation after the breathing practice. In the West in particular, tense people sometimes find relaxation an alien concept, and it may be easier after a brief neck massage, during which it is helpful for patients to focus on the experience and not feel that they have to talk or 'do' anything. Localized heat can also be helpful prior to relaxation, usually to the shoulders and neck, or to the back with the patient prone. Lying prone may facilitate relaxation, possibly because this is a less vulnerable position than supine.

Focusing on the breath itself helps relaxation, especially if patients are encouraged to gently 'breathe in the good air' and 'breathe out the tension', as if freeing the breath. Control of breathing is central to many methods of relaxation because focusing on breathing forms a mini-meditation and helps link mind and body (Gilbert 1999d). Physiotherapists should ensure that they themselves are relaxed.

Throughout treatment, a relaxed state can be maintained by bringing the patient's awareness to areas of tension, including the face, jaw, throat, neck, shoulders and abdomen.

People with HVS often have a highly developed sense of success and failure, and the relaxation session is an opportunity to remind them that there is no right or wrong way to relax.

## Abdominal Breathing

To settle the breathing pattern, the physiotherapist encourages regular and gentle speed, depth and synchrony, using a rhythmic voice. If the patient is able, breathing abdominally (p. 237) is a useful way of settling the breathing because it reduces the abnormal proprioceptive input of upper chest breathing (Bruton et al. 2011) and may reduce chest pain (Gilbert 1999c), so long as patients do not increase their depth of breathing. Abdominal breathing may be facilitated with the hands behind the head or back, while maintaining relaxation and slow gentle breaths. Occasionally abdominal breathing is easier after reducing the minute volume rather than before.

## Reducing the Minute Volume

A combination of education, relaxation and settling the breathing into an abdominal pattern may be sufficient, but patients with established HVS often require further intervention to reduce minute volume. Patients can be asked simply to 'breathe less', but very gently in order to avoid tension and exacerbation of abnormal breathing patterns. Some patients need an explanation that this means reducing the rate or depth of breathing, or both, but thinking too hard about an automatic process may be counterproductive. If the patient understands that the aim is to achieve the slight discomfort of 'air hunger', he or she can often achieve this independently without too much control by the physiotherapist. Meuret et al. (2008) found that reducing the depth of breathing contributes more to raising the $PaCO_2$ than reducing the rate.

'Low and slow' is the key. Some patients need only a pause at end-exhalation, so long as this does not go further than air hunger and cause tension. If patients tense up, they should focus on returning to smooth, gentle, steady breathing.

To help patients maintain their rhythm, it is best not to ask for verbal feedback during the practice, although they can nod or shake their head in answer to quiet questions.

Observation of the breathing pattern identifies if tension develops, which suggests that the patient has reduced the minute volume too much and needs a reminder not to allow more air hunger than is just uncomfortable. Patients are then advised to gently get their breath back.

The physiotherapist watches the patient closely and may need to give selective advice on rate or depth of breathing, or a suggestion to pause at the end of the out-breath. Patients sometimes develop manoeuvres to slip in a covert deep breath such as a subtle change in position, breathing pattern or body movement, or preceding their speech with a sharp intake of breath. The physiotherapist and patient can compete as to who notices these first! However, much of the time is in silence as the patient focuses on their breath and achieving air hunger, with occasional verbal nudges from the physiotherapist.

In the first session, when the patient feels the air hunger, he or she is congratulated and advised to start getting the breath back by allowing slightly deeper and/or slightly faster breathing, without gasping. When patients are able to tolerate the air hunger, they are asked if they can experience it for a few moments so that their respiratory centres can begin experiencing normal breathing as normal. The patient gradually learns the right balance of 'slight discomfort but no tension'. It is similar to the 'slight breathlessness' taught to respiratory patients when desensitising them to dyspnoea (p. 232). The periods of air hunger can then be gradually extended.

If this is too nebulous for the patient, more structured support can be given by pacing the patient's breathing to the physiotherapist's voice. The patient is asked to breathe in time with the physiotherapist's words, the rate of which is slightly slower than the patient's rate. Counting or pacing can be used e.g.:

- 'in-and-out, in-and-out…'
- 'in-and-out-two-three, in-and-out-two-three…'
- 'in-and-relax-out, in-and-relax-out…'
- 'in-and-let-it-out, in-and-let-it-out…'

Words and timing should be flexible to suit the patient, but instructions need to be repeated rhythmically, and the patient observed to ensure that slower breathing is not offset by deeper breathing. Some patients find that counting brings a sense of security in the early stages, the words acting as a 'breathing pacemaker'. Progression is aimed at independent control without the physiotherapist's voice.

If patients feel an irresistible need for air, they can take a conscious and controlled deeper breath, then get back gently into rhythm, sometimes with a preliminary breath-hold as compensation (but not if this causes tension). The concept of control is important for people who hyperventilate because they have felt out of control of their most fundamental physiological need. Advice can be given at intervals if necessary:

- Keep it smooth/shallow/slow.
- Swallow if you need to suppress a deep breath.
- Keep the rhythm going, you don't need to hold your breath.
- Maintain relaxation, avoid trying too hard.
- Don't fight your breath, befriend it.
- Be assured that you are in control and can stop at any time.

By establishing a lower more normal minute volume, it is thought that the normalized $PaCO_2$ resets the air hunger threshold, reducing the sensitivity to body sensations and/or desensitizing the suffocation alarm system (Meuret et al. 2008). The Buteyko technique (p. 86) is based on the principle of reducing the minute volume.

## Variations

A process as individual as breathing needs a flexible approach. Suggested variations are the following:

1. Physiotherapists may use themselves or a mirror to demonstrate the patient's breathing pattern and different options.
2. Patients can slow down by 'breathing in' to areas of muscle tension, then 'breathing out' the tension.
3. They can visualize inhalation as if going up a hill and exhalation as if coming down.
4. Feeling less cold air in their nose reminds them that they have succeeded in 'breathing less'.
5. Some patients slow down if the physiotherapist moves physically away and asks them to 'breathe from where I am'.
6. Humming may slow the breath.
7. The simple yoga technique described on p. 238 suits the most hardened workaholic because it is so brief.
8. Neurophysiological facilitation (p. 187) may be beneficial.
9. Capnography can be used as biofeedback (Meuret et al. 2012).

Examples of musculoskeletal input are:

- in prone: thoracic mobilizations;
- in supine: pectoral stretches;
- in side-lying: intercostal stretch, holding the upper elbow so that the shoulder is abducted and applying gentle pressure on the mid to lower ribs.

Johansson et al. (2017) suggest the following independent exercises:

- stretch one slightly flexed arm over your head, let the other hang relaxed by your side; after 3 s, switch arms;
- stretch arms forward, then draw each arm backwards as if single-handed rowing;
- hug yourself with both arms, then crouch, hold your breath, then breathe out as you stand up;
- 'swim' with arms upwards, to the sides and to the front.

By the nature of the syndrome, it is essential that patients are not hurried, and an undisturbed hour should be set aside for the first session and, if possible, for subsequent sessions.

## MANAGEMENT OF PANIC ATTACKS

*'I know full well that if I get panicky… it'll only get worse'*

***Patient quoted by Simon et al. 2016***

Panic attacks occur in 50% of people with HVS (Cowley 1987). Once patients understand that these episodes are not in themselves harmful, they can start gaining control over them. Breathing retraining itself can block attacks (Pappa 1993).

Coping strategies include identifying trigger factors, talking through the process, using an internal dialogue to acknowledge the fear but with a reminder that panic attacks are not damaging, behavioural strategies such as rehearsals or distraction, and a choice of the techniques used to manage breathlessness (Chapter 8) or paroxysms of coughing (p. 218). Breathing into a paper bag to retain $CO_2$ is no longer recommended because there have been occasional episodes of post-hyperventilation apnoea (Munemoto et al. 2013), but breathing into cupped hands may be beneficial.

Self-management plans that focus on regular symptom monitoring may not be beneficial for people with panic tendencies because they can reinforce preoccupation with bodily sensations (Dowson 2010). Drugs for panic disorders are sometimes associated with addictive properties, but relaxation or cognitive behavioural therapy may be helpful (NICE 2011c).

## PROGRESSION AND INTEGRATION

*The centrality of breathing in human emotion, health and consciousness is obvious from references to it in intellectual domains as wide ranging as literature, philosophy, religion and physiology.*

**Wilhelm et al. 2001**

As control is established, abdominal breathing and reducing the minute volume is repeated in sitting, standing, walking and activities that might cause breath-holding such as bending, stair-climbing or eating. Patients are also encouraged to practice selectively relaxing parts of their body during their activities.

Particular attention is required during speech. If prolonged talking brings on symptoms, slowing down speech may be practiced by reading aloud, starting with poetry in order to use the natural pauses, then reading stories to children. Tips for maintaining control during speech are to:

- check shoulder relaxation and the breathing pattern;
- take small breaths and inhale through the nose between sentences instead of gulping through the mouth;
- add mental commas (Bradley 2012).

Pacing functional activities is often beneficial, though difficult for people with a hyperactive tendency. Exercise is encouraged that is steady, rhythmic and enjoyable, with the patient avoiding either anticipatory hyperventilation or obsessive overachieving.

Posture and breathing can be affected by tense abdominal muscles, which may compress the abdomen on inspiration. Allowing outward abdominal movement needs to be balanced with patients feeling comfortable with their appearance. Tight clothes and belts should be avoided when possible.

Patients can be given recordings of advice and relaxation, sometimes including the physiotherapy session, because of the forgetfulness that sometimes accompanies HVS (Ocon 2013). If counting is used, this can be taped at fast, medium and slow speeds. If commercial relaxation tapes are used, patients are reminded to ignore instructions to breathe deeply.

Patients can also be given recordings of pacing tones with a rise in pitch to indicate inhalation and a fall for exhalation. They are advised to match their breathing to these tones for 10 min a day, preferably abdominally, followed by 5 min without auditory guidance to help the transfer to daily life. The tones are set at gradually slower rates each week (Jeter et al. 2012).

It is worth motivating patients to work hard during the first crucial week. Practice in breathing retraining should take place little and often, after brief relaxation and with the phone silenced. At first this could be around three times a day for 15 min, or mini-sessions of 3 min every hour. This is reduced for the second week, with times flexible to suit the individual. However, patients who tend to become preoccupied with a daily programme should not be burdened with excessive homework. Flexibility is particularly necessary for parents with young families, who find a tight routine impossible. One patient found that sitting beside her child as he fell asleep enabled her to slow her own breathing by pacing it to his breathing as it slowed and steadied.

Patients should maintain a steady blood sugar by ensuring that they have breakfast (including protein which is slow to metabolize), not going without a snack for more than 3–4 h, and avoiding sugar binges, which may lead to reactive hypoglycaemia. This should be emphasized for patients who are too busy to eat during the day and eat heavily at night, which can produce nocturnal or early morning symptoms. Meals should be slow (if possible) and enjoyable, avoiding excessive caffeine because of its respiratory stimulant and vasoconstrictive effects (Tal 2013). If patients must smoke, deep inhalations are to be avoided.

Spot checks throughout the day can be assisted by memory aids and use of opportunities such as red traffic lights, sitting on the bus and coffee breaks. Gradually the practice sessions can be less defined as the correct minute volume becomes automatic.

Vocal cord dysfunction, in which there is abnormal closure of the vocal cords, usually during inspiration, may respond to rapid shallow sniffing and pursed lips breathing (Barker & Everard 2015) or speech–language therapy. Other multidisciplinary input can include activity analysis and pacing from the occupational therapist, and sometimes extra relaxation. If patients ask for advice on complementary therapies, many techniques are helpful for relaxation, so long as they exclude deep breathing. Acupuncture may be beneficial by reducing symptom severity and anxiety levels (Gibson et al. 2007). Rhythmic dance techniques aimed at improving body awareness, stretching, relaxation and free flow of breathing have shown improvements in energy levels and hyperventilation symptoms (Ristiniemi et al. 2014). Hypnotherapy is unwise for people who suffer episodes of depersonalization.

Much encouragement is needed to help patients integrate their new breathing pattern and approach to life into the distractions of everyday living, but the obsessional tendencies of some patients means that adherence is usually high. If progress is slow, attention can be given to identifying individual fears and precipitating factors. Reassessment of the abnormally high demands to which patients often subject themselves may be fruitful.

Physiotherapy is needed weekly until self-management is stabilized, usually after a few sessions, then sometimes monthly for adjustment and encouragement, followed by advice that patients can ask for a review session if required. Once learned and reinforced, the new breathing pattern can be maintained automatically because there has been no physical damage, as there is with respiratory disease. Self-awareness and stress management however, must last a lifetime. Patients are advised that hyperventilation may return at stressful times, but they will recognize it and should be able to control it.

If patients do not improve after several sessions, and it becomes apparent that they are not practicing at home, or if they exhibit a 'yes but…' tendency, it is possible that they subliminally 'need' their hyperventilation to block out memories, in the same way that some patients with chronic pain express their emotional distress on a physical level (Bruera 1997). This is not a conscious process and makes the disorder no more tolerable, but if this is the case, physiotherapy is unhelpful and may just 'feed' the somatization, so referral is required.

## OUTCOMES

Reduced symptoms are the most relevant outcome. Objective outcomes include a reduced RR, stable breathing pattern, longer breath-holding, stable capnography and normalized Nijmegen score.

The following outcomes have been documented:
- ↓ respiratory symptoms, anxiety and depression, ↑ quality of life (Barker & Everard 2015);
- a doubling of breath-holding times (Maskell et al. 1999);
- ↓ symptoms, ↓ RR (Bastow 2000);

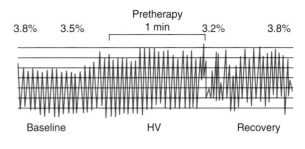

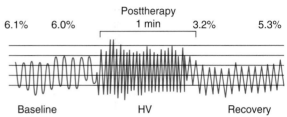

**FIGURE 17.8** End-tidal $CO_2$ trace (%) before and after physiotherapy. *HV*, Voluntary hyperventilation. (Rowbottom I and City Hospital, Edinburgh.)

- improvements in capnography (Fig. 17.8), anxiety, depression and other symptoms (Tweeddale et al. 1994);
- ↓ panic attacks (David 1985);
- ↓ Nijmegen scores, anxiety and depression in all patients audited after just two treatment sessions and a phone call (Williams 2001);
- ↓ sympathetic activity, hypertensive vasoconstriction and cardiovascular responses to physiological stress (Critchley et al. 2015);
- ↓ emergency room visits (Fig. 17.9).

Discharge letters to both general practitioner and consultant help raise awareness of the syndrome and show them the effectiveness of treatment.

*To be wholly alive is to breathe freely, move freely and to feel fully.*

**Lowen 1991**

## CASE STUDY: MS SJ

*Identify the problems of this 70-year-old woman with a 48-year history of fatigue and nonspecific symptoms.*

### Relevant medical history
- Investigated for multiple sclerosis: NAD (nothing abnormal discovered)

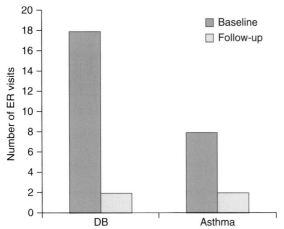

**FIGURE 17.9** Reduction in emergency room *(ER)* visits over 1 year in people with dysfunctional breathing *(DB)* and asthma after physiotherapy. (From Hagman et al. 2011.)

- Some depressive symptoms, labelled as 'abnormal illness'
- Migraine with certain foods
- Barium swallow: NAD, awaiting endoscopy
- Many other investigations but NAD

**History of present complaint**
- Since age 22: overwhelming chronic fatigue
- 4–5 years: dysphagia
- Two weeks: ↑ breathlessness

**Social history**
- Lives with husband, does not use stairs
- Only able to work part-time, took early retirement
- Spends most of the time sitting down

**Subjective**
- Fatigue since starting work, worse with stress, everything is a great effort, feels like battery going down
- Tend to drop things
- Difficulty in shops, go dizzy, need someone with me in case I fall, use a stick to help balance and keep people at a distance
- Worse since reading a book on relaxation and trying deep breathing exercises
- Always anxious, e.g. taking the iron with me in the car when I go out to ensure I've not left it on

- Difficulty sleeping
- Aches and pains since teenager, medication unhelpful
- It's like I can feel all my muscles
- Nothing but reflexology has helped
- Fed up with hospitals

**Objective**
- Nervous posture including excess hand movements
- Breathing pattern normal in sitting, tense and rapid in lying
- Sighing before speaking
- Nijmegen score 28

**Questions**
1. Analysis?
2. Patient's problems?
3. Goals?
4. Plan?

**CLINICAL REASONING**

Does this statement accurately reflect the reference to which it refers?

'...voluntary diaphragmatic movements...improve the ventilation of their lower lung zones'
   Chuter et al., 1990. Chest. 97 (5), 1110–1114

'lower lung zone ventilation...improved...during voluntary deep breathing...'.

**Response to Case Study**
1. Analysis
   - Patient has long-term poor quality of life
   - Patient using excess energy to maintain breathing pattern and avoid falling
   - Symptoms and questionnaire suggest hyperventilation syndrome
   - Original cause not explored during the session because patient is focused on improving quality of life
2. Problems
   - Fatigue
   - Anxiety
   - Poor sleep
   - Poor exercise tolerance

3. Goals
   - Shop independently and without anxiety
   - Visit friends
4. Plan
   - Educate on interrelation of symptoms, breathing, anxiety and quality of life
   - Relaxation and control of breathing
   - Pacing and energy conservation
   - Stairs
   - ↑ Exercise tolerance

### Outcomes: sequence

1. No change in symptoms, but 'husband says less huffing and puffing'
2. No change in symptoms, but 'I'm a little more in control of my breathing'
3. Able to control nightly chest pain with shallow breathing
4. Improved symptoms
5. Improved function including stairs
6. Visiting friends and distant family (without taking the iron!)
7. On discharge – some fatigue still present but not preventing activities, Nijmegen score 12
8. Christmas card 9 months later indicated that improvement was maintained

### RESPONSE TO CLINICAL REASONING

Deep breathing is not the same as diaphragmatic breathing.

## RECOMMENDED READING

Chenivesse, C., Similowski, T., Bautin, N., et al., 2014. Severely impaired health-related quality of life in chronic hyperventilation patients. Respir. Med. 108 (3), 517–523.

Decuyper, M., De Bolle, M., Boone, E., et al., 2012. The relevance of personality assessment in patients with hyperventilation symptoms. Health Psychol. 31 (3), 316–322.

Freire, R., Perna, G., Nardi, A.E., 2010. Panic disorder respiratory subtype: psychopathology, laboratory challenge tests, and response to treatment. Harv. Rev. Psych. 18, 220–229.

Han, J., Zhu, Y., Li, S., 2008. The language of medically unexplained dyspnea. Chest 133 (4), 961–968.

Kox, M., Stoffels, M., Smeekens, S.P., et al., 2012. The influence of concentration/meditation on autonomic nervous system activity and the innate immune response. Psychosom. Med. 74, 489–494.

Lung, F.W., Lee, T.H., Huang, M.F., 2012. Parental bonding in males with adjustment disorder and hyperventilation syndrome. BMC Psych. 12, 56.

Munemoto, T., Masuda, A., Nagai, N., et al., 2013. Prolonged post-hyperventilation apnea in two young adults with hyperventilation syndrome. Bio. Psych. Soc. Med. 7, 9.

Nishino, T., 2012. Lung/chest expansion contributes to generation of pleasantness associated with dyspnoea relief. Resp. Physiol. Neurobiol. 184 (1), 27–34.

Ravanbakhsh, M., Nargesi, M., Raji, H., et al., 2013. Reliability and validity of the Iranian version of Nijmegen questionnaire in Iranians with asthma. Tanaffos, 14 (2), 121–127.

Sardinha, A., Freire, R.C., Zin, W.A., et al., 2009. Respiratory manifestations of panic disorder: causes, consequences and therapeutic implications. J. Bras. Pneumol. 35 (7), 698–708.

Yoon, H.-K., Kang, J., Kwon, D.-Y., et al., 2016. Frontoparietal cortical thinning in respiratory-type panic disorder: a preliminary report. Psych. Invest. 13 (1), 146–151.

# 18

# Elderly People With Cardiorespiratory Disease

## LEARNING OBJECTIVES

*On completion of this chapter the reader should be able to:*
- differentiate the changes with ageing that are inevitable and those that are modifiable;
- identify suitable strategies for communicating with patients who are confused or have dementia;
- plan the management of elderly people with cardiorespiratory disease, including liaison with the multidisciplinary team.

## OUTLINE

*Almost every disease that primarily affects the lung is more common in older people.*

***Tyler & Stevenson 2016***

Age is the dominant risk factor for cardiovascular disease (Chantler 2012), and people aged >80 years are the fastest growing segment of the population (Scuteri 2016). Older people account for 60% of hospitalized people (Manning & Cefalu 2017), and rehabilitation helps reduce the dependency and anxiety to which they are susceptible in this environment. Both in and outside hospital, rehabilitation also helps maintain dignity, autonomy and inclusion in decision-making (Woolhead et al. 2004).

## NORMAL EFFECTS OF AGEING

The normal age-related decline in lung function starts from around age 25 (DoH 2010a), after which it is all downhill (Fig. 18.1). Changes relevant to cardiorespiratory physiotherapy include the following:

- ↓ exercise tolerance by approximately 10% per decade (Strait 2013);
- ↓ regulation of blood pressure (BP) during postural change (Agnoletti et al. 2016);
- ↑ systolic BP due to vascular stiffness (Guo et al. 2016b);
- ↓ balance and coordination, ↑ falls (Jacobs 2016);
- ↓ elasticity of lung tissue and the chest wall, ↓ gas exchange surface area, ↓ ventilatory response to hypoxaemia and hypercapnia, ↓ cough reflex (Lalley 2013);
- ventilation/perfusion mismatch and ↑ closing volume, which reaches functional residual capacity (FRC) (see Fig. 1.10) at average age 44 in supine and 65 in sitting (Olsén 2005);
- ↓ cough strength and slower mucociliary clearance (Lowery 2013);
- ↓ perception of dyspnoea (Ebihara et al. 2012), which may delay patients seeking assistance when required;
- ↑ stoicism (Abdulla et al. 2013);

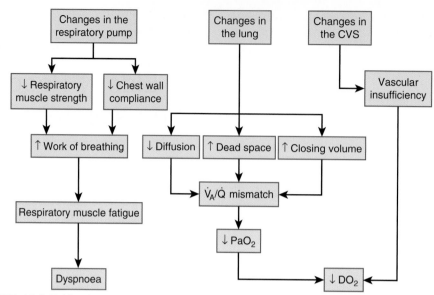

**FIGURE 18.1** Subjective and objective effects of ageing on the cardiorespiratory system. *CVS*, Cardiovascular system; *DO₂*, oxygen delivery to the tissues; $\dot{V}_A/\dot{Q}$, ventilation/perfusion.

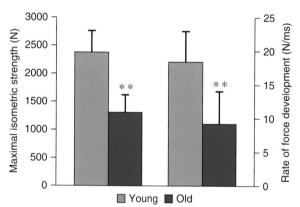

**FIGURE 18.2** Age-related reduction in strength, as shown by maximal isometric strength and force development. **, $P < .01$. (From Granacher et al. 2010.)

- altered absorption, distribution and metabolism of drugs (Schofield 2014);
- ↓ muscle mass (Fig. 18.2) at 1%–2% per year after age 50 and ↓ bone density (Abdelhamid et al. 2016);
- Immunosenescence, thus increasing vulnerability to disease (Manning & Cefalu 2017).

## PREVENTABLE EFFECTS OF AGEING

The majority of patients admitted acutely to hospital are elderly, frail and cognitively impaired (McMurdo &

Witham 2013), the strongest predictor of frailty being shortness of breath (Valenza et al. 2016). If not sensitively handled on admission, **confusion** may develop, increased by sleep fragmentation, lack of hearing aid or glasses, or relocation stress due to hospitalization.

'Hospital-acquired **delirium**' can be set off by poor communication, unnecessary transfer between wards or a history of falls (Otremba et al. 2016). It leads to cognitive deterioration at twice the rate in the year after discharge compared with those who do not develop delirium, sometimes because of the continuation of psychotropic drugs (Bell 2013). Delirium may develop into posttraumatic stress disorder (Cunningham 2013), and Collier (2012) considers delirium to be an emergency. Preventing delirium on admission is cost effective (Akunne 2012), e.g. by avoiding dehydration, constipation, polypharmacy, pain or sleep disturbance, by the patient having access to clocks with large numbers, by meals at central locations rather than in bed, and using toilets rather than bedpans. All team members, including the family, can be involved in orientation and preventive strategies (Martinez et al. 2012).

Delirium predisposes to **dementia** (NICE 2010c). Only half of demented patients are diagnosed (Russ et al. 2012), but at the same time, a label of confusion or delirium should not be accepted without investigation by a specialist. Whittamore (2014) found that, in acute elderly patients admitted to hospital, 27% had delirium, 41% had dementia and 19% had both. Dementia is less likely in people of African ancestry (Schlesinger 2013) but more likely in people with respiratory disease (Pivi 2012). Confusion differs from dementia in its acute course and reversibility. Approximately a third of Alzheimer dementia cases could be attributed to potentially modifiable risk factors such as smoking, diabetes, obesity, hypertension, depression and cognitive inactivity (Killin et al. 2016).

Dementia is associated with dysphagia and **aspiration** (Sura et al. 2012), which predisposes to pneumonia and may influence the course of chronic obstructive pulmonary disease (COPD), especially if there is poor oral health (Scannapieco 2016). A bidirectional relationship between pneumonia and cognition explains how a single episode of infection may cause a person to lose functional independence (Shah et al. 2013). Exercises aimed at vocal cord adduction and glottal closure can reduce the risk of aspiration pneumonia (Fujimaki et al. 2017).

**Adverse drug events** are more likely with ageing, along with inappropriate prescription. Overuse of psychotropic drugs increases cognitive decline and falls (Cammen 2014), along with underuse of drugs for bone health (Conroy et al. 2010).

---

**KEY POINT**

*Older people are underrepresented in clinical trials, even though they receive the majority of drug prescriptions. The safety and efficacy of medicines for this population is therefore unclear.*

Schlender et al. 2016

---

**Depression** can accelerate the ageing process (Garcia-Rizo 2013) and hinder rehabilitation (Vieira et al. 2014). It is common in later life, particularly in people who are institutionalized or suffer bereavement, isolation or functional impairment (Weyerer et al. 2013). It increases the risk of falls (Casteran et al. 2016) and predisposes to dementia. Dementia also impairs the diagnosis of depression, but depression is treatable within dementia (Katona 2004) and these must be distinguished because some antidepressants aggravate delirium (Meagher 2001). Depression should always be considered in the presence of comments such as 'she's forgetful', or 'he's beginning to dement'.

**Sleep disturbance** is common and increases the risk of coronary heart disease (Zhuang et al. 2016). It overlaps with depression, fatigue and poor concentration (Corfield et al. 2016) but can be ameliorated by exercise (Dzierzewski et al. 2013).

**Postural hypotension** is a drop in systolic BP of 20 mmHg or more on moving from sitting or lying to standing, and in older people is usually due to vascular insufficiency. It increases the risk of falls and is worsened by dehydration and diuretics (Zhu et al. 2016). **Dehydration** is common because of ageing kidneys and blunted thirst (Arai et al. 2013). Reduced mobility may inhibit fluid intake because of anxiety about incontinence.

**Urinary incontinence** affects 15%–50% of older women and is also associated with falls (Hunter 2013). An assumption that incontinence is inevitable may lead to mopping-up taking precedence over preventive action such as maintenance of mobility and ensuring access to the toilet.

---

**MINI CLINICAL REASONING**

*'The management of urinary incontinence … seems to … improve care workers' quality of life'.*

Suzuki et al. 2016

**Response**

… and the patients' quality of life?

---

**Constipation** is common and may be due to dehydration, medication, change of diet, dementia, immobility or anxiety that someone will open the curtains when they are on the commode.

**Breathlessness** affects one in four adults aged 70 and older (Smith et al. 2016c) which may be why respiratory disease is often overlooked, especially as many patients do not report the symptom. Reversible components of dyspnoea may not be treated even if a diagnosis is made (Sherman et al. 1992).

**Aerobic capacity** declines with age but can be attenuated by regular endurance exercise training (Wilson et al. 2016), even in very elderly people (Krist et al. 2013) and in those with dementia (Garuffi 2013).

**Poor mobility** is exacerbated by treatable conditions such as anaemia, painful feet or fear of exercise. One study found that gardening was the most significant predictor to mobility among all the health characteristics and social factors studied (Lêng et al. 2013).

The risk of **osteoporosis** increases with coronary artery disease (Alan et al. 2016), age, immobility, diseases such as COPD and its medication and, for people who have difficulty with food preparation, a diet deficient in musculoskeletal nutrients (Sharkey 2013). Vertebral fractures have been found in 51% of elderly patients (Jagt-Willems 2012). The role of the physiotherapist in prevention is to adapt impact exercises to the patient's lifestyle, to refer to a dietician if required, and sometimes refer to the general practitioner (GP) because of widespread underdiagnosis, especially in men (Frost et al. 2012).

**Contractures** are frequent in institutionalized elders (Müller et al. 2013), where formal exercise is often absent. Families can be enrolled, with the help of exercise diaries, to ensure the basics of mobility.

**Aches and pains** are pathological and to be investigated, not accepted as part of ageing.

## NEEDS OF OLDER PEOPLE

*Dignity refers to self respect and being valued by others. Autonomy refers to control of decision making.*

*BMJ 2001*

Patients may accept unnecessary symptoms with comments such as 'what can I expect at my age?' They should, however, be encouraged to ask for symptoms to be investigated, rather than acquiesce to the ageist attitudes that are common in the health system, e.g.:

- Asthma is often unmanaged or underdiagnosed, and is more often fatal, in elderly people (Arjona 2015).
- Fewer elderly people hospitalized with an exacerbation of COPD see a respiratory specialist, even though they have greater comorbidity and higher mortality than younger people, and they are more likely to receive a 'do-not-resuscitate' order, irrespective of comorbidities (Stone et al. (2012).
- Elderly people experience poorer access to surgery (White 2014) and problems accessing pain relief (Fig. 18.3).
- For elders with depression, 94% of junior hospital doctors miss the diagnosis, and GPs treat only 10% of their depressed elderly patients (Katona 2004).
- In hospital, curtains are less likely to be pulled round older patients left exposed than younger patients (Turnock & Kelleher 2001).

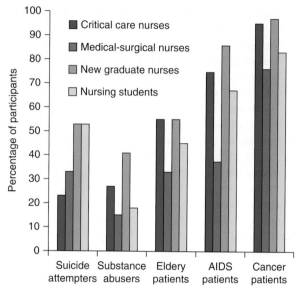

**FIGURE 18.3** Percentage of health staff who would expend maximum time and energy on patients' pain. (From Brockopp et al. 2003.)

Both ageing and cardiovascular disease are associated with oxidative stress and chronic inflammation (Sallam 2016). This can be ameliorated by little-and-often exercise, recommended by Taylor (2014) to be 150 min of moderate intensity or 75 min of vigorous intensity, in bouts of at least 10 min duration. Other benefits of exercise in elderly people are:

- a partial reversion of age-related physiological decline, ↑ work capacity and bone health and ↓ risk of cardiovascular mortality (Mendonca et al. 2016);
- ↑ cognition, balance, strength and vision, and ↓ falls, using 'exergames' at home (Gschwind et al. 2015);
- ↓ depression (Hallgren et al. 2016), agitation (Ballard et al. 2016) and urinary incontinence (Vinsnes et al. 2012);
- ↓ morbidity and mortality (Ikezoe et al. 2013).

In hospital, coloured wristbands on walking frames are useful to identify how far a patient can walk and the assistance required, e.g. red for two staff, yellow for one and green for the patient being independently mobile. In the community, exercising in groups is particularly enjoyed by elderly people, with walking a popular activity (Victor et al. 2016) preferably to the level of 'breathless but not speechless'.

Fear of falls impedes confidence. The risk of falls is increased by:

- respiratory and swallowing problems (Higashijima 2010);
- cardiovascular disease (Al-Momani et al. 2016);
- dyspnoea, pain, ↓ balance, inadequate footwear, environmental hazards or postural hypotension (NICE 2013c);
- malnutrition (Misu et al. 2016) and weakness, especially of the quadriceps (Regterschot et al. 2014);
- anxiety, which triples the likelihood of falls in elderly men (Holloway et al. 2016);
- urinary frequency, sensory impairment, dizziness, ↓ cognition, and both depression or antidepressants (Deandrea et al. 2013);
- polypharmacy (Watanabe 2016).

One study found that up to 30% of hospital admissions in elders are related to adverse drug reactions (Campbell 2014).

---

### KEY POINT

*Use psychology before drugs.*

Sharpe & Hanning 1999

---

Enjoyable ways to improve balance in older adults include Wii (Bieryla & Dold 2013), T'ai Chi (Hwang et al. 2016), yoga (Nick et al. 2016) and dance (Balingit et al. 2013). People with dementia respond particularly well to salsa dancing (Abreu & Hartley 2013).

Autonomy is central to rehabilitation. This can be facilitated by respecting patients' senior status, experience and wishes, including allowing them to return to bed when they request rather than enforcing unhappy hours slumped in a hospital chair, where discomfort may be reducing their depth of breathing.

Another limitation to rehabilitation is pain, which is undertreated in this age group, possibly because of a strange belief that it is an inevitable part of aging (Prostran et al. 2016). In care homes, pain has been identified in 66% of residents and 80% of those with dementia (Bauer et al. 2016). Methods are available for assessing pain in people who are very old (Abdulla et al. 2013) or have dementia (Herr et al. 2016). People with dementia may express their pain by agitation or aggression (Ahn 2013), but antipsychotics tend to be considered before analgesia in agitated patients (Mędrzycka et al. 2016). Dementia should not exclude a person from exercise training, which brings improvements in physical function and well-being (Zasadzka et al. 2016).

Rehabilitation is also hindered by:
- hidden malnutrition, which is associated with falls, sleep disturbance, immobility, agitation, dysphagia, insomnia and incontinence (Yildiz et al. 2015);
- memory loss, which requires physiotherapy advice and exercise programmes to be written down and explained to the patient and family.

Rehabilitation is facilitated by:
- ensuring that patients know that they are heard;
- providing information consistently;
- avoiding the use of first names uninvited, because for older generations this may be seen as a sign of disrespect rather than friendliness;
- encouraging patients to bring to hospital their personal possessions and photos;
- encouraging patients to wear their own clothes when possible;
- involving patients in goal setting;
- ensuring communication between all parties, including the family, when patients are transferred to and from acute care (Lane et al. 2013).

Some suggestions to assist communication are in Box 18.1.

A demented person's ability to feel emotions remains intact even as aphasia sets in, and it is thought that most patients are aware of, and feel distressed by, their limitations (Zimmermann 1998).

---

### MINI CLINICAL REASONING

*When washing patients, distress was ameliorated by keeping them covered, using the right water temperature, patting rather than rubbing dry and talking quietly. This approach was found to reduce crying out and the need for drugs.*

Adams et al. 2012

**Response**
It is perplexing that we need research to tell us this.

---

## Specific Environments

On the surgical wards, preoperative assessment should address function, social support, cognition and frailty (Wozniak et al. 2016), and nutrition should be checked because it has a direct effect on postoperative physical function (Ogawa et al. 2016). Postoperative delirium is reduced by adequate oxygenation, visual and hearing aids, early mobilization and avoidance of sleep

---

**BOX 18.1   Strategies to Adopt When Working With People Who Are Confused or Demented**

1   Minimize noise including loud conversation, TV, radio and bleeps
2   Walk slowly towards the patient from the foot of the bed, with eye contact and without the lighting obscuring your face
3   Before speaking, check that you have the patient's attention
4   Speak slowly and calmly, using short sentences and avoiding two questions in one sentence
5   With dementia, you may need to introduce yourself each time you speak
6   Gentle physical contact is normally beneficial, but not if the patient withdraws
7   Positive communications are more productive, e.g. 'rest in the chair' rather than 'don't get up yet'
8   Questions may need to be repeated, first in the same way and then in a different way, e.g. 'are you in pain?' a couple of times, then 'does anything hurt?'
9   Echo the patient's input, e.g. 'you're cold, I'll get you a blanket'
10  With dementia, avoid unnecessary questions

Adapted from Zimmermann 1998.

---

deprivation, dehydration and certain drugs (Brown 2010). Communication and orientation are a priority, especially following emergency surgery (Stoneham et al. 2014).

On the medical wards, early rehabilitation reduces symptoms (Liao et al. 2016a), length of stay and likelihood of discharge to a nursing home (Kosse et al. 2013). The importance of checking the fluid balance chart is underlined by a study by McCrow et al. (2016), which found a 29% incidence of dehydration on admission.

On the cardiac ward, malnutrition can reach 50% in patients aged >75, hindering rehabilitation and affecting respiratory drive, the immune system and length of stay (Brogi et al. 2016). Cardiac rehabilitation in the oldest patients after surgery or a cardiac event brings improvement in all domains of physical performance (Baldasseroni et al. 2016).

In the ICU, prediction models can detect delirium, which may be improved by re-orientation, adequate sleep and early mobilization (Slooter et al. 2017), thus limiting the risk of long-term cognitive decline (Wolters et al. 2017).

In care homes, respiratory disease is associated with low quality of life (Carreiro et al. 2016). One study found that the majority of residents were taking inaccurate medications (Lima et al. 2013).

At the end of life, patients tend to receive undesired and burdensome interventions and at the same time are underassessed and undertreated for symptoms (Verhofstede et al. 2016). Dementia is a terminal disorder and patients need the option to make an advance directive at an early stage (Steen et al. 2013). Physiotherapists can take the initiative in referring patients to the palliative team when required.

## OUTCOMES

Exercise capacity in elders can be measured by a sit-to-stand test (Bohannon 2011), shuttle test (Dyer et al. 2002) or shortened walking tests of 10 m (Fritz 2013) or 3 m (Worsfold & Simpson 2001). Valid instruments include those for quality of life (Makai 2013, Wu et al. 2013), physical activity (White et al. 2012b), activities of daily living (Huiszoon 2014) and seven screening tools for functional ability (Beaton & Grimmer 2013). A robust model for breathless older people is the above combined with the modified Medical Research Council dyspnoea scale (DePew et al. 2013). For older people with dementia, the 6-min walk test is valid for exercise, as are the Figure-of-Eight Walk test, the 'TUG' test, the 'FICSIT' balance test, the Chair Rise test (Blankevoort et al. 2012) and the Comprehensive Geriatric Assessment (Bernabei 2010).

Discharge requires multidisciplinary coordination and often a home visit.

*All unnecessary (and perhaps even some indicated) medications must be discontinued before discharge, thereby adhering to the tenets of geriatric pharmacology by prescribing as few drugs as possible.*
**Green & Maurer 2013**

## CASE STUDY: MR MM[a]

*Analyse the problems of this 82-year-old patient from Brighton who has COPD and was visited at home after a fall.*

---

[a]AS, Added sounds; BS, breath sounds; L, left; R, right; SOB, shortness of breath.

## Social history

- Former professional singer
- Lives with daughter and adolescent grandchildren, tends to 'hibernate in my room to avoid them'

## Subjective

- Recent pneumonia, continuous fatigue since then
- Don't use stairs or go into garden, can't go out, just want to sit down all the time
- Saw GP for swollen ankles, told to restrict fluid intake
- Given oxygen by GP. Seem to get headaches when use oxygen
- Not breathless at rest but main reason for limited activity is SOB, with some limitation due to fatigue, anxiety, loss of confidence after fall and avoidance of grandchildren.

On questioning about falls, Mr MM is unable to identify preceding dizziness or other cause

## Objective

- Apart from headache, no other signs of $CO_2$ retention such as flapping tremor or warm hands
- $SpO_2$ 95% on room air
- Patient leaning forwards and clutching arms of chair
- Rapid shallow rhythmic breathing pattern
- Auscultation: BS reduced but present and R = L, no AS
- No obvious environmental fall hazards
- No standby antibiotics or steroids

## Questions

1. Analysis?
2. Problems?
3. Plan?
4. Progression?

## Response to Case Study

1. Analysis
   - Mr MM has not returned to normal function since pneumonia.

- He is unsure about when to take oxygen and has not been assessed for this.
- Headache may relate to $CO_2$ retention, possibly related to uncontrolled oxygen therapy.
- Multiple reasons for reduced exercise tolerance are physical, emotional and social.
- Falls may relate to fatigue, weakness and/or loss of confidence.
- Requires overall management plan, to include GP.

2. Problems
   - Falls risk
   - Inaccurate oxygen prescription
   - Fatigue
   - Breathlessness
   - Anxiety and loss of confidence
   - Exercise intolerance

3. Plan
   - Explanation about oxygen, leaflet provided.
   - Explanation about COPD, leaflet provided.
   - Explanation of possible heart failure. Advice on ankle exercises and leg elevation when resting. Patient agrees on referral to community heart failure team.
   - Explanation about breathlessness, advice on forward lean sitting with relaxed arms.
   - Discussion on possible causes of fatigue, e.g. post-viral, loss of fitness.
   - Discussion on possible triggers for pneumonia, possibly stress contributing.
   - Advice on building up immune system.
   - SOB management strategies, Provide leaflet on SOB and exercise.
   - Demonstration of quadriceps exercises and leaflet provided.
   - Stretchy bands and leaflet provided.
   - Walk into garden, with pacing. Patient chooses to exercise at 'breathless but not speechless' level.
   - Climb bottom three steps on stairs.
   - Discussion on lifestyle and building up exercise. Walking aid declined.
   - Discussion on pulmonary rehabilitation (PR) programme. Mr MM prefers home exercise.
   - Discussion on singing and breathing. Mr MM to contact the singing teacher associated with the PR programme.
   - Advice on when to take antibiotics and/or steroids, when to call community respiratory service, GP or ambulance.

- Continuous oximetry throughout session, including exercise: no desaturation. Advised to avoid oxygen until assessment.
- Patient agrees on referral to falls clinic and oxygen clinic.
- Email to GP: information on referrals, request for advice on heart failure diagnosis, request for standby antibiotics and steroids, information provided on discontinuation of oxygen and advice requested.

4. Progression
   - Personalized exercise diary
   - Check headaches
   - Check breathing pattern, review if this has not normalized
   - Follow-up communication with GP, liaise with falls clinic
   - Build up exercise tolerance, including full flight of stairs and going out with friends

## RESPONSE TO CLINICAL REASONING

Not surprising: Training is specific. Exercise performance would not be expected to improve with postural drainage. Exercise performance may or may not improve with inspiratory muscle training, depending on the factors causing inspiratory muscle weakness.

*It is an error of youth to think that with age comes a readiness to accept the consequences of ageing and to tolerate its attendant illnesses.*

**Gems 2011b**

## RECOMMENDED READING

Baijens, L.W., Clavé, P., Cras, P.L.C., et al., 2016. European Society for Swallowing Disorders – European Union Geriatric Medicine Society white paper: oropharyngeal dysphagia as a geriatric syndrome. Clin. Interv. Aging 11, 1403–1428.

Bone, A.E., Hepgul, N., Kon, S., et al., 2017. Sarcopenia and frailty in chronic respiratory disease: lessons from gerontology. Chron. Respir. Dis. 14 (1), 85–99.

Dongen, E.J.I., Leerlooijer, J.N., Steijns, J.M., et al., 2016. Translation of a tailored nutrition and resistance exercise intervention for elderly people to a real-life setting. BMC Geriatr. 17, 25.

Huang, S.H., Lin, L.F., Chou, L.C., et al., 2016. Feasibility of using the International Classification of Functioning, Disability and Health Core Set for evaluation of fall-related risk factors in acute rehabilitation settings. Eur. J. Phys. Rehabil. Med. 52 (2), 152–158.

Hwang, U., Carpenter, C., 2016. Assessing geriatric vulnerability for post emergency department adverse outcomes. Emerg. Med. J. 33, 2–3.

Koeneman, M.A., Chorus, A., Hopman-Rock, M., 2017. A novel method to promote physical activity among older adults in residential care. BMC Geriatr. 17, 8.

McDermid, R.C., Bagshaw, S.M., 2011. Octogenarians in the ICU. Crit. Care 15 (1), 125–128.

NICE, 2015. Transition between inpatient hospital settings and community or care home settings for adults with social care needs [NG27].

NICE, 2016. Multimorbidity: clinical assessment and management [NG56].

Pieper, M.J., Francke, A.L., van der Steen, J.T., et al., 2016. Effects of a stepwise multidisciplinary intervention for challenging behavior in advanced dementia: a cluster randomized controlled trial. J. Am. Geriatr. Soc. 64 (2), 261–269.

Qin, J., Li, G., Zhou, J., 2016. Characteristics of elderly patients with COPD and newly diagnosed lung cancer, and factors associated with treatment decision. Int. J. Chron. Obstruct. Pulmon. Dis. 11, 1515–1520.

Silva, C.G., Franklin, B.A., Forman, D.E., et al., 2016. Influence of age in estimating maximal oxygen uptake. J. Geriatr. Cardiol. 13 (2), 126–131.

Suffoletto, B., Miller, T., Shah, R., et al., 2016. Predicting older adults who return to the hospital or die within 30 days of emergency department care using the ISAR tool. Emerg. Med. J. 33, 4–9.

Tyler, K., Stevenson, D., 2016. Respiratory emergencies in geriatric patients. Emerg. Med. Clin. North Am. 34 (1), 39–49.

# 19

# Palliative Respiratory Physiotherapy

## LEARNING OBJECTIVES

*On completion of this chapter the reader should be able to:*
- recognize, as part of the team, when the goals of management shift from cure of disease to control of symptoms;
- ensure that the patient's wishes drive these goals;
- use clinical reasoning to identify physiotherapy strategies to suit these goals;
- develop empathetic communication skills, including adaptation to different cultures.

## INTRODUCTION

> *It begins with an easy voice saying,*
> *just a routine examination;*
> *as October sunlight pierces the heavy velvet curtains.*
> *Later it is the friends who write but do not visit…*
> *it is doctors who no longer stop by your bed…*
> *it is terror every minute of conscious night and day to a background of pop music.*
>
> **Wilkes 1983**

Physiotherapists are suited to working with people at the end of their lives because patients often have similar needs to those with disabilities (Purtilo 1976). End-stage disease is not a time to withdraw physiotherapy because there is much that can be done to ease the passage towards a good death.

Palliative care focuses on patient-determined quality of life (QoL) and involves a multidisciplinary team including the patient and family. Symptom control and psychosocial care are required, which may need to be prolonged.

In developed countries, most people die in old age, and slowly. A proactive integrated system helps ensure early initiation of palliative care, starting from diagnosis (Fig. 19.1). Terminal cardiopulmonary diseases include chronic obstructive pulmonary disease (COPD), which traditionally lacks advance care planning and integrated palliative care (Lilly 2016) and heart failure (Ziehm et al. 2016).

Palliative care rehabilitation concentrates on the functional consequences of end-stage disease, the need increasing with disease progression (Runacres et al. 2017). This has been studied mostly in cancer patients

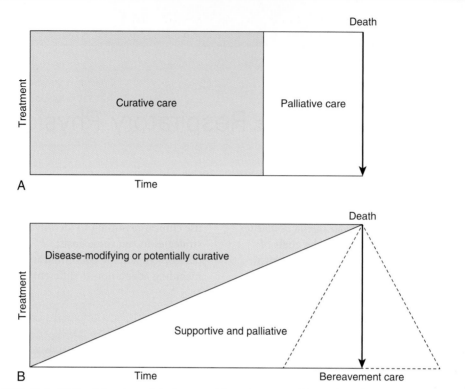

**FIGURE 19.1** (A) Traditional model of care with a clear transition point. (B) Model of care with palliation starting from diagnosis. (From Pinnock 2011.)

who find that rehabilitation reduces anxiety, increases satisfaction and feelings of control, and may enable them to be discharged home (Fu 2012), sometimes with mobile or web-based support (Hochstenbach et al. 2016).

## REACTIONS OF PATIENTS

*Accepting loss of control and loss of movement is not something I want to come to terms with.*
                                          ***Soundy et al. 2012***

When informed that they are dying, most patients feel overwhelmed and experience a variety of reactions. Disbelief and then fear usually predominate at first, though not primarily fear of death itself. Patients may be frightened of symptoms and the dying process, of isolation, of being a burden or of the unknown.

Many cardiorespiratory deaths, and 21% of global cancer deaths, are caused by smoking (Rom 2013), and guilt may be an extra burden. Anger is also an ever-ready emotion that may arise from feelings of helplessness or

act as a defence against the lonely experience of grief. Grief can develop into depression, which amplifies pain, distresses relatives and erodes the patient's ability to do the emotional work of separating and saying goodbye. Patients should be allowed to express sorrow, anger, guilt, unusual humour or any other feeling, for which they do not need to apologize. As one patient said, 'I laugh because I don't want to cry' (Soundy et al. 2012).

Many patients deny reality in order to avoid the pain of grief or fear, acting and talking as if they expect to get better. Denial may be a necessary cushion and is a defence mechanism to be respected. When and if patients are ready to confront the truth, they may sink into a dark place that can paradoxically be a creative process by which they begin to take responsibility for the way they respond to change. They may accept their loss and allow fear to dissolve.

These reactions are not stages that occur with defined boundaries, but may weave in and out of a patient's awareness, so that a moment of anger may open into acceptance, followed by the mind curling back into the darkness of fear. Time is needed, and patients with cardiorespiratory disease often have time. With support, time can be used wisely.

The media's focus on 'fighting' at the end of life does not support patients who prefer to seek peace and comfort in their last weeks. They and their family may feel stigmatized if they 'lose the battle'.

## REACTIONS OF RELATIVES

*'When someone you love dies, you pay for the sin of outliving them with a thousand piercing regrets'*
**Simone de Beauvoir 1966**

Family and friends can feel a kaleidoscope of emotions before and after a patient dies, e.g. remorse, relief, impotence at being unable to help, and similar reactions to those of the patient. 'Anticipatory grief' can be more difficult because the patient is physically present and the family needs to be functional and sometimes inhibit grief expression (Coelho & Barbosa 2017).

Patient and family may try to 'protect' each other from reality, occasionally with the collusion of health staff. Just when they need each other the most, they may be separated by a conspiracy of silence. Patients and relatives usually need the opportunity to share the truth with each other.

A third of older spouses experience bereavement complicated by difficulties beyond those associated with 'normal' grief (Acierno 2012). Risk factors include:

- prior ambiguous or dependent relationship with the deceased person;
- families from a culture who are unable to follow their own customs;
- relatives who have learning disabilities or dementia.

People with learning difficulties may manifest grief as behaviour change or self harm. If a bereaved person has dementia, they may repeatedly forget, feeling shocked each time they are told. Complicated grief may lead to posttraumatic stress disorder, especially after a death in the intensive care unit (ICU) (Bournival 2017).

The death of someone close to a child often has life-long effects on the child (Schonfeld & Demaria 2016). Children need to be seen and acknowledged, and to spend time with their sick relative (Alvariza et al. 2017). They know their own limitations and may simply want to pop in and out of the sick room. Children often fantasize that they are to blame for the death of a parent or sibling, or they may feel that they must not distress the family and so avoid talking about it.

Assistance for families includes involving them in decisions when patients are unable do this themselves, helping them to provide physical comforts for their loved one, advice on support groups, a communication diary (McEvoy 2012) and, after the death, telephone contact and anniversary cards (Goebel et al. 2017).

Widowhood increases mortality, with the majority of respiratory deaths in bereaved people being from pneumonia (Brenn & Ytterstad 2016).

## REACTIONS OF STAFF

*To be ethically engaged is to be … mindful of their needs, values and goals, attuned to their illness experiences, and emotionally open to their suffering.*
**Jensen & Greenfield 2012**

Once a patient's condition is known to preclude recovery, this is sometimes interpreted as a failure by health staff and has been described as an 'institutional liability' (Risse & Balboni 2013). Reactions may include avoidance, heroic measures to prolong life, unsuitable bonhomie, the use of drugs to suppress patients' expression of emotion, inaccurate optimism or inappropriate reassurance. Reassurance has been criticized as 'social bromide' aimed at making staff feel better rather than the patient (Fareed 1996).

Health staff working with people at the end of life require support themselves. They need access to their own feelings because expression of feelings by staff, when appropriate, has been found therapeutic for patients, who can find professional detachment unhelpful and occasionally offensive (Fallowfield 1993).

## WHERE TO DIE?

*The end of a life in the critical care environment can become one of the most powerfully uncomfortable and inhumane experiences that any human will endure.*

**Angood 2003**

Most patients prefer to die at home, but the majority die in hospital (Stilos et al. 2016) or care homes, where symptoms tend to be poorly managed (Brooke 2012). In any of these locations, patients need to be under the care of a palliative team. Hospice-at-home services are well established, including physiotherapy input (Cobbe et al. 2013), which enable patients to achieve a similar

QoL as in a hospice (Leppert 2012). People with heart failure can be managed at home even if they require inotropic infusions (Taitel et al. 2012).

For those who have to die in the ICU, this usually follows a decision to withdraw or withhold treatment, in which case alarms and electronic monitoring are disconnected, and if a tracheal tube is to be removed, plans made in case of secretions or gasping. As with dying patients outside the ICU, patients with lung disease tend to receive fewer elements of palliative care than those with cancer (Brown et al. 2016b).

Palliative services tend to be accessed late, especially for patients with end-stage respiratory disease (Landers et al. 2016), who have symptoms of similar severity to cancer but with a less predictable prognosis (Chadwick 2012). Information on advance care planning should be provided early and systematically, but Carlucci et al. (2016) found that only 50% of patients are treated according to their wishes. Different levels of support should be offered to patients, bearing in mind that their wishes may not be those of their family or their doctor (Cook et al. 2003). If the choice is for home care, information should include preparation for untoward or frightening events.

## COMMUNICATING WITH DYING PEOPLE

*His yellow eyes watched us being taught at the bedside of each patient and when we came to his bed we all walked directly past him to the patient on his other side. Not a word was said. Not a greeting. Not even a nod... Dismay turned to guilt with the thought that I, too, had no idea how to approach or comfort a dying patient.*

**Carmichael (medical student) 1981**

It is not easy to find the right words to say to people who are facing death. The key is to listen. Patients find relief if they feel that it is acceptable to talk, and the astute listener can pick up indirect questions. Patients may drop hints that they would like to talk by mentioning other people who have died, joking about their future or asking how long before they get better. We can indicate a willingness to listen by sitting down, maintaining eye contact (in Western cultures) and asking non-threatening questions such as:

- how do you feel in yourself?
- What is your understanding of what has happened?

- What have the doctors told you about your condition?
- Is there anything that you're worried about?
- Is there anyone you can rely on who can help you make important decisions?
- What are your goals?

If a patient has just received a distressing prognosis, they are unlikely to focus on their physiotherapy, but may need some space to ask questions that were not asked when receiving the information. As one patient said, 'The second the doctor told me I had cancer, the rest of the conversation was over; I don't remember anything' (Burt 2000). It is useful to ask how they understand what they have heard, and be guided by their response. Clarity of words is required, e.g. patients may understand the word 'severe' more clearly than the word 'advanced', or they may assume that the word 'cancer' equates to an inevitable or distressing death.

During and after talking, patients need time to process their thoughts, and silence can be used constructively. It is not helpful to rationalize patients out of their feelings, tell them what to do, or say that we know how they feel (we don't). It is however, helpful to provide information that reduces anxiety and increases the ability to cope, and discussion itself helps to divest death of its power. Fear of the unknown is usually a heavier burden than the truth, and patients who are left in ignorance tend to feel a loss of control that shackles their coping strategies. This is illustrated in a study in which patients who were given specific information had reduced anxiety and improved QoL (Nakajima et al. 2013), and another finding that patients who knew their cancer to be incurable experienced less fatigue, anxiety and physical symptoms than those unaware of their disease status (Lee et al. 2013c). Dewar (1995) says that 'bearing the agony of knowing one has a life-threatening condition is not as problematic as not being given adequate information'. We might also find it useful to ponder our own reactions: 'Am I feeling uncomfortable? Am I helping or hindering her flow of thought? Am I responding to his needs or mine?'

Communication is sometimes hindered by people with COPD seeing their illness as a way of life rather than a life-threatening illness: their story has no beginning, no entry point and the thought of an exit point has no context. However, significant milestones can facilitate communication:

- exacerbations
- home oxygen

- panic attacks
- need for assistance with personal care (Landers et al. 2016)

When patients ask questions about their prognosis, however, indirect, it is unethical to avoid giving information, and keeps patients in a subordinate position. This may be due to a false assumption that distress equals harm, or uncertainty about who should take the initiative. Physiotherapists have as much right and responsibility to inform patients as other health staff (Sim 1986) but it is acceptable for physiotherapists to refer difficult communications to other appropriate staff, ensuring that patients' questions are then addressed and that issues of power about who 'owns' the truth do not hinder this.

Although most patients would like end-of-life discussions, these conversations do not usually take place, leading to discordant care (Reinke et al. 2013). Patients should also decide who else is told (Buckman 1996); to reveal the diagnosis to a family without the patient's knowledge creates tension and mistrust, and is unethical. Other family requests, e.g. that the patient should be suctioned, should be respected and discussed, but must not take precedence over the rights of the patient. Some individuals and cultures favour family-based decisions, and patients can be asked about the family's role in the decision-making process.

Reaction to bad news is varied and sometimes irrational, including regression to childlike behaviour, relief, despair at the loss of fulfilment, or projection of hostility. Patients should be left with some realistic hope, even if directed towards a minor achievement. And it is always worth casting a backward glance when leaving the bedside, because it is sometimes necessary to return and pick up the pieces.

*In 1672 a French physician considered the idea of telling the truth to patients, but concluded that it would not catch on.*

**Buckman 1996**

## MANAGEMENT OF SYMPTOMS

*The tendency toward "either/or" thinking (either cure or comfort) in traditional biomedical care does little to optimize care in advancing chronic lung disease.*

**Rocker et al. 2015**

End-of-life care at home tends to be associated with less of the aggressive medical care that focuses on disease-modifying treatments at the expense of symptom management (Henson et al. 2016). At the same time, people dying from cardiorespiratory diseases are twice as likely to be admitted to ICUs at the end of life than those with cancer, and the majority of people with interstitial lung disease (ILD) die in hospital with ongoing life-prolonging procedures until death (Rajala et al. 2016), reinforcing the lack of recognition of the need for palliation in noncancer patients (Lyngaa et al. 2015). In fact, engagement of the palliative care team comes too late for a wide spectrum of patients, suggesting a need for automatic referral (Waite et al. 2017).

Patients want to maintain control of breathing and personal care, and their wishes in relation to physiotherapy are usually aimed at rehabilitation to maximize independence in these areas, with if possible a choice in the method and timing of their treatment. For people with cancer, exercise can improve sleep, body image and QoL, and reduce anxiety, fatigue and pain (Mishra et al. 2012). In people with end-stage COPD, pulmonary rehabilitation improves exercise tolerance (Ngaage 2004) and a home-based walking programme can improve QoL (Lowe et al. 2013). Supplemental oxygen, if indicated, maintains cerebral oxygenation (Fig. 19.2).

Symptoms may respond to complementary techniques practiced by physiotherapists, e.g. acupuncture for pain and fatigue (Lau et al. 2016), reflexology for dyspnoea (Wyatt 2012), massage for pain (Mitchinson 2014), or home-based yoga for QoL (Carr et al. 2016).

Symptoms suggesting that death is imminent include:

- changes in communication, social withdrawal;
- reluctance to eat or drink;
- agitation, Cheyne–Stokes breathing, reduced consciousness, mottled skin, death rattle (NICE 2015b).

## Breathlessness

*Ms. A avoided any activity that made her aware of her breathing because she believed that being breathless would make her cancer spread.*

**Bailey 1995**

Shortness of breath (SOB) is experienced by the majority of patients (Johnson. 2016 and Table 19.1). It engenders fear in patients and helplessness and anxiety in their carers, but is often undertreated at the end of life. With cancer, SOB indicates a short prognosis (Booth

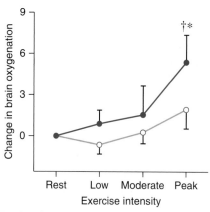

FIGURE 19.2 Increase in brain oxygen saturation in patients with end-stage lung disease during exercise, with and without added oxygen. (Adapted from Jensen et al. 2002.)

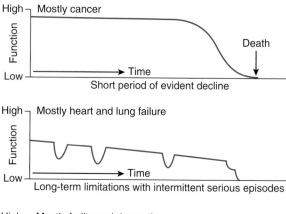
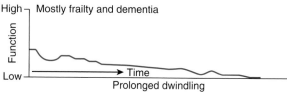

FIGURE 19.3 Trajectory of the effect of dyspnoea on function with different conditions. (From Booth et al. 2008.)

TABLE 19.1   **Estimated prevalence of breathlessness in advanced disease**

| Disease | Prevalence of breathlessness |
|---|---|
| COPD | 90%–95% |
| Heart disease | 60%–88% |
| Chronic kidney disease | 11%–62% |
| AIDS | 11%–62% |
| Cancer | 10%–70% |

*AIDS,* Acquired immune deficiency disease; *COPD,* chronic obstructive pulmonary disease.
From Fardy 2016.

et al. 2008), but with COPD it is slowly progressive (Fig. 19.3), allowing patients to develop some of their own coping strategies. However, it tends to feel worse with COPD (Javadzadeh et al. 2016) and is more frequent with ILD (Matsunuma et al. 2016) than with end-stage lung cancer. The sensation may signal to patients the beginning of a loss of control, and in end-stage disease the symbolism of not getting enough breath is an ever present reminder of approaching death.

Dyspnoea may be caused by cachexia, a tumour, lung fibrosis due to radiotherapy or a coexisting condition. Treatable causes of SOB should be identified, e.g. pleural effusion, ascites, anxiety or anaemia. Anxiety is strongly correlated with SOB because of unfounded fears of dying from suffocation (Mahler et al. 2010). Disentangling this concept is aided by desensitization

(p. 232), and respiratory panic can be reduced by slowing the breathing to its normal minute volume (Landers et al. 2016).

A physiotherapy-led breathless management programme is able to improve functional capacity and coping strategies (Wood et al. 2013) as are other measures discussed in Chapter 8. In the later stages, rocking can aid relaxation and stabilize breathing (Omlin et al. 2016), possibly due to mechanical input to chest wall receptors. Neck massage may also help.

Opioids are the drug of choice (p. 169). Fear of the side effect of respiratory depression is largely unfounded at the end of life (Kamal 2012), but if tolerance prompts increased dosing, depression of ventilation may become relevant (Emery et al. 2016). Transmucosal fentanyl may produce faster and greater relief of episodic breathlessness than morphine (Simon et al. 2016), with other modes of delivery being transdermal (Takakuwa et al. 2015), nasal (Hui et al. 2016b) subcutaneous or by nebulizer (Xu et al. 2012a). The reassuring presence of a nebulizer can help reduce respiratory panic.

Breathlessness may be eased by noninvasive ventilation (Nava et al. 2016) or sometimes high-flow oxygen (Roca et al. 2016). Other forms of oxygen are rarely

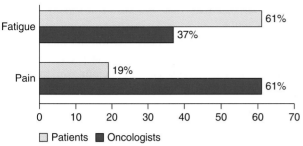

Fatigue — 61% (Patients), 37% (Oncologists)
Pain — 19% (Patients), 61% (Oncologists)

☐ Patients   ■ Oncologists

**FIGURE 19.4** Proportion of patients and oncologists reporting whether fatigue or pain most affects daily life. (From Vogelsang 1997.)

beneficial objectively for normoxaemic patients (Fardy 2016) and tend to set up a barrier between patient and family. However, they carry a strong placebo effect; if it is prescribed for this purpose, the patient needs to be informed that this is probably its mode of bringing relief, and a fan should be tried first (Wong et al. 2017).

## Fatigue

*'I was too tired to think'*

**Patient quoted by Eustace 2002**

Fatigue is under-recognized, underassessed and under-treated (Radbruch 2008), with more importance being ascribed to it by patients than by health staff (Fig. 19.4). It is reported in 80% of cancer patients, or up to 99% following radiotherapy or chemotherapy (EAPC 2016). It can be aggravated by steroids (Matsuo & Yomiya 2013) and may not be relieved by rest.

Pharmacological management is limited, but modafinil or methylphenidate may be beneficial (Mücke et al. 2015), the latter also helping depression (Kerr 2012). The exhaustion of cachexia can be eased by organ-specific nutrition (Zadák et al. 2013) and sometimes by nonsteroidal antiinflammatory drugs (Reid et al. 2013). Physical management is by energy conservation and paced multimodal exercise (Kassab 2013).

## Weakness

Weakness and the resulting lack of function are high on the 'unbearable suffering' spectrum (Ruijs et al. 2012). Causes include immobility, cachexia or some drugs, in particular steroids, which may be essential to treat raised intracranial pressure or spinal cord compression (Lo

et al. 2013). Anorexia and cachexia may cause distress to the patient, but often more so for the family (Amano et al. 2016). For people with advanced cancer, handgrip strength predicts survival (Kilgour et al. 2016), but the quadriceps are the most severely affected muscles (Brown 1999), indicating the need for little-and-often strengthening exercises. Group exercise is popular (Malcolm et al. 2017), best related to activities of daily living, with always an awareness of potential osteoporosis from radiotherapy, chemotherapy or bony secondaries. Autonomic dysfunction may be present in advanced cancer (Stone 2012), indicating a need to check for postural hypotension before mobilization. Neuromuscular electrical stimulation may be acceptable to some patients (Jones et al. 2016a).

## Immobility

The physiotherapist works with the family and staff to assist the patient with mobility, balance and transfers, and to reduce the fear of falling. This may lessen anxiety, decrease injuries and restore dignity. Other reported outcomes include improved emotional functioning, reduced fatigue for people with cancer, and, for those with spinal cord compression, less depression and pain (Turner et al. 2013).

## Cough

In the last year of life, 57% of patients complain of coughing (Leach 2010). When persistent, it can precipitate vomiting, chest or abdominal pain, rib fracture, syncope, insomnia or exhaustion. If pulmonary oedema, infection or bronchospasm contribute, they can be dealt with pharmacologically. For coughs with a neural origin, codeine and the opioids may suppress the central nervous system input (Yorke et al. 2012), whereas peripheral influences such as a lung mass compressing mediastinal structures may be eased by gabapentin (Atreya et al, 2016). Nebulized local anaesthetics can relieve an intractable cough (Truesdale 2013), but eating and drinking are banned for an hour afterwards. Physical management depends on whether the cough is productive or not (Chapter 7).

## Difficulty Swallowing

Dysphagia, often due to weak mouth or throat muscles, may cause silent aspiration, in which ingested material ends up in the lungs without signs of swallowing difficulty or coughing. This may be first identified by the physiotherapist, who can then make a speech–language referral.

## Dehydration and Thirst

Some patients escape the symptoms of dehydration such as headache, nausea and cramps, but 36% of patients are reported to experience thirst (Arai 2013). In the UK it is illegal to withhold food or fluids before coma ensues, unless rejected by the patient (Dimond 2009). Cohen (2012) found that patients who can communicate their wishes prefer to be hydrated because it improves their comfort, reduces pain and nourishes their body and mind. However, artificial nutrition and hydration does not appear to increase comfort, improve quality of life or prolong survival in people with dementia (Ackermann 2016).

To coax a patient to accept oral hydration, the best option is often physical assistance using a spoon or feeding cup, with instruction to the patient on when to swallow. This usually requires the time and patience of a relative. If the patient does not accept this, the relative can be reassured that a drink is probably not needed at that time, along with information that this is part of the natural process of dying (Hui et al. 2015).

A coated tongue or dry mouth can be relieved by some of the measures in Table 7.2, by semifrozen gin and tonic or unsweetened pineapple chunks (Regnard 1997).

## Stridor

Treatment of stridor is by upright positioning, steroids, heliox, insertion of a stent or radiotherapy (McGrath et al. 2011).

## Depression

Depression should not be accepted as a normal grief response. It may be accompanied by fatigue, guilt or thoughts of suicide, yet is often undetected and poorly managed in palliative care settings (Mellor et al. 2013). The majority of patients who express a wish to hasten their death are depressed, which may relate to feelings of helplessness or being a burden on their family (Billings 2000).

Several measuring tools for cancer are available (Johns et al. 2013) but for physiotherapists a two-question screening tool identifies depression by first asking the simple question 'are you depressed?' followed by, 'have you experienced loss of interest in things or activities that you would normally enjoy?' (Payne 2007).

A palliative team is usually able to offer medication, counselling or both, or the patient may prefer to talk to friends. Psychotherapy can be helpful for patients expected to live more than 6 months, and a 'life review' can be helpful for those expecting to die earlier (Stagg & Lazenby 2012). This records patients as they reflect on their lives, which is then transcribed and given to the patient to share with whom they like. Benefits include affirmation of the patient's life, resolution of conflicts, comfort for the family, and help with closure for both patient and family (Csikai 2013).

## Anxiety

Anxiety can be underestimated by both patient and physiotherapist (Taylor 2007). Information is always the first approach, as reflected in anxious patients being more likely to want information about end-of-life care (Fakhri et al. 2016). After information, palliative sedation may be suitable, provided at different levels:

1. Conscious sedation is a patient-controlled state achieved after initial relief of symptoms, when sedatives are reduced to a level at which communication allows patients to continue to express their wishes.
2. Intermittent sedation is provided at night, on request of the patient (Song et al. 2015).
3. Respite sedation is used for 24–48 h and then reduced for reassessment (Mazzotta 2012).
4. Deep sedation renders patients unconscious more abruptly than during the process of natural dying but does not necessarily prevent awareness or distress (Rady et al. 2013). It may be used preemptively if, for example, ventilatory support is to be removed (Berger 2012) and its effects can be monitored by observational scales (Brinkkemper 2013).

The use of sedation for existential suffering is more controversial, and addressing the root cause may be preferable, followed by strategies such as spiritual support, friendship or psychotherapy (Rosenfeld et al. 2016).

For both depression and anxiety, the physiotherapist's contribution is to maximize independence, if and when required by the patient, and to lend an ear.

## Discomfort

Regular turning and positioning to suit the individual eases the discomfort of immobility. Some patients like to be propped up with their head well supported, whereas others like to be curled up on their side with generous quantities of pillows. The skin needs meticulous attention. Simple brief exercises are usually helpful, sometimes demonstrated to the relatives.

## Pain

*No one should die while experiencing pain, for it obliterates all composure and the quiet business of the commendation of the soul.*

**Sewell 2012**

Pain is a malevolent adversary of dying patients, but undertreatment is common, especially for those in hospital (Yao 2013). Assessment is available for people of all nationalities (Huang et al. 2012) and for those with special needs (p. 298).

Fear that opioids hasten death contributes to their underuse (Fromme et al. 2008). Prescribers can be reassured that physical dependence is not the same as addiction (Hanks et al. 2010), that there is no upper limit (Silvestri 2000), that one patient who takes regular analgesics may need 100 times more than another, and that addiction when using opioids for pain relief occurs in less than 1% of patients (McCaffery 2001). Coprescription of laxatives and antiemetics are needed for side effects, but tolerance to the side effect of sedation usually develops. Delirium can occur if opioids are used for anxiety, and a multidimensional approach that includes rotation of drugs and psychosocial support can reduce both intractable pain and delirium (Mori et al. 2012). Morphine clearance is reduced near the end of life, as it is in critically ill patients (Franken et al. 2016). Anaesthetic patches should be used for venepuncture (Filbet 2017).

Despite the frequent inadequacy of pain relief, Micco et al. (2009) caution against 'knee-jerk symptom relief that can dull or remove whatever subjective experience someone may have'. Patients should be able to make a choice.

*Many patients with end-stage lung disease still die in pain after much suffering.*

**Sorenson 2013**

## Intractable Hiccups

This sudden contraction of the inspiratory muscles can exacerbate insomnia, pain, fatigue and problems with eating, drinking and speaking. Strategies are:

- sugar and/or lemon, or peppermint water;
- baclofen, chlorpromazine, metoclopramide, omeprazole or, to avoid sedation, amantadine (Hernandez et al. 2015);
- interruption of the respiratory cycle through coughing, breath-holding, hyperventilation, breathing into a paper bag or gargling;
- vagal stimulation using carotid massage or the Valsalva manoeuvre;
- interruption of phrenic nerve transmission by rubbing over the 5th cervical vertebra;
- diaphragmatic pacing electrodes;
- ultrasound-guided left phrenic nerve block (Arsanious et al. 2016).

## Nausea or Vomiting

Causes should first be checked, e.g. medication, recent chemotherapy or radiotherapy, electrolyte imbalance, raised intracranial pressure or gut problems. Drugs (Glare et al. 2012) need to be carefully chosen for frail elderly patients because of interactions and often a failing kidney and liver.

## Agitation

Possible reasons should first be identified, e.g. unrelieved symptoms such as pain or a full bladder or rectum. Questioning the patient or family may find the cause. Medication is usually based on a benzodiazepine.

## Delirium

The risk of delirium in the later stages mandates that screening for delirium is routine (Porteous 2016). Causes such as insomnia should be identified (Kerr et al. 2013), and transfer to a psychiatric unit avoided if possible because of relocation stress (Kratz 2016).

## Insomnia

Over half of patients experience sleep fragmentation (Mercadante et al, 2015). Any symptoms or environmental factors that disturb sleep need to be addressed. The patient can then choose from a variety of measures (pp. 171 and 433), or, specifically for end-stage disease, acupressure (Tsay 2003), relaxation or cognitive behaviour therapy, the latter sometimes being more sustainable than medication (Dambrosio 2013). Drugs include trazodone, which may also control nightmares (Tanimukai et al. 2013), and there is now a tentative reemergence of thalidomide, which also helps appetite (Davis et al. 2012).

## Secretions and the Death Rattle

Half of patients develop secretions in their throat at the end of life when they are too weak to expectorate or swallow (Heisler 2013). Once the patient is unconscious, audible secretions are usually called a death rattle, heralding death within an average of 16 h (Bickel & Arnold 2008). Campbell et al. (2013) claim that the secretions do not cause respiratory distress, and relatives can be reassured that the noise is a common occurrence at this stage. The term 'lung congestion' is kinder for the patient and relatives.

Position change, decreased fluid intake and drugs such as scopolamine or glycopyrrolate may be effective (Baralatei 2016). Attempted chest clearance by percussion is unhelpful and unsafe because of the risk of fracture from bony secondaries.

> **PRACTICE TIP**
>
> Suction is not indicated for the death rattle, even if the patient is unable to express distress, because it may cause distress which the patient cannot articulate, and its effect is transient.

## Terminal Restlessness

In the last few days of life, delirium is called terminal restlessness and may be more related to anguish and spiritual pain, occurring in up to 85% of patients and complicating bereavement for the family. Risk factors are unfinished business, positional pain, physical restraint, SOB, thirst, urine retention, constipation, sensory loss, pain, anxiety, fear, toxic levels of narcotics (Papadimos et al. 2011) or the withdrawal of nicotine or alcohol, these last being avoidable by substitution (pp. 170 and 478).

Even for patients who are unconscious shortly before death, quiet familiar music, a hearing aid if required and the presence of chosen family members are thought to be beneficial. Bright lights and strong environmental stimuli should be avoided. Medication may be helpful (Irwin et al. 2013).

## Deathbed Phenomena

A fifth of family members observe apparent deathbed communications by the patient, usually with a dead relative and sometimes with visionary language related to travel (Morita et al. 2016). Occurring within a month of death, these are more serene accompaniments to dying, with clear consciousness and twice the chance of a peaceful end (Lawrence & Repede 2013).

## ON DYING WELL

*'All I want to know is that there will be someone there to hold my hand when I need it. I am afraid. Death may be routine to you, but it is new to me… I've never died before'*

*Gallagher & Trenchar 1986*

This message from a dying student nurse advises her colleagues on how they can best help her towards a good death. When patients are free from fears, they are more able to live their remaining life to the full. Conscious dying is possible when a balance of minimum symptoms without undue sedation has been achieved, so that patients are not trapped between perpetual pain and perpetual somnolence, and are able to take decisions on how much they may or may not want to experience the process. Dying is an event that not all cultures, nor all individuals, want to be sedated out of experiencing. Indeed, some patients find that life in the face of death allows for a more intense existence and awareness of the present, or as described by one author 'Dying had quickened his own livingness' (Brennan 2013).

There is no 'right' way to die, but death can be a positive achievement when patients are not consumed by anxiety about symptoms and have stopped fighting for life. Through the many little deaths of dying, they have plumbed the depths of their being, but fear has dissolved, there is peace without defeatism and they are free to look for some meaning in the experience. Open communication, on the patient's terms, is thought to contribute to acceptance of dying and the quality of the dying process (Lokker et al. 2012).

Working with dying people is demanding and requires us to be emotionally healthy. It means sharing anguish, absorbing misdirected anger and providing comfort and dignity for people who are totally dependent. It includes emotional involvement, wherein lies its challenge and reward.

## OUTCOMES

*That's the trouble with death, all the loose ends.*

*Rousseau 2013*

Multiple-symptom evaluation is recommended to assess the effects of treatment. The Good Death Scale and Palliative Outcome Scale are examples (Cheng 2013, Saleem et al. 2013). For SOB in lung cancer, there is the Dyspnoea-12 questionnaire (Tan et al. 2016), and for advanced cancer there are the Cancer Dyspnea Scale (Uronis 2012), Edmonton Functional Assessment Tool (Cobbe et al. 2013) and Advanced Cancer Patients' Distress Scale (Fischbeck et al. 2013). For patients unable to self-report, a behavioural test assesses respiratory distress (Campbell et al. 2010). Carer burden is assessed using the Zarit Burden Inventory (Bausewein 2012), and after bereavement is the Care Evaluation Scale (Miyashita et al. 2017).

## CASE STUDY: MS IU

*You are called in to see a 69-year-old woman with an exacerbation of COPD.*

There was no noninvasive ventilation service in the hospital at the time.

### Social history

- Lives alone and independently
- Supportive son lives in nearby town

### Subjective

- Can't breathe
- Dry mouth

### Objective

- Medical notes state that a decision has been made not to ventilate the patient.
- $PaO_2$ 9.5 kPa (71.4 mmHg), $PaCO_2$ 11.3 kPa (85 mmHg), pH 7.21, $HCO_3^-$ 32, BE 1.4
- $SpO_2$ 85% and fluctuating
- On 24% dry oxygen
- Temperature 36°C
- On infusion of salbutamol and doxapram (respiratory stimulant)
- Propped up in bed
- Rapid shallow breathing
- Body shaking continuously
- Difficulty speaking
- Appears fearful ++

### Questions

1. Is the goal of medical treatment palliative or curative?

2. Give three possible reasons for Ms IU's shaking.
3. Problems?
4. What teamwork is needed?
5. Plan?

---

### CLINICAL REASONING

*Could the following signs and symptoms indicate anything else?*

*'Signs and symptoms which indicate a need for suctioning include: patient restlessness or anxiety, diaphoresis, increased blood pressure and heart rate.'*

*Acc Emerg Nurs* (1997) 5, 92–98

*Diaphoresis*: sweating

---

### Response to Case Study

1. There appear to be conflicting goals. With this level of respiratory acidosis, Ms. IU will die without supported ventilation, indicating that the goal is palliative. However, doxapram is a distressing drug, does not palliate symptoms and is normally aimed at keeping patients alive.
2. Fear, hypercapnia, side effects of doxapram.
3. Anxiety
   - Dyspnoea and fatigue
   - Dry mouth
   - Hypoxaemia
   - Hypercapnia and acidosis
4. Liaise with referring doctor to revisit decision not to ventilate (declined).
   - Liaise with nurse to contact son.
5. Fear: the patient was unable to speak, so she was reassured that her son was being contacted, that she would not be left alone and that her needs would be attended to. She was also told that one of the drugs in her drip was likely to be causing her shakes.

   Dyspnoea: fan, gentle back rubbing, positioning sitting over the edge of the bed, feet on the floor and leaning forward over a pillow on a table, with manual support.

   Dry mouth: mouth care, sips of water offered, mask changed to nasal cannulae; humidification was not attempted because the patient could not be left and the nurse was unable to fetch the equipment (it was 3:00 a.m. and only one nurse was on duty).

Hypoxaemia: $FiO_2$ titrated using oximetry.

Hypercapnia and acidosis: intermittent positive pressure breathing attempted but the patient was too weak to trigger the machine.

The patient died quietly 2 h later.

---

**RESPONSE TO CLINICAL REASONING**

There are many possible causes of restlessness, anxiety, sweating and disturbed vital signs. If not identified and remedied, these could be increased by suctioning.

---

## RECOMMENDED READING

Bajwah, S., Higginson, I.J., Ross, J.R., et al., 2013. The palliative care needs for fibrotic interstitial lung disease. Palliat. Med. 27 (9), 877.

Barawid, E.L., 2013. Rehabilitation modalities in palliative care. Crit. Rev. Phys. Rehab. Med. 25 (1-2), 77–100.

Baxter, S.K., Baird, W.O., Thompson, S., et al., 2013. Use of non-invasive ventilation at end of life. Palliat. Med. 27 (9), 878.

Billings, J.A., 2012. Humane terminal extubation reconsidered. Crit. Care Med. 40 (2), 625–630.

Brown-Saltzman, K., Upadhya, D., Larner, L., et al., 2010. An intervention to improve respiratory therapists' comfort with end-of-life care. Respir. Care 55 (7), 858–865.

Carson, K., McIlfatrick, S., 2013. More than physical function? Exploring physiotherapists' experiences in delivering rehabilitation to patients requiring palliative care in the community. J. Palliat. Care 29 (1), 36–44.

Davis, C., Guyer, C., 2013. Integrated care pathways for dying patients – myths, misunderstandings and realities in clinical practice. Eur. J. Palliat. Care 20 (1), 112–119.

Druml, C., Ballmer, P.E., Druml, W., 2016. ESPEN guideline on ethical aspects of artificial nutrition and hydration. Clin. Nutr. 35 (3), 545–556.

Ernecoff, N.C., Cox, C.E., 2017. Spirituality, palliative care, and the intensive care unit. A new approach. Am. J. Respir. Crit. Care Med. 195 (2), 150–152.

Gerber, L.H., 2017. Cancer-related fatigue: persistent, pervasive, and problematic. Phys. Med. Rehab. Clin. 28 (1), 65–88.

Guo, Q., Cann, B., 2017. Keep in Touch (KIT): feasibility of using internet-based communication and information technology in palliative care. BMC Palliat. Care 16 (1), 29.

Horton, R., Rocker, G., Dale, A., et al., 2013. Implementing a palliative care trial in advanced COPD. J. Palliat. Med. 16 (11), 67–73.

Jacobe, S., 2015. Diagnosing death. J. Paediatr. Child Health 51 (6), 573–576.

Kehl, K.A., Kowalkowski, J.A., 2013. A systematic review of the prevalence of signs of impending death and symptoms in the last 2 weeks of life. Am. J. Hosp. Palliat. Med. 30 (6), 601–616.

Killick, S., 2013. Managing the conflicting wishes of a woman on ventilatory support and her family. Eur. J. Palliat. Care 20 (4), 172–173.

Mitchell, G., Agnelli, J., McGreevy, J., et al., 2016. Palliative and end-of-life care for people living with dementia in care homes: part 1. Nurs. Stand. 30 (43), 54–63.

Mitchell, G., Agnelli, J., McGreevy, J., et al., 2016. Palliative and end-of-life care for people living with dementia in care homes: part 2. Nurs. Stand. 30 (44), 54–63.

Mols, A., 2013. Palliative surgery in cancer patients. Eur. J. Palliat. Care 20 (1), 9–13.

Morgan, D.D., White, K.M., 2012. Occupational therapy interventions for breathlessness at the end of life. Curr. Opin. Supp. Palliat. Care 6 (2), 138–143.

Muecke, R., Paul, M., Conrad, C., et al., 2016. Complementary and alternative medicine in palliative care. Integr. Cancer Ther. 15 (1), 10–16.

Nelson, J.E., Hope, A.A., 2012. Integration of palliative care in chronic critical illness. Respir. Care 57 (6), 1004–1013.

NICE Guideline, 2013. Opioids in palliative care [CG140].

Nogler, A.F., 2014. Hoping for the best, preparing for the worst: strategies to promote honesty and prevent medical futility at end-of-life. Dimens. Crit. Care Nurs. 33 (1), 22–27.

Orellana-Rios, C.L., Radbruch, L., Kern, M., et al., 2017. Mindfulness and compassion-oriented practices at work reduce distress and enhance self-care of palliative care teams: a mixed-method evaluation of an "on the job" program. BMC Palliat. Care 17 (1), 3.

Payne, C., Wiffen, P.J., Martin, S., 2012. Interventions for fatigue and weight loss in adults with advanced progressive illness. Cochrane Syst. Rev. (1), CD008427.

Peereboom, K., Coyle, N., 2012. Facilitating goals-of-care discussions for patients with life-limiting disease. J. Hosp. Palliat. Nurs. 14 (4), 251–258.

Primus, C.P., Flett, A.S., Cheung, C.C., et al., 2013. Palliative care provision in an advanced heart failure clinic: patients' experiences. Eur. J. Palliat. Care 20 (3), 127–129.

Raj, V.S., Silver, J.K., Pugh, T.M., et al., 2017. Palliative care and physiatry in the oncology care spectrum: an opportunity for distinct and collaborative approaches. Phys. Med. Rehab. Clin. 28 (1), 35–47.

Read, S., 2013. Palliative care for people with intellectual disabilities. Palliat. Med. 27 (1), 3–4.

Rush, B., Hertz, P., Bond, A., et al., 2017. Use of palliative care in patients with end-stage COPD and receiving home oxygen. Chest 151 (1), 41–46.

Sakhri, L., Saint-Raymond, C., Quetant, S., et al., 2016. Limitations of active therapeutic and palliative care in chronic respiratory disease. Rev. Mal. Respir. 34 (2), 102–120.

Simon, S.T., Bausewein, C., Schildmann, E., et al., 2013. Episodic breathlessness in patients with advanced disease. J. Pain Sympt. Manag. 45 (3), 561–578.

Simpson, C., 2012. Advance care planning in COPD. Chron. Respir. Dis. 9 (3), 193–204.

Singer, A.E., Meeker, D., Teno, J.M., et al., 2016. Factors associated with family reports of pain, dyspnea, and depression in the last year of life. J. Palliat. Med. 19 (10), 1066–1073.

Tan, L., 2017. Advance care planning. Am. J. Hospice Palliat. Med. 34 (1), 26–33.

Tripodoro, V.A., De Vito, E.L., 2016. What does end stage in neuromuscular diseases mean? Key approach-based transitions. Curr. Opin. Supp. Palliat. Care 9 (4), 361–368.

Twomey, S., Dowling, M., 2013. Management of death rattle at end of life. Br. J. Nurs. 22 (2), 81–85.

Ullrich, A., Asgherfeld, L., Marx, G., et al., 2017. Quality of life, psychological burden, needs, and satisfaction during specialized inpatient palliative care in family caregivers of advanced cancer patients. BMC Palliat. Care 16 (1), 31.

Van der Steen, J.T., Dekker, N.L., Gijsberts, M.-J.H.E., et al., 2017. Palliative care for people with dementia in the terminal phase: a mixed-methods qualitative study to inform service development. BMC Palliat. Care 16 (1), 28.

Verberkt, C.A., 2016. A randomized controlled trial on the benefits and respiratory adverse effects of morphine for refractory dyspnea in patients with COPD. Contemp. Clin. Trials 47, 228–234.

Vicent, L., Nuñez Olarte, J.M., Puente-Maestu, L., 2017. Degree of dyspnoea at admission and discharge in patients with heart failure and respiratory diseases. BMC Palliat. Care 16 (1), 35.

Waller, A., Dodd, N., Tattersall, H.N., et al., 2017. Improving hospital-based end of life care processes and outcomes: a systematic review of research output, quality and effectiveness. BMC Palliat. Care 16 (1), 34.

Weathers, E., O'Caoimh, R., Cornally, N., et al., 2016. Advance care planning: a systematic review of randomised controlled trials conducted with older adults. Maturitas 91, 101–109.

20

# Critical Care, Support and Monitoring

*David McWilliams, Alexandra Hough*

## LEARNING OBJECTIVES

*On completion of this chapter the reader should be able to:*
- understand how the ICU environment affects the patient;
- describe the principles and complications of mechanical ventilation;
- understand the relevance of fluids, nutrition and medication to patient stability and their relation to physiotherapy treatment;
- understand how advanced life support systems modify physiotherapy;
- interpret monitor readings.

## OUTLINE

## INTRODUCTION

> *He may cry out for rest, peace, dignity, but…he will get a dozen people around the clock, all busily preoccupied with his heart rate, pulse, secretions or excretions, but not with him as a human being.*
>
> ***Kübler-Ross 1973***

Critical care is for patients who require intensive therapy, intensive monitoring and/or intensive support. They are not necessarily critically ill (and the term 'critical care' can be worrying for relatives) but they are at risk of failure of one or more major organs. Their needs range from observation of vital signs after major surgery, to total support of physiological systems. There is a growing awareness that survival alone is not enough to demonstrate success, and physiotherapy is playing an increasing role in enabling patients to return to a meaningful life.

Level of care in the UK is allocated according to clinical need:
1. Level 3 is provided in the intensive care unit (ICU), where patients require one-to-one nursing and either mechanical ventilation or support of two or more organ systems.
2. Level 2 involves monitoring or support of a single system and acts as step-down or step-up between levels of care. Patients are nursed in an ICU or high dependency unit.

**TABLE 20.1 Typical call criteria for a critical care outreach team**

| Vital sign | Criteria |
|---|---|
| Airway | Threatened airway, e.g. excessive secretions or stridor |
| Breathing | RR <8 or >25 breaths/min |
| Circulation | HR <50 or >150 beats/min |
| | Systolic BP <90 mmHg, >200 mmHg or drop of >40 mmHg |
| | Systolic BP less than patient's normal value |
| Consciousness | Sustained drop or fluctuation in GCS of >2 in past hour |
| Oxygen | $SpO_2$ <90% on >.50 $FiO_2$ |
| Urine output | <30 mL/h for more than 2 h (unless normal for patient) |
| General | Clinically causing concern |
| | Not responding to treatment |

*BP*, Blood pressure; *$FiO_2$*, fraction of inspired oxygen; *GCS*, Glasgow Coma Scale; *HR*, heart rate; *RR*, respiratory rate.

3. Level 1 is 'intensive care without walls' for those at risk of their condition deteriorating or who have recently relocated from a higher level. Their needs are met on an acute ward with support from a proactive 24-h multidisciplinary outreach team (Table 20.1).
4. Level 0 is for patients whose needs can be met through normal ward care in an acute hospital.

Noninvasive ventilation is provided at Level 1 or 2.

## ENVIRONMENT

*The environment was interpreted as 'being in the middle of an uncontrollable barrage of noise, unable to take cover'.*

***Johansson & Bergbom 2013***

### Effects on the Patient

*'[The staff] were looking at something in the magazine together and they were laughing, and I thought they were laughing at me'.*

***Darbyshire et al. 2016***

Patients describe feeling 'trapped, terrified and alone', with recurring themes being a sensation of dissociation and lack of control, or 'an unsettling window to the edges of life' (Darbyshire et al. 2016). It is not an optional extra to give attention to the human aspect of patient management, but an integral part of physiotherapy. The physiological effects of stress are on p. 23.

Pain, lack of sleep and intubation are the three main causes of ICU stress (Kamdar et al. 2012), the severity of the stress response varying with the patient's ability to control his or her situation. Autonomy is enhanced by shared decision-making (Kon et al. 2016) and hindered by dependence on others for the most basic care decisions, leading to anxiety and sometimes nightmares that may last for years (Schelling et al. 2003). Sensory and sleep deprivation, psychotropic drugs, prolonged immobility, isolation and reduced communication are classified as psychological torture by Amnesty International. These conditions are found in the ICU, albeit without intent. Examples are listed in the following:

1. **Communication difficulty.** Inability to communicate leads to a high level of frustration because of intubation and, for some patients, loss of concentration and short-term memory due to sedation.

*'...I couldn't make anybody understand. I couldn't make my family understand. I tried to tell them, I couldn't talk'.*

***Darbyshire et al. 2016***

2. **Uncertainty and anxiety.** Communication problems lead to patients 'not knowing what is going to happen', or 'if they will make it or not' (Cypress 2016), exacerbated by problems with short-term memory and recall. Anxiety is associated with ongoing problems 6 months after ICU discharge (Castillo et al. 2016). Empathy with patients' experiences helps staff anticipate and identify these needs, along with regular reorientation.

3. **Sleep fragmentation** (Fig. 20.1). Most patients lack sleep, with the following outcomes:
   • impaired rehabilitation and physical recovery (Kamdar 2012);
   • ↓ immune response and wound healing, ↑ perception of pain and mortality, chronic insomnia after discharge (Shaw 2016);
   • ↑ severity of illness and cardiovascular problems (Schulman 2016);
   • risk of multisystem failure (Allen et al. 2012);
   • ↑ energy consumption, delirium and memory loss, ↓ respiratory response to hypercapnia and hypoxaemia, compromised weaning (Stevens et al. 2014).

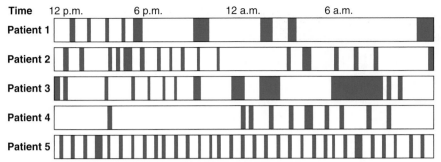

**FIGURE 20.1** Sleep fragmentation in five critically ill patients. Purple areas represent sleep and white areas represent wakefulness. (From Freedman et al. 2001.)

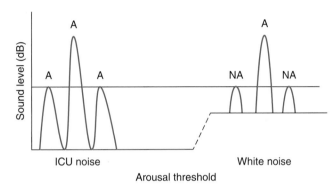

**FIGURE 20.2** Arousals from sleep without and with white noise. *A*, Arousals; *ICU*, intensive care unit; *NA*, no arousals. (From Stanchina et al. 2005.)

Lack of sleep has a greater influence on posttraumatic stress symptoms than the severity of illness (Weiner & Sprenkle 2008).

A full sleep cycle (p. 24) is needed to achieve the restorative benefits of sleep, but this is rare in the ICU (Kamdar 2012). The more ill the patient, the more sleep they need and the less they are likely to get. Sleep disruption is due to lights, anxiety, pain, reversal of the day–night cycle, difficulty in finding a comfortable position, fear of falling asleep and not waking again, and noise, which is consistently above recommended levels (Tainter et al. 2016).

Suggested strategies are:
- noise reduction, diurnal lighting, clustering of nocturnal activities and relaxation (Porter & McClure 2013);
- the optimizing of ventilatory settings (Rittayamai et al. 2016);
- a background of white noise such as ocean sounds (Fig. 20.2).

- eye masks, earplugs, noise-cancelling head phones or the patient's favourite music, played softly (Mofredj et al. 2016);

Earplugs can also reduce the incidence of delirium (Litton et al. 2016).

4. **Fear**. Patients face fears which are compounded by helplessness and the confusing effect of some drugs. They try to assess their progress by watching the reactions of staff and family, and by comparing themselves to others on the unit. Anxiety has been found highest in patients with respiratory disease (Chlan 2008). Involving patients in decisions about their rehabilitation reduces fear and anxiety.

*'I remember one of the doctors who I really thought was trying to kill me… if he came anywhere near me, I thought he was trying to switch the tubes off [then] the nurse got a gun to me head trying to kill me'.*

***Darbyshire et al. 2016***

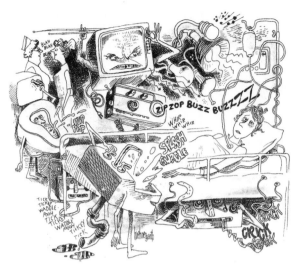

**FIGURE 20.3** Sensory overload. (From Lindenmuth et al. 1990.)

5. **Sensory deprivation**. A form of emotional solitary confinement may be caused by social isolation, immobilization, certain drugs, a limited visual field, loss of social media, lack of nonclinical touch and removal of hearing aid or glasses. This can leave patients feeling intense loneliness despite constant attention. Sensory deprivation is amplified threefold in the absence of windows (Criner & Isaac 1995). It is ameliorated by 24-h clocks, ambient lighting (Oldham et al. 2016) or virtual reality systems to provide implied environments (Turon 2013).

6. **Sensory overload** (Fig. 20.3). Patients find themselves lost in a sea of electronic wizardry, bombarded by unfamiliar beeps, alarms, confining equipment, painful procedures (sometimes without warning), tubes in various orifices and incomprehensible conversation over their heads. Noise can lead to physiological damage (Alway 2013) and, along with too much light and not enough sleep, predisposes to delirium (Blot et al. 2015).

*'Sometimes the fear is worse than the pain, and the combination of fear with pain... there came a time when I already wanted to die'.*
**Alonso-Ovies & La Calle 2016**

7. **Disorientation, depersonalization** and **delirium**. Combined sensory deprivation and overload can cause perceptual distortion, in which hallucinations arise from false perceptions of sensory input, often after the first 2 or 3 lucid days. Hallucinations lead to some patients perceiving their body boundaries as permeable and the equipment as part of their body (Johansson 2005). Over half of patients develop delirium, which increases morbidity, mortality, length of stay and long-term cognitive decline (Darbyshire et al. 2016), but up to 75% of cases are missed, partly because the majority manifest the hypoactive rather than the hyperactive form (Hipp & Ely 2012). The main experience for patients is fear (Van Rompaey et al. 2016), with patients reporting nightmares of being trapped and delusional memories of people trying to kill them (Garrouste-Orgeas et al. 2012). These persist longer than factual memories (Carr 2007) and worsen the experience of pain (Azzam & Alam 2013). Delirium, unlike agitation, may trigger the reemergence of fearful memories of past events such as wartime bombing or being sent to boarding school (Hazzard 2002). Delusions should be neither challenged nor agreed with, but the cause of agitation should be identified when possible because it may precede delirium (Blot et al. 2015). Depersonalization may be eased by using personal information provided by the family, to be used when communicating with the patient (Fig. 20.4). It is worsened by inappropriate joking between staff, which can be misunderstood by patients or relatives. Appropriate joking is fine, indeed often welcomed, so long as the patient is included. Delirium can be reduced by early mobilization, ensuring full sleep cycles, reduced sedation (Vincent et al. 2016), opening/closing of blinds, repeated orientation, cognitive stimulation (Rivosecchi et al. 2016) and nicotine replacement if indicated (Park et al. 2016b).

*'...once I was convinced I was in hospital I did start to feel a bit more secure'.*
**Darbyshire et al. 2016**

8. **Sensory monotony** and **loss of time sense**. Patients struggle to keep track of time through a tranquillized haze, which is worse when there is no day–night sequence in lighting or routine. This compounds disorientation, or, for more alert patients, causes boredom. Occasionally the empty time gives patients an opportunity for reflection, and some emerge with a sharpened perception of what is important in their life.

Patient profile of ...........................................................................

Completed by ....................................................................

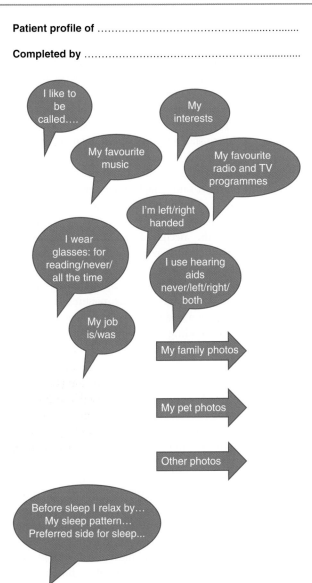

I like to be called....

My interests

My favourite music

My favourite radio and TV programmes

I'm left/right handed

I wear glasses: for reading/never/all the time

I use hearing aids never/left/right/both

My job is/was

My family photos

My pet photos

Other photos

Before sleep I relax by...
My sleep pattern...
Preferred side for sleep...

**FIGURE 20.4** Patient profile to be kept at front of confidential folder at the bedside, then returned to patient on discharge.

9. **Discomfort**. Patients may experience immobility, gagging on the endotracheal tube, dribbling, a dry mouth, distended abdomen, unscratchable itches and asynchrony with the ventilator. Discomfort is increased with paralysis or other forms of restraint. Physical restraints can stimulate inflammation (Tymen et al. 2013), impede communication,

increase both anxiety and depression (Happ 2008), predispose to delirium (Porter & McClure 2013) and in the UK may only be used if is necessary to prevent harm to a patient who lacks capacity (ICS 2005).

10. **Pain**. Pain intensity and pain distress are significantly greater than reported at the time (Puntillo et al. 2016). Preemptive analgesia is mandated prior to invasive and potentially painful procedures (Krupp & Balas 2016).

11. **Helplessness, dependency** and **depression**. The less patients are able to do for themselves, the more frustrated they feel. This may become internalized as depression, especially as they feel inhibited in expressing feelings when dependent on those who care for them. Depression can hinder rehabilitation, especially as, on average, it continues in 28% of patients over the following year (Kamdar 2012).

12. **Loss of privacy, dignity** and **identity**. It is easy for us to forget how people feel when they lose their clothes, teeth, personal space and surname. Patients who are elderly or from a different culture are particularly vulnerable to this form of depersonalization. Sometimes patients want privacy from their own relatives, and their permission should be obtained before visitors are ushered in willy-nilly.

Patients' preferences for visiting varies. Gonzalez (2004) found that a third of patients preferred unlimited visiting, a third once a day, and many did not want visitors during procedures, when needing to rest, or either early or late in the day.

**KEY POINT**

Unless we nurture empathy in understanding a patient's experience, we will not be fully effective with our treatment.

Long-term effects vary. Granja (2005) found nearly half of ICU survivors experienced sleep disturbance 6 months later, a third reported poor concentration and memory, and over half suffered fatigue. All experienced reduced quality of life (McKinley et al. 2016). ICU-related posttraumatic stress disorder (PTSD) has been found in 10% of survivors in the year after hospitalization (Patel et al. 2016). This can lead to years of memory dysfunction, panic attacks and depression, as well as the re-experiencing of traumatic ICU events (Carr 2007). Cognitive impairment has been found in up to 70% of ICU patients (Hopkins et al. 2012).

Use of a diary to maintain a detailed narrative of events, with contributions from staff and relatives, helps link memories with reality, improve quality of life and reduce PTSD (Perier 2013). Anxiety, depression and PTSD symptoms can also be reduced with a clinical psychologist on the team (Peris et al. 2011).

*Knowing what to expect gives some control back to a vulnerable person who feels like everything is happening in a haphazard fashion.*

**Hipp & Ely 2012**

## Effects on Relatives

*'They were constantly seeing to Sam, doing things and writing things down, but I actually felt really alone'.*
**Mother of ICU patient, 24 Hours in A&E,**
***Channel 4, 2015***

Relatives can do much to ease a patient's stress, so long as they in turn are given support. Many feel bewildered, daunted by the environment, and reluctant to voice their concerns, with a significant number developing anxiety, depression and PTSD symptoms (Petrinec & Daly 2016). They benefit from:

- information about the patient's condition, equipment and the reason for physiotherapy, especially as family understanding of physiotherapy is limited in this setting (Latchem et al. 2016);
- 24-hour visiting, and visible evidence that staff care about the patient (Board 2016);
- a share in decision-making (Kon et al. 2016);
- advice that children usually benefit from visiting, especially if they can be involved (Knutsson & Bergbom 2016), e.g. with hair-brushing;
- the opportunity to say what they are thinking or feeling;
- reassurance that touch and conversation are welcomed by most patients;
- a leaflet describing the ICU layout, machines, terminology and different staff responsibilities;
- encouragement to become involved in patient care, e.g. foot massage, certain passive movements, mouth

care and writing in the diary (Nielsen & Angel 2015).

Families can provide useful information on patients' likes and hobbies so that rehabilitation can be focused on these goals. Family involvement in early mobility has shown adherence increase from 66% to 94% (Rukstele & Gagnon 2013).

If acceptable to staff and the patient, relatives may be allowed to join ward rounds or witness resuscitation attempts (Jabre et al. 2013), with appropriate support. One family member said, 'Maybe they were a little more gentle because they knew someone else was watching' (Eichhorn 2001).

Occasionally the needs of patients and relatives diverge, as illustrated by two opposing examples for the same patient:

- 'My mother…cries and gets all dramatic. She grabbed my hand and I got angry and the machine started to go beep beep beep and they took her away…'
- '…Laurie was holding my hand. She was talking to me… she is strong and calm' (Chlan 1995).

## Effects on Staff

Emotional responses can become dulled by the frequency with which they are elicited. People working in an ICU need defences against the suffering around them, but these are not incompatible with sensitive patient care.

Staff who become stressed are not only less able to identify with the experience of the patient, but they may also compromise patient safety (Welp et al. 2016). Reactions to working in the ICU include overdetachment, exhaustion, anxiety due to the responsibility, frustration at communication difficulties or inability to relieve suffering, and burnout (Papadimos et al. 2011).

Strategies to reduce stress include:

- involvement of all staff in decision-making;
- multidisciplinary training to increase confidence;
- feedback, sharing of ideas, debriefing after traumatic incidents and recognition that doubts are acceptable;
- consistent attention to communication (Henrich et al. 2016).

Relatives can be asked to bring photographs of patients from when they were well, which are put on the locker to remind staff of the human side of the patient. Shared information on the patient's likes, dislikes, interests and hobbies also help the humanizing process.

# Patients' Rights

## Consent

The following are currently valid in Britain and are taken from CSP (2016), ICS (2005), Richardson (2013), Dimond (2009), Delany & Frawley (2012), White (2014) and the Mental Capacity Act 2005. They relate to treatment, teaching and research in all areas of physiotherapy.

A patient is assumed to have the capacity to refuse treatment even if the treatment is life-saving or the reason for withholding consent is unwise, irrational, unknown or nonexistent. If a patient cannot gesture his or her wishes, a communication aid is required. It is illegal to force physiotherapy on patients who resist or who are unable to resist but have made their wishes clear by word or gesture, or have made their wishes clear prior to losing capacity. Patients may withdraw consent during treatment.

The elements of informed consent are:

- explanations, to include risks and alternative options, and anything that the patient wants to know, including answers to all questions, or signposts to someone who can answer the questions;
- voluntariness: patients to take their decision without undue influence;
- capacity: the patient's ability matches the required decision-making;
- consent itself: a voluntary agreement based on relevant understanding.

Consent should be reaffirmed if there are significant changes to the treatment plan, the patient's condition or new information from the patient. Believing that the patient may become upset and refuse treatment is not a reason to withhold information.

If patients do not know that they have these rights, they should be informed. In the face of refusal, physiotherapists should seek a change of mind but must not use duress or deceit. The following allow treatment without consent:

- emergencies
- statutory authorization (Mental Health Act 2007)
- lack of capacity

A patient is considered to lack capacity if they cannot understand and/or remember and/or use the information provided. Panic, indecisiveness, irrationality, mental illness or intellectual disability do not themselves amount to incapacity. However, if mental incapacity from medication or illness renders patients incapable of understanding or retaining information so that they are unable to assess risks and make a decision, this constitutes incapacity. Unless granted lasting power of attorney, relatives cannot give or withhold consent for adults even if the patient is unconscious, but their opinion must be taken into account.

The medical notes should provide information on the patient's wishes, 'presumed consent', difficult decisions discussed with the team, refusal of treatment and subsequent action. Each hospital and ICU will have their own protocol, and decisions on individual capacity should be taken by the multidisciplinary team.

Physiotherapists must be able to justify their decisions, which have to be acceptable to the majority of their peers.

## Moral rights

*'I could think and I could hear. But I could not move and I could not talk or open my eyes'.*

*Lawrence 1995*

Patients have the right to know the truth, to participate in decision-making, to refuse to be used for teaching, and to be given full care even when their choice differs from ours. These rights should not be violated if the patient is young or has learning disabilities.

## End-of-life decisions

*Ethics is the exercise of moral reasoning in circumstances where strong feeling is not always the surest guide to action nor procedural powers the surest way to justice.*

*Dunstan quoted by Branthwaite 1996*

It has been argued that ICU admission at the end of life should be a 'never event' (Angus & Truog 2016). However, it is often not easy to tell if a patient is dying, and there are advantages in the ICU of one-to-one nursing and access to accurate pain management. If a patient is already on the ICU when imminent death is identified, transition to a ward and unfamiliar staff may be disruptive, and the palliative team can contribute.

The notes need to be checked for a 'do not attempt resuscitation' (DNAR) order, which is based on medical judgment that resuscitation would lead to a high probability of death or severe brain damage, plus if possible the patient's judgment on their quality of life. The British Medical Association directs that DNAR orders be made in consultation with the patient, unless this is impossible, because physicians rarely predict accurately a patient's perception of their quality of life (Papa-Kanaan et al. 2001). Patients often want their families involved in the decision. Physiotherapists need to be included in the team discussion of end-of-life decisions in order to avoid possible legal complications (Raper & Fisher 2009).

Advance directives, or living wills, allow individuals, when competent, to express a wish to be spared life-sustaining treatment in case of intractable or terminal illness. These are not legally binding in many countries, and may not be available, retrieved or honoured during acute hospital care, but they reduce the likelihood of unnecessary cardiopulmonary resuscitation (Karnik & Kanekar 2016).

A decision to withdraw mechanical ventilation from a dying patient usually begins a process of 'terminal weaning', in the knowledge that it will be followed by death. This should be accompanied by titrated narcotics and noninvasive monitoring (Billings 2012), in close liaison with the palliative care team (Braus et al. 2016) and with extra support for the bereaved family (Bournival 2017).

## Infection Control

Critically ill patients, often in a state of immune exhaustion, may have their upper airways bypassed, multiple catheters inserted and their ventilator circuit opened, contributing to hospital-acquired infection being the primary cause of preventable death and disability among hospitalized patients (Boev 2017). Measures to reduce this risk include:

- hand cleaning, because gloves frequently have undetectable holes, one study finding that anaesthetists' gloved finger tips were contaminated in 83% of cases (Kocent et al. 2002);
- colour-coded plastic aprons to ensure a change between patients;
- fastidious attention to sterile suction technique, e.g. resting the disconnected catheter mount on the glove paper to avoid it touching the sheets;
- respect for tracheostomies as the surgical wounds that they are;
- doors to the ICU opening only on activation of the handwash dispenser.

## Teamwork

Communication problems, along with hierarchical barriers, are major causes of errors (McCulloch et al. 2011), augmented by what has been termed 'the tyranny of busyness' (Manias 2000). Teamwork is enhanced by mutual respect and assertiveness, mutual teaching and learning, flexibility, and multidisciplinary rounds, to include physiotherapists, occupational therapists and speech–language therapists (Brown 2013). The Intensive Care Society stipulates that a physiotherapist attend ward rounds, and that one physiotherapist be provided for every four beds (ICS 2013).

Problems may arise over boundaries and autonomy. If physiotherapists would like to ask for review of a medical therapy that is not their direct responsibility, they can raise the subject diplomatically by asking for advice about it, or by clarifying the link between medical management and rehabilitation. If physiotherapy is medically prescribed, physiotherapists can thank the doctor for their advice and explain that the patient will be assessed and treated as appropriate. Results are likely to be positive when communicating in a way that makes it easy for others to agree.

Communication between physiotherapists and nurses is facilitated by the physiotherapist offering to help change sheets when it fits in with turning the patient during treatment, and the nurse incorporating regimens such as hourly incentive spirometry into the nursing plan. Turning for physiotherapy should be coordinated with turning for pressure area care.

## MECHANICAL VENTILATION

*Some patients… resented health professionals touching their ventilators… others perceived the surrounding machinery as reassuring. Patients reported a need for repeated explanations.*

**Jablonski 1994**

The need for invasive mechanical ventilation is the commonest cause of admission to the ICU, with respiratory disease accounting for 79% of patients (Crooks et al. 2012). The ventilator augments or replaces the function of the inspiratory muscles by delivering gas to the lungs under positive pressure. This substitutes for the respiratory pump but is not beneficial for lung tissue, and there is a narrow range of pressures and volumes within which the lungs are safe from either overdistension or atelectasis/derecruitment.

Mechanical ventilation (MV) is supportive, not curative. It helps control gas exchange and acid–base balance by manipulating inspired oxygen, minute ventilation ($V_E$), inspiratory:expiratory (I:E) ratio, positive end-expiratory pressure (PEEP) and either pressure or volume. It is less about the application of a machine to a passive patient and more about the complex interaction between patient and machine.

## Indications

Whether or not patients have respiratory disease, they are usually in impending or established respiratory failure, i.e.:

• they are unable to ventilate adequately, oxygenate adequately, or both; examples are inspiratory muscle weakness due to neurological impairment, severe hypoxaemia due to lung parenchymal disease, or inspiratory muscle fatigue due to exacerbation of COPD;

• they are able to breathe adequately but this is deemed inadvisable, e.g. patients with acute brain injury may be sedated to the point of requiring ventilatory assistance;

• they require intubation for airway protection or to overcome upper airway obstruction and need added ventilatory support to compensate for the extra work of breathing (WOB) caused by the tubing and loss of expiratory resistance from the larynx.

## Airway

*'…like a toilet paper roll…a hard rubber tube…a soggy cigar…like you were gagging on something'.*
**Jablonski 1994**

Patient and ventilator are connected through a sealed tracheal tube (endotracheal or tracheostomy tube, Fig. 20.5), which reaches just beyond the vocal cords.

An **endotracheal tube** (ETT) through the mouth or nose can be used for up to 2 weeks, but causes distress and sometimes 'periods of terror' (ICS 2014a). A nasal tube causes less movement-related injury to the larynx but increases the risk of sinusitis and creates more airflow resistance, although this resistance can be counteracted

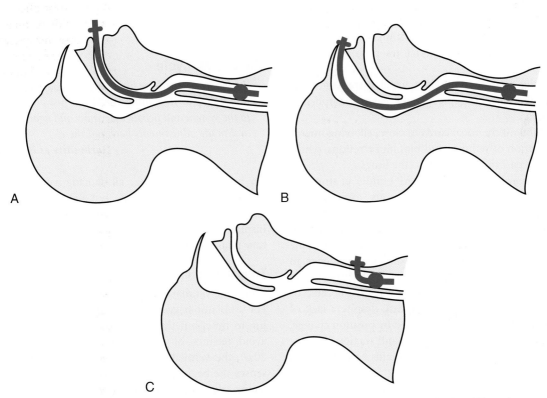

**FIGURE 20.5** Tracheal tubes: (A) oral endotracheal tube, (B) nasal endotracheal tube, (C) tracheostomy tube.

by an 'automatic tube compensation' facility in some ventilators. The process of intubation is best accompanied by nasal high-flow oxygen to reduce hypoxaemia (Ricard 2016). The patient is haemodynamically unstable immediately after intubation (Overbeck 2016).

A **tracheostomy tube** is more comfortable than an ETT, causes less resistance, is easier for suctioning, may improve oxygenation and ventilation (Bellani et al. 2013) and allows speaking and normal eating. If it becomes apparent that prolonged MV is required, early tracheotomy can reduce duration of ventilation, length of stay and sedative use (Puentes et al. 2016). A newly created tracheostomy indicates the need for extra care during patient handling and suctioning, although once established, it is more secure than an ETT and allows freer mobility. Initial tubes should not be fenestrated (p. 327) because of the risk of subcutaneous emphysema with positive pressure ventilation (Powell et al. 2011).

The main disadvantage of tracheal tubes is in providing a gateway for ventilator-associated pneumonia (VAP), which is hospital-acquired pneumonia that develops after 48 h of intubation. It is the most common complication of MV, bringing a mortality of 13% (Boev 2017). It is precipitated by the following:

- a biofilm that lines the tube within hours of intubation and acts as a bacterial reservoir (Zolfaghari 2012);
- positive pressure in the chest, which is transmitted to the abdomen and precipitates gastro-oesophageal reflux;
- inability of the vocal cords to close, allowing micro-aspiration of refluxed and biofilm secretions, which trickle past the cuff and into the lungs.

The risk may be reduced by a 'VAP bundle' of strategies such as 2-hourly turns, continuous aspiration of subglottic secretions above the cuff, tracheal and oral suction, mouth care, humidification and head elevation (Larrow & Klich-Heartt 2016). However, a Cochrane review found that there was insufficient evidence to recommend head elevation (Wang et al. 2016d), and Khan et al. (2017b) claimed that it was used because of its simplicity, ubiquity and low cost, despite a lack of evidence. VAP may also be reduced by position change, manual hyperinflation, vibrations and suction (Pattan-shetty & Gaude 2010). Ultrasound aids early detection (Mongodi et al. 2016).

The optimum cuff pressure to maximize mucosal perfusion and minimize aspiration is 20–30 cmH$_2$O,

which should be checked in different positions (Blot et al. 2015) and kept stable because fluctuations can trigger an ischaemia–reperfusion cycle (Huckle & Hughes 2010). Squeezing the external balloon to 'test' the pressure is banned.

Other complications of tracheal tubes are:

- loss of the warming and humidifying functions of the upper airway, which could cause thick secretions and ciliary damage (Chandler 2013); humidification is required for all patients (AARC 2012);
- communication difficulty, one study finding that most patients did not understand why they could not speak (Magnus 2006);
- with a tracheostomy: the complications described on p. 327;
- with an ETT: discomfort, retching, oversalivation, damage to the trachea and larynx, and post-extubation hoarseness;
- later, tracheal stenosis in 10%–22% of patients (Modrykamien 2012), dysphagia in 84% and aspiration (Macht et al. 2011); speech–language therapy and swallow-stimulation exercises can mitigate the damage (Hwang et al. 2007) but airway resection may be required (Shadmehr et al. 2017).

## The Breath Cycle

*'I felt I was something like a washing machine built into a shop or something. And I was just plugged in to the system and people every now and again came and made adjustments here and there'.*

**Darbyshire et al. 2016**

An array of all-singing, all-dancing ventilators has created a terminology jungle, but a ventilator breath is basically classified according to how it is triggered into inspiration, controlled (generated) during the inspiratory phase, then cycled into expiration.

### Trigger: start of the breath

Either the ventilator or the patient triggers inspiration. For ventilator-triggered breaths, the trigger is set according to time, but the patient can take extra breaths to avoid feelings of panic. For patient-triggering (Fig. 20.6), the ventilator delivers the breath as soon as it senses the beginning of the patient's inspiration. Ineffective triggers are the main cause of distressing ventilator asynchrony (ICS 2014a).

## Control: delivery of the breath

This driving mechanism describes how the ventilator delivers gas to the patient, remaining constant while other parameters vary according to ventilatory load. Thus the ventilator can be set as a pressure or volume controller, or a mix. A cycling pressure limit is set for safety, at about 10 cmH$_2$O above the peak inspiratory pressure.

**Volume control** (volume-constant) (VC) ventilation delivers a preset tidal volume (V$_T$) at a constant flow rate. The operator sets the V$_T$, flow, respiratory rate (RR) and inspiratory:expiratory (I:E) ratio. Airway pressure rises slowly during inspiration to a peak pressure that varies with airway resistance and lung compliance, so that if the lung stiffens or airways narrow, the pressure rises (Fig. 20.7A). VC may be used for adults because:
- it can be relied on to deliver a consistent V$_E$ regardless of lung characteristics;
- it maintains steady PaCO$_2$ levels when this is imperative, e.g. with acute brain-injured patients.

**Flow control** is similar to VC but derives volume from flow measurements and maintains a more consistent flow waveform.

**Pressure control** (pressure-constant) (PC) ventilation delivers a preset target pressure during inspiration (Fig. 20.7B). The operator sets the peak inspiratory pressure, inspiratory time and RR to achieve a target PaCO$_2$. Tidal volume varies with airway resistance, lung compliance and patient effort, leading to a risk of atelectasis, and in a supine patient, there is often little ventilation to the lung bases (Zoremba et al. 2010). However, PC ventilation delivers lower peak airway pressure and reduced risk of barotrauma (Sen et al. 2016) and is useful in patients with acute respiratory distress syndrome (ARDS) to control the amount of pressure delivered to damaged alveoli, or for children to compensate for the leak through their uncuffed ETT.

**Dual control** provides the advantage of PC ventilation (limiting peak inspiratory pressure to protect the alveoli) while maintaining the advantage of VC (delivering a constant volume even if lung mechanics vary). It switches between the two as required, varying between breaths or within a breath, but can only control one variable at a time. A variety of confusing names are used:
- Volume Support, which pressure-controls inspiration but adjusts the pressure limit to achieve a target V$_T$ at each breath;

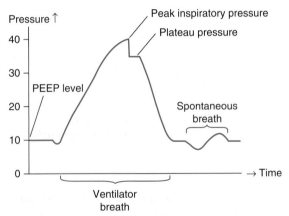

FIGURE 20.6 Pressure–time waveform showing a ventilator breath and a spontaneous breath, both being patient-triggered as identified by the negative pressure deflection. The ventilator breath is larger to make up for the V̇$_A$/Q̇ mismatch inherent in a positive pressure breath. A high positive end-expiratory pressure (PEEP) level of 10 cmH$_2$O is shown.

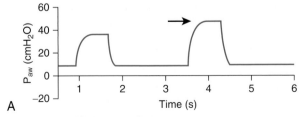
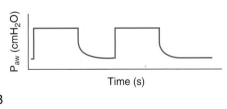

FIGURE 20.7 Pressure–time waveforms. (A) Volume control ventilation, the second breath showing increased pressure (arrow), indicating the development of airflow obstruction or stiff lungs. (B) Pressure control ventilation. Lack of negative pressure deflection in both waveforms at the start of inspiration indicates ventilator triggering rather than patient triggering. P$_{aw}$, mean airway pressure.

- Adaptive Support Ventilation, which adjusts $V_T$ and RR to achieve a preset $V_E$;
- Volume Assured Pressure Support, which automatically adjusts pressure in order to provide a consistent $V_T$.

Other names are Autoflow, Pressure Regulated Volume Control and Volume Control Plus.

The above control parameters are sometimes called modes of ventilation in the literature, which can cause confusion because they are actually different variables within a mode. Modes (below) are maintained independently of the control mechanism.

### Cycle: end of the breath

Cycling into expiration occurs according to time, flow, volume or a mix. **Time-cycling** is used for PC ventilation, gas delivery being maintained until a preset pressure is reached and then maintained for a preset time. **Flow-cycling** is used in pressure support mode (p. 443), when a reduction in peak inspiratory flow cycles the ventilator into expiration. **Volume-cycling** causes the ventilator to cycle at a preset $V_T$, but if an inspiratory pause is added, the breath will be classified as both volume- and time-cycled.

## Modes of Ventilation

*The new clinician is assaulted with a list of acronyms that sound impressively similar but can mean the difference between a calm, well-oxygenated patient and an agitated, hypoxic one struggling to breathe.*

*Robertson 2016*

---

**Mandatory breath**: triggered and cycled by the ventilator
**Assisted breath**: triggered by the patient, cycled by the ventilator
**Spontaneous breath**: triggered and cycled by the patient

---

With spontaneous breathing, the WOB normally represents less than 5% of total oxygen consumption ($\dot{V}O_2$), but it can rise to 30% in a catabolic critically ill patient (Leach & Treacher 2002). A ventilator can take over all the work with controlled mandatory ventilation (CMV) or it can be shared between ventilator and patient using a variety of ventilatory modes. These create the pressure, flow and volume that allow ventilatory support to be adjusted to the individual so that less sedation is required and less complications ensue than with full CMV.

Modes have to be matched skilfully to the patient because asynchrony is common, leading to unnecessary WOB, discomfort, prolonged weaning and sometimes a tug of war between patient and machine (Ramirez et al. 2017). At night, a mode should be chosen that provides extra support (Andréjak et al. 2013).

---

**KEY POINT**

Too much support leads to muscle atrophy, too little leads to fatigue.

---

Names for each mode vary with country and manufacturer, each new machine seeming to further stir up the terminology soup, leading to a 'calamity for ventilation research' because of the lack of accurate definition (Henzler 2011). Robertson (2016) has identified 47 mode names on just 4 ventilators. However, the terms described in the following sections are generally recognized.

### Controlled mandatory ventilation (CMV)

This fully controlled mode is ventilator-triggered and only used for patients who are unable to breathe or for whom complete control is necessary (Fig. 20.8). It is an unforgiving mode that mandates the depth and frequency of each breath and time-cycles into exhalation. Patients do not like to be controlled, and heavy sedation is required. Risk of intrinsic PEEP (p. 450) and other complications is significant. Minute volume is set high enough to maintain a mild respiratory alkalosis so that spontaneous breathing is inhibited.

### Assist-control

Assist-control is patient-triggered CMV. Breaths are triggered or imposed according to patient effort so that spontaneous breaths are assisted in the same way as controlled breaths. With some ventilators the only difference with CMV is the trigger sensitivity. Hyperventilation and respiratory alkalosis are risks.

### Intermittent mandatory ventilation (IMV)

The IMV mode allows patients to breathe spontaneously between a preset number of mandatory breaths, without regard to the patient's breathing pattern. Its nickname 'intermittent respiratory failure' reflects its lack of popularity (Kacmarek & Branson 2016).

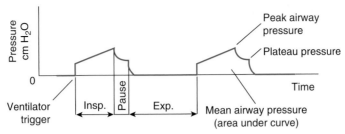

**FIGURE 20.8** Pressure–time waveform representing controlled mandatory ventilation.

## Synchronized intermittent mandatory ventilation (SIMV)

SIMV breaths are mandatory or spontaneous according to the stage of the cycle. If patients do not breathe after a preset time interval, a mandatory breath is delivered. SIMV has largely superseded IMV because synchrony with inspiratory effort is more comfortable and breath-stacking is avoided, but asynchrony may still develop. Preset variables include minute volume and I:E ratio. Cycling is by pressure or time, whichever comes first. The spontaneous breaths of SIMV are usually pressure-supported (see below) in order to overcome the resistance of the tubing (Fig. 20.9A).

## Pressure support ventilation (PSV)

Also known as assisted spontaneous breathing (ASB), PSV is a patient-triggered mode that provides a pressure boost to each inspiratory effort, the pressure support level (above PEEP) reducing WOB in proportion to the pressure delivered. Various pressures have been advised:

- Epstein (2002) claims that 3–14 $cmH_2O$ offsets the work of breathing through the tubing;
- Tobin (2012) states that pressures of 5–10 $cmH_2O$ decrease WOB by 31%–60%;
- Aliverti et al. (2006) make the sensible suggestion of fine tuning the pressure by titrating it to the most synchronous breathing pattern.

Even better, the patient could be asked what pressure suits him or her best.

The preset pressure continues on a plateau until flow reaches between 10% and 40% of peak inspiratory flow (Chang 2014, p. 67), at which point cycling into expiration occurs. Patients must be able to reliably trigger the ventilator and determine their own RR, $V_T$ and I:E ratio (Fig. 20.9B). The preset variables are trigger sensitivity and pressure support level.

PSV is relatively comfortable and facilitates synchrony because the patient is in control. It acts like IPPB (p. 193) but is flow triggered rather than pressure triggered, thus eliminating extra work to trigger the breath. It is also similar to the BiPAP mode in noninvasive ventilation, where IPAP relates to the pressure support level and EPAP equates to PEEP (p. 240).

The terms 'assist mode' or 'continuous spontaneous ventilation' are sometimes used for this mode.

## Proportional assist ventilation

This is similar to PSV but the supporting pressure provides a positive feedback system by varying in proportion to patient effort, delivering a form of 'power steering' so that the harder the patient pulls, the more the ventilator pushes (Fig. 20.9C). It brings the added bonus of improving both sleep and exercise tolerance (Robertson 2016).

## Assist mode

This is also similar to PSV and the terms are sometimes used interchangeably, but the breathing pattern is more dependent on the characteristics of the machine.

## Neurally adjusted ventilatory assist (NAVA)

This mode detects electrical signals from the diaphragm in order to coordinate the inspiratory trigger with spontaneous breathing, the ventilator acting like a muscle under patient neural command, leading to improved patient-ventilator synchrony. Pressures of 0.5–2.5 $cmH_2O$ are comparable to PSV levels of 7–25 $cmH_2O$ in terms of respiratory muscle unloading, but the mode can be sometimes excessively sensitive to electrical activity of the diaphragm for triggering (Carteaux et al. 2016).

## Bilevel positive airway pressure (BiPAP)

BiPAP through the ventilator is equivalent to the support provided by noninvasive ventilation used with spontaneously breathing patients (p. 240).

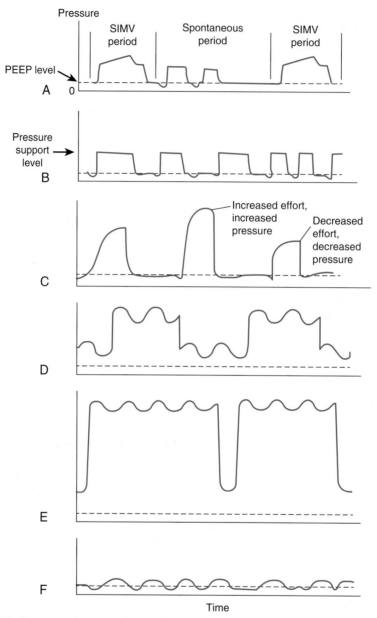

**FIGURE 20.9** Pressure–time waveforms showing (A) synchronized intermittent mandatory ventilation *(SIMV)*, (B) pressure support ventilation, (C) proportional assist ventilation, (D) biphasic positive airways pressure, (E) airway pressure release ventilation, (F) CPAP.

## Biphasic positive airway pressure (BIPAP)

The term BIPAP, with a capital 'I', was invented by someone with an interesting sense of humour. It is not BiPAP with a small 'i', as above, but allows spontaneous breathing at preset high and low positive pressure levels (Fig. 20.9D). For further confusion, some research studies do not use a capital 'I'. The mode has some similarities to airway pressure release ventilation, see below.

## Airway pressure release ventilation (APRV)

Also called Bi-Vent, APRV is pressure-controlled and time-cycled, with the benefit of unrestricted spontaneous breathing throughout the cycle. High and low pressure levels are preset, as with BIPAP, but the low level pressure lasts for just a second or so to allow $CO_2$ to escape and fresh gas to fill the alveoli (Fig. 20.9E). This leads to an inverse I:E ratio of about 8:1 and an open lung strategy of near-continuous positive pressure to help prevent derecruitment in ARDS lungs. A lower PEEP is able to deliver the same $V_T$ with less risk of overdistension (Fig. 20.10).

Preset parameters are the high and low pressures, and the time at each pressure level, with expiratory release time set short enough to prevent alveolar derecruitment. Unlike BIPAP, the I:E ratio is always inverted and there is rarely time for spontaneous breathing to occur at the lower level. Problems include:

- long inspiratory time, which inhibits venous return so the mode is unsuited to haemodynamically unstable patients;
- the short expiratory time, which facilitates gas trapping;
- sometimes excessive WOB, tidal volume and atelec-trauma (Chatburn et al. 2016).

### Continuous positive airway pressure (CPAP)

CPAP (see Fig. 20.9F) provides a level of positive pressure, devoid of mandatory breaths, within which the patient breathes spontaneously. For intubated patients, CPAP follows the same principle as noninvasive CPAP (p. 191) but without the complications of a mask.

CPAP is suited to patients who have poor gas exchange, as with mask CPAP. It also helps reduce intrinsic PEEP because it splints open the airways throughout the cycle to allow trapped gas to escape. Some ventilators confusingly use the term CPAP when inspiratory pressures are greater than expiratory pressures, which is actually BiPAP.

### Mandatory minute ventilation

This mode provides a guaranteed preset minute volume if spontaneous breathing drops below a preset level. Pressure support may be added to ensure an adequate $V_T$ for patients with rapid shallow breathing.

### Variable ventilation

The intrinsic fluctuations of healthy spontaneous breathing are mimicked by this mode in order to dampen inflammation in vulnerable lungs (Huhle et al. 2016).

> *The choice of which ventilator mode to use is based on which is the most comfortable for your patients.*
> *Robertson 2016*

## Strategies of Ventilation
### Inverse-ratio ventilation

For patients with refractory hypoxaemia and high airway pressures, peak pressure can be reduced and mean airway pressure raised by prolonging inspiratory time to the point of reversing the I:E ratio (Fig. 20.11). This is achieved by slowing inspiratory flow or increasing inspiratory pause.

Benefits are recruitment of collapsed alveoli and 'expiratory flow bias', the faster expiratory time encouraging mucus to move towards the mouth (Volpe et al. 2008). Disadvantages are the risk of intrinsic PEEP,

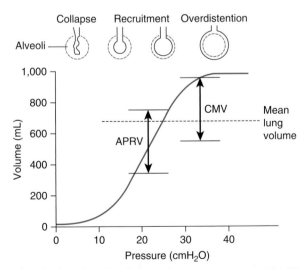

FIGURE 20.10 Controlled mandatory ventilation *(CMV)* and airway pressure release ventilation *(APRV)* superimposed on a compliance curve, showing how CMV requires a higher pressure to achieve the same mean lung volume, thus increasing the risk of injury by overdistension. (From Mireles-Cabodevila et al. 2016.)

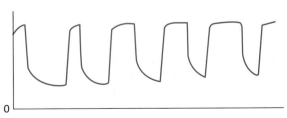

FIGURE 20.11 Pressure–time waveform showing increasing degrees of inverse-ratio ventilation.

overstretched alveoli, compromised cardiac output and the discomfort of an unnatural breathing pattern during which the patient is often unable to fully exhale. Heavy sedation is used and no spontaneous breathing allowed.

### Lung protective ventilation

Deliberately underventilating a patient reduces the pressure and volume risks of MV. Blood gas targets are modified and a low minute volume allows $PaCO_2$ to rise as far as 8 kPa (60 $cmH_2O$), with pH and oxygenation closely monitored. Acid–base compensation restores pH in the brain and myocardium over several hours. Guo et al. (2016c) found the following outcomes:

- low $V_T$ + high PEEP – highest $PaO_2/FiO_2$ ratio, although high PEEP still causes a parallel increase in alveolar stress and strain at a different end-inspiration (Retamal et al. 2013);
- high $V_T$ + low PEEP – highest pulmonary compliance;
- low $V_T$ + lower PEEP – shortest length of ICU stay;
- lower $V_T$ + zero PEEP – lowest $PaO_2/FiO_2$ ratio and pulmonary compliance.

Some acidosis brings the unexpected benefit of attenuating ventilator-induced lung injury (Contreras et al. 2012) and diaphragm atrophy (Schellekens et al. 2014). Hypercapnia is normally tolerated so long as the kidneys are functioning well enough to stabilize acid–base status. $SpO_2$ may be allowed to drop to 88% so long as tissue oxygenation is monitored (Macintyre 2013a).

This 'permissive hypercapnia' is used for people with ARDS or acute asthma, and may be used to prevent or reduce alveolar inflammation in other patients (Guo et al. 2016c).

Patients may feel breathless and suffocated if the strategy is not carefully managed (Vincent et al. 2002), and there is a risk of atelectasis (Gilbert et al. 2009). It is normally contraindicated in conditions intolerant of hypercapnia such as acute brain injury, severe pulmonary hypertension or congestive heart failure (Gattinoni et al. 2002).

Ultraprotective strategies decrease $V_T$ even further, leading to a reduction in potential damage from hyperinflation and cyclic opening and closing of alveoli. Hypercapnia is avoided by increasing RR and reducing dead space, but problems related to physiotherapy include both sputum retention (Cork et al. 2014) and atelectasis (Retamal et al. 2013). Atelectasis may be prevented by at least one normal $V_T$ every 2 min. Other

risks relate to people with ARDS, for whom this strategy is usually applied, e.g. 30%–40% of recruitable lung remains closed and newly formed atelectasis cannot be reopened (Gattinoni 2016).

---

### PRACTICE TIP FOR STUDENTS

Find out which ventilator is used in your ICU, research it online to clarify the terminology, consult Robertson (2016), then ask if you can go in pairs to the ICU and sit in front of a spare ventilator with the handbook to correlate what you have learned.

---

### Settings

*'Sometimes it's going too fast for you, so instead of the machine synchronizing with you, you have to synchronize with the machine'.*

**Jablonski 1994**

Ventilation and oxygenation are matched to the patient according to $PaCO_2$ and $PaO_2$ respectively. Minute ventilation ($\dot{V}_E$) is adjusted according to $PaCO_2$, $V_T$ being adjusted for a small change and RR adjusted for a larger change, with equilibrium reached in an average 30 min (Retamal et al. 2013). Normal values for $\dot{V}_E$ vary widely: a COPD patient with chronic hypercapnia requires a great deal less than a hypermetabolic septic patient. Ventilator settings can be adjusted to reduce the dyspnoea experienced by 35% of patients (Schmidt et al. 2011) or to influence flow bias by manipulating flow rate, I:E ratio and PEEP (Graf & Marini 2008). The trend is towards low tidal volume lung protective strategies to minimize complications. As with the mode of ventilation, ventilator settings impact patient synchrony and comfort.

**Inspired oxygen concentration** ($FiO_2$) is adjusted according to $PaO_2$, although the relationship between $FiO_2$ and $PaO_2$ is less direct than that between $\dot{V}_E$ and $PaCO_2$ because $PaO_2$ is subject to more variables.

**Inspiratory flow rate** is set from about 40 L/min (e.g. with ARDS in order to prolong inspiration and the time for gas exchange) to about 100 L/min (e.g. with COPD in order to increase expiratory time and limit hyperinflation). **I:E ratio** is normally 1:2 to allow adequate expiratory time for $CO_2$ clearance and to facilitate venous return. Levels as low as 1:4 are used to help prevent intrinsic PEEP and as high as 4:1 (inverse-ratio ventilation) to recruit alveoli. It is manipulated by the flow rate, RR, $\dot{V}_E$ and/or inspiratory time.

**Inspiratory pause** (plateau) provides an end-inspiratory hold that enhances gas distribution by allowing time for recruitment of poorly ventilated alveoli.

The **100% oxygen** button can be used freely by physiotherapists and has a timed cut off. Experienced physiotherapists may use other buttons, e.g. for ventilator hyperinflation, as part of the team.

**Alarms** are set for pressure, volume, flow, and levels of oxygen and $CO_2$. It is useful to learn the characteristics of the alarms for each machine, including reset time.

## Complications

The adverse effects of MV are of particular interest to the physiotherapist because some are increased further by the extra positive pressure of manual hyperinflation. Added to the complications of intubation (p. 439) are those described in the following sections.

### Impaired cardiac output

The heart is a pressure chamber within a pressure chamber. Positive pressure in the chest displaces approximately 15%–20% of pulmonary blood volume to the systemic circulation (Chang 2014, p. 34), impeding venous return, leading to decreased cardiac output and sometimes reduced blood flow to voracious organs such as the kidney, liver and brain (De Beer 2013). Compensatory peripheral vasoconstriction normally maintains BP, but this is less viable in patients who are elderly, or who suffer autonomic neuropathy such as with Guillain-Barré syndrome, or are hypovolaemic, either absolutely, or functionally due to the vasodilation of septic shock. These patients may become hypotensive at the initiation of MV or on repositioning (Vollman 2013).

Haemodynamic compromise is most likely with high mean airway pressures, prolonged inspiratory time or high PEEP levels. Haemodynamic stability can be facilitated by fluids, inotropic drugs or reduced I:E ratio so that expiratory time is longer and the heart has more time to fill. Patients with poorly compliant lungs suffer less haemodynamic compromise because pressure is transmitted less easily through stiff lungs (Chang 2014).

### Barotrauma

Barotrauma is air in the wrong place, e.g. pneumothorax, subcutaneous emphysema, pneumopericardium or pneumomediastinum. The prefix 'baro-' arose from the

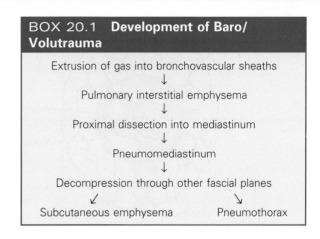

**BOX 20.1   Development of Baro/Volutrauma**

Extrusion of gas into bronchovascular sheaths
↓
Pulmonary interstitial emphysema
↓
Proximal dissection into mediastinum
↓
Pneumomediastinum
↓
Decompression through other fascial planes
↙              ↘
Subcutaneous emphysema        Pneumothorax

assumption that the cause was excess pressure because these complications are associated with high plateau pressures. But it is now thought that excess volume, specifically end-inspiratory volume, is the main culprit because sustained alveolar stretch overdistends the delicate alveolar–capillary membrane. This explains why coughing, when pressure increases massively but volume is stable, rarely causes barotrauma. The term 'volutrauma' rather than 'barotrauma' may therefore be used to describe extra-alveolar air in this context, but the two are linked via the pressure–volume curve (p. 8).

Box 20.1 and Fig. 20.12 indicate the process, air first squeezing out from distended alveoli, especially if the lungs are hyperinflated or unevenly damaged, then tracking centrally along the bronchovascular sheaths and into the interstitial spaces, where it is known as **pulmonary interstitial emphysema**. This is difficult to detect radiologically in adults unless contrast is provided by a background of generalized opacification, e.g. ARDS, but it shows up in infants as a mottled opacity (see Fig. 15.11A). This can lead to **pneumomediastinum**, i.e. air around the mediastinum, which can dissect up into the neck. This is rarely dangerous (Saleem et al. 2016) but may be the first visible warning to avoid manual hyperinflation. Air may then get under the skin, causing **subcutaneous emphysema** (Fig. 20.13), or into the pleura, causing **pneumothorax.**

**Pneumopericardium**, when air accumulates in the pericardium, is a less common form of barotrauma but may occur after heart surgery, chest trauma, with recreational drug use or in neonates with stiff lungs. An upright X-ray shows as a dark outline contouring the heart and crossing the midline above the diaphragm, the

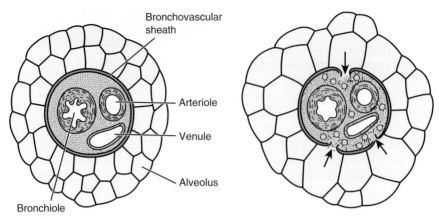

FIGURE 20.12 Development of barotrauma. Left: cross-section of normal alveoli and vessels. Right: overdistended alveoli rupturing through the delicate alveolar–capillary membranes. (From Maunder et al. 1984.)

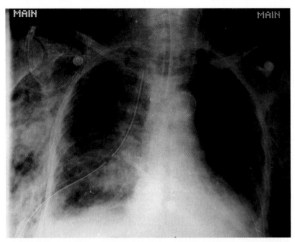

FIGURE 20.13 Intubated patient with soft tissue shadowing under the skin bilaterally, R > L, indicating subcutaneous emphysema. The patient also has a R chest drain, suggesting a recent pneumothorax. He also has a partially calcified aorta, representing advanced age.

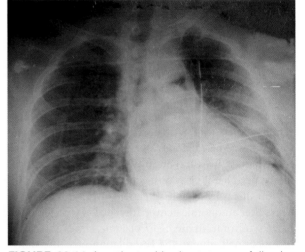

FIGURE 20.14 A patient with chest trauma following a car accident, showing a continuous diaphragm sign indicating pneumopericardium, fractured L ribs, and a kinked L chest drain.

'continuous diaphragm' sign (Fig. 20.14), and on CT the heart is partially or completely surrounded by air (Uluçam 2013). The air does not dissect up into the neck.

### Ventilator-induced lung injury

Injury to the alveoli can be caused by the abrasive stress of cyclic opening (recruitment) and closing (derecruitment), particularly at low lung volumes (Fig. 20.15). Healthy lung can usually withstand this, but repetitive stretch and collapse of alveoli in patients with injured lungs can provoke inflammation, pulmonary oedema and ventilator-induced lung injury, also known as atelectrauma (Miles & Cook 2017). Smokers fare worse because of their extra neutrophils (Hirsch et al. 2014) and insult may be added to injury by the process increasing the risk of critical illness myopathy (Musch 2010) and multisystem failure, especially when a chest infection increases bacterial translocation (Fletcher & Cuthbertson 2010).

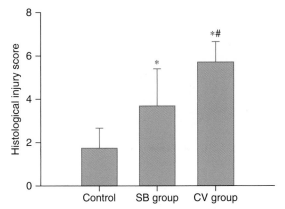

**FIGURE 20.15** Degree of lung injury with increasing ventilator support. *CV*, Controlled mandatory ventilation; *SB*, spontaneous breathing. (From Xia et al. 2011.)

The risk is reduced by incorporating spontaneous breaths into the breathing cycle, limiting plateau pressure, ensuring adequate PEEP to minimize derecruitment, modifying the waveform to increase surfactant (Amin & Suki 2012), using lung protective strategies or turning the patient prone to reduce stretch on ventral lung tissue (Gattinoni et al. 2013).

### Gastro-oesophageal reflux

The more positive the pressure, the more the stomach contents can be forced up into the oesophagus. Positioning reduces the risk of gastro-oesophageal reflux (p. 125).

### Weakness and muscle damage

Unlike an actively contracting diaphragm, the passive displacement caused by MV reduces perfusion to the diaphragm, contributing to atelectasis (Chen et al. 2016f), diaphragmatic injury (Hussain et al. 2016b) and greater atrophy than is explained by disuse (Berger et al. 2016). This occurs most rapidly in the first 72 h (Schepens et al. 2015), but full CMV leads to diaphragmatic dysfunction in 6–24 h (Martin et al. 2013), leading to increasing mortality (Medrinal et al. 2016). The generalized muscle weakness caused by patient immobility augments this.

### Perfusion gradient

Positive pressure accentuates the perfusion gradient from non-dependent to dependent regions (Fig. 20.16), leaving nondependent regions cyclically without blood

flow (West 2016), and displacing blood overall from the chest. The degree to which perfusion is affected depends on the proportion of positive pressure generated by the ventilator compared to the negative pressure generated by patient effort.

### Ventilation gradient

Positive pressure in the chest directs inspired gas to take the path of least resistance, which is to the more open non-dependent regions (Fig. 20.16). This is because:
- the diaphragm is inactive so that the more stretched dependent fibres are no longer drawing air downwards;
- dependent lung is less compliant due to compression by the increased perfusion.

Dependent areas therefore receive the least ventilation and are vulnerable to progressive atelectasis. This is ameliorated by positioning or a mode of ventilation in which spontaneous breathing is encouraged.

### Atelectasis

Risk factors for volume loss are immobility, reversed ventilation gradient, low tidal volume and impaired surfactant secretion (Miles & Cook 2017). This can lead to atelectasis and ventilator-associated pneumonia (Ntoumenopoulos & Glickman 2012).

> **KEY POINT**
>
> The main physiotherapy contribution to prevention of atelectasis is regular and accurate position change, plus as much activity that is subjectively and objectively feasible.

### Increased dead space

Dead space increases because of reduced overall perfusion, and to a lesser extent because of the ventilator tubing.

### Ventilation/perfusion ($\dot{V}_A/\dot{Q}$) mismatch

The above complications lead to $\dot{V}_A/\dot{Q}$ mismatch and increased shunt (Vimláti 2012), which would lead to hypoxaemia if not offset by ventilator settings such as PEEP, inspiratory pause and supplemental oxygen.

### Discomfort

If ventilation is not matched synchronously to the patient, and if full explanations are not given, sometimes

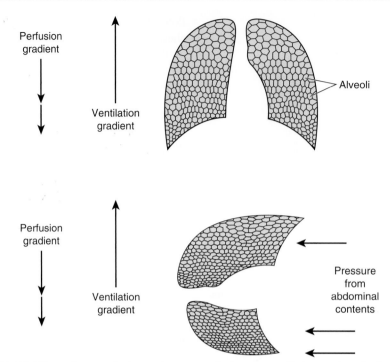

**FIGURE 20.16** Effect of controlled mandatory ventilation on ventilation and perfusion gradients. The perfusion gradient increases downwards and (compared to healthy young subjects) the ventilation gradient is reversed. (See also Fig. 1.9.)

repeatedly, MV can be anything from 'grossly uncomfortable' to 'the most inhumane treatment ever experienced' (Chlan 2011).

### Breathlessness

Dyspnoea is frequent and strongly associated with anxiety (Schmidt et al. 2011). Causes are feeling out of control, abnormal stimulation of lung stretch receptors and asynchrony with the ventilator. Asynchrony can prolong MV and increase morbidity and mortality (Rittayamai et al. 2016). It is suggested by flow or pressure waveforms (Branson et al. 2013), but is often missed if the patient is unable to communicate this, and monitoring is advised (Dres et al. 2016). After checking for anxiety, secretions and the adequacy of ventilation (by minute volume or $PaCO_2$), the intensivist should be informed so that ventilator settings can be adjusted.

### Gut and kidney dysfunction

Splanchnic blood flow does not have autoregulation capabilities and is dependent on BP. It is therefore vulnerable to haemodynamic upset, as well as the abdominal distension that is common in ventilated patients. Hypoperfusion risks the gut mucosal barrier becoming permeable, facilitating multisystem failure, paralytic ileus, bleeding and ulceration. The kidney is also vulnerable to hypoperfusion, receiving 25% of the circulating blood volume at any one time (Chang 2014, p. 35). Haemodynamic compromise triples the risk of acute kidney injury (Akker et al. 2013).

### Excess secretions and sputum retention

Bronchial secretions are increased due to irritation from the tracheal tube. Retention of these secretions then occurs if there is an absent cough, high ventilatory pressures or inadequate humidification.

### Intrinsic PEEP

Gas trapping can be quantified in terms of volume (hyperinflation) or pressure (intrinsic PEEP or PEEPi), though the terms are interchangeable in practice. PEEPi is unwelcome PEEP, which occurs unintentionally when exhalation has not finished before the next breath triggers into inspiration (see Fig. 3.4). It is commonest with

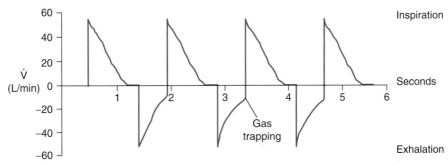

**FIGURE 20.17** Flow–time waveform of inverse-ratio ventilation with gas trapping as the gas starts flowing in before exhalation is finished. $\dot{V}$, Flow.

hyperinflation caused by airflow obstruction, such as occurs with COPD or acute asthma, or in unevenly damaged ARDS lungs. Lung emptying is also impeded by a narrow endotracheal tube or rapid breathing, which may not allow enough time for expiration. The flow–time curve shows persistent flow at end-expiration (Fig. 20.17) and distal airway pressures can reach 15 $cmH_2O$ (Chang 2014). The results are discomfort, overdistended alveoli, heightened risk of barotrauma, compromised haemodynamics, ventilator asynchrony and extra work of breathing to reach the trigger threshold at each breath (Ku 2016).

PEEPi can be mitigated by:
- strategies to offset the resistance of the ETT (Haberthür 2009);
- reducing RR, prolonging expiratory time and if necessary instigating lung protective strategies;
- adding normal (extrinsic) PEEP at no more than 85% of the PEEPi level (Chang 2014) to splint open the airways and allow trapped gas to escape, similar to people with hyperinflation finding relief in pursed-lips breathing;
- airway clearance to reduce airflow resistance.

## Positive End-Expiratory Pressure (PEEP)

There are several ways to boost $SpO_2$:
- ↑ $FiO_2$
- prolong the plateau
- ↑ the I:E ratio
- ↑ PEEP

For all practical purposes, PEEP is CPAP, but the term is used for ventilated patients only. PEEP raises functional residual capacity (FRC) and maintains constant positive pressure throughout the respiratory cycle so that airway pressure does not fall to atmospheric

pressure at end-exhalation. It cannot itself increase lung volume without using excessively high pressures (Hess & Bigatello 2002) and if recruitment potential is low, increasing PEEP may simply overdistend already open alveoli (Hess 2011b).

This helpful PEEP is termed 'extrinsic PEEP' when it needs to be distinguished from unhelpful intrinsic PEEP. It is used with all modes of ventilation, averaging 5 $cmH_2O$ but varying from 3 to over 20 $cmH_2O$. It is shown on the pressure–time waveform as the pressure to which the breath returns at end-exhalation (see Figs 20.6 and 20.7).

### Benefits

Positive effects are:
- to help prevent collapse of alveoli and airways (Chen et al. 2016f);
- ↑ lung compliance by raising resting lung volume out of the range of airway closure and derecruitment;
- ↑ alveolar–capillary surface area for gas exchange;
- ↑ stability of alveoli, conservation of surfactant, ↓ risk of atelectrauma;
- ↓ muscle effort to negate the expiratory gradient if intrinsic PEEP is present (Peigang & Marini 2002);
- ↑ recruitment of compressed alveoli in acute respiratory distress syndrome.

### Complications

Excess PEEP can lead to exaggerations of the complications of MV:
1. The continuous positive pressure impairs venous return and cardiac output, the effect being greater with PEEP than with CPAP (Chang 2014). This can offset the beneficial effects of PEEP by causing a net decrease in oxygen delivery to the tissues (Mendéz

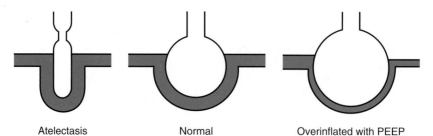

Atelectasis                    Normal                  Overinflated with PEEP

**FIGURE 20.18** Alveoli and their capillaries. *Left,* Inadequate positive end-expiratory pressure *(PEEP); right,* excess PEEP. (From Pilbeam & Cairo 2006.)

2017). Haemodynamic compromise usually occurs at >15 cmH₂O PEEP in normovolaemic patients, at higher pressures in patients with stiff lungs and at lower pressures in hypovolaemic patients. Fluid administration can stabilize cardiac output, but may incur pulmonary oedema when PEEP is discontinued. PEEP above 5 cmH₂O should be applied in small increments and titrated against oxygen delivery.

2. High PEEP may disrupt the alveolar–capillary barrier and redistribute alveolar fluid, leading to pulmonary oedema.
3. Excessive PEEP compresses pulmonary capillaries and decreases compliance by overdistending alveoli (Fig. 20.18).

Raised pressure in the chest increases central venous pressure (CVP) and pulmonary artery wedge pressure (PAWP) readings (p. 467) at the same time as the ventricular filling pressure that they represent is declining because of impaired venous return. This is not a complication but allowance is made for this during assessment.

### Best PEEP

Optimum PEEP is achieved when it is titrated to ventilation homogeneity through electrical impedance tomography (Chang 2014), or to maximum tissue oxygenation (Bikker et al. 2013), or to a balance of SpO₂ and cardiac output. Fig. 20.19 shows how best PEEP improves ventilation to the lung bases. When PEEP is reduced, the effect on oxygenation shows in minutes, but compliance can take an hour to reach equilibrium. On increasing PEEP, time to equilibrium is longer (Chiumello 2013).

### Precautions

High-pressure PEEP is a risk if there is intracranial hypertension or an undrained pneumothorax, and may

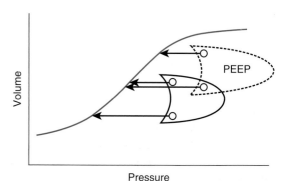

**FIGURE 20.19** Effect of positive end-expiratory pressure *(PEEP)* on regional pressure and volume relationships, showing how it raises dependent lung onto a steep part of the compliance curve, thereby encouraging basal ventilation. (From Lumb 2000.)

be detrimental for patients who have subcutaneous emphysema, bullae, bronchopleural fistula or following lung surgery. Hypovolaemia is a relative contraindication, but if high PEEP is necessary, cardiac output can be supported with fluids and inotropes. At high PEEP levels, manual hyperinflation requires modifications (p. 492).

Disconnecting the ventilator circuit for suction is detrimental in PEEP-dependent patients but this risk is eliminated with an inline suction catheter.

### High-Frequency Ventilation

How does the Himalayan mountain shrew maintain oxygenation during copulation? With a RR up to 600 breaths/min, its tidal volume (V_T) is less than its dead space, but it manages to achieve gas exchange for this important task by a mechanism similar to the intriguing phenomenon of high-frequency ventilation (HFV). High RR and low $V_T$ are achieved by the following:

1. High-frequency positive pressure ventilation uses time-cycled conventional ventilation at rates of 50–100 b/min.
2. High-frequency jet ventilation (HFJV) directs short rapid jets of gas through a nozzle into the airways and entrains air by the Venturi principle. Expiration is by passive recoil and rates of 100–600 b/m are achieved.
3. High-frequency oscillation (HFO) forces minibursts of gas in and out of the airway at 3–20 breaths/s so that both inspiration and expiration are active. This brings extra benefits of helping clear secretions (Morgan et al. 2016), but it can be damaging for those with vulnerable lungs because high volumes are sometimes generated (Nguyen et al. 2016). Spontaneous breathing during HFO is encouraged and helps to preserve lung volume.
4. High-frequency percussive ventilation delivers equivalent or improved oxygenation at lower peak pressures than conventional ventilation, and also helps mobilize secretions (Kunugiyama 2013).

## Mechanism

With such a meagre $V_T$, gas exchange cannot rely on bulk flow of gas. The classic concept of 'dead' space is no longer applicable, and this space is in fact thought to play an active part in gas exchange by the following mechanisms:

- High-velocity flow creates turbulent mixing in the central airways, which is propagated peripherally by convective inspiratory flow.
- Gas mixing may occur by filling and emptying alveoli independent of each other, an effect known merrily as 'disco lung'.
- Molecular diffusion, the primary mechanism of normal gas exchange in terminal lung units, is augmented, especially by the vibrating gas of HFO.

## Advantages

1. 'Lung rest' for people with ARDS is afforded by some forms of HFV because of minimal volume and pressure changes (Michaels et al. 2015).
2. Spontaneous respiration is inhibited and little sedation is needed. Most patients find the sensation comfortable, as if being massaged from inside.

3. HFV provides an even distribution of ventilation because diffusion is independent of regional compliance and gas flow does not take the path of least resistance.
4. HFJV via minitracheostomy allows spontaneous breathing through the natural airway.

## Disadvantages

1. High levels of sedation may be required.
2. Except with HFO, high inspiratory flows and limited exhalation time risk generating intrinsic PEEP.
3. Some machines are noisy.

## Indications

HFV tends to be used as a rescue mode when other techniques have failed. The following may benefit:

- patients with bronchopleural fistula, large air leak, flail chest or those with vulnerable lungs such as neonatal respiratory distress syndrome;
- patients who are unable to tolerate large pressure swings in the chest, e.g. those with acute brain injury or unstable cardiovascular status;
- patients with severe ARDS who have reached the maximum safe levels of conventional ventilation.

## Physiotherapy

Suction can be performed without interruption of ventilation, and causes less adverse effects on oxygenation or heart rhythm than with conventional MV. $FiO_2$ must be increased by about 20% for 3 minutes before and after suction because manual hyperinflation is usually not possible, although a system has been created for its use with HFO (Hickey 2006). Jet ventilation through a minitracheostomy allows patients to take deep breaths and cough.

## Weaning

*'I was sure I would not be able to breathe on my own. The machine was put to a setting which gave me a couple of breaths and the rest was up to me. I hated that, I never knew when to take my breaths'.*
**Ludwig (patient and physiotherapist) 1984**

Multidisciplinary teamwork speeds weaning and can increase survival for long-term patients (Black et al. 2012b). Various procedures are balanced between patient, clinician and machine, for example:

- Automated weaning recognizes deviations from the patient's expected activity and enforces rapid compliance with a standardized weaning strategy, but is unable to address individual problems causing patient distress (Holets et al. 2016).
- A physiotherapy-driven weaning plan can decrease weaning time compared to an automated system because it takes into account individual difficulties (Taniguchi et al. 2015).
- MacIntyre (2013b) claims that some comfortable interactive ventilator modes eliminate the need for a weaning process.

The proportion of patients experiencing difficulty in weaning is 25% and rising (Martin et al. 2013), especially those with chronic lung disease or neuropathies, and anyone after prolonged ventilatory support. They may benefit from inspiratory muscle training (Chung et al. 2016d). Ventilator manipulations may not provide an effective training stimulus (Cader et al. 2012), but the physiotherapist can negotiate a protocol that ensures adequate rest and appropriate inspiratory muscle activity through the ventilator, or attach an inspiratory muscle trainer to the tracheal tube (Fig. 20.20).

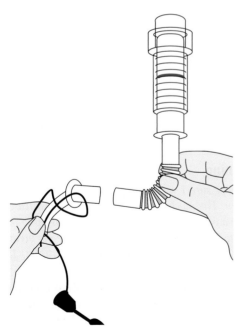

**FIGURE 20.20** Connection of threshold inspiratory muscle trainer to tracheal tube.

Weaning should be seamless, and the physiotherapist starts as soon as the patient is intubated, the process being integral to the rehabilitation programme. The first step is a preliminary rest and good night's sleep, then little-and-often exercise as the patient is able, e.g. squeezing a ball and quadriceps contractions. A graduated exercise programme is then developed, which can shorten weaning time (Chen & Lin 2012).

Liberation from the ventilator entails:

- progressive and intermittent reduction in support until the patient is able to sustain spontaneous breathing;
- a trial of spontaneous breathing through the tracheal tube;
- extubation.

**KEY POINT**

The physiotherapist's contribution to the team management of weaning is to advise on the balance of rest and exercise, to assess the breathing pattern, and sometimes to extubate the patient.

## Intermittent Reduction in Ventilatory Support

*It is surprising that respiratory muscle dysfunction largely develops without being noticed.*

**Heunks et al. 2015**

Reduction in ventilatory support involves periods of decreasing pressure on PSV or decreasing number of breaths in SIMV mode, the latter being considered less effective (Tanaka 2013). This is interspersed with rest, including sometimes full ventilator support at night (Chang 2014), because if the respiratory muscles become fatigued (Fig. 20.21) they steal blood supply from the skeletal muscles, which themselves are needed for rehabilitation (Ramsook et al. 2016) and the diaphragm may then need 24 h to recover (Laghi et al. 2002). Clear explanations and autonomy are the first priority, and a fan is often helpful. Relaxation facilitated by guided imagery can shorten weaning time and improve oxygenation (Spiva et al. 2015).

Options for monitoring include ultrasound or airway flow/pressure waveforms to identify the effort and work of breathing (Bellani & Pesenti 2014), respiratory muscle monitoring to help prevent muscle damage caused by overusing fatigued muscles (Heunks et al.

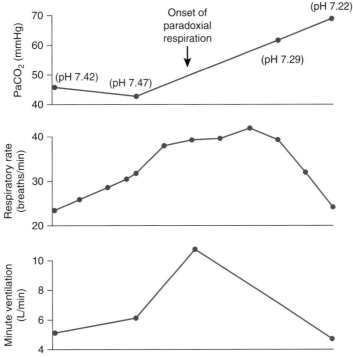

**FIGURE 20.21** Failed weaning attempt. Fatigue develops at first, represented by ↑ RR, ↓ PaCO$_2$ and alkalosis. Then exhaustion supervenes, represented by ↓ RR, ↑ PaCO$_2$ and acidosis. *RR*, Respiratory rate. (From Cohen et al. 1982.)

2015), and a daily sedation break to enable screening for consciousness, oxygenation, ventilation, airway patency and cardiovascular stability. The following then identify readiness to proceed:

- correction of the underlying reason for MV;
- optimum nutrition, fluid, metabolic and cardiovascular status, including adequate haemoglobin;
- elimination of unnecessary work of breathing (WOB), including clear airways, minimum intrinsic PEEP and no abdominal distension;
- restoration of normal diurnal rhythm;
- minimum pain and balanced reversal of sedation (Lu et al. 2016);
- good sleep quality, adequate diaphragm strength and generalized strength, the latter assessed by handgrip strength, absence of abdominal paradox or rapid shallow breathing and adequate cough.

Typical criteria for weaning would be minimum need for sedatives, vasopressors or inotropes, no neuromuscular-blocking drugs, stable cardiovascular status (HR <140, haemoglobin >8 g/100 mL, systolic BP 90–160 mmHg), normal temperature, V$_T$ >5 mL/kg, vital capacity >10 mL/kg, RR <35/min, SpO$_2$ >90% on FiO$_2$ <0.4 (or PaO$_2$/FiO$_2$ >200), PaO$_2$ >8 kPa (60 mmHg) and PaCO$_2$ <8 kPa (60 mmHg), pH >7.30, PEEP <8 cmH$_2$O, maximal inspiratory pressure below −20 to −25 cmH$_2$O and rapid shallow breathing index (RR/ V$_T$) <105 (Zein et al. 2016b).

## Spontaneous Breathing Trial (SBT)

A hot-water humidifier should normally be used because a heat moisture exchanger causes significant airflow resistance (Uchiyama et al. 2013). The patient takes up his or her preferred position (usually sitting upright), suction is applied if required, and spontaneous breathing encouraged, with support from PSV equivalent to spontaneous breathing without the tracheal tube, e.g. 5–8 cmH$_2$O.

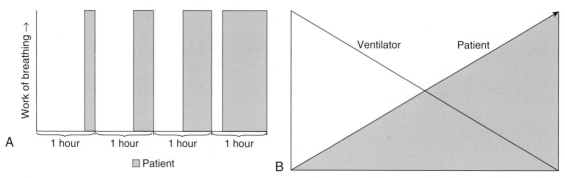

**FIGURE 20.22** (A) Intermittent weaning with periods of complete rest for muscle recovery and periods of maximal work for muscle training. (B) Gradual weaning without periods of rest to replenish the respiratory muscles.

CPAP and T-piece weaning are no longer recommended (Schmidt et al. 2017). T-piece breathing entails connecting high-flow humidified oxygen to the inspiratory limb of a T-piece attached to the tracheal tube. The patient is no longer connected to the bells and whistles of the ventilator for monitoring and it is hard work, especially with an inflated cuff (Ceriana et al. 2006) and can activate the stress response if prolonged (Koksal 2003).

Increasing periods of spontaneous breathing are encouraged (Fig. 20.22A), up to a maximum 2 h (Zein et al. 2016), while questioning the patient to ensure that fatigue is avoided, and observing for laboured breathing, desaturation, rising $PaCO_2$ or drowsiness. Motivation is helped by liberal praise and the 'exercise' part of the process lasting no longer than promised. A dyspnoea visual analogue scale enables patients to contribute to weaning decisions, and they need a 'day off' if a setback such as infection or diarrhoea occurs.

Continuing problems may be due to weaning strategies that provide neither sufficient muscle work nor sufficient rest (Fig. 20.22B), leading to muscle atrophy and/or fatigue. Fatigued muscles cannot be trained, and patients are unable to rest their respiratory muscles as they can other skeletal muscles.

Difficulties may be undetected, e.g. diaphragmatic paralysis, obstructive sleep apnoea or fear of suffocation. Fears are managed by providing information and extra ventilatory support when requested. Patients unable to wean should be referred to a specialist weaning centre (Bonnici et al. 2016).

**PRACTICE TIP**

Patients have reported that their primary experience during weaning is exhaustion (Twibell et al. 2003), which reinforces the importance of taking their views into account throughout.

### Extubation

*'A single, memorable moment of relief'.*
                        ***Karlsson & Forsberg 2008***

Weaning indices are limited as predictors for extubation (Savi et al. 2012) but this is usually feasible if the reason for intubation has been alleviated, there is a stable breathing pattern, the patient can perform an adequate peak cough flow (Su et al. 2010), pressure support level is <12 $cmH_2O$ and PEEP <7 $cmH_2O$.

There should be a leak when the cuff is deflated, indicating adequate patency. Inflammation may cause swelling in the upper airway, which only becomes apparent by the development of stridor after extubation.

Another problem is the haemodynamic decompensation that can occur with removal of PEEP. Loaded spontaneous inspiration, in particular, can lead to increased venous return and possible pulmonary oedema in people with COPD and a cardiac history (Porhomayon et al. 2012). It has been suggested that patients at risk are given 30 min unsupported spontaneous breathing through a T-piece before extubation, to ensure that they can cope with the extra cardiac load (Tobin 2012), but longer than this can risk atelectasis

(Singer & Webb 2009) as well as exhaustion, and other authors have advised maintaining a degree of CPAP for this (Vitacca et al. 2014).

The steps for extubation are described by Cooper et al. (2012) and Chang (2014) p. 179. Reintubation is required in up to 25% of high-risk patients, and is associated with high mortality. This may be avoided by suction and a recruitment manoeuvre before extubation (Craig 2017) or support after extubation with high-flow nasal oxygen (Hernández 2016) or noninvasive ventilation (NIV) (Schmidt et al. 2017). If sputum retention is anticipated, it is sometimes better to request a minitracheotomy than await respiratory distress.

Dysphagia is common and Scheel et al. (2016) found that 22% of patients aspirate after prolonged intubation.

## Decannulation of Tracheostomy

Weaning for tracheostomied patients incorporates an intermediate step of replacing the cuffed with an uncuffed tube (Powell et al. 2011), which is then plugged for increasing periods to test for adequate breathing around the tube, with the inner cannula removed. The tracheostomy tube is not usually downsized because this increases resistance to airflow and increases WOB (Valentini 2012). Adjuncts are a Passy-Muir valve to encourage air flow around the tube (Engels et al. 2009) or intermittent NIV (Pu et al. 2015).

The tube can be removed when there is a satisfactory cough reflex, cough strength and oxygenation, and minimum secretions. Neurological patients require peak cough flow testing (McKim 2012) and sometimes mechanical insufflation–exsufflation.

Once the tube is removed, the patient is taught to hold a sterile dressing over the stoma when coughing. For those leaving the ICU with a tracheostomy, a removable inner tube is essential in case of blockage.

## SUPPORT SYSTEMS

### Oxygen

Oxygen delivered through the ventilator follows the same principles as in Chapter 5. For spontaneously breathing patients, high-flow nasal cannulae demonstrate benefits such as humidification, improved mucociliary clearance, positive pressure generation and alveolar recruitment (Zhang et al. 2016d).

Oxygen has to be closely monitored because there is a direct association between hypoxia and mortality in ventilated patients (Eastwood et al. 2012), but excessive hyperoxaemia causes vasoconstriction and may lead to atelectasis, reduced bacterial clearance and ventilator-associated pneumonia (Six et al. 2016).

### Fluids

- **Dehydration**: intracellular and interstitial water deficit, as shown by a dry tongue and low skin turgor.
- **Hypovolaemia** or **volume depletion**: intravascular fluid depletion, due, for example, to severe dehydration or haemorrhage, sufficient to affect haemodynamic stability.
- **Preload**: pressure of blood in the ventricles just before systole, which stretches the myocardium and assists contraction:
  - determined by venous return and blood volume
  - increased in heart failure or fluid overload, decreased in hypovolaemic shock
  - left preload is monitored by PAWP, right preload by CVP (p. 467).
- **Afterload**: pressure in the aorta/pulmonary artery, against which the ventricles must work during systole, as if opening the door against a wind:
  - increased with systemic/pulmonary hypertension or vasoconstriction, decreased with vasodilation, e.g. with septic or neurogenic shock
  - left ventricular afterload is monitored by systolic BP, right by pulmonary artery pressure.

Fluid imbalance can arise from hypovolaemia, hypervolaemia or normovolaemia with maldistribution of fluid. Blood volume determines preload and is the basis of haemodynamic stability, so an adequate circulating volume is the primary consideration before drugs or other forms of support are provided. Manual hyperinflation and suction are risky in hypovolaemic patients.

Plasma fluid in the intravascular space (Fig. 20.23) is the only fluid compartment accessible therapeutically. Greater than 10% loss of blood volume reduces cardiac output, and more than 20% can reduce BP (Kreimeier 2000). Fluid therapy must be balanced in order to avoid fluid overload or, conversely, allow the kidneys to run dry, and is usually guided by the response of the stroke volume to a fluid bolus. Fluids may be isotonic, hypotonic or hypertonic in relation to plasma, and electrolytes play an integral role. Administered fluids are either crystalloid or colloid, and perfusion-sensitive organs such as the kidney and gut respond differently to diverse fluids (Wu et al. 2015a).

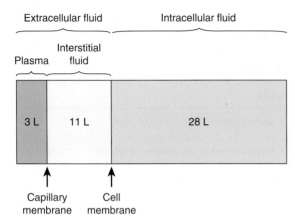

**FIGURE 20.23** Body fluid compartments in an average adult, showing 3 L in blood vessels, 11 L in the interstitial space and the rest in tissue cells.

**Crystalloids** are salt solutions such as dextrose or saline that freely cross capillary walls. They are mostly isotonic (e.g. normal saline) but may be hypotonic (e.g. dextrose in water) or hypertonic (e.g. hypertonic saline). Most infused crystalloid escapes from the vascular space within 30 min (Vercueil et al. 2006). Too much escaped fluid can cause pulmonary oedema, which impairs gas exchange in the lungs, and interstitial oedema, which impairs oxygen delivery into tissue cells. Enthusiastic crystalloid infusion is particularly risky in patients with leaky capillaries, e.g. in multisystem failure, and excess normal saline can upset the kidney and acid–base balance (Li et al. 2016c). Hartmann solution and Ringer-Lactate solution are buffered solutions similar to saline but more closely replicate plasma because they contain lactate, potassium, calcium and bicarbonate.

**Colloids** are thick fluids such as plasma, dextran, gelatins and albumin, which have molecules large enough to exert oncotic pressure across the microvascular membrane so that they are retained in the circulation and stabilize cardiovascular function. Colloids that have an oncotic pressure greater than plasma are called *plasma expanders*, e.g. hypertonic saline-dextran, which allows small-volume resuscitation. Complications of colloids include atelectasis, chest infection, bronchospasm and arrhythmias (Canet et al. 2013). However, the type of fluid used for resuscitation does not appear to affect outcome (Pierce et al. 2016).

## Nutrition

*The combination of nutrition and exercise may have the greatest impact on physical recovery of survivors of critical illness.*

**Heyland et al. 2016**

Nutrition has changed from being an adjunct in critical care to definitive therapy, but malnutrition is common even today, with a direct effect on mortality (Abdelhamid et al. 2016). Undernutrition may be due to a hypermetabolic state, not inadequate calories, but rehabilitation is directly affected, one study showing how extra postoperative nutrition in orthopaedic patients enabled them to be rehabilitated 5 days earlier than controls (Bastow et al. 1983).

### Causes of malnutrition

Many critically ill patients face a cumulative calorie debt during hospitalization because of:

- impaired perfusion to the liver or kidney;
- gut stasis due to critical illness or surgery, leading to reduced food tolerance, malabsorption, reflux or aspiration (Chapman et al. 2011);
- lack of recognition of a process as undramatic as malnourishment;
- lack of a dietician on ward rounds (Soguel et al. 2012);
- the patient's lack of hunger, ability to express hunger or capacity to eat normally;
- systemic inflammation, hypermetabolism or a catabolically stressed state, in which protein reserves are stripped first from skeletal muscle and then from the viscera, at up to 1% of total body protein per day, particularly with burns or acute brain injury (Hill 2011).

### Effects of malnutrition

**Underfeeding** is associated with muscle weakness, increased length of stay (Hill 2011), infection, impaired wound healing and mortality (Merriweather et al. 2014). Of particular interest to the physiotherapist are reduced surfactant predisposing to atelectasis, and reduced albumin leading to pulmonary oedema and muscle weakness (Visser et al. 2005).

**Overfeeding** with carbohydrate can destabilize blood sugar and increase $CO_2$ production, which may precipitate respiratory distress during weaning for patients who have little respiratory reserve (Chang 2014).

**Inappropriate feeding** contributes to oxidative stress, diaphragmatic atrophy and vitamin deficiency (Jaber et al. 2011). 'Refeeding syndrome' is caused by overfeeding after starvation, identified first at the liberation of Auschwitz and recently in the anorexia nervosa population. This can occur 2–5 days after excess nutrients are administered to patients who have been starved for over 48 h, leading to cardiopulmonary or neurological complications (Skipper 2012).

## Management

Malnutrition affects clinical outcomes (Lew et al. 2016) and all patients require nutritional assessment on admission (Rahman et al. 2016), with early nutrition support to reduce the risk of myopathies and aid physical rehabilitation (Confer et al. 2013). Severe illness requires extra protein replenishment, and major surgery or other trauma indicates the need for immunonutrition to strengthen the body's defences and dampen inflammation (Abdelhamid et al. 2016). A stable blood sugar is required with critical illness, particularly sepsis, because of the risk of developing diabetes (Hsu et al. 2016b).

If patients are able, they should sit out of bed and eat orally at normal times, maintaining head and chest elevation at 30 degrees for an hour afterwards. Mastication releases hormones that facilitate gut motility. If patients cannot swallow, direct feeding beyond the stomach is advised because this has shown a 30% lower rate of pneumonia than a gastric tube (Alkhawaja et al. 2015).

The gut is one of the largest immune systems in the body and needs regular bathing in nutrients to maintain its structural and functional integrity. Parenteral feeding leads to atrophy of the gut lining, which may allow intestinal flora access to the systemic circulation, whence to wreak havoc and risk multisystem failure (Anastasilakis et al. 2013). Enteral feeding reduces the risk of infections and length of ICU stay (Elke et al. 2016).

To optimize rehabilitation, nutritional support needs to continue after discharge from the ICU (Merriweather et al. 2014).

## Critical Care Drugs

*'They put that many drugs in to me that I'm tripping, like hallucinating things and I don't know what's what'.*

*Darbyshire et al. 2016*

Infusion pumps are used to titrate drug dosage because:
- some ICU drugs have a narrow window between effective and toxic doses;
- individuals respond differently to complex interactions of multiple drugs;
- physiological processing may be affected by the stress response;
- ICU delirium has been associated with opiates, anticholinergics, antibiotics, steroids and sedatives (Hipp & Ely 2012) so the dosage must be accurate for the balance of risk and benefit;
- drugs may have to rely on a failing organ for processing and excretion.

### Cardiovascular drugs

Cardiac output (CO) depends on heart rate (HR), contractility, preload and afterload. The relationship between heart function, vascular tone and fluid volume can be manipulated to augment CO, reduce myocardial oxygen demand or redistribute blood flow to vital organs. This forms part of 'goal-directed therapy', which is the haemodynamic regulation of oxygen delivery to meet oxygen consumption.

*Diuretics.* Blood volume and preload are reduced by diuretics (p. 139).

*Inotropes.* Inotropes boost cardiac output. Fluid status should first be optimized to ensure adequate preload so that the drug is not stimulating an empty heart. Some inotropes have been called a 'necessary evil' because of their association with neurological complications (Bryan et al. 2013), arrhythmias, hypotension and mortality (Aljundi et al. 2016). They are often given alongside vasodilators to reduce the extra work imposed on the heart.

**Dopamine** activates the same brain mechanism as does falling in love (Xu 2012), but its less agreeable side effect of peripheral vasoconstriction limits its use, although a small 'renal dose' may selectively vasodilate vessels to the vulnerable kidney (Xing et al. 2016). **Dobutamine** gives a greater boost to oxygen delivery, but can cause myocardial damage, tissue hypoxia, bacterial growth and immunosuppression (Singer & Brealey 2011). **Dopexamine** increases renal and splanchnic blood flow and has some antiinflammatory properties (Hollenberg 2013).

**Adrenaline** is a stress hormone that stimulates the sympathetic system and increases the speed and force of cardiac contraction, dilating coronary and skeletal muscle vessels. When given as medication it constricts other vessels and risks organ injury (Tarvasmäki et al. 2016). **Noradrenaline** causes more generalized vasoconstriction.

**Digoxin** is a mild inotrope that has been in and out of fashion for two centuries. It helps control atrial fibrillation by strengthening and slowing the HR, but increases the risk of stroke in some patients (Chang et al. 2013), appears to increase mortality in patients with incident heart failure (Freeman 2013) and in one study was found to be used inappropriately in nearly 60% of patients (Biteker et al. 2016).

*Vasodilators.* Arterial dilators such as hydralazine reduce afterload and are used for hypertension. Venodilators such as the nitrates predominantly reduce preload.

*Vasoconstrictors.* Vasoconstrictors boost BP. High doses can reduce CO and sometimes impair brain and kidney perfusion (Müller et al. 2008).

*Beta-blockers.* Beta-adrenoceptor blocking agents, or β-blockers, have a negative inotropic effect by blocking some heart activity (p. 139). They are also used for anxiety, migraine and glaucoma.

*Pulmonary vasodilators.* **Inhaled nitric oxide** (iNO) has an unpromising history as a corrosive gas in bus exhausts, cigarette smoke and welding fumes, but more helpfully it dilates vessels adjacent to ventilated alveoli and reduces $\dot{V}_A/\dot{Q}$ caused by pulmonary hypertension (Teman et al. 2015). When inhaled, its effects are limited to the pulmonary vasculature because it is inactivated by haemoglobin and is powerless by the time it reaches the systemic circulation. Patients should not be removed from their nitric oxide during physiotherapy. If manual hyperinflation is necessary, the gas can be entrained through a hyperinflation bag, or ventilator hyperinflation can be used. However, many of these patients are critically ill and PEEP-dependent, and manual hyperinflation may be contraindicated.

**Prostacycline** is administered by nebulizer or intravenously and is less toxic than iNO, but it has a half-life of 5 min and is not metabolized by the lung so it can affect the systemic vasculature and cause hypotension.

## Sedatives

*The truth may be that we are transitioning some patients from an unpleasant reality to a terrifying delusion by undermining their ability to rationalize their thoughts as unreal.*

*Intensive Care Society 2014*

Sedation should not be used for the first line management of anxiety or asynchrony with the ventilator, for which explanations or ventilator manipulations are required. Drugs that cloud consciousness cause delusions if anxiety stems from the patient's realistic perception of their situation. Factual memories, even if disagreeable, assist patients to anchor their ICU experience in reality rather than in a fog of confusion and anxiety, with sometimes the legacy of PTSD (ICS 2014a). Sedation blocks conscious but not unconscious memory (Lundeberg 2015), which can cause misinterpretation of events, hallucinations, nightmares, delirium and sleep disturbance (ICS 2014a).

Other side effects include reduced sputum clearance (ICS 2014a), prolonged weaning, pneumonia, hypotension (Gurudatt 2012) and cognitive dysfunction (Porhomayon et al. 2015). These are worsened by early deep sedation, which limits the opportunity for orientation (Balzer et al. 2015), and continuous sedation, which abolishes melatonin secretion (Rittayamai et al. 2016). However, sedation is less damaging than physical restraint, and many sedatives have antiinflammatory properties (ICS 2014a). The optimal dose is that which allows verbal communication (ICS 2014a), and when possible, is controlled by the patient in order to reduce cardiorespiratory adverse effects (Jokelainen et al. 2016). Few sedatives have analgesic properties.

Commonly prescribed anxiolytics are:
- **benzodiazepines** such as diazepam or midazolam, which have a variable half-life and can lead to tolerance (ICS 2014a) or, with heavy dosing, delirium (Fig. 20.24);
- **propofol**, with its advantages of reduced nausea and intracranial pressure, and its disadvantages of diaphragm dysfunction (Bruells et al. 2014), hypotension, respiratory depression (ICS 2014a), risk of aspiration in nonintubated patients (Gemma et al. 2016), suppression of REM sleep and poor sleep quality (Kondili et al. 2012);
- **isoflurane**, which appears to produce better control of sedation than midazolam or propofol (Bellgardt et al. 2016);

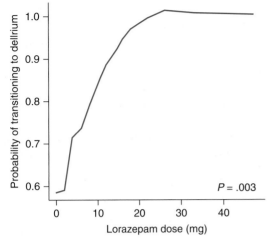

**FIGURE 20.24** Probability of delirium with increasing dose of benzodiazepine. (From Pandharipande et al. 2006.)

- **dexmedetomidine**, which induces analgesia as well as sedation, speeds weaning (Reade et al. 2016), does not cause respiratory depression (Zhao 2015) or sleep disruption (Rittayamai et al. 2016), and shows some neuroprotective effects (Zhang et al. 2016e);
- **ketamine**, which is useful for facilitating painful procedures, and has some bronchodilating effects, but as a sedative can cause hallucinations (ICS 2014a);
- **chlormethiazole**, which can increase bronchial secretions.

Deep sedation can be differentiated from neurological damage by an assay method described by McKenzie et al. (2005).

*'Have I dreamt that or did it happen?'*
**Darbyshire et al. 2016**

## Analgesics

*The principle that patients require more analgesia than sedation is probably not a bad starting point.*
**Intensive Care Society 2014**

Flexible multimodal analgesia is recommended (Vincent et al. 2016). Prior to physiotherapy, a bolus of intravenous analgesia is often indicated, using a short-acting drug such as fentanyl or alfentanil.

## Muscle relaxants

*'You can't scratch your arm if it itches. You can't do nothing. Except lay there in one position. That's very, very uncomfortable'.*
**Jablonski 1994**

Neuromuscular blocking agents are paralysing drugs which are used if communication or deep sedation are inadequate, e.g. to reduce oxygen consumption in hypoxic patients, to prevent patients moving after acute brain injury or, as a last resort, for patients who are resisting ventilation.

These drugs dissociate responsiveness from consciousness and may feel to patients as if they are 'being tied down' (ICS 2014a). They are frightening if patients have not been told that they are receiving a drug that will make them feel weak, and they must not be used as chemical restraints. Patients should be sedated to the point of unrousability beforehand (Oh 2009) and appropriate analgesia administered because muscle relaxants may obliterate the only means by which patients can indicate distress.

Neuromuscular blockade may lead to persistent myopathy (Piriyapatsom et al. 2013), but an unexpected benefit is less painful postoperative suction because patients cannot cough.

## Inhaled drugs

Inhaled bronchodilators are only indicated if there is demonstrable evidence of airflow obstruction, but Ari et al. (2012) found that they are often used in ventilated patients without obstructed airways.

An advantage of inhaled drugs in the ICU is that, in supine patients, distribution is more homogenous than the upright position (Dhanani et al. 2016).

Complications of bronchodilators include:
- tachycardia from $\beta_2$-agonists, leading to haemodynamic compromise in unstable patients;
- disconnection to attach the delivery device, leading to derecruitment, swings in oxygenation and infection risk (Grivans et al. 2009);
- impaction of the inhaled drug on the artificial airway, reducing deposition to an average 2.9% (Kallet 2013).

Benefit should be identified by decreased wheeze on auscultation, reduced peak airway pressure (with VC ventilation), a normalized flow curve (see Fig. 20.31C) or decreased intrinsic PEEP. If improvement is not evident, it is worth removing the inline suction catheter, which may impede delivery, and trying again, before abandoning the drug. People with severe asthma invariably benefit from inhaled bronchodilators, those with COPD often benefit, but those with parenchymal disorders such as ARDS do not (Matthay et al. 2011).

Bronchodilators or steroids can be delivered to ventilated patients by small-volume nebulizer or, for greater efficiency, metered-dose inhaler (Ari et al. 2015b), after removal of any heat–moisture exchanger in the ventilator circuit or removal/bypass of a humidifier (Dhanani et al. 2016). Advantages of nebulizer delivery are near-continuous bronchodilation for status asthmaticus, and no need for coordinated administration with the patient's breath. Disadvantages are that higher doses are needed, along with more equipment and staff time, and there is greater potential for errors and risk of infection than an inhaler (Khoo et al. 2009).

If an inhaler is used, a spacer is required and the following advised (Ari 2015c):
- ensure that the ventilator tidal volume is more than 500 mL and that inspiratory time (excluding the pause) is over a third of the total breath time;
- shake the inhaler;
- insert the canister into the spacer and then into the inspiratory limb of the ventilator circuit (Fig. 20.25);
- fire the inhaler at the onset of inspiration;
- allow passive exhalation;
- repeat after 15- to 60-s intervals or until the total dose is delivered, usually after four puffs;
- leave the spacer in the ventilator circuit, but check that moisture does not accumulate.

Dry powder inhalers cannot be used (AARC 1999b).

A nebulizer should be connected to the inspiratory limb of the circuit, and for tracheostomied patients, after removing the inner cannula. These and many other practical tips, such as decreasing the flow from the ventilator, are described comprehensively by Ari (2015c).

Nebulized antibiotics can show a greater effect than intravenous delivery (Fig. 20.26), but 'very few' ICUs follow the recommendations (Dhanani et al. 2016).

## Advanced Life Support

*'You hear something bleeping and you think what – what's happening, but you couldn't do anything about it'.*

**Darbyshire et al. 2016**

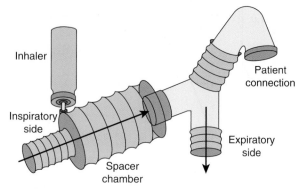

**FIGURE 20.25** Metered-dose inhaler and spacer.

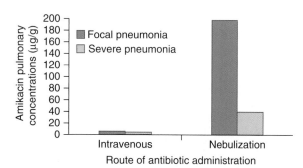

**FIGURE 20.26** Relationship of route of drug administration to lung concentration of antibiotic for different severities of pneumonia. (From Dhanani et al. 2016.)

## Advanced cardiac support

When the heart's conducting pathways are damaged, an artificial **pacemaker** can deliver an electrical stimulus to the heart muscle. For temporary use, pacing wires connect the patient's myocardium to an external pacing box. For permanent support, the energy source is implanted under the skin. Indications are third-degree heart block, arrhythmias refractory to medication, or prophylactic support in the days after heart surgery. Insertion of a permanent pacemaker requires the patient to rest afterwards, the length of time depending on the patient and surgeon.

An implanted **cardioverter defibrillator** recognizes ventricular fibrillation or arrhythmias and delivers corrective defibrillatory discharges for patients at risk. Aerobic training is safe and can improve quality of life (Isaksen et al. 2016).

For hospitalized patients in profound heart failure, for whom vasopressor and inotropic support are inadequate, temporary assistance with an **intraaortic balloon**

damage, embolism and lower limb ischaemia, with a leg amputation rate of 2%–10% (Segesser et al. 2016). Heparinization lessens the risk of thrombosis but increases the risk of bleeding.

Indications for the balloon pump are critically impaired cardiac output, e.g. cardiogenic shock, inability to wean from cardiopulmonary bypass, and occasionally prophylactic use for high-risk surgical patients. As patients recover, assistance is reduced gradually from every beat (1:1) to every 8th beat (1:8).

Implications for physiotherapy are the following:
1. The augmented BP should be monitored throughout.
2. With a femoral catheter, hip flexion should be avoided on the cannulated side, and sitting up is limited.
3. If the patient is stable enough for turning, care is required to avoid disconnection of the cannula.
4. If manual hyperinflation is necessary, cardiac output should be closely monitored.
5. Manual percussion or vibrations are unwise because of interference with the ECG, and mechanical percussors and vibrators are contraindicated. If vibrations are needed, a supporting hand under the patient minimizes movement.
6. Coughing should be avoided for 4–6 h after removal of a femoral catheter, to prevent pressure on the healing femoral artery.

A **ventricular assist device** is a supplementary pump implanted in the abdomen and used for permanent circulatory support or as a bridge to recovery or transplantation. Precautions for physiotherapy relate to the complications of bleeding or thrombosis.

### Advanced pulmonary support

**Liquid ventilation** emerged as a concept in the First World War, when it was found that gas-poisoned lungs tolerated large quantities of saline lavage. It is now used in neonates to eliminate the gas–liquid interface in dependent lung regions, which are most susceptible to collapse, and sometimes in adults with ARDS to prevent further damage to alveoli and dampening inflammation (Cao et al. 2016b).

A heavy inert liquid called perfluorocarbon, through which the patient is able to breathe, fills the lungs to FRC, eliminating surface tension, reducing ventilatory pressures and recruiting dependent alveoli by a 'liquid PEEP' effect. Radioopacity makes densities such as consolidation undetectable on X-ray, although pneumothoraces are crystal clear. Mucus cannot mix with

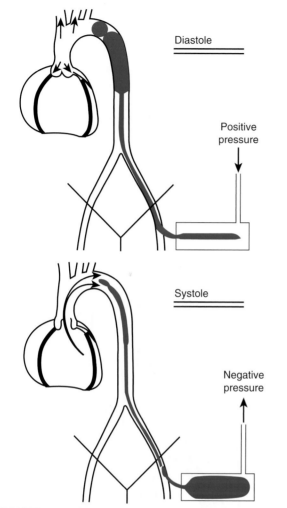

**FIGURE 20.27** Intraaortic balloon pump system. (From Collier & Dohoo 1980.)

**pump** provides mechanical support for cardiac output. The pump is connected to a catheter with a deflated balloon at its tip. This is threaded through the femoral or radial artery and up into the aorta (Fig. 20.27), from where it is triggered by the heart's own electrical activity. Diastole triggers balloon inflation, which assists aortic valve closure and diverts blood to the myocardium, increasing cardiac output by up to 40% (Macauley 2012). In systole, the balloon deflates, decreasing afterload and assisting cardiac output (Fig. 20.28).

The effect is similar to combined inotropic and vasodilator therapy, increasing myocardial perfusion and reducing workload. Complications include vascular

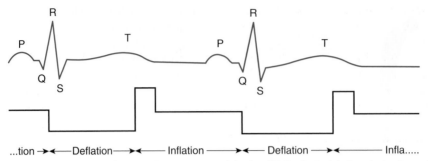

**FIGURE 20.28** Synchrony of the balloon pump with the ECG. *P,* Atrial depolarization; *Q,* ventricular depolarization; *R,* first positive deflection during ventricular depolarization; *S,* first negative deflection during ventricular depolarization; *T,* ventricular repolarization (recovery period). (From Parissis et al. 2016.)

perfluorocarbon and tends to float on top, from where it can be debrided by saline lavage. Normal suction is forbidden.

### Advanced cardiopulmonary support

For severe but potentially reversible cardiopulmonary failure, extracorporeal gas exchange acts as a form of cardiopulmonary bypass and buys time for an injured lung to recover.

**Extracorporeal membrane oxygenation** (ECMO) supports cardiorespiratory function via cannulae connected to a circuit that pumps blood through an oxygenator and then back into the patient, either into the arterial system (venoarterial [VA] circuit) or venous system (venovenous [VV] circuit). The VA system requires 80% of the cardiac output to be drained, pumped, oxygenated, rewarmed and returned to the internal carotid artery, with $CO_2$ transferring back as a secondary effect (Fig. 20.29). The VV system relies on some heart function and requires 20% of the circulating volume to be outside the body at one time, removing desaturated blood from the vena cava, oxygenating it outside the body and returning it to the venous system.

ECMO is well-established in specialist neonatal units, though there is concern about neurological damage from cannulation of the carotid artery. For adults with ARDS, it may be used to facilitate low-volume, low-pressure ultraprotective mechanical ventilation (Fanelli et al. 2016) but acute kidney injury is a risk. Renal replacement therapy can be integrated into the main extracorporeal circuit (Villa et al. 2015).

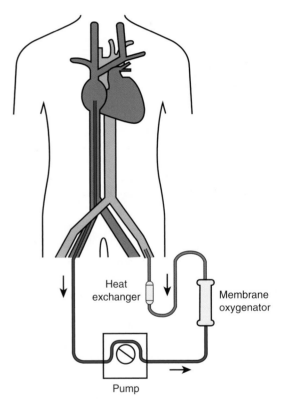

**FIGURE 20.29** Extracorporeal membrane oxygenation via venoarterial circuit. Venous blood passes through a membrane oxygenator to substitute for lung function and a pump to substitute for heart function, then returns to the arterial system.

Implications for physiotherapy are the following:

1. Reliance cannot be placed on auscultation because of the reduced ventilation.
2. Physiotherapy is not likely to cause hypoxaemia because oxygenation is maintained outside the lungs.
3. Analgesic doses should be increased to compensate for loss of the drug through the circuit (Shekar et al. 2012).
4. Bleeding during suction is a risk if there is not tight heparin control.
5. Mobilization is feasible (Abrams & Brodie 2016) but the ECMO cannulae require careful handling and a technician should stand by in case the machinery needs attention.

Mobilization is extra important if ECMO is being used as a bridge to lung transplantation (Rahimi et al. 2013), and brings the added benefit of reducing costs (Bain et al. 2016).

Support systems such as haemodialysis, plasmapheresis and surfactant replacement are discussed with the relevant pathologies.

# MONITORING

*'Frankly it feels quite awful to be connected to machines through every available orifice, plus several new medically made ones, in spite of feeling thankful for all the life-sustaining help and healing ministrations'.*

**Brooks 1990**

Monitoring differs from measuring: it implies regular observation and a systematic response if there is deviation from a specified range. It is complementary to clinical observation and is necessary to record sudden or subtle changes in a patient's status. False alarms are frequent and can lead to 'crying-wolf syndrome' (Zong et al. 2016).

## Ventilator Waveforms

The relationship between patient effort and mechanical support is represented by pressure, volume and flow, measured relative to their values at end-expiration (Fig. 20.30). Pressure levels are relative to PEEP, volume is measured as lung volume above FRC, and flow is measured relative to its end-expiratory value. Details are described in Cairo 2012, p. 148, Chang 2014, p. 309, or the ventilator manufacturer's handbook. The following is an outline.

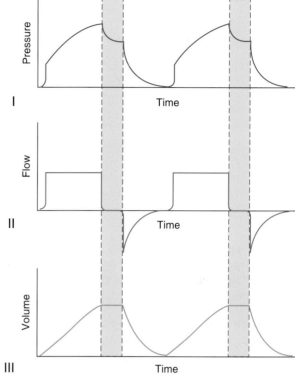

**FIGURE 20.30** Pressure, flow and volume waveforms, with the end-inspiratory hold shaded. (From Mellema 2015.)

The **pressure time curve** shows pressures throughout the respiratory cycle (see Figs 20.6–20.9) and is useful when volume control is used. Peak airway pressure (peak inspiratory pressure) is the highest pressure. This settles down to the end-inspiratory 'plateau pressure', termed 'inflation hold' or 'inspiratory pause' on some ventilators, and reflects alveolar pressure. Mean airway pressure is represented by the space under the curve and is associated positively with oxygenation and negatively with the haemodynamic side effects of MV.

The **flow time curve** is useful to verify the presence of intrinsic PEEP, as shown by inadequate expiratory time, and the effect of bronchodilators (Fig. 20.31). Both curves can identify asynchrony (Ramire et al. 2017).

## Gas Exchange

Each step of the oxygen cascade can be monitored, as described in the following section for gas exchange in the lungs and on p. 471 for oxygen delivery to the tissues.

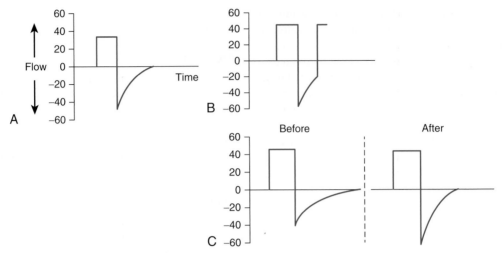

**FIGURE 20.31** Flow–time curves. (A) Normal inspiratory flow above the line and normal expiration below. (B) Intrinsic PEEP, as indicated by expiratory flow not returning to zero before the next inspiration begins. (C) Before and after bronchodilation, shown as prolonged and then normal expiratory flow.

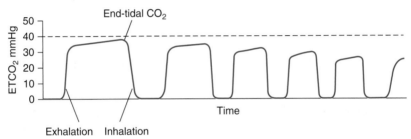

**FIGURE 20.32** Capnography waveform, with $ETCO_2$ plotted against time during progressive hyperventilation.

**Arterial blood gas** measurements (p. 14) are taken continually from an indwelling arterial catheter rather than by intermittent arterial puncture.

**Arterial oxygen saturation** ($SaO_2$) is also monitored continuously, using pulse oximetry ($SpO_2$). If desaturation occurs during physiotherapy, treatment should normally stop and the '100% oxygen' button on the ventilator activated. If $SpO_2$ does not return to its baseline within a minute, remedial action should be taken such as repositioning the patient, increasing $FiO_2$, or initiating manual hyperventilation or suction. An ear probe or forehead sensor may be used if there is low cardiac output or poor perfusion, and in the most severely ill patients there may be discrepancy between $SaO_2$ and $SpO_2$.

**PRACTICE TIP**

Physiotherapists may need to activate the '100% oxygen' facility throughout treatment.

**Capnography** is the measurement of inspired and expired $CO_2$ concentration and should be provided for all ventilated patients (ICS 2014b). Exhaled end-tidal $CO_2$ ($ETCO_2$) continuously assesses the adequacy of ventilation (Fig. 20.32) via a sensor between the tracheal tube and ventilator tubing. It shows good correlation with $PaCO_2$ (Overbeck 2016), the normal value being 1 mmHg below, with an acceptable range of up to 5 mmHg difference. Values decrease during manual hyperinflation because this usually incorporates hyperventilation.

**Transcutaneous monitoring** ($PtcO_2$ and $PtcCO_2$) measures oxygen and $CO_2$ noninvasively as they diffuse through the skin, using a heated sensor to increase gas permeability across the skin barrier. Measurements vary with cardiac output and capillary blood flow, but $PtcCO_2$ is more accurate than $ETCO_2$ and can be used to monitor hypercapnic patients at night (Stieglitz et al. 2016). Neonates show good correlation with arterial measurements, but adults have varying skin thicknesses and results are less reliable.

## Haemodynamic Monitoring

*'They would come round and fiddle with things behind you, but you couldn't see what was there and you weren't actually told what was there'.*

**Darbyshire et al. 2016**

The heart and vascular systems act as a continuous loop in which pressure gradients keep the blood moving. In many patients, cardiovascular function can be gauged from BP, HR, urine output and mental status, but these may be unreliable in critical illness, and invasive monitoring is then required to identify vascular pressures and assume volumes. These can be affected by varying degrees of hypovolemia, left and right ventricular dysfunction, abnormalities of vascular tone, and microvascular dysfunction.

### Fluid status

The term 'resuscitation' in the ICU usually relates to fluid resuscitation. Haemodynamic stability depends on the volume and responsiveness of intravascular fluids, especially during and after surgery and in the 'golden hour' after trauma. Fluid volume in the vasculature affects all aspects of the haemodynamic system, i.e. HR, BP, cardiac output, left and right atrial pressures (below), and, representing the kidney's sensitivity to perfusion, urine output. Fluids in the interstitial and intracellular spaces are more difficult to assess, but dehydration is suggested by thirst and dry mucous membranes, and overhydration may cause increased weight and peripheral/pulmonary oedema. Fluid balance is monitored by the fluid chart, weight change, electrolyte concentration or fluid responsiveness, measured by stroke volume variation, pulse pressure variation or passive leg raising, which transfers venous blood from the lower body towards the right heart (Monnet & Teboul 2015).

### Blood pressure

A continuous BP display is provided by an arterial line in the radial, femoral or brachial artery, so long as the transducer is in line with the patient's heart, and the line is not kinked, as represented by a dampened trace on the monitor. The most relevant reading is mean arterial pressure, which represents perfusion pressure over the cardiac cycle.

### Cardiac output (CO)

Reduced urine output may be the first indication of impaired CO. Monitoring is by invasive and noninvasive methods such as arterial pulse waveform analysis (Sawa et al. 2016), which is integrated with physical examination and vital signs. Cardiac output usually reflects BP, but peripheral vasoconstriction may maintain BP in the face of a falling CO. Conversely, a septic patient in a hyperdynamic state may have a high CO but vasodilation reduces BP.

### Central venous pressure (CVP)

An extension of the patient's vascular system is created by passing a radio-opaque catheter through a large central vein, usually via the neck or arm, until it is in the superior vena cava just outside the right atrium. All venous blood passes through this system, and the pressure within it (the CVP) reflects right atrial pressure (RAP), which indicates the preload of the right ventricle. CVP is a pressure but relates to circulating blood volume and the ability of the heart to handle that volume. It is similar to the jugular venous pressure and is affected by the interaction between blood volume, right heart function, peripheral venous tone, posture and the pressure changes of breathing, thus limiting its utility. High-pressure MV or high PEEP levels increase intrathoracic pressure, leading to higher CVP readings, but the trend is still relevant.

Single values are less pertinent than the trend, but a high value might indicate heart failure, pulmonary embolism, COPD, pneumothorax or overtransfusion of fluid. The CVP also provides early warning of cardiac tamponade, which causes a sudden rise in CVP, or haemorrhage, which causes a sudden drop. CVP is more sensitive to haemorrhage than BP because arterial pressure can be maintained for longer by vasoconstriction.

Numerous functions are serviced by multilumen catheters in a central vein, infusing fluids, drugs, blood and nutrition while maintaining continuous pressure monitoring. Thick hyperosmolar feeds are needed for patients who need nutrition without too much volume, and these require central rather than peripheral veins for delivery.

Implications for physiotherapy are the following:

1. Cannulation of a large vein near the pleura may cause a pneumothorax, haemothorax or subcutaneous emphysema. After placement of a central line, the X-ray should be examined before positive pressure treatments such as manual hyperinflation.

2. A high CVP may indicate pulmonary oedema, which impairs gas exchange. A low CVP may indicate hypovolaemia, which can lead to adverse haemodynamic responses to positioning, manual hyperinflation or suction.

## Pulmonary artery wedge pressure (PAWP)

The CVP usually reflects filling pressures for both sides of the heart. However, left atrial pressure may need to be measured separately because:

• it takes time for the CVP to rise in response to left ventricular failure because the pressure has to back up through the pulmonary circulation, and the right ventricle may initially compensate;

• the CVP does not reflect left atrial pressure if the compliance of either ventricle is affected by septic shock, ischaemia, vasopressors or vasodilators;

• the CVP does not reflect left atrial pressure if pulmonary hypertension pushes up the CVP while the patient is systemically hypovolaemic.

To measure left atrial pressure, a balloon-tipped pulmonary artery catheter is used, sometimes called a Swan-Ganz. It is passed along the CVP catheter route, then swishes through the right ventricle into the pulmonary artery, assisted by the inflated balloon at its tip. Here it measures pulmonary artery pressure (PAP), which reflects the pressure that needs to be generated by the right ventricle to pump blood through the pulmonary vasculature. A raised PAP indicates pulmonary hypertension, pulmonary embolism or fluid overload.

The catheter is then carried into ever smaller pulmonary vessels until it becomes wedged (Fig. 20.33).

Once wedged, the catheter tip is isolated from pressure fluctuations in the right side of the heart and is in communication with the left atrium via the pulmonary capillary bed, so long as there is a continuous column of blood between the two (Fig. 20.34). The pressure monitored at this point is the PAWP or left atrial pressure, reflecting pressure in the left atrium via the lung vasculature. The balloon acts as a form of pulmonary embolus so is deflated when not needed.

The continuous column of blood in the pulmonary vascular bed is tenuous if the catheter is in the upper zone of the lung (p. 13) where there may be no perfusion under the positive pressure of MV. Measurements are also affected by position change, hypovolaemia, high inflation pressures from the ventilator,

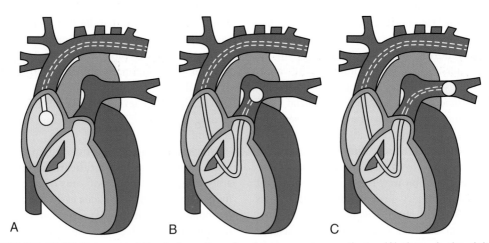

**FIGURE 20.33** Passage of the balloon-tipped pulmonary artery catheter (A) through the right atrium, (B) into the pulmonary artery and (C) wedged into the pulmonary vasculature.

valve stenosis floppy ventricles following serial myocardial infarction or sepsis, or stiff ventricles following sympathetic stimulation caused by hypovolaemic shock. The more ill the patient, the less accurate are single measurements.

PAWP can also calculate cardiac output and systemic vascular resistance, allow fine tuning when establishing

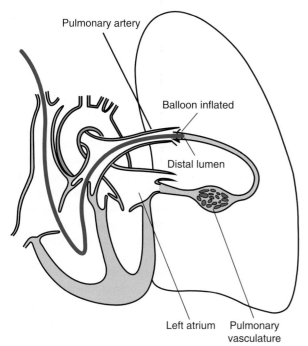

FIGURE 20.34 Pulmonary artery catheter wedged into a branch of the pulmonary artery, where it is isolated from pressure in the right side of the heart and now transmits pressure from the left atrium.

optimum PEEP, help to rationalize fluid and drug therapy, and distinguish hypovolaemia (↓ PAWP) from left ventricular failure (↑ PAWP). Implications for physiotherapy are similar to those with CVP.

PAWP is also known as pulmonary artery occlusion pressure, pulmonary capillary wedge pressure or, on ward rounds, simply wedge pressure. Noninvasive measurements are becoming available, thus reducing the complications of vascular catheters such as thrombosis, sepsis, arrhythmias, air embolism, trauma to the delicate pulmonary vessels (resulting in blood stained secretions) and pulmonary ischaemia or infarction. It has been claimed that these catheters are associated with no improvement for patients, and, in some studies, worse patient outcomes (Durbin 2016).

Table 20.2 compares vascular pressures for different conditions.

## Electrocardiography (ECG)

Disturbances such as hypoxia, physiotherapy, electrolyte imbalance, anxiety or myocardial ischaemia can cause disorders of heart rate (HR) or rhythm. The effects are significant if they affect cardiac output (CO). They are picked up on the ECG (Fig. 20.35), which represents electrical activity in the heart, recorded from the body surface and comprising waves, complexes and intervals.

**Sinus rhythm** is normal heart rhythm originating from the sinoatrial (SA) node. Supraventricular arrhythmias originate from above or in the atrioventricular (AV) node and are known as atrial or nodal dysrhythmias respectively. **Sinus tachycardia,** or **supraventricular tachycardia,** is HR over 100 beats/min, recognized by a rapid rate, regular rhythm and normal QRS

| TABLE 20.2 | Vascular pressures | | |
|---|---|---|---|
| | **CVP** | **PAP** | **PAWP** |
| Normal | 0–8 mmHg | Systolic 15–30 Diastolic 4–12 | 2–15 mmHg |
| Advanced COPD | ↑ | ↑ ↑↑ during sleep | N |
| ARDS | N (but manipulated by treatment) | ↑ | N (but manipulated by treatment) |
| Hypervolaemia | ↑ | ↑ | ↑ |
| Hypovolaemia | ↓ | ↓ | ↓ |
| Pulmonary oedema/LVF | ↑ | ↑ | ↑ (>20 mmHg) |
| Right-sided heart failure | ↑ | ↓ | ↓ |

*ARDS,* Acute respiratory distress syndrome; *COPD,* chronic obstructive pulmonary disease; *CVP,* central venous pressure; *LVF,* left ventricular failure; *N,* normal; *PAP,* pulmonary artery pressure; *PAWP,* pulmonary artery wedge pressure.

complex. Causes include sympathetic activity, electrolyte imbalance or excess $\beta_2$-agonist medication. CO is rarely compromised. **Sinus bradycardia** is HR under 60 bpm with normal rhythm. **Ventricular tachycardia** is distinguished from supraventricular tachycardia by a lost P wave and a broad and bizarre QRS complex. It usually impairs CO, BP and tissue perfusion, and can lead to pulmonary oedema or ventricular fibrillation.

**Nodal rhythm** occurs when the AV node takes over from a nonfunctioning or slow SA node. This causes lost P waves and a variable or absent PR interval. CO may fall because atrial contraction is out of synchrony with the ventricle, which loses its atrial kick.

The SA node is the natural pacemaker, but if it does not initiate an impulse at correct intervals, an ectopic (abnormal) focus outside the SA node may take the initiative. These 'ectopics' are seen as premature beats followed by a compensatory pause, sometimes felt as missed heart beats by the patient. They are common and do not contraindicate physiotherapy unless they increase in number or cause haemodynamic disturbance. However, they may signal the onset of more significant arrhythmias.

**Atrial ectopics** manifest as occasional abnormal P waves or an early normal beat, and are of little significance unless frequent. **Ventricular ectopics** are caused by an irritable focus in the ventricle, producing an absent P wave, wide and wayward QRS complex and inverted T wave. They occur in smokers, in those who have hypoxia or low potassium, or following heart surgery or myocardial infarction (MI). **Bigeminy** means that every other heart beat is ectopic, and **trigeminy** means that every third beat is ectopic.

**ST segment elevation** suggests pericarditis, coronary artery spasm or MI which will respond to thrombolytic drugs. **ST segment depression** indicates myocardial ischaemia or infarction which is unresponsive to thrombolytic therapy.

**Atrial fibrillation** (AF) occurs when ectopic foci throughout the atria discharge too fast for the atrial muscle to respond other than by disorganized twitching out of sequence with ventricular activity. It appears as a rapid rate, irregular rhythm and the replacing of P waves with a chaotic baseline (Fig. 20.36A). It may

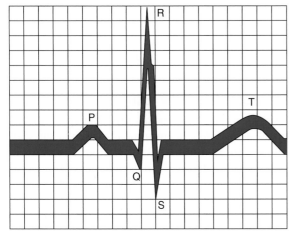

**FIGURE 20.35** Normal ECG trace of one heart beat. *P wave,* Atrial depolarization; *PR interval,* atrioventricular conduction time; *Q,* ventricular depolarization; *QRS complex,* total ventricular depolarization; *R,* first positive deflection during ventricular depolarization; *S,* first negative deflection during ventricular depolarization; *T,* ventricular repolarization (recovery period).

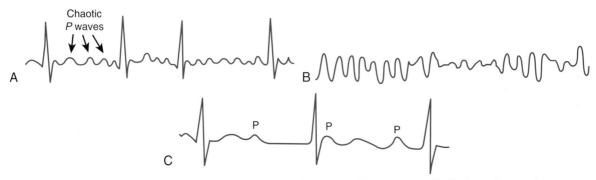

**FIGURE 20.36** ECG traces indicating (A) atrial fibrillation, (B) ventricular fibrillation, (C) complete (third-degree) heart block. *P,* Atrial depolarization.

be triggered by sympathetic stimulation, hypoxia, overhydration or underhydration, theophylline toxicity, pulmonary embolism, low potassium or magnesium levels, myocardial ischaemia, heart surgery, heart failure or advanced age. The ventricles may be unable to sustain normal CO. Patients may have no symptoms or they may suffer palpitations, dyspnoea, fatigue, angina, hypotension or stroke. Treatment is by correction of the cause when possible, conversion to sinus rhythm using antiarrhythmic drugs, or cardioversion by DC shock. Slow AF does not contraindicate physiotherapy.

**Atrial flutter** is less common than AF and is short lived. It causes regular sawtooth undulations on the ECG, and either deteriorates to AF or spontaneously recovers.

**Ventricular fibrillation** (VF) is the commonest cause of cardiac arrest. Breakdown of ordered electrical activity causes an ineffectual quivering of the ventricles, appearing as a chaotic line and providing no CO (Fig. 20.36B). **Asystole** is ventricular standstill, i.e. cardiac arrest. It is caused by VF which has burnt itself out, or a bradyarrhythmia that grinds to a halt. It shows as a straight line with occasional minor fluctuations. VF and asystole can be misdiagnosed when similar traces are produced by manual techniques to the chest or disconnected electrodes respectively.

**Heart block** (HB) is an anatomic or functional interruption in the conduction of an impulse, shown as a disrupted relationship between the P wave and QRS complex. Causes are hypoxia, MI, digoxin therapy, heart disease or complications from heart surgery. First-degree HB shows a prolonged PR interval, but there are no symptoms or need for treatment. Second-degree HB shows dropped beats, and if it causes dizziness, fainting or reduced CO, a pacemaker is required. In third-degree HB, atrial and ventricular rhythms are independent of one another (Fig. 20.36C). This requires a pacemaker to avoid a form of syncope called a Stokes Adams attack. **Bundle branch block** disturbs intraventricular conduction and widens the QRS complex.

Changes in rhythm that occur during physiotherapy indicate that treatment should be stopped until it settles or until action is taken by the team to stabilize it.

## Tissue Oxygenation

Oxygen delivery to the tissues ($DO_2$) relates to $SpO_2$ and CO, with contributions from haemoglobin and blood vessel integrity.

## Mixed venous oxygenation ($S\overline{v}O_2$)

Directly related to patient outcome is the oxygen saturation of haemoglobin in the pulmonary artery ($S\overline{v}O_2$), which indicates the amount of oxygen left in the blood at the end of its journey. It reflects the extent to which oxygen supply (CO, haemoglobin and $SpO_2$) meets demand (oxygen extraction at tissue level), thus including both haemodynamic and gas exchange components of the oxygen cascade.

The oxygen saturation of venous blood leaving different organs varies, but the mixed venous blood in the pulmonary artery comprises an average of the individual streams from a multitude of capillary beds that, having been mixed further in the right ventricle, now return to the lungs for refuelling (Fig. 20.37). Although in the pulmonary artery, it is venous blood because it has given up all the oxygen required for metabolism.

$S\overline{v}O_2$ values are on average 65%–75%, and should be more than 10% below $SpO_2$ to show that oxygen has been delivered to the tissues.

A low $S\overline{v}O_2$ suggests:
- ↓ $DO_2$, e.g. from suction, anaemia, low CO or hypoxaemia
- ↑ $\dot{V}O_2$ (oxygen consumption), e.g. from agitation, anxiety, laboured breathing Fig. 20.38), suction, excess exercise in a compromised patient, pain, fever or hypermetabolic states.

$S\overline{v}O_2$ does not pinpoint which variable is responsible for any change, and is increased by a high $PaO_2$ (Ho 2016) so acts more as an early warning system. Cardiac output and $SpO_2$ are simultaneously monitored in order to identify their contributions.

Values below 50% are associated with anaerobic metabolism, and those below 40% are incompatible with life. People with chronic heart failure are more tolerant of low levels. Excessively high values above 85% are, paradoxically, not a good sign. This 'luxury perfusion' means that sepsis has released inflammatory mediators that have damaged the microvasculature so that capillary beds are bypassed and oxygen not supplied to the tissues (Tánczos 2013).

$S\overline{v}O_2$ can be improved by increasing $FiO_2$ or CO, reducing stress, or addressing other factors hindering $DO_2$. During physiotherapy, if $S\overline{v}O_2$ varies by more than 10% from baseline for more than 3 minutes, treatment should be stopped (Hayden 1993).

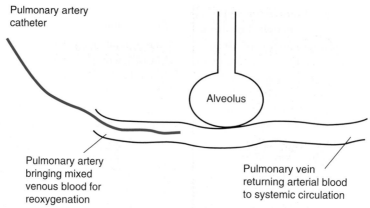

FIGURE 20.37 Measurement of oxygen saturation of haemoglobin in mixed venous blood via the pulmonary artery catheter.

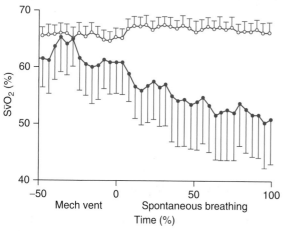

FIGURE 20.38 S$\bar{v}O_2$ during successful *(open symbols, top)* and unsuccessful *(closed symbols, bottom)* weaning. (From Tobin 2000.)

## Central venous oxygenation (ScvO₂)

Oxygen in blood from the vena cava represents central venous oxygenation, which reads slightly higher than S$\bar{v}O_2$, with normal values at 73%–82% (Kocsi et al. 2012). Both S$\bar{v}O_2$ and ScvO₂ show significant variability among patients (Squara 2015).

## Cerebral oximetry

Monitoring the brain noninvasively by cerebral oximetry has shown improved outcomes in both neurologic and major organ morbidity (Moerman & De Hert 2015).

## CASE STUDY: MR FA

*Identify the problems of this patient from London who collapsed in the emergency department, requiring intubation and ventilation.*

### Relevant medical history

- Alcoholism
- Epilepsy

### On examination

- On SIMV and PSV with 5 cmH₂O PEEP
- Heavily sedated
- Stable

### Questions

1. Auscultation and percussion note (Fig. 20.39A)?
2. Analysis?
3. Problems?
4. Goals?
5. Precaution?
6. Plan?
7. Passive movements?
8. Outcome (Fig. 20.39B)?

### CLINICAL REASONING

'Chest physiotherapy may cause cardiac arrhythmias, bronchospasm, and transient hypoxemia, and may prolong the duration of mechanical ventilation [references 126–128].'

*Crit Care* (2008) 12(2): 209

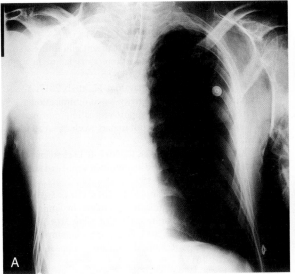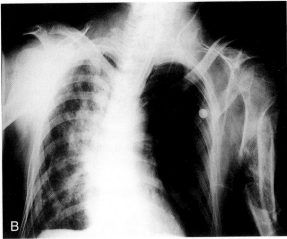

**FIGURE 20.39** (A) Mr FA before physiotherapy, (B) Mr FA after physiotherapy.

## Response to Case Study

1. Auscultation and percussion note
   - Absent breath sounds on right, percussion note dull on right.
2. Analysis
   - Patient collapse probably due to a seizure.
   - Fig. 20.32A suggests aspiration to right lung, which subsequently collapsed.
   - Possible alcohol intake increased the risk of aspiration.
3. Problem
   - Patient has loss of lung volume on the right.
4. Goals
   - Short term: restore functioning lung volume
   - Medium term: mobilize
   - Long term: team management of follow-up support and rehabilitation
5. Precaution
   - No head-down postural drainage due to recent seizure.
6. Plan
   Review radiologist report in case of hidden rib fractures due to fall. If all clear:

   - Optimize analgesia
   - Position in left side-lying
   - Manual hyperinflation
   - Percussion and vibrations
   - Suction
   Continue until breath sounds are clear, adding saline instillation if required.
7. Passive movements
   - Unsafe until patient is able to report pain and orthopaedic team has assessed fractured left humerus, head of right humerus and right clavicle (fractures were identified by a student physiotherapist and not picked up by the ICU medical team, indicating the problems of the 'medical model' approach, and the importance of physiotherapists taking responsibility for the safety of their treatments). Fractures turned out to be old and pain free, and were nonunited due to malnutrition related to alcoholism.
8. Outcome
   - Fig. 20.39B: short- and medium-term goals achieved.
   - Long-term goal: patient agreed to alcohol and physical rehabilitation.

## RESPONSE TO CLINICAL REASONING

Ref. 126 – Cardiac arrhythmias during postural drainage and chest percussion of critically ill patients. *Chest* (1992) 102: 1836–1841.

- The authors persuaded their physical therapists to treat haemodynamically unstable patients who had pulmonary emboli, pulmonary oedema and ARDS (none of which are hypersecretory disorders) using head-down postural drainage and 10 min of percussion (described as 'a chest thump given to convert asystole'). The outcome, unsurprisingly, was further haemodynamic instability. This is an oft-quoted study 'proving' the dangers of physiotherapy in the ICU.

Ref. 127 – Chest physiotherapy. *BMJ* (1989) 298: 541–542.

- This did not relate to ventilated patients.

Ref. 128 – Chest physiotherapy prolongs duration of ventilation in the critically ill ventilated for more than 48 h. *Int Care Med* (2007) 33(11): 1938–1945.

- This study compared patients who did and did not receive physiotherapy. 'Physiotherapy' was not standardized and included undefined 'respiratory muscle exercise'.
- Half the control patients required 'rescue physiotherapy', thus invalidating the results and, incidentally, showing the benefit of physiotherapy.
- The value of physiotherapy was confirmed by more patients in the control group being reventilated or dying, but this was noted quietly in a Table in the article and not discussed in the text.
- 'Overwhelming illness' was described as a contraindication for 'physiotherapy', without either being defined.
- The authors could not spell 'physiotherapist'.

## RECOMMENDED READING

ACCCM, 2013. Clinical practice guidelines for the management of pain, agitation, and delirium in adult patients in the intensive care unit. Crit. Care Med. 41 (1), 263–306.

Ari, A., Harwood, R., Sheard, M., et al., 2016. Quantifying aerosol delivery in simulated spontaneously breathing patients with tracheostomy using different humidification systems with or without exhaled humidity. Respir. Care 61 (5), 600–606.

Aubron, C., 2017. Is platelet transfusion associated with hospital-acquired infections in critically ill patients? Crit. Care 21, 2.

Ball, L., Sutherasan, Y., Caratto, V.C., et al., 2016. Effects of nebulizer position, gas flow, and CPAP on aerosol bronchodilator delivery. Respir. Care 61 (3), 263–268.

Bartlett, R.H., Deatrick, K.B., 2016. Current and future status of extracorporeal life support for respiratory failure in adults. Curr. Opin. Crit. Care 22 (1), 80–85.

Beloncle, F., Piquilloud, L., Rittayamai, N., et al., 2017. A diaphragmatic electrical activity-based optimization strategy during pressure support ventilation improves synchronization but does not impact work of breathing. Crit. Care 21 (1), 21.

Binks, A.P., Desjardin, S., Riker, R., 2017. ICU clinicians underestimate breathing discomfort in ventilated subjects. Respir. Care 62 (2), 150–155.

Broyles, L.M., Tate, J.A., Happ, M.B., 2012. Use of augmentative and alternative communication strategies by family members in the intensive care unit. Am. J. Crit. Care 21, e21–e32.

Calzia, E., Dembinski, R., 2013. Preserving spontaneous breathing during mechanical ventilatory support. Crit. Care 17 (6), 1013.

Castillo, M.I., Cooke, M., Macfarlane, B., et al., 2016. Factors associated with anxiety in critically ill patients. Int. J. Nurs. Stud. 60, 225–233.

Credland, N., 2016. How to remove an endotracheal tube. Nurs. Stand. 30 (36), 31–33.

De Prost, N., 2013. Effects of ventilation strategy on distribution of lung inflammatory cell activity. Crit. Care 17, R175.

Dermitzaki, D., Tzortzaki, E., Soulitzis, N., et al., 2013. Molecular response of the human diaphragm on different modes of mechanical ventilation. Respiration 85 (3), 228–235.

Duan, J., Han, X., Huang, S., et al., 2016. Noninvasive ventilation for avoidance of reintubation in patients with various cough strength. Crit. Care 20, 316.

Flaatten, H., 2014. The impact of age in intensive care. Acta Anaesthesiol. Scand. 58 (1), 3–4.

Fodor, G.H., Babik, B., Czövek, D., et al., 2016. Fluid replacement and respiratory function. Eur. J. Anaesthesiol. 33, 34–41.

Gardner, A.J., Griffiths, J., 2014. Propranolol, post-traumatic stress disorder, and intensive care. Crit. Care 18, 698.

Gingell, E., Rushton, C.Y., 2012. Ethics in critical care: preventive ethics in the intensive care unit. AACN Adv. Crit. Care 23 (2), 217–224.

Gunst, J., Van den Berghe, G., 2017. Parenteral nutrition in the critically ill. Curr. Opin. Crit. Care 23 (2), 149–158.

Gunther, A.C., 2013. Palmar skin conductance variability and the relation to stimulation, pain and the motor activity assessment scale in intensive care unit patients. Crit. Care 17, R51.

Haas, C.F., Bauser, K.A., 2010. Advanced ventilator modes and techniques. Crit. Care Nurs. Q. 35 (1), 27–38.

Henderson, W.R., Sheel, A.W., 2012. Pulmonary mechanics during mechanical ventilation. Respir. Physiol. Neurobiol. 180 (2-3), 162–172.

Ho, K.M., 2016. Pitfalls in haemodynamic monitoring in the postoperative and critical care setting. Anaesth. Intensive Care 44 (1), 14–19.

Hsieh, E., 2014. Management of autism in the adult intensive care unit. J. Intensive Care Med. 29 (1), 47–52.

Huang, H., Xu, B., Liu, G., 2017. Use of noninvasive ventilation in immunocompromised patients with acute respiratory failure: a systematic review and meta-analysis. Crit. Care 21 (1), 4.

Karnatovskaia, L.V., 2015. The spectrum of psychocognitive morbidity in the critically ill: a review of the literature and call for improvement. J. Crit. Care 30 (1), 130–137.

Kettles, L., 2013. Hypovolaemia. Anaesth. Int. Care Med. 14 (1), 5–7.

La Calle, G.H., 2016. An emotional awakening. Int. Care Med. 42 (1), 115–116.

MacIntyre, N., 2013. Patient-ventilator trigger dys-synchrony. Crit. Care 17, 157.

Magder, S., 2015. Understanding central venous pressure. Curr. Opin. Crit. Care 21 (5), 369–375.

Mahmood, N.A., Chaudry, F.A., Azam, H., 2013. Frequency of hypoxic events in patients on a mechanical ventilator. Int. J. Crit. Illn. Inj. Sci. 3 (2), 124–129.

McConnell, R.A., Kerlin, M.P., Schweickert, W.D., et al., 2016. Using a post-intubation checklist and time out to expedite mechanical ventilation monitoring. Respir. Care 61 (7), 902–912.

McKim, D., Rose, L., 2015. Efficacy of mechanical insufflation-exsufflation in extubating unweanable subjects with restrictive pulmonary disorders. Respir. Care 60 (4), 621–622.

Mireles-Cabodevila, E., Hatipoğlu, U., Chatburn, R.L., 2013. A rational framework for selecting modes of ventilation. Respir. Care 58 (2), 348–366.

Murias, G., Lucangelo, U., Blanch, L., 2016. Patient-ventilator asynchrony. Curr. Opin. Crit. Care 22 (1), 53–59.

Neto, A.S., Schultz, M.J., Festic, E., 2016. Ventilatory support of patients with sepsis or septic shock in resource-limited settings. Int. Care Med. 42 (1), 100–103.

NICE, 2016. Extracorporeal carbon dioxide removal for acute respiratory failure [IPG564].

Orlowski, J.L., 2013. Hyperglycemia in critical illness. Adv. Emerg. Nurs. J. 35 (3), 209–216.

Pinsky, M., Clermont, G., Hravnak, M., 2016. Predicting cardiorespiratory instability. Crit. Care 20, 70.

Pryor, L.N., Baldwin, C.E., Ward, E.C., et al., 2016. Tracheostomy tube type and inner cannula selection impact pressure and resistance to air flow. Respir. Care 61 (5), 607–614.

Puah, A.H., Sze, C.T.P., 2017. Lung herniation after positive pressure ventilation. Respir. Med. Case Rep. 20, 61–63.

Qureshi, S.I., 2016. Meta-analysis of colloids versus crystalloids in critically ill, trauma and surgical patients. Br. J. Surg. 103 (1), 14–26.

Rafiei, H., Abdar, M.E., Amiri, M., et al., 2013. The study of harmful and beneficial drug interactions in intensive care. J. Intens. Care Soc. 14 (2), 155–158.

Ramprasad, R., Kapoor, M.C., 2012. Nutrition in intensive care. J. Anaesthesiol. Clin. Pharmacol. 28 (1), 1–3.

Ramsingh, D., 2013. Clinical review: does it matter which hemodynamic monitoring system is used? Crit. Care 17, 208.

Rittayamai, N., Wilcox, E., Drouot, X., et al., 2016. Positive and negative effects of mechanical ventilation on sleep in the ICU. Int. Care Med. 42 (4), 531–541.

Rose, L., Adhikari, N.K., Leasa, D., et al., 2017. Cough augmentation techniques for extubation or weaning critically ill patients from mechanical ventilation. Cochrane Database Syst. Rev. (1), CD011833.

Schindler, A.W., 2013. ICU personnel have inaccurate perceptions of their patients' experiences. Acta Anaesthesiol. Scand. 57, 1032–1040.

Schwaiberger, D., Karcz, M., Menk, M., et al., 2016. Respiratory failure and mechanical ventilation in the pregnant patient. Crit. Care Clin. 32 (1), 85–95.

Sjöberg, F., Svanborg, E., 2013. How do we know when patients sleep properly or why they do not? Crit. Care 17, 145.

Smith, C.D., Grami, P., 2017. Feasibility and effectiveness of a delirium prevention bundle in critically ill patients. Am. J. Crit. Care 26 (1), 19–27.

Spiegel, R., Haney Mallemat, H., 2016. Emergency department treatment of the mechanically ventilated patient. Emerg. Med. Clin. North Am. 34 (1), 63–75.

Stocchetti, N., Roux, P.L., Vespa, P., 2013. Clinical review: neuromonitoring. Crit. Care 17, 201.

Turner-Cobb, J.M., 2016. The acute psychobiological impact of the intensive care experience on relatives. Psychol. Health Med. 21 (1), 20–26.

Tusman, G., Bohm, S.H., Suarez-Sipmann, F., 2016. Advanced uses of pulse oximetry for monitoring mechanically ventilated patients. Anesth. Analg. 124 (1), 62–71.

Van Rompaey, B., Van Hoofemail, A., van Bogaertemail, P., et al., 2016. The patient's perception of a delirium. Intensive Crit. Care Nurs. 32, 66–74.

Vassilakopoulos, T., 2016. Respiratory muscle wasting in the ICU: is it time to protect the diaphragm? Thorax 71 (5), 397–398.

Vincent, J.L., 2008. Understanding cardiac output. Crit. Care 12 (4), 174.

Volpe, M.S., Adams, A.B., Amato, M.B.P., 2008. Ventilation patterns influence airway secretion movement. Respir. Care 53 (10), 1287–1294.

# 21

# Physiotherapy for Critically Ill Patients

*David McWilliams, Alexandra Hough*

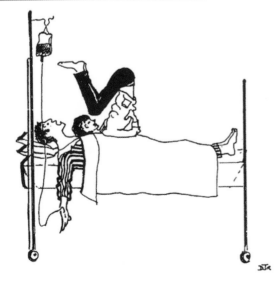

'The physiotherapist will come and do exercises on his chest'. From *ACPRC Newsletter*, 11, 1987, with permission.

## INTRODUCTION

Pulmonary complications are the most common causes of morbidity and mortality in the intensive care unit (ICU) (Kuyrukluyildiz et al. 2016). Physiotherapy counters these by clearing secretions, reversing atelectasis, reducing the need for intubation, facilitating weaning (Gosselink et al. 2008) and moderating brain dysfunction (Girard 2012). Physiotherapy combined with occupational therapy leads to less delirium, shorter time on mechanical ventilation (MV) and increased return to independent function (Piriyapatsom et al. 2013). Hanekom et al. (2012) show how a specialist physiotherapist allocated to the ICU improves patient outcomes. The more frequent the treatments, the shorter the average length of stay (Castro et al. 2013).

# ASSESSMENT

Modifications to the assessment described in Chapter 2 are below, with assessment scales on p. 507.

## Notes and Charts

White cell count, blood sugar, lactate and urea/electrolyte levels can affect treatment. The implications of abnormal values are shown on p. 32 and in the Glossary, with some ICU examples below.

1. Low or high potassium levels predispose to arrhythmias, as does low magnesium (Parikh 2012), with significantly abnormal readings contraindicating most forms of physiotherapy.
2. Low albumin is common in ICU patients because of fluid and membrane permeability problems, leading to metabolic alkalosis and systemic and pulmonary oedema.
3. Neutropaenia can be caused by malnutrition, immune deficiency or anticancer drugs, leaving a patient vulnerable to infection (Dale 2016).
4. Anaemia is found in up to 95% of patients, compromising oxygen delivery (Kocsi et al. 2012) and indicating a need for careful consideration before mobilization.
5. High creatinine levels suggest failing kidneys (Connor 2016), usually reflecting global hypoxia.
6. Impaired clotting occurs with disseminated intravascular coagulation (p. 537), or, less drastically, if a patient is on anticoagulants. This increases the risk of bleeding with suction. Conversely, enhanced clotting increases the risk of deep vein thrombosis.

The notes identify patients who are dependent on tobacco or alcohol. This is not a time for cold turkey and patients should be given nicotine replacement or medication respectively (ICS 2014a).

For patients with pyrexia, some conditions require surface cooling, e.g. sepsis, and some not necessarily so, e.g. septic shock (Doyle 2016). Peripheral temperature is normally 2°C lower than core temperature, but if the difference is more than 5°C, poor perfusion is implicated, with an effect on oxygen delivery if there is little reserve.

The chart may incorporate scales for mobility (Kasotakis et al. 2012), thirst (Puntillo 2014), agitation, organ failure (Vasilevskis et al. 2016), sedation, delirium (Darbyshire et al. 2016), sleep and pain. Pain should not rely on vital signs for assessment (Reinke et al. 2014).

Scales have been validated for mechanically ventilated patients unable to report pain (Marra et al. 2017).

Multimodal analgesia is advised (Ehieli et al. 2017) because severe pain occurs in 50%–65% of patients and its legacy can impair quality of life even after discharge (Payen & Chanques 2012). It is worth checking that analgesia and not sedatives are given for pain relief (Vincent et al. 2016).

There is no reliable scale for assessing awareness, so it is assumed that patients can hear and understand conversation. A rough test for comprehension is to ask patients to poke out their tongue, which patients with profound polyneuropathy and most forms of paralysis are physically still able to do.

Blood pressure (BP) should be checked on the chart for its response to turning or previous sessions of manual hyperinflation (MH). If BP is low, unstable or sags on inspiration, or if mean arterial pressure is <65 mmHg, the patient may be unable to maintain cardiac output during turning or MH. A drop in systolic BP by more than 40 mmHg suggests sepsis (Sevransky 2010). A labile BP can cause emboli to travel to the brain, heart or lungs (Monroe 2013).

Electrolyte and haematocrit concentration are decreased with fluid excess and increased with fluid loss. Fluid status is disturbed by diuretics, diabetes, vomiting, diarrhoea, heart or kidney failure, burns, ascites or large open wounds. Dehydration is difficult to assess clinically because oedema or overhydration can coexist with intravascular depletion in critically ill people, so reliance is best placed on the fluid balance chart and nurse report.

Signs of hypovolaemia or reduced cardiac output are:

- ↑ heart rate (HR)
- ↑ respiratory rate (RR)
- ↓ systolic BP
- ↓ urine output
- dizziness with position change
- sweating
- confusion or altered consciousness.
- ↓ peripheral temperature

Hypovolaemia alone is distinguished by:

- dark coloured urine
- ↓ pulse pressure because compensation by vasoconstriction assists venous return and helps maintain diastolic pressure

Decreased cardiac output alone is distinguished by:

- pallor
- cold extremities

A typical chart is shown in Appendix A.

## The Patient

*Inability to report symptom distress is not synonymous with inability to experience suffering.*

***Campbell 2010***

What channels of communication are available? Is the patient conscious, confused, agitated, sedated, in pain or paralysed? Paralysis, whether pathological or pharmacological, indicates the importance of clarity in communication because patients may be trying to make sense of sounds and sensations but cannot give feedback. Agitation, which is associated with a higher rate of infection and longer hospital stay, may be due to lack of information, discomfort from the endotracheal tube, fear, awkward positioning, immobility, thirst, hunger, constipation, a full bladder or, most commonly, pain (ICS 2014a).

However unconscious a patient appears, it is worth remembering the 'unconscious' survivor of the 7/7 London bombings who later reported that he had heard paramedics pass him by with the comment that he could not be saved.

Thirst is reported by 70% of patients (Arai et al. 2014), but is not routinely assessed, partly staff often do not perceive that mechanically ventilated patients could be thirsty (Puntillo et al. 2010).

For patients who can indicate yes or no, breathlessness may be measured by two standardized questions (Karampela et al. 2002):

- Are you feeling short of breath right now?
- Is your shortness of breath mild, moderate or severe?

For other patients, observation scales incorporating respiratory and behavioural signs can be used (Persichini et al. 2016). Breathlessness may be due to patient–ventilator asynchrony (Branson et al. 2013) or it may reflect anxiety.

Table 21.1 shows that unrelieved and distressing symptoms are present for the majority of critically ill patients.

Other points to note are the following:

1. Accessory muscle activity suggests excess work of breathing (WOB), while laboured breathing may indicate excess WOB or an obstructed airway.

### TABLE 21.1 Prevalence of symptoms reported by intensive care unit patients

| Symptom | Percentage of patients |
|---|---|
| Fatigue | 74.7 |
| Thirst | 70.8 |
| Anxiety | 57.9 |
| Restlessness | 49.0 |
| Hunger | 44.8 |
| Breathlessness | 43.9 |
| Pain | 40.4 |
| Sadness | 33.9 |
| Fear | 32.8 |
| Confusion | 26.6 |

From Puntillo et al. 2010.

2. A distended abdomen is common; constipation has been found in 83.3% of patients, which reduces lung volume, delays weaning and enteral feeding (Mostafa et al. 2003) and predisposes to delirium (Smonig et al. 2016).
3. Lines and tubes, especially femoral lines, haemofiltration lines, pacing wires, chest drains and lines in the feet, should be kept in view throughout treatment.
4. Muscle atrophy may be masked by limb oedema.
5. A wheezelike sound at the mouth may indicate air leaking around the cuff of the tracheal tube.
6. An acoustic detector is available which can identify airway secretions (Lucchini et al. 2011).
7. If MH is anticipated, breath sounds can be heard more clearly when the bag is squeezed, and sometimes crackles can be elicited with a sharp release on expiration.
8. Absent or reduced breath sounds over the left lung may indicate right lung intubation (Fig. 21.1).

## Monitors

Monitors (p. 465) should be observed before, during and after treatment. The arterial line allows continuous monitoring of BP and blood gases. Oxygen levels must be maintained throughout, low levels being a risk factor for subsequent cognitive dysfunction (Modrykamien 2012). Pulse oximetry is less accurate with low perfusion conditions such as poor cardiac output, vasoconstriction and hypothermia, and an $SpO_2$ above 94% appears necessary to ensure arterial oxygen saturation ($SaO_2$) of 90% (Louw et al. 2001).

## Ventilator

The charts indicate ventilator settings and trends in the patient's response, while the ventilator screen shows events in real time. Interaction between patient and ventilator are represented as waveforms (p. 465) and loops (Fig. 21.2). Erratic readings may indicate a patient fighting the ventilator or coughing, confirmed by observation of the patient. A high level of positive end-expiratory pressure (PEEP) means that patients are at risk of hypoxaemia if they are disconnected from the ventilator. A sawtooth pattern on the expiratory portion of the waveform indicates excess secretions (Fig. 21.3).

In volume-control ventilation, airway pressure provides the following information:
1. Peak pressure below normal is usually due to a leak in the circuit.
2. End-expiratory pressure below the baseline suggests excess WOB.

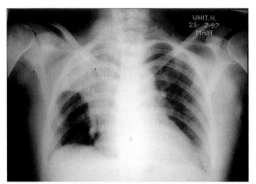

**FIGURE 21.1** The ETT has passed into the right main bronchus and beyond the RUL bronchus, leading to absorption of gas in the nonventilated RUL and atelectasis. The left lung would also have collapsed if the ETT had not been removed. *ETT*, endotracheal tube; *RUL*, right upper lobe.

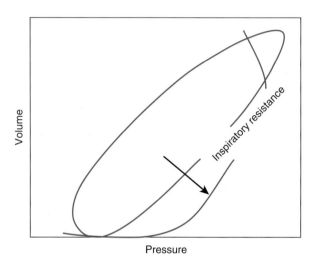

**FIGURE 21.2** Downward widening of pressure–volume loop indicating impedance in the system anywhere from the ventilator to the patient's abdomen, e.g. patient biting the ETT or raised intraabdominal pressure. (From Robertson 2016.)

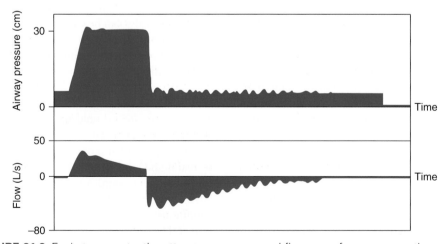

**FIGURE 21.3** Expiratory sawtooth pattern on pressure and flow waveforms, suggesting a need for suction. (From Branson 2007.)

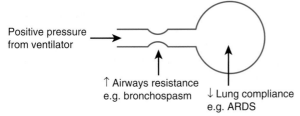

FIGURE 21.4 Increased peak airway pressure in patients on volume-control ventilation. *ARDS*, Acute respiratory distress syndrome.

3. Oscillations in airway pressure signify spontaneous breaths between ventilator breaths.
4. Peak pressures >30 cmH$_2$O above PEEP may be due to airflow obstruction, stiff lungs, pulmonary oedema, pneumothorax, obstruction by upper airway secretions, a kinked tube or clenched teeth (Fig. 21.4).

An alarmed pressure limit is set for safety.

Alveolar pressure is more negative than airway pressure during patient triggering and more positive during a positive pressure breath.

## Imaging

Portable X-rays are taken with the patient supine or sitting up as they are able. Pleural effusions are common because of fluid imbalance or leaky membranes, but a supine or slumped position causes it to lose its clear boundary (Fig. 21.5) and appear as a generalized opacity with no air bronchograms (Fig. 21.6). Ultrasound scans improve diagnosis and are increasingly used by physiotherapists (Leech et al. 2015).

A pneumothorax caused by blunt trauma can be identified in up to 55% of patients (Richter & Ragaller 2011), but it is difficult to identify on a portable X-ray because the classic apicolateral location is less common and sometimes the boundary between air and lung is lost.

Close scrutiny of the X-ray is required:
- after unexpected loss of consciousness, in case of aspiration;
- after trauma or cardiopulmonary resuscitation, in case of rib or sternal fracture;
- after neck line insertion, in case of haemothorax or an apical pneumothorax;
- after intubation.

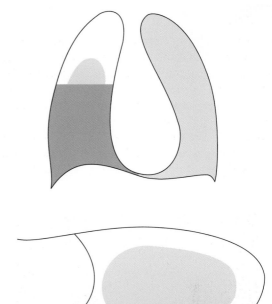

FIGURE 21.5 Representation of pleural effusion upright and supine.

Hardware is deliberately radiopaque. The tracheal (endotracheal or tracheostomy) tube is identified by its opaque line and shows up inside the tracheal air column, stopping about 5–7 cm from the carina. If the tube goes past the carina, unventilated areas collapse (Fig. 21.1). If it is too short, the patient's head should be moved as little as possible because it may become dislodged. A central venous line is usually traceable to the vena cava. A pulmonary artery catheter passes through the heart in a loop, with its tip in a branch of the pulmonary artery.

A clinical decision-making tool for ICU patients is shown in Box 21.1.

## HANDLING PEOPLE WHO ARE CRITICALLY ILL

*Who am I?*
*Where am I?*
*Why do I hurt so much?*

**Nursing Times** *1981*

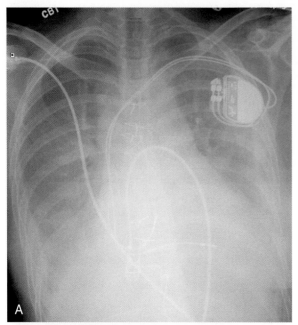

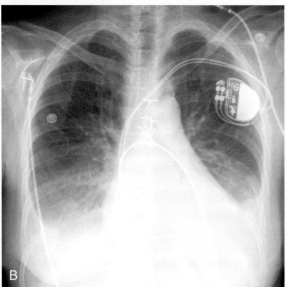

**FIGURE 21.6** Pleural effusion in (A) supine, showing diffuse opacities and visible vascular markings and (B) upright, showing blunted costophrenic angles and dense lower zone opacities. (From Elicker et al. 2016.)

## Minimizing Oxygen Consumption

*'I heard a lot more than I think they think I heard'.*
**Jablonski 1994**

### Preliminaries

*'Someone would come near me and would just be working and not saying anything to me. That would be frightening because I didn't know what they were going to do next'.*
**Parker et al. 1984**

Patients are often scared, disorientated and sleep deprived. Medication may prevent the creation of new memories and they will often not remember information about previous treatments or even where they are. They need regular explanations about treatment, and even when unconscious or paralysed, they need to be told before any physical touch, otherwise anxiety increases oxygen consumption ($\dot{V}O_2$).

Increased oxygen, fluids or medication may be required to maintain oxygenation while ensuring stable haemodynamics and minimum pain. If sedation is needed, a bolus of propofol before treatment is suitable because of its short recovery time. The traditional regimen of percussion, vibrations and suction can, if done inappropriately, destabilize cardiac output, raise BP and HR, increase $\dot{V}O_2$ and reduce $SpO_2$ (Weissman 1993). However, Berney et al. (2012) state that appropriate and sensitive physiotherapy creates no greater metabolic demands than turning the patient into side-lying.

---

**KEY POINT**

Stress increases oxygen consumption and reduces motivation. Treatment is most effective in a motivated patient. Stress is therefore better prevented than treated.

---

### Orientation

*'When the link to life seems tenuous, the immediate world is clung to desperately … I had a passionate need to make that corner of the world a home'.*
**Moore 1991**

Most patients need a visible clock, calendar, family photographs and personal belongings in an area that they

**BOX 21.1  Intensive Care Unit Clinical Reasoning Model**

**Precautions**

Clotting status

Other

**Assessment**

Nurse comments

Subjective assessment

Charts

| Pain score | Breathlessness | Sedation | Delirium | GCS |
|---|---|---|---|---|
| CVS stable Y / N | BP | | HR | |
| Temp. | Fluid balance   +ve...........   -ve........... | | $SpO_2$ | |

| ABGs on $F_1O_2$ of..... | pH | $PaO_2$ | $PaCO_2$ | $HCO_3^-$ | BE |
|---|---|---|---|---|---|

| Normal ☐ | Acidosis ☐  Alkalosis ☐ | Respiratory ☐  Metabolic ☐ | Acute ☐  Compensated ☐ |
|---|---|---|---|

Relevant medication

**Ventilation**

| Self-ventilating | $FiO_2$ | CPAP Y / N | RR | Breathing pattern |
|---|---|---|---|---|
| NIV | $FiO_2$ | Mode | | |
| MV | $FiO_2$ | VC / PC / dual | Mode | |
| | VC: peak pressure | | PC: $V_T$ | |
| | PEEP level | Patient triggering Y / N | Humidifier / HME | |

CXR: date

Radiology report ☐
Own interpretation ☐

Clinical assessment

Appearance

| Auscultation: | Breath sounds | Added sounds |
|---|---|---|
| Palpation: | Abdominal distension Y / N | Percussion note |

Additional respiratory information

Additional nonrespiratory information

*Continued*

## BOX 21.1   Intensive Care Unit Clinical Reasoning Model—cont'd

**Physiotherapy problems**

**Goals**

| Short term | Medium term | Long term |
|---|---|---|
| | | |

**Plan** (including instructions for patient/family/staff

**Treatment**

None ☐

Education (patient/family)

| Positioning: | R s.ly. | L s.ly. | Prone | Long sitting | Other |
|---|---|---|---|---|---|

| SR: to ↑ volume: | Deep breathing | Incentive spirometry | IPPB |
|---|---|---|---|

| SR: to clear sputum: | ACBT | PD/perc/vibs | Devices | Cough |
|---|---|---|---|---|

| Mechanical vent: | MH | PD/perc/vibs | Suction x ............ Quality of sputum | Saline instillation ........ml. |
|---|---|---|---|---|

| Passive movements | Active exs | SOEB | SOOB |
|---|---|---|---|

Walk

Exercise diary

Other

**Outcomes**

| Lung volume ↑: | BS ↑ | Bronchial breathing cleared | PN resonant | X-ray cleared |
|---|---|---|---|---|

| Secretions mobilised: | Crackles cleared. | Sawtooth on waveform cleared. |
|---|---|---|

| Both the above | SpO$_2$ ↑ | PIP ↓    V$_T$ ↑ | Other |
|---|---|---|---|

| Full ROM | |
|---|---|
| Mobility | |
| Function | |
| Other | |

| Goals achieved | Short term | Medium term | Long term |
|---|---|---|---|

*ABG,* Arterial blood gas; *CPAP,* continuous positive airway pressure; *HME,* heat–moisture exchanger; *IPPB,* intermittent positive pressure breathing; *L s.ly,* left side-lying; *MV,* mechanical ventilation; *NIV,* noninvasive ventilation; *PIP,* peak inspiratory pressure; *R s.ly,* right side-lying; *ROM,* range of movement; *SOEB,* sitting over edge of bed; *SOOB,* sitting out of bed; *SR,* spontaneous respiration.
(Modified from Veronica Bastow.)

can control, if they are able. They also need information on progress, interpretation of noises and voices, attendance to alarms promptly, explanation of neighbours' alarms, their phone if they are able to talk, and treatment with the same physiotherapist before, during and after admission to the ICU when feasible. We should enter the patient's space gently, introduce ourselves and explain our purpose.

## Sleep and rest

Patients should not, if possible, be woken if asleep, especially when flickering eyelids indicate that they are in the REM phase of the sleep cycle, when tissue regeneration is at its maximum. Sleep is an essential component of rehabilitation in its function of resting muscles so that they are fit for exercise.

## Family

If visitors are present, they can either be invited to stay or asked to leave during treatment, depending on the patient's wish. The presence of relatives means that they can become involved in patient care and are reassured that physiotherapy is not distressing. However, if the patient's wish cannot be ascertained, it is usually best that visitors are asked to leave.

## Communication

'Do not deny the patient their experience. The most helpful conversation I had was with a physician who acknowledged that I was in a 'dark' place … Immediately, I believed she knew I was suffering … I trusted this physician'.

*Hipp & Ely 2012*

The priority is to establish communication, including:
- clear and explicit explanations, repeated as necessary, including why physiotherapy is necessary, what it will feel like, how long it will last and instructions on how to ask for it to stop;
- hearing aid or glasses if used, which reduces the incidence of delirium (Allen et al. 2012);
- a speaking valve (Sutt 2017) or a speaking tracheostomy tube, which also facilitates protective expiration after swallowing to help prevent aspiration (Prigent et al. 2012);
- referral to speech–language therapy (Radtke et al. 2011) a lip-reading interpreter (Meltzer et al. 2012) or translator, if required;

- communication aids such as word or picture charts (Fig. 21.7), smartphone (Fig. 21.8), paper and clipboard, a magic slate or computer systems (Koszalinski et al. 2012);
- if unable to write or use picture charts, yes/no questions asked one at a time, e.g.: 'Are you hot? cold? itchy? thirsty? worried? tired? sleepy? nauseous? in pain? Do you have cramp? Is your mouth dry? Is the tube bothering you? Do you want to turn? raise or lower your head? Do you need more air? less light? less noise? more information? bottle or bedpan?'

Communication should be aimed *at* patients rather than *over* them. Chatting over patients can increase stress more than suction (Lynch 1978). One patient said 'it didn't matter what they talked about, so long as they talked to me' (Villaire 1995).

Anxious patients are not usually helped by being told to relax. The source of anxiety needs to be identified and information provided.

If a patient wishes not to communicate, this should also be respected.

## Helplessness

*What do you do when you can't bear it? What are the alternatives?*

*Rollin 1976*

Helplessness can lead to depression, so the more helpless the patient, the more important is autonomy. Patients can choose whether they would like treatment now or later, if possible, and their preferred position to be left in after treatment, if this fits in with nursing needs. If they request, patients should be turned before the allotted time. They can have charge of the television remote and radio channel, if available, and decide whether they would like to regain their day/night rhythm by being woken in the day or having a sleeping pill at night. Autonomy is particularly important in this situation of unequal power.

Anxiety is reduced by combining factual information with advice that enables patients to be proactive, as much as they are able. Depression is eased by allowing expression of emotion, encouraging independence, using imaginative interventions such as pet visitation schemes (Miracle 2009) and initiating rehabilitation from the start (Gosselink et al. 2008). Clinicians also need to identify how much each patient would like to

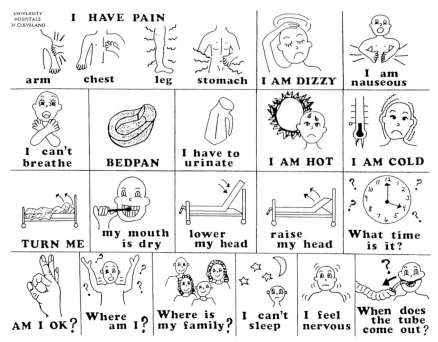

**FIGURE 21.7** Communication chart.

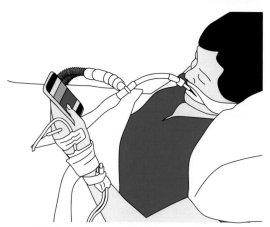

**FIGURE 21.8** Texting. (From Bell 2016.)

take their own decisions and how much they cede decision-making to staff (Kon et al. 2016).

## Touch

ICU patients are extra sensitive to human physical contact as a contrast to the cold clinical procedures to which they are subjected. Therapeutic touch reduces anxiety (Zare et al. 2010), massage decreases stress

(Waldmann 2009, p. 71) and reflexology can lessen the need for sedation (Akin et al. 2014). As always, it should be remembered that individuals and cultures vary and some dislike touch, particularly male-to-female touch.

## Handling Unconscious or Paralysed People

*'I was imprisoned and people were sitting on me and I just couldn't get out, because I was restricted where I was and I couldn't move'.*

**Darbyshire et al. 2016**

One study has found that one-third of handling procedures are accompanied by cardiac instability, desaturation or ventilatory distress (Jong et al. 2013). Repositioning and suctioning have been identified as the two procedures causing the most pain in ventilated patients (Ayasrah 2016). Forewarning is always required, and a bolus of morphine often needed (Ahlers et al. 2012).

## Turning

*'To be talked frankly through a complete procedure would help curb the deadly effects of uninformed anticipation'.*

**Brooks 1990**

The longer a patient has been immobile, the more sensitive their cardiovascular system is to position change. A lateral turn in a critically ill patient can cause haemodynamic instability (Shannan et al. 2015) or reduce tissue oxygenation by 8%–22%, with increased $\dot{V}O_2$ bearing a greater responsibility than reduced oxygen delivery ($DO_2$) (Vollman 2013). A suggested sequence is the following:

1. Turn off continuous tube feed.
2. Inform the patient, then talk them through each step.
3. Ensure sufficient slack in lines and tubes.
4. Ensure that glide sheets are in place, the team is following the same manual handling protocol and an individual is responsible for the airway and vulnerable lines.
5. Ensure that the team is coordinated in relation to care of the skin and joints, e.g. protect heels from friction, avoid using the leg as a lever.
6. Suction oral secretions, as far as above the cuff, to minimize the risk of aspiration (Gentile & Siobal 2010).
7. Support the tracheal tube. Some patients like to hold an endotracheal tube briefly with their teeth during the turn.
8. Say clearly, so that the team and patient can hear, previously agreed instructions e.g. 'ready, steady, turn'.
9. Turn smoothly, ensuring that the shoulder joints and head are supported if the patient is paralysed, and that creases in the sheet are smoothed out.
10. Check lines, patient comfort, monitors, joint positions, ensure there is no cuff leak.
11. Reattach continuous tube feed.
12. Check tracheal tube cuff pressure (Lizy et al. 2014).

## Pressure Area Care

Pressure sores distress patients and are avoidable. Risk factors are malnutrition, obesity, steroids, diabetes, advanced age, immobility, hypovolaemia and vasopressor drugs (Smit et al. 2016).

Anything can be put on a pressure sore except the patient. Hospitals are full of concoctions, but better still is prevention by:

- adequate nutrition (Miller et al. 2015), especially vitamin C and protein
- regular turning, without friction, and judicious positioning
- specialized beds
- keeping pressure areas dry

A sacral pressure sore that has developed in supine does not preclude sitting out in a chair, so long as a pressure cushion is used and an upright position maintained to prevent pressure on the sacrum. A time limit should be set and there must be meticulous monitoring of the wound before and after.

## TECHNIQUES TO INCREASE LUNG VOLUME

*'No-one explained … all they said was not to worry about it'.*

                        ***Thomson 1973***

For spontaneously breathing patients, lung volume may be increased by the techniques in Chapter 6. For ventilated patients, the following modifications can be used.

### Positioning

*There is no single 'ideal' position for all pulmonary disorders.*

                        ***Bein et al. 2015***

Positioning is the main physiotherapy intervention for critically ill patients, and may be the only treatment for some patients. Spending too long in supine encourages basal atelectasis, especially of the left lower lobe because the heart compresses its bronchus (Khan et al. 2009b). Turning from supine to side-lying helps reverse lower lobe atelectasis, reduce the risk of pneumonia, promote patient comfort, safeguard pressure areas and increase cardiac output (Thomas et al. 2007). If the patient is side-lying well forward (Berney et al. 2012), the abdominal contents are prevented from encroaching on lung volume.

Other effects of positioning have been documented:

1. As with spontaneously breathing patients, ventilated patients with unilateral lung pathology normally show optimal gas exchange when lying with the affected lung uppermost (Ng & Ong 2010).
2. Automated turning modestly improves outcomes compared with manual turning (Hanneman et al. 2015).
3. Side-lying can also improve gas exchange, respiratory mechanics and secretion clearance, shorten duration

of MV and, so long as the tracheal tube is kept horizontal, reduce aspiration (Mauri et al. 2010).

4. With the patient horizontal, mucus may be prevented from flowing distally; Bassi et al. (2008) claim that the head-up position may act as a form of reverse postural drainage, facilitating colonization of the airways and possibly pneumonia.

However, evidence for head-of-bed elevation is conflicted (Metheny 2013). Raising the head of the bed is generally considered to prevent ventilator-associated pneumonia by minimizing gastro-oesophageal reflux, especially in supine, but the semirecumbent position encourages pooling of secretions above the cuff, and one study investigating a head-up position of 45 degrees found this to be achieved only 15% of the time (Michetti 2017). Unless the whole bed is tipped head-up, skin integrity is put at risk and head elevation tends to become the slumped position (Davis & Kotowski 2015), with abdominal pressure restricting lung volume and, for patients receiving enteral feeding, increasing gastro-oesophageal reflux (Leng et al. 2011). Head-of-bed elevation to 45 degrees may also reduce BP and oxygen delivery (Gocze et al. 2013) and monitoring must be continuous.

Factors which may limit positioning are abnormal muscle tone, pain, neurological instability such as brain or spinal cord injury, fractures, pressure sores and unstable BP. Some invasive support systems such as haemofiltration are a reminder to be extra vigilant.

For rehabilitation, patients with a degree of postural hypotension benefit from the tilt table, usually increasing in 10-degree increments as tolerated. Neurological patients require close observation and haemodynamic monitoring during this process.

## Deep Breathing on the Ventilator

Most patients are on a mode of ventilation that incorporates spontaneous breathing and they may be able to take deep breaths voluntarily. Deep breathing is particularly successful when patients are motivated by watching the results of their endeavours on the tidal volume ($V_T$) monitor. Neurophysiological facilitation of respiration (p. 187) can also be rewarding.

## Manual Hyperinflation

> 'It was by far the most frightening thing that happened to me'.
>
> **Patient, quoted by Rowbotham 1990**

MH delivers extra volume and oxygen to the lungs by, for example, a rebreathe bag. Compared with positioning, which is accepted as preventive care for most ICU patients, MH is not used routinely because prophylaxis has not been substantiated, and the procedure comes with complications.

## Terminology

- **Manual ventilation** means squeezing gas into a patient's lungs at tidal volume, for example when changing ventilator tubing.
- **Manual hyperventilation** delivers rapid breaths, for example if the patient is breathless, hypoxaemic or hypercapnic.
- **Manual hyperinflation** provides deep breaths in order to increase lung volume, e.g. when treating a person with atelectasis or sputum retention.

Physiotherapy is associated with MH. The words 'bag-squeezing' or 'bagging' are also used, but not in front of patients as they can be misinterpreted, e.g. that the patient is to go into a body bag.

## Effects

Benefits of MH are:
- reversal of atelectasis (Berney et al. 2012)
- sputum clearance (van Aswegen et al. 2013)
- improved oxygen levels (Fig. 21.9) and temporary improvement in lung compliance (Choi & Jones 2005)

## Complications

The complications of MH are an exaggeration of the complications of MV, particularly barotrauma and haemodynamic compromise (Leatherman 2015).

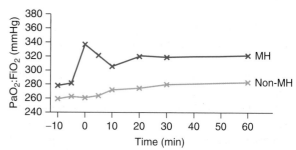

**FIGURE 21.9** Improved gas exchange immediately after MH and at 10-min intervals afterwards. $PaO_2$:$FiO_2$, oxygen tension in relation to inspired oxygen; *MH*, manual hyperinflation. (From Patman et al. 2006.)

Mean arterial pressure may rise (Grap et al. 1994) or fall (Paulus et al. 2010), either of which can reduce cardiac output even in people with normal cardiac function (Anning et al. 2003). Hypotension is caused by reduced venous return to the heart and is more pronounced in patients who are hypovolaemic or vasodilated.

If not explained adequately, MH may cause anxiety, and if minute ventilation is not maintained, $PaCO_2$ may rise (Paulus et al. 2010), along with further anxiety.

For patients on high PEEP, disconnection from the ventilator to attach the bag may not be offset by the benefits of the procedure. In this case, the options are to use ventilator hyperinflation or to modify the technique as on p. 492.

### MINI CLINICAL REASONING

'Five patients developed anxiety/agitation during or shortly after MH, mandating additional sedation in four patients'
Minerva Anestesiol (2010) 76 (12), 1036–1042

**Response**
- Explanation and accurate technique should ensure that MH is neither uncomfortable nor worrisome.
- Sedation blocks memory but not the experience, which may remain as a distorted recollection.

### Equipment

A rebreathe Mapleson-C or Water's bag (Fig. 21.10A) is inflated with wall oxygen and comes in 1–3 L sizes, the 2 L being used for most adults. It incorporates an expiratory valve, which is used to adjust pressure to the patient, and its compliance allows the clinician to feel the ease of inflation.

Semi-rigid units such as the self-inflating Ambu or Laerdal bag (Fig. 21.10B), use room air with added oxygen, and contain inbuilt one-way valves that prevent rebreathing. The flow and pressure are not easily controlled and they are less responsive to techniques such as the end-inspiratory hold. They have a lower peak expiratory flow and do not appear to clear secretions as effectively as the Mapleson-C bag (van Aswegen et al. 2013). It is also suggested that they are less able to improve respiratory mechanics than ventilator hyperinflation (Savian et al. 2006). High pressures are avoided by a pressure release valve rather than controlled by the

operator. Both bags can be used with a PEEP valve so that pressure is not lost during treatment.

The gas delivered to the patient is usually 100% oxygen. This is safe for patients during the brief period of treatment, but for hypercapnic COPD patients who might be dependent on their hypoxic drive to breathe (p. 158), and who are breathing spontaneously with no synchronized intermittent mandatory ventilation (SIMV) backup, an air source and oxygen entrainment might be preferable, with continuous observation of $SpO_2$ and end-tidal $CO_2$.

A heat–moisture exchanger (HME) incorporating a bacterial filter is added to the circuit to ameliorate the inrush of cold air, causing discomfort and sometimes bronchospasm.

### Technique

1. Ensure that the patient's cardiovascular status is optimum.
2. Explain to the patient the purpose of the procedure and that it involves several deep breaths; ensure that they know how to communicate if they want the procedure to stop, and obtain consent. Ask if they would like extra analgesia.
3. Ensure that a manometer and HME are connected.
4. Position the patient well forward in side-lying (Fig. 21.11). In supine the bases are unlikely to be responsive to hyperinflation because positive pressure favours the more compliant nondependent regions, especially in the larger right lung (van Aswegen et al. 2013). For patients who cannot turn, close attention to technique (especially nos.10–11, below) may deliver some extra volume to the lung bases in supine. If a different lung region is to be targeted, it is best placed uppermost if possible.
5. Check monitors after the turn. MH should not be started until cardiovascular stability is assured in the new position.
6. Observe chest expansion.
7. Ensure that the patient is free of distractions or nursing interventions.
8. Connect the bag to the oxygen with a flow rate at a minimum 15 L/min (the flow received by the patient is governed by squeezing the bag, not by the flowmeter), turn off the low pressure alarm, turn the ventilator and humidifier to standby, disconnect the patient from the ventilator and connect to the bagging circuit.

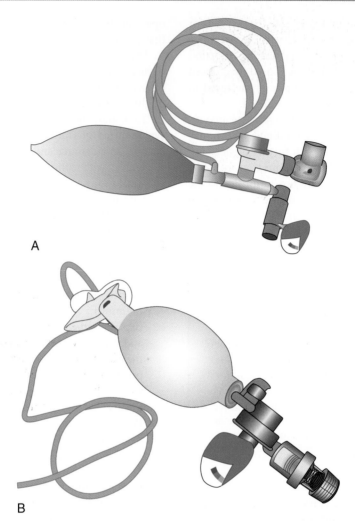

A

B

**FIGURE 21.10** Mapleson-C (A) and Laerdal (B) circuits with pressure manometers and positive end-expiratory pressure valves. (From van Aswegen et al. 2013.)

9. Rest tubing on the sheet to avoid pulling on the tracheal tube, tell the patient when to expect ordinary breaths and when deep breaths. Using two hands, squeeze the bag twice at $V_T$ to acclimatize the patient and to assess lung compliance.

10. Then give slow, smooth deep breaths, adjusting the valve to increase pressure until expansion is greater than on MV. It is suggested that a breath at 150% of $V_T$ reverses the adverse effects of suction, and twice $V_T$ reverses atelectasis (Maxwell & Ellis 2002). Slow steady inspiration minimizes circulatory depression (Odenstedt et al. 2005), turbulence and

the risk of alveolar damage (Silva et al. 2012). Inspiratory times of at least 3 s are required to avoid excessive peak inspiratory pressures (Bennett et al. 2015b). Watch the manometer to ensure a safe and effective pressure (see below).

11. Hold maximum pressure at end-inspiration for 1 or 2 s in to encourage the filling of poorly ventilated alveoli, especially if atelectasis is the problem. This is similar to the plateau pressure in Fig. 20.6. Haemodynamically unstable patients should not receive this end-inspiratory hold, and are best given one deep breath interspersed with several

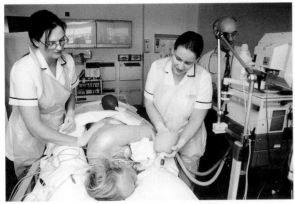

FIGURE 21.11 Manual hyperinflation targeting the left lower lobe, which is being palpated to check for optimum expansion.

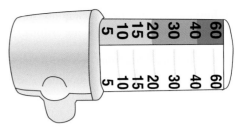

FIGURE 21.12 Manometer.

tidal breaths, or if the patient is able, spontaneous breaths.

12. Release the bag sharply to simulate a huff, especially if sputum retention is the problem.

13. Ensure adequate time before the next inflation, to avoid build up of intrinsic PEEP or cardiovascular instability, while watching the $SpO_2$ monitor.

14. Throughout, watch the chest for expansion, the face for distress and the abdomen for signs of unwanted active expiration. The more alert the patient, the greater is the need to co-ordinate with their own breathing. Stop if the patient's facial expression or the monitors indicate distress, or if crackles indicate that secretions have been mobilized and suction is required. If crackles are heard or the patient coughs, give tidal volume breaths until the patient is suctioned, to avoid pushing the secretions back down. If MH causes no change, stop after about six breaths for reassessment.

15. Reset the ventilator, advise the patient and reconnect to the ventilator. Observe chest movement and monitors, auscultate the chest. Suction if required.

16. Repeat the cycles until auscultation indicates that volume is restored or secretions cleared. If this is not achieved within 5–10 min of accurate MH, it is unlikely to occur in this session.

17. To maintain the benefits of MH, the side-lying position should be maintained for a period afterwards,

ensuring that the tracheal tube is kept horizontal, so long as this position is comfortable for the patient and compliant with unit policy.

## Pressures

Each bed space should be supplied with its own manometer (Fig. 21.12) to ensure effective and safe pressures (Davies & Igo 2004) and to reduce complications (Hila & Ellis 2002). The following are suggestions:

1. For MH to be effective in normal lungs, inflation to $40$ $cmH_2O$ is required to reverse atelectasis (Novak et al. 1987, Rothen et al. 1999).

2. For MH to be safe in normal lungs, inflation to $50$ $cmH_2O$ has been considered safe so long as PEEP is maintained to stabilize the alveoli (García-Fernández et al. 2013). Khanna et al. (2013) maintain that two hyperinflations to a maximum $60$ $cmH_2O$ are safe, but few physiotherapists would be willing to go up to this pressure on the basis of one study.

3. For MH to be safe in diseased or damaged lungs, there is no guaranteed safe pressure. For people with acute respiratory distress syndrome (ARDS) a maximum $30$ $cmH_2O$ has been suggested (Das et al. 2015), although Oczenski et al. (2005) found no evidence of complications using continuous positive airway pressure (CPAP) at $50$ $cmH_2O$ for $30$ s, so long as the prone position was used to protect vulnerable lung regions. However, most physiotherapists would avoid using MHI in people with such damaged lungs.

All the above studies had limitations, and efficacy should be monitored throughout, to ensure that no more than the minimum effective pressure is used.

## Contraindications

MH should be avoided with the following:

- extra-alveolar air, e.g. undrained pneumothorax, subcutaneous emphysema or bulla;

- bronchospasm causing peak airway pressures above 40 cmH$_2$O, in particular with acute asthma.

## Precautions and modifications

MH should be avoided or modified with the following:

- patients at risk of barotrauma, e.g. those with emphysema, fibrosis, pneumocystis pneumonia or ARDS;
- rib fracture because an accompanying pneumothorax may be difficult to pick up on X-ray; if MH is essential, a scan should be requested and/or a radiologist's opinion sought;
- pneumothorax with a chest drain, because positive pressure might slow the sealing of the pleura;
- air leak, as demonstrated by air bubbling through a chest drain bottle;
- hyperinflated lungs with intrinsic PEEP; if MH is essential, a longer expiratory time may reduce the risk of further gas trapping;
- bronchopleural fistula;
- recent pneumonectomy because of the risk of a hidden bronchopleural fistula;
- BP that is low, high or unstable; if MH is essential in hypotensive patients, they should be maximally stabilized first and the technique should be brief, with prolonged expiration and no end-inspiratory hold, in order to facilitate venous return;
- hypovolaemia; if MH is necessary, the above modifications are advised;
- arrhythmias or frequent ectopics;
- during renal dialysis if this destabilizes BP;
- acute brain injury, especially if there is no intracranial pressure monitoring;
- haemoptysis of unknown cause;
- severe hypoxaemia with PEEP above 10 mmHg because disconnection from the ventilator entails loss of PEEP; if MH is essential, desaturation can be minimized by:
  - incorporating a PEEP valve in the circuit (Fig. 21.13), though this may slow expiratory flow;
  - manually preventing the bag fully deflating at end-expiration;
  - increasing the flow rate, and increasing the speed of the procedure to augment oxygenation and prevent deflation, but only if the patient is haemodynamically stable;
  - ventilator hyperinflation (VH).

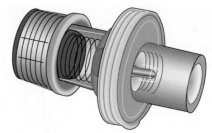

**FIGURE 21.13** Positive end-expiratory pressure valve.

## Ventilator Hyperinflation or Recruitment Manoeuvre

To reduce some of the complications of MH, alveolar recruitment can be aided by hyperinflation through the ventilator. Hartland et al. (2015) claim that these recruitment manoeuvres open collapsed alveoli and improve gas exchange, although the benefits may not be sustained unless high PEEP levels are maintained (Hess & Bigatello 2002). The following have been described:

1. In volume control, V$_T$ is gradually increased until peak airway pressure reaches 40 cmH$_2$O, then six breaths are delivered before returning the ventilator to its previous settings. After 30 s rest, the process is repeated until the desired outcome is achieved, or complications such as patient distress or haemodynamic instability supervene. This can improve lung compliance and clear secretions, with the assumption that it would also increase lung volume. The technique allows the flow pattern to be observed on the screen, to ensure full exhalation before the next breath is delivered, thus reducing the risk of intrinsic PEEP (Berney & Denehy 2002).

2. In pressure control, a stepwise increase in PEEP up to 15 cmH$_2$O and V$_T$ up to 18 mL/kg is administered until a peak inspiratory pressure of 40 cmH$_2$O is reached, then maintained for 10 cycles. This has shown improved oxygenation immediately after heart surgery, with stabilization of newly recruited alveoli by ongoing PEEP (Claxton et al. 2003).

3. The pressure and/or time of the positive pressure breath is increased, e.g. peak pressure of 45 cmH$_2$O and PEEP of 35 cmH$_2$O for 1 min followed by PEEP of 10 cmH$_2$O (Halter 2003).

4. Inflation pressure is increased to 30–40 cmH$_2$O for 30–40 s, inspiratory pause is extended, three consecutive sighs are delivered at plateau pressure 45 cmH$_2$O, or PEEP raised to 40 cmH$_2$O with

pressure control at 20 cmH$_2$O above this level for 2 min, followed by ongoing PEEP at 25 cmH$_2$O (Hess & Bigatello 2002).

5. In SIMV, the fraction of inspired oxygen (FiO$_2$) is increased to 1.0, inspiratory time adjusted to 3–5 s, RR to 6–8 breaths/min and V$_T$ to 15 mL/kg body weight, increasing at first by 150 mL per breath until a peak pressure of 40 cmH$_2$O is achieved. Four sets of eight ventilator breaths per treatment are claimed to produce the same outcomes and safety profile as MH (Dennis et al. 2012).

6. Inflation pressure is increased to 40 cmH$_2$O for 10 s (Hedenstierna 2012).

Other examples are in Fig. 21.14. Thomas (2015) claims that using VH with volume control and the SIMV mode bring the best outcomes.

The following complications of VH have been identified:

- haemodynamic instability caused by sustained positive pressure, e.g. 20 s inflations at 40 cmH$_2$O for 8 min (Nunes et al. 2004);

- alveolar overdistension caused by pressure support at 50 cmH$_2$O and PEEP levels above those required for optimal compliance (Villagrá et al. 2002);

- for patients with acute lung injury: desaturations, arrhythmias and air leaks following 40 cmH$_2$O of CPAP for 40 s (Fan et al. 2012);

- gas trapping, which can be prevented by ensuring that exhaled V$_T$ is no less than inhaled V$_T$.

Monitoring by thoracic tomography has been suggested for safety (Dueck 2006).

Recruitment manoeuvres were originally developed to maintain alveolar stability and offset the lost lung volume caused by lung protective ventilation strategies for ARDS (p. 545), not primarily to expand collapsed lung units. Most studies do not report on complications, and some of the pressures are alarmingly high, especially for patients with damaged lungs. The safety of VH has been questioned (Hess 2002), particularly after 3–5 days into the course of ARDS, when the lungs are at their most fragile. Martin (2009) claims that they improve radiographic images of the lungs but not patient

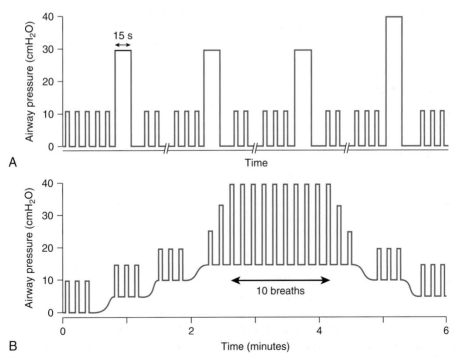

**FIGURE 21.14** Pressure–time curves of two ventilator hyperinflation breaths, showing (A) three hyperinflations to 30 cmH$_2$O followed by one at 40 cmH$_2$O, each held for 15 s, (B) progressive PEEP up to 15 cmH$_2$O, to a peak of 40 cmH$_2$O, maintained for 10 breaths. (From Lumb 2000.)

outcomes, begging the question as to whether these 'open lungs' are happy lungs or simply pretty lungs. Hess (2015) suggests that potential damage may be lessened by increasing pressure gradually.

As with MH, supine is best avoided (Fig. 21.15).

MH, which is designed to clear secretions as well as increase volume, has been described as the treatment of choice for physiotherapists (Barker & Adams 2002), and appears to produce longer lasting improvements in oxygenation than VH (Ahmed et al. 2010). However, Anderson et al. (2015) found both techniques to have similar effects on secretion clearance, oxygenation and cardiovascular stability. Physiotherapists will probably use both, depending on outcomes, and further research may tip the balance in favour of using the ventilator rather than a bag to reinflate lungs or clear secretions.

---

### PRACTICE TIP

Set up a test lung with a spare ventilator, using a spontaneous mode with high flow, and display the pressure–volume loop. Practise hyperinflation through the ventilator and relate it to $V_T$ and the pressure attained with MH, including maintenance of manual PEEP. The screen can be frozen to identify details.

---

## TECHNIQUES TO CLEAR SECRETIONS

The most effective interventions to clear thick secretions in intubated patients are hydration, humidification and mobilization (Halm 2008). For those who cannot mobilize, regular turning will help keep secretions moving. Hydration in the ICU is normally aimed at optimum haemodynamic status rather than secretion clearance, but the physiotherapist can have a say on ward rounds. Other interventions are humidification, sometimes manual techniques or MH, and suction as required.

### Humidification

Humidification is provided by a **hot water humidifier**, with temperature alarms set at maximum 37°C and minimum 30°C. An alternative is an **HME**, which may be adequate for short-term use in well-hydrated patients who do not have excessive or thick secretions. Added to the information on p. 200, the following arguments have been made about the two systems:

1. Compared with hot water humidification, HMEs provide significantly less humidity than hot water humidifiers (Lellouche et al. 2014) and even the most efficient HMEs result in a net loss of heat and moisture from the respiratory tract (Branson 2014).
2. HMEs create resistance (Fig. 21.16) and quadruple the risk of endotracheal tube (ETT) obstruction

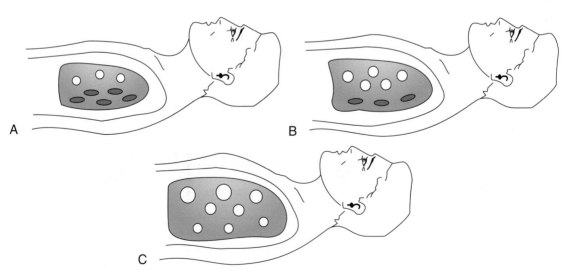

**FIGURE 21.15** Recruitment manoeuvre in supine. (A) Dependent lung closed. (B) Middle area beginning to open. (C) Overinflation of nondependent lung. (From Pilbeam & Cairo 2006.)

(Branson et al. 2014) and increase the WOB such that Hilbert (2003) suggests increasing the support level for patients on pressure support ventilation by 8–15 cmH$_2$O. Resistance in hydrophobic HMEs was found to be twice that of hygroscopic (p. 204) HMEs, and patients with excess or thick secretions need a hot water humidifier straight away (Branson 2014).

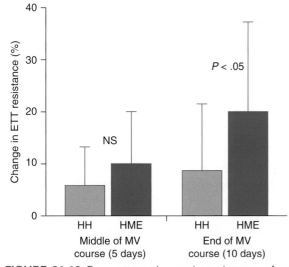

**FIGURE 21.16** Percentage change in resistance of an endotracheal tube *(ETT)* after 5 and 10 days of mechanical ventilation *(MV)* with a heated humidifier *(HH)* and a heat–moisture exchanger *(HME)*. *NS,* Nonsignificant. (From Branson 2007.)

3. HMEs increase dead space and reduce CO$_2$ clearance (AARC 2012) and allowance should be made for a drop in PaCO$_2$ when the device is removed (López et al. 2000).
4. Hot water humidifiers have the advantage of inhibiting inflammatory damage to lung tissue caused by MV itself (Jiang et al. 2015).
5. If MV is expected to last more than a few hours, a heated humidifier has been advised (Ryan et al. 2002), although one of the authors of this study was employed by a humidifier company.

Fig. 21.17 compares the risk of ETT occlusion with different HMEs and a hot water humidifier.

**Saline nebulizers** are much loved by ICU bacteria. Before reaching for these devices, attention should first be given as to why the humidification system is inadequate. A somewhat balmy scenario is to intersperse an HME with saline nebulizers, when the job could be done more safely and effectively with continuous hot water humidification.

## Postural Drainage

The side-to-side positioning applied to most patients is usually adequate for postural drainage, either manually or by a kinetic bed. It has also shown benefit by increasing sputum yield with MH (Berney et al. 2012). A head-down tilt may occasionally be required (Berney et al. 2004) but gravity is thought to have less of an effect on the movement of secretions than flow bias (Graf & Marini 2008). The position also loads the diaphragm and may compromise haemodynamic stability.

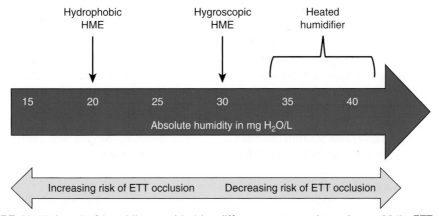

**FIGURE 21.17** Level of humidity provided by different systems (see also p. 204). *ETT,* Endotracheal tube; *HME,* heat–moisture exchanger. (From Branson 2009.)

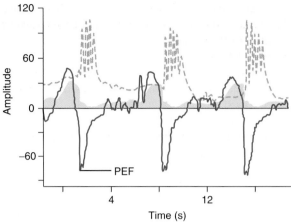

FIGURE 21.18 Manual hyperinflations with chest wall vibrations. Pressure amplitude is denoted by the shaded area ($cmH_2O$), flow by the continuous line (L/min) and force during chest wall vibrations as the dashed line. *PEF*, Peak expiratory flow. (From Shannon et al. 2010.)

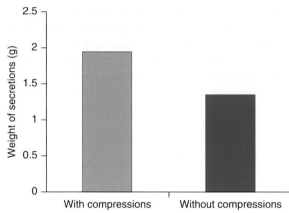

FIGURE 21.19 Mean weight of suctioned secretions with and without chest compression. (From Yousefnia et al. 2016.)

## Manual Techniques

Percussion, shaking or vibrations are not required routinely, and when combined with postural drainage they have shown mixed results in reducing ventilator-associated pneumonia (VAP) or atelectasis (Branson 2007). However, Shannon et al. (2010) found that vibrations, along with MH, can reduce intrinsic PEEP by ensuring full exhalation before the next hyperinflation, and, when started just before termination of the end-inspiratory hold (Fig. 21.18), can increase lung volume.

'Thoracic squeezing' to the lower third of the chest may improve the efficacy of suction (Fig. 21.19) and, when compression of the abdomen is included, they may clear extra secretions (Freynet et al. 2016). These procedures did not include vibrations or shaking and would need to be followed by hyperinflations, if not contraindicated, to restore lung volume.

'Rib cage compression', which may have similar effects to rib-springing, can reduce lung volume, hinder gas exchange and may actually reduce sputum clearance (Unoki et al. 2004) though this may not occur if followed by strategies to restore volume.

Literature on actual vibrations and percussion is sparse. Physiological reasoning suggests that if secretions are not cleared by humidification, position change, MH and suction, these should be tried.

## Flow Bias

Expiratory flow greater than 10% above inspiratory flow facilitates movement of mucus towards the mouth (Ntoumenopoulos et al. 2013). The physiotherapist can discuss ventilator settings with the intensivist if an extra boost to clearance of mucus is required.

## Manual and Ventilator Hyperinflation

VH may improve sputum clearance (Lemes et al. 2009), as can MH with an emphasis on rapid release to reinforce expiratory flow bias (van Aswegen et al. 2013).

## Mechanical Aids

Both bubble PEP (p. 214) and the Flutter (Jones et al. 2013, Chicayban 2011) can be slotted into the exhalation port. High frequency percussive ventilation may also be used, with both spontaneous ventilation and MV, and an insufflation–exsufflator can be connected to the tracheal tube to facilitate a cough, although disconnection from the ventilator limits its use (Kallet 2013).

## Suction

*'The coughing, gagging and choking spasms produced by the sink plunger technique were terrifying'.*
**Day et al. 2002**

Suction stops the patient breathing and may cause pain (Paulus et al. 2013) but, so long as no 'sink plunger' technique is employed, it is normally less harrowing than nasopharyngeal suction, if the patient is fully informed and then talked through the process.

Secretions in peripheral airways are unlikely to contribute to airflow obstruction because of the number of alternative airways, but if stagnant they may contribute to infection. Secretions in the large airways, where there is less collateral ventilation, may interfere with gas exchange or cause plugging.

Suction should be carried out when indicated and if secretions are accessible (AARC 2010).

## Complications

Suction may cause:
- ↓ lung volume, hypoxaemia, discomfort, bronchoconstriction, infection, mucosal injury, arrhythmias and haemodynamic upset (Rodrigues et al. 2017);
- ↑ oxygen demand (White et al. 1990);
- repeated inoculation of the lungs from the biofilm lining the tracheal tube, releasing up to 60,000 colonies of bacteria with each suction pass (Lewis 2002);
- bleeding (Maggiore et al. 2013), due to clotting disorder, heparinization or suction that is rough, frequent or performed with dry airways;
- bradycardia in certain patients, which can be attenuated by nebulized atropine (Brooks et al. 2001).

Most complications can be reduced by pre-oxygenation, postsuction hyperinflation and optimal technique.

## Catheters

The smallest effective catheter should be used, which must be no more than half the internal diameter of the tracheal tube, a larger size causing more mucosal damage than the suction pressure (AARC 2010). A size >12 FG is likely to reduce $PaO_2$ and tidal volume, while increasing pulmonary artery pressure and $PaCO_2$ (Almgren et al. 2004).

A closed-circuit inline catheter (Fig. 21.20) is sealed in a protective sleeve and becomes part of the ventilator circuit. It brings the following advantages:
- no disconnection from the ventilator, leading to less desaturation, less volume loss (Maggiore 2003), less airway collapse, maintenance of PEEP and attenuation of pressure changes (Palazzo & Soni 2013);
- less risk of cross infection (Chung et al. 2015);
- more stable HR, BP and blood gases after open heart surgery (Özden & Görgülü 2016).

Open suction requires disconnection of the patient from the ventilator but has some advantages:
- less likelihood of the preserved PEEP blowing mucus back into the lungs, which may require subsequent compensation with higher suction pressures (Branson 2014);
- ability to use the rocking thumb technique (p. 221) to relieve pressure, rather than the intermittent suction that occurs with closed-circuit catheters.

Although inline catheters can reduce cross infection, there appears to be little difference in their ability to remove secretions or prevent pneumonia (Branson 2014).

## Preliminaries

Analgesia is usually required, even if (especially if) patients are unable to express themselves or are deeply sedated (Paulus et al. 2013). Pre-oxygenation is needed to prevent hypoxaemia, at between 0.20 above baseline $FiO_2$ and $FiO_2$ 1.0, the higher level also preventing $CO_2$ retention (Vianna et al. 2017). Self-ventilating patients may find it helpful subjectively to hyperventilate beforehand.

Indications, contraindications and technique for nasopharyngeal suction are shown on p. 219, with modifications for intubated patients below.

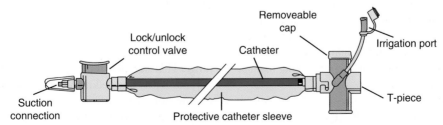

**FIGURE 21.20** Closed-circuit catheter connected to the tracheal tube via a T-piece. The irrigation port allows the passage of saline for loosening secretions or cleaning the catheter.

## Technique for closed-circuit suction

Each unit will have its own protocol, but some tips are:

1. Extra gloves are not necessary.
2. The suction pressure is checked with the vacuum on, i.e. with the vacuum control valve unlocked.
3. If the MH bag is connected during suction, its valve must be kept open.
4. The T-piece should be supported throughout.

During catheter insertion, it is standard practice to avoid suction to minimize mucosal damage, although Lewis (2002) claims that greater risk is caused without suction due to bacteria being pushed further down the airways. Standard practice is advised until further research emerges.

During catheter withdrawal, some patients hold their breath longer than necessary, in which case they can be told, once the catheter has been withdrawn back to the tracheal tube, that they can breathe again. Unlike with nasopharyngeal suction, it is not always clear to patients when they can breathe again.

If more than one suction pass is necessary, oxygenation must return to baseline before repeat suction. The procedure should be terminated if HR slows by 20 or increases by 40 bpm, if BP drops or arrhythmias develop. The final suction should be outside the endotracheal tube, with the patient's permission, to reach secretions above the cuff, which helps prevent microaspiration and VAP (Hess 2002).

Difficulty in passing the catheter may be due to kinking of the tracheal tube, herniation of the cuff over the end of the tube, or the patient biting the tube. Biting requires reassurance and sometimes insertion of a bite block or Guedel airway.

Vibrations are unnecessary during suction because, unless the patient is paralysed, the enforced coughing accompanying suction overrides outside influences. Occasionally apical vibrations may stimulate a cough.

The AARC (2010) claim that shallow suction, i.e. only as far as the end of the tracheal tube, reduces complications, but Ntoumenopoulos (2013) suggests that this is based on neonatal literature and may be counterproductive.

## Modifications for open suction

Open suction entails inserting a sterile catheter directly into the tracheal tube. Aseptic technique should be pristine: the catheter must not touch the rim of the tracheal tube on insertion and sterile gloves are mandatory. Boxed gloves are not sterile and Rossoff (1993) found that half were contaminated. The same catheter should not be used for repeat suction.

For access to the left main bronchus, Branson (2014) recommends turning the head to the right, or using an angled (coudé-tip) catheter with the tip directed towards the left main bronchus. These techniques are used by anaesthetists, but most physiotherapists do not find them necessary because secretions are usually mobilized sufficiently beforehand.

## Reducing hypoxaemia

Returning the patient to the ventilator at normal settings between suction passes is not adequate to prevent desaturation, and the following are suggested:

1. Pressing the '100% oxygen' button whenever the patient is on the ventilator helps maintain oxygenation.
2. Manual hyperventilation or hyperinflation helps reverse hypoxaemia and atelectasis respectively, if not contraindicated.
3. After suction, VH can be used, e.g. 30 s of peak inspiratory pressure at 35–40 cmH$_2$O and PEEP at 15 cmH$_2$O (Heinze et al. 2011).
4. No more than 10 s should be spent with the patient unable to breathe. If longer is needed, this can be accommodated during open suction by withdrawing the catheter sufficiently to prevent coughing, removing the thumb from the catheter port to release the vacuum, occluding the catheter mount opening (with the catheter still in situ), then giving the patient 100% oxygen by the bag or ventilator. Suction can be resumed when the patient has stabilized. This avoids unnecessary removal and reinsertion of the catheter, which increases infection risk.

## Saline instillation

The need for saline suggests that humidification is inadequate. If this has been corrected but secretions are still too thick to clear, normal saline may be instilled into the lungs. This can increase the yield of sputum (Schreuder & Jones 2004) and reduce VAP (Fig. 21.21), possibly by rinsing out bacteria from the ETT or by stimulating a cough. However, other studies have shown an increased risk of infection, so it should only be done if essential (Roberts 2009).

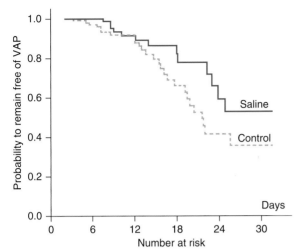

**FIGURE 21.21** Probability of remaining free of ventilator-associated pneumonia *(VAP)*. Log rank 0.02 Kaplan–Meier curve. (From Caruso et al. 2008.)

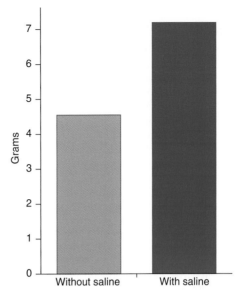

**FIGURE 21.22** Mean 'sputum weight' after suction with and without saline instillation. (From Hudak et al. 1996.)

The mode of action of saline instillation may be to physically dislodge encrusted secretions or to stimulate a cough, because mucus does not incorporate water easily (Halm 2008).

The procedure should not be prolonged, otherwise gas exchange is compromised (Young-Ra 2002) and breathlessness can persist for up to 10 min afterwards (Halm 2008). The following are suggested:

1. Warm the saline, e.g. by always keeping saline in the pocket so that it is readily available at body temperature.
2. When opening the container, the open ends must not be touched even with gloved hands.
3. Advise the patient, then administer the saline slowly to prevent them feeling as if they are drowning.
4. No more than 5 mL at a time is advised (Bostick & Wendelgass 1987), although this can be repeated so long as it is accompanied by increased ventilator $FiO_2$, sometimes interspersed with manual or ventilator hyperventilation to prevent desaturation.
5. If the aim is to loosen secretions (rather than dislodge debris at the end of the tracheal tube), the patient should be turned after instillation, so that the instilled side is uppermost, gravity can do its work and manual techniques applied if required. This may be co-ordinated with the patient's regular turns to avoid unnecessary disruption. The timing involved with the turn is such that suction is then able to clear both secretions and saline.

Tips for open suction:
- Do not allow the saline to splatter over the tracheostomy dressing, or indeed over anything.
- If saline instillation does not clear the secretions, it can be delivered more distally by injecting it through the catheter before suction.

Tip for closed-circuit suction:
- Hold the T-piece upwards to help the passage of saline, unlock the vacuum control valve, advance the catheter, and inject saline through the side port just before inspiration so it is carried distally with the next breath.

Patients should not be turned again until stable. Those who are able can use the yankauer sucker to clear their mouth afterwards.

### MINI CLINICAL REASONING

Do not forget the 'Limitations' section in the literature. Fig. 21.22 shows a 'positive' outcome from saline instillation, but the authors sensibly point out, in their Limitations paragraph, that the sputum weight included the saline.

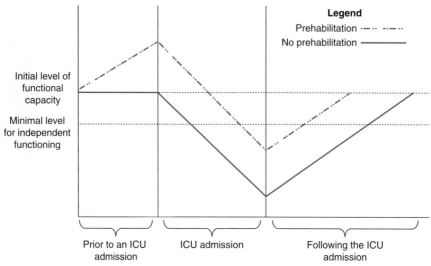

FIGURE 21.23 Proposed effect of prehabilitation. *ICU*, Intensive care unit. (From Topp et al. 2002.)

## EXERCISE AND REHABILITATION

*'Getting me out of bed has always made me feel like the team and I are working together, not against each other'.*

*Hipp & Ely 2012*

The main long-term complication of critical illness is deconditioning, which underlines the importance of early rehabilitation and the consequent reduction in readmission rates (Vollman 2013) and mortality (Rydingsward et al. 2016). Greater numbers of ICU patients now survive (Fan 2010), but the TEAM study (2015) found that less than a third had returned to their previous work after 6 months.

Low muscle mass on admission contributes to mortality (Weijs et al. 2014) and exercise should be initiated immediately (Asher 2013), or beforehand if admission is anticipated (Fig. 21.23). Rehabilitation should be facilitated by nutritional supplements (Jones et al. 2015c) and an 'animated ICU' in which sedation is minimized (Hall 2010). Exposure to steroids during critical illness is associated with reduced physical functioning (Solverson et al. 2016), which can be discussed on ward rounds.

Assessment for rehabilitation should be within 24 h of admission, and rehabilitation is then recommended for a minimum 45 min a day, as tolerated (ICS 2013). The importance of exercise is underlined by the detrimental effects of immobility (p. 24) and the reported outcomes of ICU rehabilitation:

- ↑ quality of life (QoL), ↓ critical care polyneuropathy/myopathy and mortality (Connolly et al. 2016);
- brain protection by reduction of delirium (Hopkins et al. 2012);
- lung protection by modulation of inflammation in early acute lung injury (Goncalves et al. 2012);
- faster weaning, ↑ clinical and functional outcomes (Verceles & Hager 2015);
- ↑ exercise tolerance, ↓ dyspnoea and need for sedation (Adler & Malone 2012);
- ↓ readmissions and pressure ulcers (Azuh et al. 2016);
- ↑ respiratory muscle strength, sphincter control and ventilator-free time (Porta et al. 2005);
- ↑ secretion clearance (Morris & Afifi 2010, p.228);
- ↓ cost (Corcoran et al. 2017).

Early mobilization, in particular, has shown:

- ↓ lung and vascular complications (Clark et al. 2013);
- ↓ delirium (Porter & McClure 2013);
- ↓ time on the ventilator, leading to ↓ atelectasis, pneumonia and the cognitive and functional limitations that can otherwise continue for years after discharge (Vollman 2013);

- ↓ length of stay and ↑ functional ability (McWilliams et al. 2017);
- ↓ morbidity and mortality (Hopkins et al. 2012).

An individual outcome is shown by one proud patient who converted her pre-ICU exercise tolerance of 3 metres to 37 metres during her 9-day stay (Korupolu et al. 2010).

## Passive Exercise

*The complications of bed rest can be nearly as devastating as the illness itself.*

**Rukstele & Gagnon 2013**

Clavet et al. (2008) found that a third of patients who spend more than 2 weeks in the ICU develop joint contractures sufficient to impair function. This can be prevented by passive movements, which also maintain sensory input and comfort, help preserve muscle architecture (Kress 2013) and, if done frequently, reduce the risk of myopathy (Renaud et al. 2013).

Special attention is needed for the Achilles tendon, hip joint, joints around the shoulder, two-joint muscles and, for long-term patients, the jaw and spine. A stiff chest wall may respond to stretching exercises including manual rotation of the thorax in time with the ventilatory cycle (Leelarungrayub et al. 2009), while ensuring that the tracheal tube is stabilized. Continuous passive motion may be used to reduce protein loss (Morris 2007), pain and muscle inflammation (Amidei 2013).

All ICU staff need advice on care of the joints, especially the shoulder, which is the most common joint affected by subsequent chronic pain (Battle et al. 2013). Patients with fractures, burns or altered muscle tone need input from specialist colleagues, and those with impaired peripheral circulation due to septic shock need multidisciplinary intervention. To prevent overstretch of flaccid anterior tibial muscles, a pillow at the end of the bed can be placed against a vertically placed tray to maintain plantigrade.

There is some limited evidence of benefit from neuromuscular electrical stimulation (Fischer et al. 2016) or functional electrical stimulation (Parry et al. 2012). For affluent units, whole-bed vibration helps stimulate neuromuscular activity (Wollersheim 2017).

## Active Exercise

*No modern ICU can match the body's sophisticated system for delivery of biochemical compounds during exercise.*

**Woodard & Berry 2001**

Exercise helps maintain conditioning and reduce inflammation (Winkelman et al. 2007). Benefit has been shown from resistive exercises (Gosselink et al. 2008 and Fig. 21.24), functional exercises such as turning in bed or sitting over the edge of the bed (Chiang et al. 2006), and the use of a Wii (Kho et al. 2012). Some specific effects include the following:

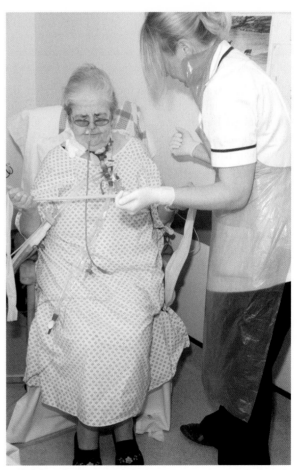

**FIGURE 21.24** Strengthening with stretchy bands (Manchester Royal Infirmary).

1. Arm strengthening for 20 min a day improves strength, mobility and dyspnoea (Porta et al. 2005).
2. Stretching, resistance and endurance exercise can improve pulmonary mechanics and functional status (Chen & Lin 2012).
3. Inspiratory muscle training is useful for patients who have limited ability for systemic exercise, who are haemodynamically stable and are using the pressure support mode of ventilation (Chung et al. 2016d); training twice daily up to Borg score 6–8 can progress exercise tolerance and ADL (Chang et al. 2005).

Inspiratory muscle endurance training occurs with progressive weaning trials and strength training with an inspiratory muscle trainer (Schellekens et al. 2016).

> **KEY POINT**
>
> Active little-and-often exercise is required for all patients who are willing and able.

The quadriceps are a particular focus for regular exercise because they have been found the weakest muscles in survivors (Solverson et al. 2016). Static bikes give a morale boost and are useful for patients who cannot move away from the bedside. Patients on renal replacement therapy can safely practise bedside exercise (Toonstra et al. 2016) and some on ECMO (p. 464) can do bed exercises (Munshi et al. 2017). Those on inotropic support can be mobilized but without vigorous activity that could tax their limited cardiovascular reserve. Patients, nurses and relatives will be motivated by an exercise diary to encourage progression.

## Mobilization

*'Getting me out of bed … helps ground me in the environment and helps my mind, which seems to work overtime to understand the stimuli that bombard it'.*

*Hipp & Ely 2012*

Early rehabilitation has enabled 59% of patients to return to independent function after discharge, as opposed to 35% of those provided with 'standard care' (Page & Casarin 2014). The decision to mobilize should be based on an assessment of cardiovascular stability and respiratory reserve (Table 21.2 and Fig. 21.25). With fastidious observation and monitoring, and solicitous attention to hardware, patients can be mobilized with tracheal tubes (Fig. 21.26), femoral catheters (Perm et al. 2013), other central lines, vasoactive drugs, renal replacement catheters, and in the presence of acute lung injury or delirium (Vollman 2013). Reduced arousal is not a contraindication to rehabilitation, and supported sitting on the edge of the bed may serve as a stimulus to aid wakening and form part of the neurological assessment. The presence of a Sengstaken tube contraindicates mobilization because of the risk of perforation.

Sitting over the edge of the bed aids assessment of sitting balance and physiological stability in response to activity and position change (Fig. 21.27). To acclimatize patients, the head of the bed should be raised before they sit up over the edge of the bed. A drawsheet can be used around the patient if they have poor trunk control. Three to five staff may be needed, depending on whether the patient is ventilated, obese, of low arousal or with profound weakness.

An individualized seating programme can then be devised, using supportive stretcher chairs for patients with limited trunk control, or more active transfers out of bed for patients with some trunk stability. This may require hoists or standing hoists to achieve standing transfers to the chair regularly throughout the day.

A programme of challenged sitting on the edge of the bed, coupled with sitting in a chair helps to prevent hypovolaemia, redistribute skin pressure, maintain muscle length, assist orientation and load vertebrae to limit calcium loss and promote cartilage nutrition. Tipping chairs are useful for patients with orthostatic intolerance, and tilt tables can benefit those with low lung volume, muscle weakness, pressure sores and venous pooling (Chang et al. 2004).

Prior to mobilization, the feed is stopped, and increased ventilatory support may be needed at first, with brief sessions to avoid fatigue. Throughout rehabilitation, the patient's colour and monitors are kept under observation, especially pallor, dizziness, unstable cardiovascular status or reduced $SpO_2$. Standing without walking should be brief to prevent venous pooling.

The following complications of mobilization have been reported in a systematic review that included mechanically ventilated patients with central lines or on haemodialysis:

- ↓ $SpO_2$ (the most common adverse event)
- unstable BP

## TABLE 21.2 Precautions when mobilizing intensive care unit patients

| System | Factors that may limit mobilization | System | Factors that may limit mobilization |
|---|---|---|---|
| **Cardiovascular** | | **Neurological** | |
| MAP | <65 mmHg or below target range >20% recent variability | Brain injury | Increased ICP or recent surgery |
| | | Spinal cord lesion | Unstable injury |
| Heart rate | <40 or >130 bpm | | |
| Cardiac | Cardiac ischaemia, new MI, unstable ECG, unstable angina Arrhythmia requiring new drug Temporary pacemaker | Seizures | Uncontrolled |
| | | **Renal** | |
| | | Haemodialysis | Unstable blood pressure Arteriovenous fistula dislodgement |
| Other haemodynamic problems | Inotropes, vasoactive drugs especially new vasopressor, β-blockers Bleeding, including oesophageal varices Platelet count <20,000 mm$^{-3}$ PE or DVT not yet medically stable Orthostatic hypotension | **Orthopaedic** | Unstable fracture |
| | | **Other** | Hb <7 g/100 mL or acute ↓ in Hb Bleeding Split skin graft, vascular surgery Blood sugar <3.5 mmol/L Recent eye surgery |
| **Respiratory** | | | |
| SpO$_2$ | <90% >4% recent decrease | **Contraindications, or factors indicating that activity should stop** | |
| FiO$_2$ | <0.6 | Request by patient to stop, or visible distress Dizziness New onset chest pain Change in colour ↓ Blood pressure or heart rate RR >35 breaths/min sustained for >60 s Change in heart rhythm SpO$_2$ <85% | |
| PaO$_2$/FiO$_2$ | <300 | | |
| Respiratory rate | <8 or >30 breaths/min | | |
| Ventilator | PEEP >10 cmH$_2$O Asynchrony with ventilator Insecure airway Pressure support >20 cmH$_2$O or SIMV >18 breaths/min FiO$_2$ >0.6 | | |

*DVT*, deep vein thrombosis; *ECG*, electrocardiogram; *Hb*, haemoglobin; *HR*, heart rate; *ICP*, intracranial pressure; *MAP*, mean arterial pressure; *MI*, myocardial infarct; *PE*, pulmonary embolism; *PEEP*, positive end-expiratory pressure; *RR*, respiratory rate; *SIMV*, synchronized intermittent mandatory ventilation.
From Chung & Mueller 2011, Hodgson et al. 2014, Kortebein 2009, Parry et al. 2012, Perme 2009, Stiller 2007, Talley et al. 2013, Vollman 2013.

- falls
- loss of nasogastric tube
- loss of arterial line
- extubation
- patient–ventilator asynchrony (Adler & Malone 2012)

This list should not prevent mobilization but is a useful reminder of the vigilance required. Although a femoral line can be managed, some physiotherapists encourage their teams to site these elsewhere when possible.

Long-term patients may be excited at the prospect of their much-awaited first expedition out of bed, and some are then disillusioned by the extent of their weakness and fatigue, especially if they have lost the comprehension as well as the ability to walk. One patient stated: 'I didn't know how to walk any more' (Strahana & Brown 2005).

For patients able to go further than walking on the spot, mobile monitoring and either a reservoir bag or portable ventilator on a trolley can be used. Adventurous patients aim to exercise to 50%–60% of maximal

| Respiratory considerations | In-bed exercises | Out-of-bed exercises |
|---|---|---|
| Endotracheal tube | ● | ● |
| Tracheostomy tube | ● | ● |
| **Fraction of inspired oxygen** | | |
| ≤0.6 | ● | ● |
| >0.6 | ▲ | ▲ |
| **Oxygen saturation** | | |
| ≥90% | ● | ● |
| <90% | ▲ | ⬣ |
| **Respiratory rate** | | |
| ≤30 bpm | ● | ● |
| >30 bpm | ▲ | ▲ |
| **Ventilation** | | |
| Mode HFOV | ▲ | ⬣ |
| **PEEP** | | |
| ≤10 cmH$_2$O | ● | ● |
| >10 cmH$_2$O | ▲ | ▲ |
| **Ventilator dysynchrony** | ▲ | ▲ |
| **Rescue therapies** | | |
| Nitric oxide | ▲ | ▲ |
| Prostacyclin | ▲ | ▲ |
| Prone positioning | ⬣ | ⬣ |

● Low risk of adverse event.

▲ Risks and benefits to be weighed up prior to mobilization. If decision to go ahead, gradual initiation of mobility.

⬣ No mobilization without agreement of intensivist, senior physiotherapist and senior nurse.

**FIGURE 21.25** Respiratory safety considerations. *HFOV,* High-frequency oscillation ventilation. (From Hodgson et al. 2016.)

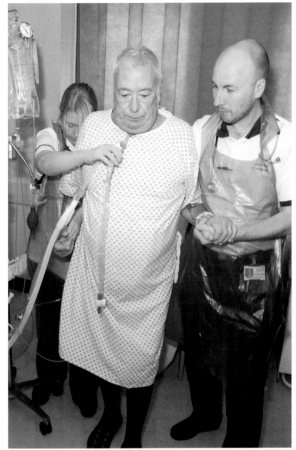

FIGURE 21.26 Mobilizing at Manchester Royal Infirmary.

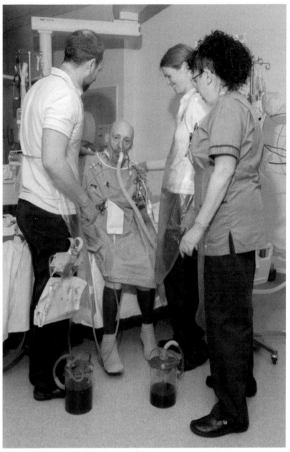

FIGURE 21.27 Sitting balance (Manchester Royal Infirmary).

HR (Stiller 2007). An assistant should follow with a wheelchair, and motivation should be provided with a progress chart and record sheet (Appendix A), both negotiated with the patient.

With these precautions, Leditschke et al. (2012) were able to mobilize their patients on most days, and Nava (1998) showed how a little-and-often but intensive rehabilitation programme led to 'dramatic improvements', even in patients unable to wean. Clark (1985) documents a patient describing how visits outside helped to 'maintain my sanity'. The gym is also a useful destination, and even the pool for some ventilated patients (Wegner 2017).

Getting dressed is a good morale booster, done in a separate session and with the aid of the occupational therapist if required. Occupational therapy is recommended from the onset of MV (Pohlman et al. 2010) because it speeds functional independence (Hodgson et al. 2012), and is particularly useful if patients are experiencing delirium (Álvarez et al. 2017).

## End of Treatment Session

After treatment, the following are suggested:
1. Check that all alarms are on.
2. Ensure that the patient's nurse, if not present, knows that treatment is finished.
3. Ensure that the call bell and other requirements are within reach of the patient.
4. Ensure that lines are in view.

5. Reassure the patient that they are not being left alone and that their lines are safe so that they do not feel inhibited from moving.

6. For a side-lying patient, check shoulder position and ensure that their ear is not folded over.

7. Check any individual concerns, e.g. anxiety about facing a wall.

8. Tell the patient the time and ask if they need further information.

9. If a rest is required, liaise with the nurse about dimming the light and using eye shades.

## Transfer From the Intensive Care Unit

*'You'd gone from this hugely protective critical care to this sort of hit and miss uncoordinated service'.*

**Field et al. 2008**

At the heart of rehabilitation is teamwork and autonomy (Reames et al. 2016), which are particularly relevant on transfer. For longer-term patients who have been under constant supervision, transfer to the ward is a vulnerable time as well as bringing relief at reaching a milestone. Strategies to minimize relocation stress include early identification of risk factors (Hosein et al. 2013), restoration of sleep patterns, information packs for the patient and family, phased reduction of bedside equipment, a visit from the ward physiotherapist, if different, an exit interview, follow-up outreach and post-ICU assessment (Appendix A). Patients may be weaker than either they or the ward staff expect, sometimes leaving them unable to pick up their tablets or press the buzzer. They may need preparation for their first use of a mirror so they are not shocked if their appearance has changed, e.g. a drastic loss of weight.

Mortality is increased by transfer being either premature (Danbury et al. 2013) or delayed, but the risk can be reduced by early warning scores (Churpek et al. 2016) and transition programs (Niven 2014). Nighttime discharge should be documented as an adverse incident (NICE 2007).

## Follow-Up

*She had offered to peel the potatoes and managed four potatoes in 40 min, then had to have an hour's rest before peeling the other four.*

**Jones & Griffiths 2002, p. 54**

Post-ICU functional status has a direct effect on mortality (Rydingsward 2016). The aftermath of an ICU stay includes persistent cognitive and emotional effects (Merbitz et al. 2016), with more than 50% of patients suffering disability (Davidson et al. 2017) and a third with neurological consequences (Sharshar et al. 2016). Three months after hospital discharge, the majority of survivors continue to experience ongoing muscle weakness (Solverson et al. 2016), and follow-up is advised for at least 6 months (Beusekom et al. 2016), with longer-term patients needing access to a multidisciplinary follow-up clinic (Bourseau et al. 2016).

Structuring rehabilitation on the ICF model (p. 29), including attention to restoring sleep patterns (Aitken et al. 2015), helps prevent 'postintensive care syndrome' (Farley et al. 2016). An individualized exercise program improves QoL (Shelly et al. 2017), and significant functional improvements can be achieved even for patients who are ventilator-dependent (Sobush et al. 2012).

Physiotherapy is aimed at a progressive programme of functional exercises, circuit and endurance training, strengthening exercises for limb and respiratory muscles, pacing, balance practice and education on the recovery process (Major et al. 2016). A dedicated gym class enables patients to find support from others who have been through a similar experience, support which neither professionals nor family can provide in the same way. For example, one young patient had not been able to come to terms with attempting to hit a nurse while hallucinating, despite reassurance from staff. 'Oh that's nothing to what I tried to do' said a fellow patient on the neighbouring exercise bike, immediately lifting the burden from the young man.

Multidisciplinary input includes dealing with fears of falling and panic attacks, healthy eating for fragile appetites, and contributions from the occupational therapist, pharmacist or nurse, and a rehabilitation psychologist (Jackson et al. 2016). A third of patients suffer depression at 12 months (Rabiee et al. 2016), and some may need help in constructing a narrative of events, facilitated by their diary. Other patients feel that they have been given a second chance in life and experience heightened spirituality (Papathanassoglou et al. 2003), each day seeming more precious than before. Follow-up gives them the chance to process this.

Ongoing rehabilitation continues to improve QoL (McWilliams et al. 2016a), and there is the opportunity to identify complications such as visual difficulties due to hypotensive episodes, sexual dysfunction, chronic fatigue syndrome and polypharmacy (Waldmann 2009, p. 70).

Late rehabilitation may also be successful, one patient describing her continued dyspnoea years later, until she hired a trainer, 'to brutalize me on the treadmill', and fully recovered after 12 sessions (Misak 2011).

Feedback from follow-up clinics helps to sensitize ICU staff to the patient experience. For example, a patient who had been described as an ICU success story told how she had experienced lying naked in bed while staff washed her, chatting to each other about their social lives. Every day for the past 3 years, she said, she 'wished she was dead' (Russell 1999).

Modest goals and exercise plans should be included in the discharge summary and sent to community physiotherapists and general practitioners, with copies to the patient.

*Surviving critical illness is only the beginning.*
**Batt et al. 2013**

## PHYSIOTHERAPY OUTCOMES

Clinical outcomes include:
1. Auscultation
   - ↑ Breath sounds, ↓ bronchial breathing, ↓ crackles
2. Radiology
   - ↑ Lung volume
3. Observations
   - ↑ $SpO_2$
   - With pressure controlled ventilation: ↑ tidal volume
   - With volume controlled ventilation: ↓ airway pressure.
   - ↑ Muscle strength (Vanpee et al. 2013)

For measuring physical function, valid tools are step tests (Anderson 2016), Manchester Mobility Score (McWilliams et al. 2016a), Functional Status Score (Huang et al. 2016d), Chelsea Critical Care Physical Assessment Tool (Corner et al. 2016), motion sensors (Beach et al. 2017) ICU Mobility Scale (Tipping 2016), Physical Function Test (Denehy et al. 2013) and the Acute Care Index of Function (Bisset et al. 2016). QoL outcomes include the Hospital Anxiety and Depression Score, Impact of Events Score and Short Form 36 (Beusekom et al. 2016).

*'I suppose it's safe to say that I'm not the same person as before'.*
**Patient, quoted by Karlsson & Forsberg 2007**

## RECOGNITION AND MANAGEMENT OF EMERGENCIES

The key to the successful management of emergencies is informed anticipation and recognition. Physiotherapists are not immersed in life-threatening events every day, so it is advisable to review protocols regularly to maintain confidence and avoid the indecision that is often evident at the scene of an emergency. It is also necessary to know if a patient has an advance directive declining a certain procedure, and if this has been changed subsequently.

Some emergencies are covered in the text:
- asphyxic asthma, p. 83
- burns, p. 535
- near-drowning, p. 537
- chest drain complications, p. 317
- fat embolism, p. 536
- laryngospasm, p. 220
- shock, p. 540
- spinal cord injuries, p. 527
- tracheostomy complications, p. 327

Local protocols should take precedence over the information in this section.

### Cardiac Arrest

Cardiac arrest is cessation of heart function. It is the normal mechanism of the old-fashioned process of death, but is occasionally reversible. It is followed within seconds by loss of consciousness and then by loss of breathing.

#### Anticipation

Before starting work on any new ward, the first task is to locate the crash trolley. When seeing a new patient, the medical history will provide evidence of Do Not Attempt Resuscitation (DNAR) status and risky conditions such as ischaemic heart disease, severe respiratory disease, drug overdose, metabolic disturbance, arrhythmias or shock. Abnormal vital signs may be present in the hours up to a cardiac arrest (Andersen 2016). Physiotherapists working in the community or out of reach of a crash trolley need to carry a pocket mask for mouth-to-mask ventilation. Teamwork is assisted by a cardiac arrest risk triage system (Churpek et al. 2012).

## Recognition

Warning signs are a change in breathing, colour, facial expression or mental function. Hypoventilation with altered consciousness is an ominous combination. The electrocardiogram (ECG) then shows pulseless electrical activity, pulseless ventricular tachycardia, ventricular fibrillation or asystole.

After cessation of the heart beat:
- the ECG flatlines
- in 15 s, the patient loses consciousness
- in 30 s, the pupils dilate fully
- in 90–300 s, cerebral damage occurs (Papastylianou 2012), though the brain stem lasts longer

The patient's colour may be pale, ashen or blue, depending on the cause. No carotid pulse can be felt in the groove between the larynx and sternomastoid muscle. Respiration may become gasping and then stop, unless respiratory arrest has been the primary event.

## Action

The time between collapse and initiation of resuscitation is critical, and a false alarm is better than a dead patient. If suspicions are raised by a change in consciousness and colour, call out to the patient, and if they are unresponsive, follow the basic life support stage of cardiopulmonary resuscitation (CPR) as in the Resuscitation Council (UK) guidelines (Appendix A, Guidelines and links for health professionals) and local training, with refinement of technique described by Riess (2016).

On arrival of the crash team, advanced life support may include defibrillation, during which staff should stand clear. When no longer needed, the physiotherapist can give attention to other patients who will be distressed at witnessing the event. Survival for inhospital cardiac arrests is about 10% (Hellenkamp et al. 2016). Most survivors report an acceptable QoL (Haydon 2017), but some sustain hypoxic brain damage and require an ICF-based rehabilitation programme (Moulaert et al. 2011).

## Respiratory Arrest

Loss of airway integrity and compromised lung function are the most rapid killers in emergency medicine (Mattu 2016). As cardiac arrest leads to respiratory arrest, so does respiratory arrest, if not reversed, lead to cardiac arrest.

## Anticipation

Predisposing factors include exacerbation of COPD, airway obstruction (e.g. foreign body, smoke inhalation, swelling or bleeding from trauma) or aspiration. Warning signs are inability to speak, and violent respiratory efforts, laboured breathing or drowsiness.

## Recognition

Respiratory arrest is indicated by absence of chest movement, loss of airflow from the mouth and nose, and sometimes cyanosis. This progresses to loss of consciousness.

## Action

1. Call for help.
2. Establish a patent airway as for CPR. Sometimes just moving the head will open the throat. If there is no airflow, continue as below.
3. If a foreign body is the likely cause and the victim is choking, attempt to dislodge it from the throat by suction or by hand. The main culprits are the tongue, vomit and blood. If unsuccessful, follow the Resuscitation Council choking algorithm (Appendix A) and local training. If the patient is still not breathing, continue as below.
4. Ventilate by a bag-valve-mask (Ambu bag) system connected to oxygen, one person maintaining the jaw thrust while the other squeezes the bag. Otherwise use a Laerdal face mask or mouth-to-mouth. Slow flow rates minimize gastric insufflation. Inspiration time is $1\frac{1}{2}$ to 2 s. Repeat once every 6 s. Continue for 1 min, then reassess.

If cardiac arrest ensues, instigate full CPR. If breathing starts, turn the patient into the recovery position because vomiting is common as consciousness lightens.

## Seizure
### Anticipation

The medical notes indicate whether a patient has a history of epilepsy. Other causes of fitting are brain injury, alcohol intoxication, or, in children, fever. Some patients sense an aura in advance, and there may be some muscle twitching.

## Recognition

Seizures vary from transient loss of consciousness to major muscle activity, followed by drowsiness and sometimes cardiac arrhythmias (Lende et al. 2016).

## Action

1. Patients subject to seizures should have the bed kept low, side rails up and padded, and oxygen and suction available.
2. If there is advance warning, insert a Guedel airway, if the patient consents. Do not attempt this once the seizure is under way.
3. Protect the patient's head and body from injury. If they are out of bed, ease them to the floor. Loosen tight clothing around the neck if possible. Clear the area of risky objects. Do not use restraints or hold the victim down.
4. If there is no pulse or breathing when the seizure is over, call the crash team and begin CPR. Otherwise put the patient in the recovery position. Suction the mouth if required. If the patient is conscious, explain what has happened. Request medical assessment.

## Haemorrhage

### Anticipation

Uncontrolled bleeding can follow surgery, arterial line disconnection or trauma.

### Recognition

External bleeding is usually apparent. Internal bleeding is suspected if there are signs of severe hypovolaemia (p. 478). BP and HR are the least reliable of these signs because BP can be maintained by vasoconstriction and HR is responsive to other variables. Bleeding into a closed space causes progressive pain.

### Action

1. Position the patient supine.
2. Apply pressure to the bleeding point if accessible.
3. Elevate the affected part if feasible.
4. Request assistance.
5. Explain to the patient what is happening.

The medical management of severe bleeding is described by Riha and Schreiber (2013).

## Massive Haemoptysis

Coughing up more than 200 mL of blood over 24 h risks hypotension or aspiration of blood.

### Anticipation

Predisposing factors are lung cancer, bronchiectasis, abscess or tuberculosis.

### Action

If the patient can protect their airway, they should sit up and expectorate the blood until bronchoscopy is ready. Other patients should be positioned with the head slightly down, and if the side of the haemorrhage is known, laid on the affected side to prevent aspiration into the healthy lung. Cough suppressants or sedatives should not be given. Patients with depressed consciousness or at risk of aspiration need intubation, suction and sometimes bronchial artery embolization (Okuda et al. 2016).

## Cardiac Tamponade

Cardiac tamponade is accumulation of gas or fluid, usually blood, in the pericardium. The pericardium is not distensible in the short term and can only accommodate 100 mL fluid rapidly without affecting cardiac output, after which an additional 40 mL doubles pericardial pressure, compressing the heart and damming back blood into the systemic veins (Fig. 21.28). If this increasing pressure is not relieved, cardiac arrest ensues.

### Anticipation

Tamponade can occur in the 24 h after heart surgery. Other predisposing factors are trauma, dissecting aneurysm, infection or malignancy.

### Recognition

Progressive compression of the heart leads to precipitate loss of cardiac output, and the following may be evident:

- $\downarrow$ BP, $S\bar{v}O_2$ and urine output
- $\uparrow$ HR, CVP and PAWP
- CVP and PAWP approximately equal
- pulsus paradoxus
- distended neck veins
- enlarged heart on X-ray
- restlessness, fear or, typically, feelings of impending doom (Ikematsu & Kloos 2012)

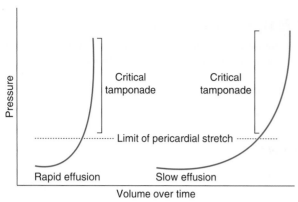

**FIGURE 21.28** Pressure–volume curves showing cardiac tamponade. The left curve shows the fluid quickly exceeding the limit of pericardial stretch. The right curve shows a slower rate of pericardial filling which takes longer to reach this limit. (From Spodick 2003.)

### Action

Alert the doctor, who will aspirate the fluid or take the patient to theatre.

### Tension Pneumothorax

Gas entering the pleural space on inspiration but unable to escape on expiration causes a tension pneumothorax. Cardiac arrest normally follows within 20 min.

### Anticipation

In ventilated patients, pneumothoraces may be under tension at the following times:
- immediately after intubation, if inadvertent tube placement into the right main bronchus causes hyperinflation of the right lung;
- in the hours following initiation of MV, when air is forced through a previously unknown leak in the pleura.

Predisposing factors are emphysema, and surgery or other trauma to the chest. Subcutaneous emphysema in the neck can be a warning sign.

### Recognition

Tension pneumothorax is sufficiently rare to be sometimes mistaken for severe bronchospasm. Both of these conditions cause respiratory distress, wheeze, increased airway pressure and laboured breathing. The added features of a tension pneumothorax are:
- ↓ amplitude in ECG (often the first sign)
- ↓ chest movement and ↑ expansion on the affected side
- hyperresonant percussion note on the affected side
- ↓ breath sounds on the affected side, or both sides if severe
- ↓ $SpO_2$
- cyanosis
- distended neck veins and ↑ CVP (unless the patient is hypovolaemic)
- displaced apex beat
- in self-ventilating patients, dyspnoea and tracheal deviation away from the affected side
- in ventilated patients, high airway pressure (in volume-control ventilation), and expired minute volume less than preset minute volume
- ↓ BP, ↑ HR, progressing to cardiovascular collapse
- X-ray as in Fig. 21.29.

### Action

Alert the doctor, who will insert a 7 cm needle into the pleura at the second intercostal space in the midclavicular line to release the pressure (Hecker et al. 2016). While waiting, give 100% oxygen, and an experienced physiotherapist can disconnect the patient from the ventilator, connect to a bag and manually ventilate with 100% oxygen, using high flow and low pressure. Otherwise $FiO_2$ through the ventilator should be maximized. A few patients may be able to breathe spontaneously, which will reduce the positive pressure in the chest. These decisions are usually taken by the team.

## Air Embolism
### Anticipation

Air may enter the circulation after cardiac or neurosurgery, with a pneumothorax or during insertion or removal of a pulmonary artery catheter or vascath.

### Recognition

A large air embolus causes respiratory distress, palpitations, dizziness, weakness and pallor or cyanosis.

### Action

Summon help. Place the patient head-down in left side-lying, which diverts air away from the right heart and pulmonary circulation. Give 100% oxygen. An embolus

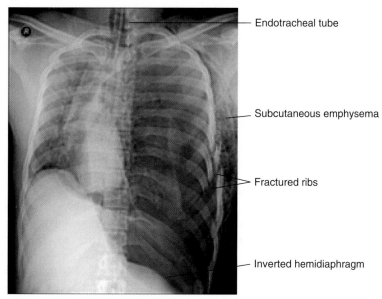

Endotracheal tube

Subcutaneous emphysema

Fractured ribs

Inverted hemidiaphragm

**FIGURE 21.29** Left tension pneumothorax, as indicated by a black area devoid of lung markings on the patient's left, and mediastinal shift to the right. This is an X-ray that should never be seen because there is usually no time to obtain a film.

>100 mL may cause cardiac arrest, which requires the supine head-down tilt and cardiac compression with heavy and deep pressure to disperse air bubbles to peripheral segments of the pulmonary artery. Venous gas embolism may require surgical removal, while arterial embolism may benefit from hyperbaric oxygen.

## Anaphylaxis

Anaphylaxis often manifests as respiratory distress or, with anaphylactic shock, hypotension, occurring minutes to hours after exposure to an allergen. After summoning assistance, the patient should be positioned with legs raised. In hospital they need high-percentage oxygen (Ninchoji et al. 2016). Outside hospital, they may self-administer adrenalin.

## Ventilator Malfunction or Disconnection

Astute eyes and ears pick up the slight hiss of an air leak, identify from an orchestra of alarms which is the offending malfunction, or notice the subtle change in a drowsy patient's demeanour signifying that something is amiss. Prevention includes reading the ventilator handbook to understand its workings and distinguish what each alarm signifies.

## Alarms

The most relevant alarms for the physiotherapist are the high and low pressure alarms, and those for BP, $FiO_2$ and the humidifier heater. The high pressure alarm is set at about 5–10 $cmH_2O$ higher than peak airway pressure and may be activated if there is:

- major atelectasis
- sputum retention in a large airway
- patient coughing or fighting the ventilator
- bronchospasm
- pneumothorax
- partial extubation
- right main bronchus intubation
- cuff herniation over the end of the tracheal tube
- patient biting the ETT

If the patient bites the ETT, this requires dissuasion or a bite block. For a displaced ETT, the doctor will deflate the cuff, reposition the tube, inflate the cuff, listen for equal breath sounds and request a check X-ray.

The low pressure alarm means that pressure has fallen more than 5–10 $cmH_2O$ below the desired limit and indicates that there is a leak in the system, confirmed by reduced expired minute volume and/or airway pressure. A disconnected ventilator circuit should be reconnected, after a quick alcohol wipe if it has touched anything. The patient's condition should be checked, the cause determined, appropriate adjustments made and the nurse informed.

Alarms are fallible. Patient observation comes first.

## Arterial Line or Central Line Disconnection

If a major line becomes disconnected at a junction, the patient requires reassurance because of the amount of blood loss, and the nurse may need assistance in reconnecting the line, while ensuring that no air is present in the line.

If a major line comes out of the patient, firm pressure to the site is required and the doctor informed so that it can be reinserted.

## Unplanned Extubation

Accidental endotracheal extubation can destabilize a patient haemodynamically and compromise ventilation. Prevention is assisted by using weaning protocols and avoiding restraints (Bouza et al. 2007). If extubation occurs, call for help, apply oxygen, optimize the patient's position to assist breathing, and advise him/her to breathe steadily. Bag/mask ventilation may be required.

## Distress in a Ventilated Patient

Patient problems causing distress include:
- subjective problems (p. 479);
- objective problems (Fig. 21.30);
- pneumothorax, pulmonary oedema, bronchospasm, abdominal distension or excessive secretions;
- biting the tube.

Ventilator problems include:
- kink (high pressure alarm) or leak (low pressure alarm) in the circuit;
- intrinsic PEEP;
- inaccurate settings for flow rate, tidal volume, I:E ratio or trigger sensitivity.

## Action

Call for assistance. Check airway pressure or tidal volume, and monitors. Ask the patient if they want more air. If the answer is a nod, or the patient is unable to respond, disconnect the patient from the ventilator, after informing them, and connect to the bag with oxygen. Either manually ventilate or allow the patient to self-ventilate through the bag, with the valve open for minimal resistance and a high flow rate for comfort.

If distress continues, it is probably a patient-based problem (Fig. 21.31), to be sorted with yes/no questions

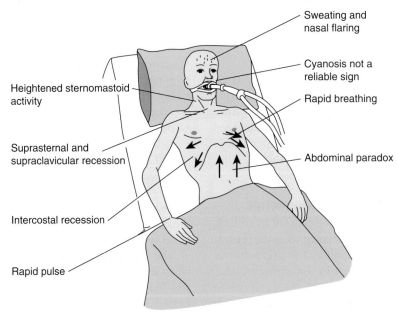

Sweating and nasal flaring

Cyanosis not a reliable sign

Rapid breathing

Heightened sternomastoid activity

Suprasternal and supraclavicular recession

Abdominal paradox

Intercostal recession

Rapid pulse

**FIGURE 21.30** Physical signs of patient distress. (Adapted from Tobin 1991.)

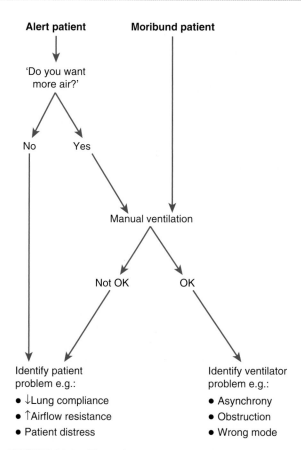

**FIGURE 21.31** Flow chart to manage distress in a ventilated patient.

(p. 486) or suctioning the airway. Unilateral air entry raises suspicions of a malpositioned tracheal tube, pneumothorax or mucous plug.

If manual ventilation resolves the distress, it is probably a ventilator problem, to be dealt with as follows:

- leaking tracheal tube cuff: inflate the cuff with air from a syringe, just enough to eliminate the leak, inform the nurse who will measure and record the cuff pressure;
- tube disconnection: reconnect after cleaning the disconnected ends;
- inability to identify problem: inform the nurse;
- tracheal tube malfunction, bronchospasm, ventilator asynchrony unresolved by talking to the patient: inform the doctor.

## ON CALLS

A well managed on-call system can sustain many a sick patient through a difficult night. The key to success is education, so that all parties understand the scope and limitations of physiotherapy.

### Education of Medical Staff

All levels of medical staff need information on the indications for out-of-hours physiotherapy, with particular attention to juniors starting a new rotation. Young doctors in a new environment can become anxious with an unfamiliar event and call out the physiotherapist unnecessarily, or not call when it is indicated. Education can be through informal talks, involvement in doctors' continuing education programmes and ensuring that the junior doctors' induction pack contains on-call information. Medical training hardly brushes the subject of physiotherapy and this is an educational opportunity to be grasped gladly.

### Education of Nursing Staff

Nurses and physiotherapists work closely and have an understanding of each others' roles. Day-to-day exchange of information lays the foundation for co-operation, and this can be developed into teaching sessions so that nursing staff know when to advise doctors that the physiotherapist should be called.

### Education of Physiotherapists

Junior and non-respiratory senior staff need confidence in making respiratory decisions. Useful time can be spent going through equipment and practising problem-solving with case studies. Competency tools are available (Thomas et al. 2008) and several steps can be taken to facilitate a sound night's sleep for those on call:

- shadowing a senior colleague on a call-out;
- time set aside the preceding afternoon for the on-call physiotherapist to see any borderline patients with the respiratory physiotherapist;
- a respiratory physiotherapist available at the end of the phone for advice;
- after a call-out, discussing with a mentor the clinical reasoning and treatment of the patient;
- a handout to include switchboard arrangements, location of equipment, bleep information and who is authorized to call out the physiotherapist.

If called to the emergency department, it is advisable to check when the patient will be available for treatment and not immersed in tests and investigations.

The interests of the patient and good relations with other disciplines can be fostered by the physiotherapist pre-arranging call-outs when appropriate. The physiotherapist can also give advice over the phone.

Many departments organize evening physiotherapy shifts because there is evidence that this can prevent deterioration in patients after major surgery (Ntoumenopoulos & Greenwood 1996). Seven-day working has also improved clinical outcomes (Smith & Coup 2011).

An on-call service is particularly helpful for patients with acute COPD (Babu et al. 2010). Box 21.2 provides suggestions for the alleviation of dyspnoea in these and other acutely unwell patients.

## CASE STUDY: MS CM

*Identify the problems of this 58-year-old woman from Chichester who has been admitted for MV due to apnoea of unknown cause.*

### Background

•   Several admissions for MV

### Nurse report

•   Patient needs regular reminders to breathe at night

### Subjective

•   I hate this tube in my throat
•   Tired, not sleeping well

### Objective

•   Intubated, on CPAP via the ventilator
•   Patient alert, in side-lying
•   Vital signs, $SpO_2$, auscultation and X-ray normal

### Day 2

•   Diagnosed with Ondine's curse

### Questions

1. Does the patient have a problem with impaired oxygenation?
2. Does the patient have a problem with impaired ventilation?

3. Does the patient have a problem with her inspiratory muscles?
4. Does the patient have a problem with her respiratory pump?
5. Is the mode of ventilation suitable?
6. Goals?
7. Plan?

*Ondine's curse:* apnoea caused by loss of automatic control of respiration, usually due to defective chemoreceptor responsiveness secondary to neurological or other disorder.

---

### CLINICAL REASONING

Re. intubated patients:

*'Although published guidelines recommend that these catheters be used once only when employing an open technique, this recommendation does not appear to be research based'.*

**Effect of reusing suction catheters,**
*Heart Lung* (2001) 30: 225–233

---

### Response to Case Study

1. No, $SpO_2$ is normal.
2. Yes, Ms M requires regular reminders to breathe at night.
3. No, she is not complaining of breathlessness and is able to breathe when prompted.
4. Yes, the diagnosis implicates the neurological component of her respiratory pump.
5. No, CPAP supports oxygenation, not ventilation. Ms M needs a mode that provides mandatory breaths at night for when she does not breathe, e.g. SIMV. No ventilation is required in the day when she can initiate breaths consciously.
6. Goals: maintain function while short and long-term management are organized.
7. Plan:
    •   liaise with team about mode of ventilation; suggest nocturnal noninvasive ventilation (NIV);
    •   check patient's understanding of diagnosis and agree plan of action;
    •   mobilize patient as able while ventilated; when weaned, give clothes and advise on self-mobility;

## BOX 21.2   Management of the Acutely Breathless Patient

**Tips**
- Avoid noise, bright lights and crowding.
- Do not enter the patient's personal space until after introductions.
- Avoid chatter, be specific, talk gently and steadily.
- Offer questions with yes/no answers.
- Identify the patient's view of the cause of their dyspnoea.
- Relatives may have information on what normally helps their family member.
- Patients may find curtains claustrophobic or need the window open.

**Management of symptoms**
- Fatigue and SOB: rest, positioning and SOB techniques (Chapter 8).
- Feeling out of control: identify patient's own strategies, suggest others, ensure autonomy.
- Anxiety: identify cause, provide information.
- Lack of sleep: liaise with team re. environment, check physical discomfort and positioning.
- Pain: identify cause. If due to coughing, educate on selective cough facilitation and suppression (Chapter 7) as and when appropriate, or wound support. If due to muscle tension, relieve by positioning and relaxation.
- Exhaustion: monitor $PaCO_2$ and pH to identify need for noninvasive ventilation (NIV).

**Management of objective signs**

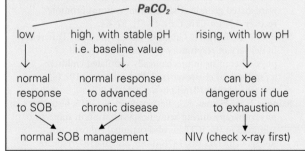

If $PaCO_2$ is not available:
- monitor $SpO_2$ which is less sensitive to $V_E$ but will decrease if ↓ $V_E$ is severe;
- monitor signs of rising $CO_2$: headache, flapping tremor, warm hands.

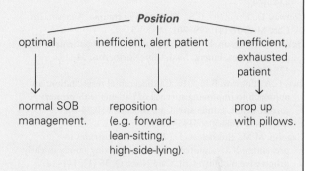

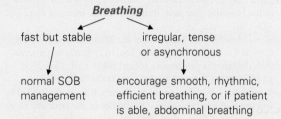

**Management of secretions in a breathless patient**
- Hydration
- Humidification (warm if bronchospasm)
- Slow rhythmic percussion
- AD or modified ACBT (without slowing RR)
- Cough suppression until secretions are accessible, then cough facilitation

*ACBT*, Active cycle of breathing; *AD*, autogenic drainage; *RR*, respiratory rate; *SOB*, shortness of breath; *V_E*, minute volume.

- liaise with physiotherapist at referral centre to which patient will be sent for initiation of long-term home nocturnal NIV.

Footnote – dolphins are also 'conscious breathers' and can only allow half of their brain to sleep at a time.

### RESPONSE TO CLINICAL REASONING

If there is no research to justify a technique, then physiological reasoning would suggest that reinserting a used catheter into a sterile airway is likely to introduce infection.

# RECOMMENDED READING

Asher, A., 2013. Equipment used for safe mobilization of the ICU patient. Crit. Care Nurs. Q. 36 (1), 101–108.

Baldwin, C.E., Paratz, J.D., Bersten, A.D., 2013. Muscle strength assessment in critically ill patients with handheld dynamometry. J. Crit. Care 1, 77–86.

Connors, G.R., Siner, J.M., 2015. Clinical reasoning and risk in the Intensive Care Unit. Clin. Chest Med. 36 (3), 449–459.

Conway, D., Urquhart, C.S., 2017. Airway trauma. Anaesth. Int. Care Med. 18 (4), 199–201.

DeVos, E., Jacobson, L., 2016. Approach to adult patients with acute dyspnea. Emerg. Med. Clin. North. Am. 34 (1), 129–149.

Ewy, G.A., Bobrow, B.J., 2016. Cardiocerebral resuscitation: an approach to improving survival of patients with primary cardiac arrest. J. Intensive. Care Med. 31 (1), 24–33. doi:10.1177/0885066614544450.

Gagnon, M.M., Rukstele, C.D., 2013. Making strides in preventing ICU-acquired weakness: involving family in early progressive mobility. Crit. Care Nurs. Q. 36 (1), 141–147.

Gudzenko, V., Bittner, E.A., Schmidt, U.H., 2010. Emergency airway management. Respir. Care 55 (8), 10–35.

Jain, S.N., 2011. A pictorial essay: Radiology of lines and tubes in the intensive care unit. Indian J. Radiol. Imaging 21 (3), 182–190.

Kanji, S., MacPhee, H., Singh, A., et al., 2016. Validation of the Critical Care Pain Observation Tool in critically ill patients with delirium: a prospective cohort study. Crit. Care Med. 44 (5), 943–947. doi:10.1097/CCM.0000000000001522.

Karnatovskaia, L.V., Johnson, M.M., Benzo, R.P., et al., 2015. The spectrum of psychocognitive morbidity in the critically ill: a review of the literature and call for improvement. J. Crit. Care 30 (1), 130–137. doi:10.1016/j.jcrc.2014.09.024.

Kaul, T.K., Mittal, G., 2013. Mapleson's breathing systems. Indian J. Anaesth. 57 (5), 507–515. doi:10.4103/0019-5049.120148.

Kelly, F.E., Hommers, C., Jackson, R., et al., 2013. Algorithm for management of tracheostomy emergencies on intensive care. Anaesthesia 68 (2), 217–219.

Khan, A.N., Al-Jahdali, H., Al-Ghanem, H., 2009. Reading chest radiographs in the critically ill. Ann. Thorac. Med. 4 (2), 75–87.

Lieberman, P.L., 2014. Recognition and first-line treatment of anaphylaxis. Am. J. Med. 127 (1 Suppl.), S6–S11. doi:10.1016/j.amjmed.2013.09.008.

Mattu, S., 2016. Pulmonary emergencies. Emerg. Med. Clin. North Am. 34 (1), xi–xii.

NICE, 2016. Therapy Support Workers in critical care: improving physical and cognitive rehabilitation. National Institute for Health and Care Excellence, United Kingdom.

Nievera, R.A., Fick, A., 2017. Effects of ambulation and nondependent transfers on vital signs in patients receiving norepinephrine. Am. J. Crit. Care 26 (1), 31–36.

Ntoumenopoulos, G., Glickman, Y., 2012. Computerised lung sound monitoring to assess effectiveness of chest physiotherapy and secretion removal. Physiotherapy 98 (3), 250–255. doi:10.1016/j.physio.2011.12.003.

Ohtake, P.J., 2017. Impairments, activity limitations and participation restrictions experienced in the first year following a critical illness: protocol for a systematic review. BMJ Open 7 (1), e013847.

Olkowski, B.F., Devine, M.A., Slotnick, L.E., et al., 2013. Safety and feasibility of an early mobilization program for patients with aneurysmal subarachnoid hemorrhage. Phys. Ther. 93 (2), 208–215.

Overbeck, M.C., 2016. Airway management of respiratory failure. Emerg. Med. Clin. North Am. 34 (1), 97–127.

Parry, S.M., 2017. Factors influencing physical activity and rehabilitation in survivors of critical illness: a systematic review of quantitative and qualitative studies. Int. Care Med. 43 (4), 531–542.

Rahu, M.A., Grap, M.J., Cohn, J.F., 2013. Facial expression as an indicator of pain in critically ill intubated adults during endotracheal suctioning. Am. J. Crit. Care 22 (5), 412–422. doi:10.4037/ajcc2013705. http://www.ncbi.nlm.nih.gov/pmc/articles/PMC3913066/.

Richards, A.M., 2016. Pediatric respiratory emergencies. Emerg. Med. Clin. 34 (1), 77–96.

Richardson, V., 2013. Patient comprehension of informed consent. J. Perioper. Pract. 23 (1/2), 26–30.

Robertson, L.C., 2013. Recognizing the critically ill patient. Anaesth. Int. Care Med. 14 (1), 11–14.

Rose, L., Adhikari, N.K., Poon, J., 2016. Cough augmentation techniques in the critically ill: a Canadian national survey. Respir. Care 61 (10), 1360–1368. doi:10.4187/respcare.04775.

Russian, C.J., Gonzales, J.F., Henry, N.R., et al., 2014. Suction catheter size: an assessment and comparison of 3 different calculation methods. Respir. Care 59 (1), 32–38.

Salisbury, L.G., 2010. Rehabilitation after critical illness: could a ward-based generic rehabilitation assistant promote recovery? Nurs. Crit. Care 15 (2), 57–64.

Shannon, H., Stocks, J., Gregson, R.K., et al., 2015. Differences in delivery of respiratory treatments by on-call physiotherapists in mechanically ventilated children: a randomised crossover trial. Physiotherapy 101 (4), 357–363. doi:10.1016/j.physio.2014.12.001.

Skinner, E.H., Haines, K.J., Berney, S., et al., 2015. Usual care physiotherapy during acute hospitalization in subjects admitted to the ICU: an observational cohort study. Respir. Care 60 (10), 1476–1485. doi:10.4187/respcare.04064.

Sokolovs, D., Tan, K.W., 2017. Ear, nose and throat emergencies. Anaesth. Int. Care Med. 18 (4), 190–194.

Snelson, C., Jones, C., Atkins, G., et al., 2017. A comparison of earlier and enhanced rehabilitation of mechanically ventilated patients in critical care compared to standard care: study protocol for a single-site randomised controlled feasibility trial. Pilot Feasibility Stud. 3, 19.

Suau, S.J., DeBlieux, M.C., 2016. Management of acute exacerbation of asthma and chronic obstructive pulmonary disease in the emergency department. Emerg. Med. Clin. North Am. 34 (1), 15–37.

Tipping, C.J., Harrold, M., Holland, A., et al., 2017. The effects of active mobilisation and rehabilitation in ICU on mortality and function: a systematic review. Int. Care Med. 43 (2), 171–183.

Tonnelier, A., 2013. Impact of humidification and nebulization during expiratory limb protection. Respir. Care 58 (8), 1315–1322.

Voepel-Lewis, T., 2010. Reliability and validity of the face, legs, activity, cry, consolability behavioral tool in assessing acute pain in critically ill patients. Am. J. Crit. Care 19 (1), 55–61.

Whyte, J., 2013. Medical complications during inpatient rehabilitation among patients with traumatic disorders of consciousness. Arch. Phys. Med. Rehabil. 94 (10), 1877–1883.

Wilson, J.G., Epstein, S.M., Wang, R., et al., 2013. Cardiac tamponade. West J. Emerg. Med. 14 (2), 152.

Worrell, S.G., Demeester, S.R., 2014. Thoracic emergencies. Surg. Clin. North Am. 94 (1), 183–191.

# 22

# Modifications for Different Disorders

*David McWilliams, Tammy Lea, Alexandra Hough*

## LEARNING OBJECTIVES

*On completion of this chapter the reader should be able to:*
- understand the pathology of lung conditions, neurological conditions, trauma and multisystem failure in critical care;
- modify treatment according to this pathology;
- contribute to the multidisciplinary management of critically ill patients.

## OUTLINE

This chapter covers mostly nonsurgical patients who are mechanically ventilated and require a specific physiotherapy approach to maintain oxygenation and promote rehabilitation.

## LUNG DISEASE

### Chronic Obstructive Pulmonary Disease

For people with chronic obstructive pulmonary disease in ventilatory failure, noninvasive ventilation (NIV) is used when possible. If invasive mechanical ventilation (MV) is required, it brings high mortality (Hajizadeh et al. 2015), one culprit being intrinsic PEEP (p. 450), which disrupts synchrony with the ventilator, increases inspiratory effort and disturbs haemodynamics (Liu 2015). Normally the pressure support mode is used, with PEEP at about 80% of intrinsic PEEP to offset hyperinflation. Patients with chronic hypercapnia have their minute volume titrated to pH rather than to partial pressure of $CO_2$ in arterial blood ($PaCO_2$) so that compensatory renal bicarbonate retention is adequate for buffering during weaning. A patient who has acclimatized to complex acid–base compensations may find the sudden change to MV destabilizing, leading to hypotension in 25% of cases (Schumaker 2004), as well as arrhythmias and the unmasking of hypovolaemia. If physiotherapy is needed within 30 min of starting MV, the monitors must be watched closely.

Rest and sleep are required for 24 h after initiation of MV for as much time as possible, interspersed with specialized nutritional support (Hsieh et al. 2016), orientation, chest clearance and very modest exercise. Bed exercises should be demonstrated to the patient, nurse and family, written down and left with the nursing notes. Once the patient has fully rested, daily standing and walking on the spot are added to progressive bed exercises, unless contraindicated or declined. Manual hyperinflation is not advisable because of the vulnerability of hyperinflated alveoli. Infection control measures must be immaculate because of the extra risk of ventilator-associated pneumonia (Toney 2016).

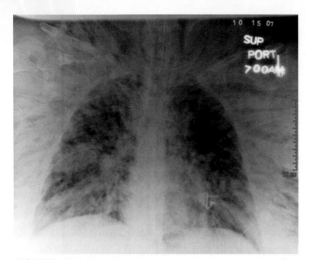

**FIGURE 22.1** Ventilated patient with asthma, showing widespread subcutaneous emphysema.

Work of breathing may be 10 times normal (Chang 2014, p. 41), and weaning can be tiring, protracted and frightening. This is minimized with balanced rest and exercise and, if required, NIV after extubation.

## Asthma

MV is a perilous venture for people with acute asthma, bringing a mortality rate of nearly 10% (Kaur et al. 2015), but is required if noninvasive support is unsuccessful and their condition is life-threatening. High-volume positive pressure risks dangerous levels of intrinsic PEEP, barotrauma (Fig. 22.1), impaired venous return, hypotension, arrhythmias and right heart failure due to compressed pulmonary capillaries. Dehydrated patients are particularly vulnerable, and adequate fluid resuscitation and correction of hypokalaemia are required. Other difficulties are refractory bronchospasm or mucous plugging.

Patients will be exhausted from the effort of maintaining hyperinflation to keep their obstructed airways open. A hyperinflated chest means that MV does not necessarily relieve the distressing sensation of breathlessness.

High levels of oxygen and bronchodilators are required, the latter delivered by continuous infusion or instillation (Johnston et al. 2015).

The risks of hyperinflation and barotrauma may be reduced by:

- lung-protective ventilation, long exhalation times and sufficient extrinsic PEEP to counteract intrinsic PEEP (Jungblut et al. 2014);
- heliox, anaesthetic agents, hypothermia or extracorporeal support (Lee et al. 2017);
- brief disconnection from the ventilator by the intensivist to allow the trapped gas to escape, which can be facilitated by the physiotherapist briefly performing strong bilateral expiratory manual compressions on the chest (Phipps 2003) during several successive exhalations, using two people in synchrony, or, for one person, applying sustained pressure over the eighth to tenth ribs.

Other forms of physiotherapy are inadvisable immediately after initiation of MV because the combination of anaesthesia, hypovolaemia and high airway pressures can cause profound hypotension. $\beta_2$-Agonists may reduce potassium and further destabilize the cardiovascular system.

However, when pressure or volume has settled, treatment to clear mucous plugs may be required. Airway mucus in severe acute asthma is associated with abnormal mucin structure, and fatalities are usually associated with mucous plugging (Rubin & Pohanka 2012). Benefit has been shown with nebulized DNase (Chia 2013) or instillation of 2 mL warmed sterile saline every 15 min (Branthwaite 1985), along with regular position change and manual techniques if required, with close attention to any increase in bronchospasm. Manual hyperinflation is dangerous because of the overinflated chest.

Any sudden deterioration should raise suspicions of a tension pneumothorax. The usual signs (p. 510) may be obliterated in a hyperinflated patient on MV.

## NEUROLOGICAL CONDITIONS

### Traumatic Brain Injury

> **CSF**: cerebrospinal fluid
> **ICP**: intracranial pressure: normal 0–15 mmHg, critical >20 mmHg
> **CPP**: cerebral perfusion pressure: normal >70 mmHg, critical <50 mmHg
> **GCS**: Glasgow Coma Scale (Table 22.1)
> **MAP**: mean arterial pressure (reflects blood pressure): normal 90 mmHg, critical <80 mmHg

Traumatic brain injury (TBI) is the leading cause of death in children and young adults (Eytan et al. 2016)

| TABLE 22.1 | Glasgow coma scale | |
|---|---|---|
| Best eye-opening response | Spontaneous | 4 |
| | To voice | 3 |
| | To pain | 2 |
| | None | 1 |
| Best verbal response | Oriented | 5 |
| | Confused | 4 |
| | Inappropriate words | 3 |
| | Incoherent | 2 |
| | None | 1 |
| Best motor response | Obeys commands | 6 |
| | Localizes pain | 5 |
| | Withdraws from pain | 4 |
| | Flexes to pain | 3 |
| | Extends to pain | 2 |
| | None | 1 |
| Maximum score | | 15 |

and a contributing factor in 30% of injury-related deaths (Gottlieb 2016). Nowhere is accurate assessment and finely tuned clinical judgement more vital. Methods to control ICP and prevent lung problems may be in conflict, and are often complicated by other injuries.

The effect of most injuries is maximal at onset, but TBI may precipitate a process that converts a moderate injury into a life-threatening condition. Primary brain damage at impact is irreversible, but secondary damage affects 35% of patients within minutes, hours or days (Çelik 2004).

Oxygen delivery to the injured brain is hampered by any of the following (Haddad & Arabi 2012):

- partial pressure of oxygen in arterial blood ($PaO_2$) <8 kPa (60 mmHg) or peripheral arterial oxygen saturation ($SpO_2$) <90%
- partial pressure of $CO_2$ in arterial blood ($PaCO_2$) <4.66 kPa (35 mmHg) or >6 kPa (45 mmHg)
- systolic BP <90 mmHg or >160 mmHg, or MAP >110 mmHg
- haemoglobin <100 g/L or haematocrit <0.30
- serum sodium <142 mEq/L
- blood sugar >10 mmol/L or <4.6 mmol/L
- pH <7.35 or >7.45
- fever, or temperature <35.5°C.

### Effect on oxygen delivery

'Brain–lung crosstalk' via complex pathways leads to both organs exacerbating each other's troubles. On average, pneumonia occurs in 40% of patients, and acute respiratory distress syndrome (ARDS) in 35%, the latter tripling mortality and signifying that protective lung ventilation may be advisable from the start. A 'double hit' may occur, noradrenaline being released and creating a sympathetic storm of systemic vasoconstriction. Fluid rushes into the pulmonary circulation, causing neurogenic pulmonary oedema, and an acute inflammatory response in both brain and lungs leading to a 'blast injury' effect from systemic inflammation (Mrozek et al. 2015). Neuroinflammation can persist for years and may contribute to neurodegeneration (Russo & McGavern 2016).

Damage to the respiratory centres may upset the breathing pattern: hyperventilation reduces $PaCO_2$ and cerebral blood flow (Lund et al. 2016), and hypoventilation increases $PaCO_2$, causing vasodilation and raised ICP, usually as a terminal event. Cheyne-Stokes and ataxic breathing are also signs of severe TBI.

Associated trauma such as facial injury, fractured ribs, haemopneumothorax or lung contusion may compromise the airway or impair gas exchange. Immobility, recumbency and depressed consciousness leads to shallow breathing and may impair cough (Fig. 22.2).

Further injury can be added by:

- severe fluid restriction in an attempt to reduce cerebral oedema, leading to hypotension, reduced oxygen delivery and thick secretions, or
- lavish fluid administration in an attempt to maintain cerebral perfusion, worsening pulmonary oedema and cerebral oedema.

### Effect on the brain

The brain is a hungry organ, requiring 20% of the body's energy to function (Magistretti & Allaman 2015). Primary injury is caused by bleeding, contusion or shearing forces when the oscillating brain distracts nerve fibres from their bodies. Secondary damage includes cerebral oedema, raised ICP, unstable BP and hypoxia.

The contents of the skull comprise 80% brain tissue, 10% CSF and 10% blood. When damaged, swelling within this rigid container reaches a maximum 3 to 5 days post injury (Shakur et al. 2009). Initially, swelling can be accommodated by displacement of CSF and venous blood into the spinal subarachnoid space and jugular veins (Fig. 22.3). When these compensating mechanisms have reached their limit, a small increase in cerebral oedema causes a disproportionate upsurge in

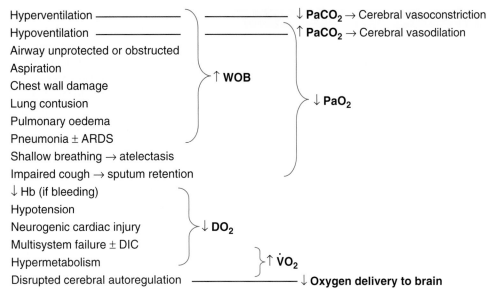

Hyperventilation ——————————— ——————————— ↓ PaCO$_2$ → Cerebral vasoconstriction
Hypoventilation ——————————— ——————————— ↑ PaCO$_2$ → Cerebral vasodilation
Airway unprotected or obstructed
Aspiration
Chest wall damage          ↑ WOB
Lung contusion                                      ↓ PaO$_2$
Pulmonary oedema
Pneumonia ± ARDS
Shallow breathing → atelectasis
Impaired cough → sputum retention
↓ Hb (if bleeding)
Hypotension
Neurogenic cardiac injury     ↓ DO$_2$
Multisystem failure ± DIC
Hypermetabolism               ↑ V̇O$_2$
Disrupted cerebral autoregulation ——————————— ↓ Oxygen delivery to brain

**FIGURE 22.2** Effects of acute brain injury on oxygen delivery. *ARDS*, Acute respiratory distress syndrome; *DIC*, disseminated intravascular coagulation; *DO$_2$*, oxygen delivery to the tissues; *Hb*, haemoglobin; *VO$_2$*, oxygen consumption; *WOB*, work of breathing.

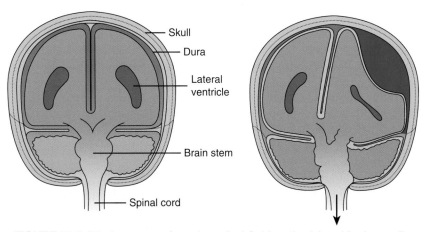

Skull
Dura
Lateral ventricle
Brain stem
Spinal cord

**FIGURE 22.3** Displacement of cerebrospinal fluid as the injured brain swells.

ICP (Fig. 22.4) and may persist for several days (Oddo et al. 2016). Extreme intracranial hypertension may cause coning, in which the brainstem herniates down through the foramen magnum.

Cerebral perfusion pressure is the driving force of cerebral circulation. Reduced CPP is the principal mechanism by which elevated ICP exerts secondary damage. MAP and ICP are, in effect, competing for space:

$$CPP = MAP - ICP$$

CPP is therefore compromised by a high ICP, which prevents perfusion even with high MAP. Fig. 22.5 shows how a rise in the nonperfusing ICP, without a compensating increase in BP, impairs the perfusing CPP.

The picture is further complicated if the autoregulation that normally stabilizes cerebral blood flow is lost (Trofimov et al. 2016). This generally remains constant over a CPP of 50–150 mmHg, due to compensatory vasodilation in response to hypoxia or hypotension. If this mechanism is damaged by brain injury, ICP follows

MAP passively rather than remaining independent. BP must therefore be tightly controlled therapeutically.

Intracranial dynamics are reflected in a vicious cycle that exacerbates the secondary effects of TBI (Fig. 22.6). Lung complications can cause hypoxia, to which brain tissue is already sensitive because of its high oxygen requirements and dependence on aerobic glucose metabolism. Hypoxia swells the brain further, and disturbances in $PaCO_2$ add to this woeful picture. It is no wonder that TBI has a reputation for being treacherous.

### Factors which increase intracranial pressure or decrease cerebral perfusion pressure

*Arterial hypotension is a major risk factor for secondary brain injury.*

*Kinoshita 2016*

1. Either hypertension or hypotension increases mortality (Krishnamoorthy et al. 2016). The following carry particular risk:
   - on admission, when a patient may be quietly bleeding into the abdomen and losing consciousness because of hypotension rather than TBI;
   - during surgery, when BP may be deliberately kept low to minimize the risk of bleeding;
   - if head elevation is too high, when cerebral desaturation can occur if blood flow autoregulation is impaired and MAP not maintained (Zheng et al. 2015).
2. Head-down postural drainage increases arterial, venous and intracranial pressures because cerebral veins have no valves. It also impairs compensatory

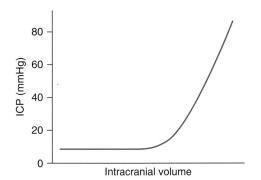

**FIGURE 22.4** Intracranial compliance curve. Intracranial pressure *(ICP)* is stable at first, but when spatial compensation is exhausted, shown by the inflection point, further swelling causes a steep rise.

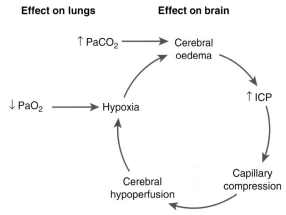

**FIGURE 22.6** Vicious cycle set up by acute brain injury. *ICP,* Intracranial pressure.

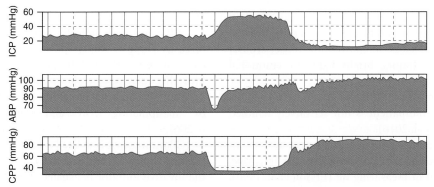

**FIGURE 22.5** Effect of increased intracranial pressure *(ICP)* and decreased arterial blood pressure *(ABP)* on cerebral perfusion pressure *(CPP)*. (Adapted from Lu et al. 2012.)

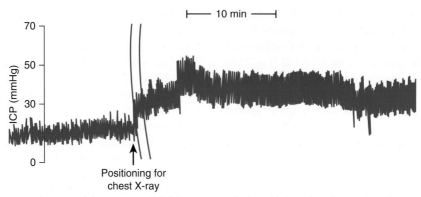

**FIGURE 22.7** Intracranial pressure *(ICP)* in a severely head-injured patient, showing prolonged elevation after position change. (From Shalit & Umansky 1977.)

venous outflow and is contraindicated in the acute stage (Petersen et al. 2016).

3. Head movement, coughing, suction, manual hyper-inflation and sometimes manual techniques can impede outflow from the brain and raise ICP (Paratz 1993). Outflow may also be obstructed by tight tracheal tube tape or a cervical collar.

4. Turning the patient increases ICP if head movement is allowed to obstruct drainage from the brain (Fig. 22.7).

5. Even deeply comatosed patients show a surprising sensitivity to conversation over their beds. Discussion about their condition increases ICP more than general discussion (Mitchell & Mauss 1978). However, when relatives talk to patients, a reduction in ICP may be seen (Chudley 1994).

6. Continuous sedation must not be interrupted for neurological assessment because this can cause spikes in ICP (Prisco & Citerio 2012).

7. Brain-injured people show an exaggerated response to the pain of associated injuries (Mirski 1995). ICP also increases with injections, movement of the tracheal tube, yankauer in the mouth, noise, arousal from sleep, restraints, bright lights or emotional upset (Yanko & Mitcho 2001).

8. Transfer, even within the hospital, can have a significant effect if the patient is not sensitively handled (Kleffmann et al. 2016).

9. Supposedly minor stressors can cause a spike in ICP, e.g. knocking the bed, using a cold stethoscope, fitting a splint or measuring BP (Ersson et al. 1990).

Most of these factors warn physiotherapists to keep their distance, but the importance of maintaining gas exchange is a cogent reminder not to stray too far.

### General management

*Immediate management.* All acutely brain-injured people are handled on the assumption that they have an unstable spine until proven otherwise. A CT scan can be transmitted electronically from a general intensive care unit (ICU) to a neurosurgical unit for advice. Patients with a GCS score below 8 should be resuscitated, intubated, ventilated, stabilized, scanned and transferred to a neurosurgical unit, accompanied by a doctor trained in the handling of such patients, so long as the cause of any unexplained hypotension has been identified (NICE 2014b).

Respiratory and haemodynamic stabilization are required because these systems contribute as much to brain hypoxia as intracranial upset (Kinoshita 2016).

*Monitoring.* Clinical examination is often clouded by coma, sedatives or encephalopathy. Monitoring is therefore relied on, preferably with noninvasive devices to minimize stimuli that might stir up ICP (Robba et al. 2015).

CPP is the main indicator of brain perfusion, monitored by Doppler sonography, cerebrovascular reactivity or indirectly by MAP and ICP (Aries et al. 2012). Mortality increases by about 20% for each 10 mmHg drop in CPP, and the aim is to keep it at 70–80 mmHg by manipulating MAP and fluids (Chang 2014, p. 266).

ICP monitoring is needed if GCS falls below 8 or the CT scan shows cerebral oedema. Unless contraindicated, the invasive monitor is usually placed in the right side because this hemisphere is nondominant in 80% of people. Risks of ICP elevation should be predicted and managed while still within normal limits. Clinical signs of cranial hypertension are not apparent in a patient on paralysing drugs, but even if evident they indicate that secondary damage has already occurred.

Other monitors are:

- end-tidal $CO_2$ ($ETCO_2$) as a surrogate for vasomotor stability;
- electroencephalogram (EEG) power spectral analysis to identify awareness (Goldfine et al. 2012);
- direct monitoring of brain tissue oxygenation (Ngwenya et al. 2016);
- cerebrovascular haemodynamic monitoring, which is particularly useful to fine tune head elevation (Kim et al. 2013).

**Head elevation.** Raising the head of the bed tends to reduce ICP but may also reduce CPP, especially in hypovolaemic patients. Head position should be established individually according to the monitors, but 10–15 degrees of elevation is commonly advised (Cowley 2008), with no neck flexion, the reverse Trendelenberg position being used if a suitable bed is available.

**Fluid management.** Normovolaemia is the usual target so that excess fluid does not rush into the injured brain nor dehydration reduce brain perfusion. Small changes in blood osmolality exert a strong effect on brain water, and initial fluid resuscitation is probably best achieved with hypertonic saline (Diringer 2016), the sodium ions of which do not cross the blood–brain barrier or risk brain swelling, or cause the renal dysfunction seen with repeated mannitol administration. Fluids and drugs aim to keep MAP at >80 mmHg (NICE 2007).

**Sleep.** Inadequate sleep in the acute period correlates with a poor functional outcome (Sandsmark et al. 2016).

**Nutrition.** Patients are hypermetabolic, hypercatabolic and hyperglycaemic. Specialist nutritional support is needed because diet modifies brain plasticity (Gomez-Pinilla et al. 2011), vitamin D reduces brain inflammation (Cekic et al. 2011) and immunonutrition boosts antioxidents (Khalid & Selim 2012). Resting energy expenditure is 40%–200% above normal for about 3 weeks, and a degree of hypermetabolism can last for a year (Yanko & Mitcho 2001), but patients have been found to receive just 56% of their requirements, with signs of malnutrition evident in two-thirds of patients 2 months after admission (Chapple et al. 2016). Paralytic ileus may be a hindrance for the first fortnight, and over half the patients have impaired swallow (Bremare et al. 2016) so early speech–language referral

is advised. Enteral feeding is preferable because intravenous (IV) feeding risks infection and can cause neuronal damage from hyperglycaemia (Yanko & Mitcho 2001). Almost half of patients are injured while inebriated (Bombardier 2013) and alcohol dependence may require vitamin B supplements to avoid encephalopathy (Guerrini 2013).

**Temperature control.** Temperature must be tightly regulated. Damage to the hypothalamus may cause a fever, raising oxygen consumption by 10% for each 1°C rise in temperature (Yanko & Mitcho 2001). Hypothermia can cause arrhythmias, shift the oxygen dissociation curve to the left and, if it causes shivering, increase oxygen consumption. However, short-term therapeutic hypothermia delivered transarterially may benefit some patients (Kurisu et al. 2016).

**Drug therapy.** The following may be used:

1. Judicious doses of the osmotic diuretic mannitol temporarily reduce intracellular volume, with a transient improvement in cerebral blood flow and oxygenation. Side effects may include dehydration, hypotension and a delayed increase in ICP, after the drug crosses the blood–brain barrier (Gottlieb 2016).
2. Hypotensive patients who are normovolaemic need systemic vasoconstrictors, which do not cause damaging vasoconstriction in the brain because cerebral vessels have few adrenergic receptors.
3. Brain hypermetabolism is reduced by anaesthetic agents, β-blockers (Murry et al. 2016) and sedatives, although sedatives may also reduce cerebral blood flow (Oddo et al. 2016).
4. Neuromuscular blocking agents are not recommended unless necessary for refractory intracranial hypertension because they increase the risk of pneumonia (Haddad & Arabi 2012).
5. Melatonin has neuroprotective effects (Dong et al. 2015).
6. Anticoagulation reduces the risk of thromboembolism, after preexisting medication has been checked (Prinz et al. 2016).
7. Laxatives may be required because pressure from constipation affects intrathoracic pressure and inhibits outflow from a swelling brain.
8. High percentage oxygen delivered through the ventilator can resuscitate stunned neurons, inhibit neural ischaemia, maintain CPP and improve long-term outcomes (Taher 2016).

Entonox is contraindicated.

***Mechanical ventilation.*** Intubation may be needed to maintain a clear airway and assisted ventilation to regulate an unstable breathing pattern, deliver high percentage oxygen, control ICP or manage chest complications. If prolonged ventilation is anticipated, Siddiqui et al. (2015) recommend early tracheotomy to reduce the incidence of pneumonia. NICE (2007) advises that $PaO_2$ is kept above 13 kPa (97.5 mmHg) and $PaCO_2$ kept low to normal at 4.5–5.0 kPa (33.8–37.5 mmHg), but hyperventilation should not be initiated in the first 24 h because it may cause cerebral ischaemia (Haddad & Arabi 2012), and $PaCO_2$ levels need to be balanced with lung-protective ventilation. High PEEP impedes outflow from the brain.

## Physiotherapy

> **KEY POINT**
>
> The hallmark of physiotherapy is maximum involvement and minimum intervention.

Physiotherapy involvement in the early stages is by:
- frequent assessment to assist delicate risk–benefit decisions
- supervision of handling to minimize ICP disturbance

Physical intervention is unwise in the presence of cardiovascular instability, hypotension or ICP above 15 mmHg (Paratz 1993). If it is essential for gas exchange, a drug to stabilize ICP should be given beforehand. Quiet explanations are required for all patients, however deeply comatose.

### Assessment

*Unresponsiveness is an inadequate proxy for unconsciousness.*

***Sanders et al. 2016c***

Any reduction in $SpO_2$ or other signs of impending chest complications requires preventive action. BP, ICP and $ETCO_2$ should be monitored throughout treatment. In the absence of ICP monitoring, clinical signs of intracranial hypertension are:
- ↑ pupil size
- pupil unresponsive to light
- change in GCS
- change in vital signs, breathing pattern or muscle tone
- vomiting

If the patient is not intubated, a minitracheostomy is advisable if suction is necessary. Nasal suction is contraindicated in the presence of:
- watery CSF leaking from the nose or ear, indicating a connection between the subarachnoid space and nasal passages, risking infection;
- severe epistaxis.

***Positioning.*** Turning is safe with ICP <15 mmHg (Chudley 1994), one person being responsible for maintaining head alignment. Accurate positioning in side-lying with neutral head position aids prophylactic chest care, so long as pressure on any postoperative bone flap is avoided. However, for patients with unstable ICP and low risk of lung complications, it is best to leave the patient supine in the early stages if there is a suitable mattress to prevent pressure sores. Neck flexion must be prevented by using a thin pillow or none.

***Manual hyperinflation.*** Both manual and ventilator hyperinflation could impede outflow from the brain (Mrozek et al. 2015) and are inadvisable unless essential, in which case they must follow sedation, be brief, and avoid disturbing $PaCO_2$. The $ETCO_2$ monitor should be transferred to the manual hyperinflation circuit, and the endotracheal tube kept stable throughout.

***Manual techniques.*** Paratz (1993) claims that vibrations and percussion can impede compensatory outflow from the brain and increase ICP, but Neto et al. (2013) and Fig. 22.8 show that careful technique, if required, can avoid this complication. Percussion is likely to cause less pressure change than vibrations.

***Suction.*** Elevation of ICP during suction is inevitable (Neto et al. 2013) and sometimes prolonged. If suction is indicated, the following precautions are advised:
- the patient rested from previous activity
- 100% oxygen delivered before and after
- head kept strictly in alignment
- tracheal tube stabilized throughout
- contact with the carina avoided
- no more than one suction pass at a time, and use of hyperventilation to reduce ICP if necessary

A systematic review has found that combined manual techniques and suction transiently increase ICP but not CPP (Ferreira et al. 2013).

## Exercise

If spasticity develops, appropriate positioning must be maintained and factors that increase tone avoided, e.g. pain, anxiety or pressure under the feet. If clonus or

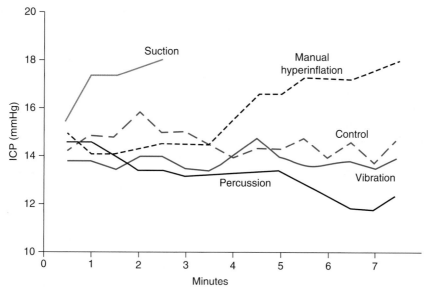

**FIGURE 22.8** Effect of physiotherapy on intracranial pressure *(ICP)*, showing suction to be the most damaging intervention, followed by manual hyperinflation. (From Garradd et al. 1986.)

increased tone in the calf is identified, immediate stretching and splinting to maintain dorsiflexion has been recommended (Moseley 2008), while ensuring some periods with the splint off.

If there is no altered muscle tone, it may be best to avoid any movements in the first 72 h while the brain may be swelling. Thereafter, comfortable passive movements can actually reduce ICP (Thelandersson et al. 2010) and help promote neural plasticity (Kocan & Lietz 2013), but hip flexion of more than 90 degrees should be avoided in the early stages because it can raise ICP by increasing vena cava pressure (Yanko & Mitcho 2001). Once ICP is stable, patients can sit over the edge of the bed and start active rehabilitation. A graded exercise programme also helps improve mood (Bognor 2012), with particular attention to minimizing fatigue (Juengst et al. 2013). Bone mineral density needs to be checked (Banham-Hall et al. 2013).

Close assessment continues to be important after discharge from the ICU, when 10% of patients suffer a serious adverse event (Tirkkonen et al. 2013) at the same time as monitoring is reduced.

### Teamwork

Co-ordinated teamwork is especially important in the vulnerable first week. Preplanning is needed to avoid a cumulative rise in ICP, e.g. to stagger physiotherapy,

nursing and other interventions as far apart as possible to minimize the stress response (Genzler et al. 2013).

Brain injury can impair the assessment of pain, which increases ICP, limits rehabilitation and may impair recovery of consciousness (Lanzillo et al. 2016). The physiotherapist may be the first to detect pain.

Studies have identified progressively increasing depression in the majority of patients (Fann & Hart 2013) and a 50%–80% incidence of fatigue that does not resolve spontaneously (Juengst et al. 2013). Posttraumatic stress disorder can develop even after mild brain injury (Hoffman et al. 2012), and skill in motivation and encouragement of autonomy are required. Early rehabilitation and goal-planning are best based on the contextual factors of the ICF model (Ptyushkin 2012), and integrating neurorehabilitation into the ICU can benefit patients even if they are in a vegetative state (Eifert et al. 2013). Recovery of consciousness in patients who survive their coma but evolve to a vegetative state can be identified (Bodart & Laureys 2014), and absence of consciousness should not preclude referral for specialized rehabilitation (Sommer et al. 2013).

### Acute Quadriplegia

*'The big things you get used to easier, like not getting up and walking around. The trivial things – like not being able to scratch your nose or feed yourself – they hurt'.*
**Stewart & Rossier 1978**

| Quadriplegia: paralysis of limbs and trunk |
|---|
| Tetraplegia: paralysis of limbs |

People whose lives have been devastated by disease or trauma to the cervical spine are overwhelmed at first and find it difficult to comprehend how savagely their life has been curtailed. Physiotherapists who care for people with acute quadriplegia need to allow them to work through their grief at their own pace, while endeavouring to prevent respiratory complications which are the leading cause of death (Jia et al. 2013).

## Pathophysiology, clinical features and medical treatment

Primary injury is the direct damage sustained from trauma, tumour, infection or vascular lesion, while secondary injury relates to release of a cascade of inflammatory chemicals that can be toxic to neuronal tissue (Allison & Ditor 2015). Respiratory function may be compromised by ascending oedema of the damaged spinal cord, or neurogenic pulmonary oedema caused by vasoconstriction, sometimes exacerbated by overhydration in an attempt to treat shock.

The first few hours are when the accuracy, adequacy and speed of management may have an effect on the final outcome (Wing et al. 2008). Log rolling, for example, should be avoided (Conrad et al. 2012). If a halo vest is used to stabilize a fracture, all those involved must know how to open or adjust it in case of cardiac arrest. As with TBI, the first 72 h are when the maintenance of blood flow and oxygenation are the primary goals (Cook 2003). Cardiovascular instability due to sympathetic dysfunction is most pronounced in the first 1–2 weeks (Casha & Christie 2011). Patients who cannot be transferred immediately to a spinal unit need specialist assessment by an outreach team. Prehospital management is described by NICE (2016e).

Complications include mucous plugging, atelectasis, pneumonia (Galeiras 2013) and, with trauma, a high incidence of acute brain injury. Later complications include neuropathic pain (Norrbrink & Löfgren 2016), bladder and gut problems, pressure sores, cardiopulmonary disease (Cristante et al. 2012) and, in the majority of patients, obstructive sleep apnoea (Bauman et al. 2016).

Lesions above T6–L1 paralyse the abdominal muscles and impair coughing. Higher lesions paralyse the intercostals so that they are unable to buttress the rib cage on inspiration, causing paradoxical inward motion as negative pressure sucks in the chest. Lesions above C4 denervate the diaphragm, leaving only the sternomastoid and trapezius muscles to shift a trace of air into the lungs.

Paralysed abdominal muscles also impair venous return and risk an exaggerated response to hypovolaemia. Lesions above T6 remove sympathetic control to the splanchnic bed, which is a major reservoir for controlling BP. Hypotension and bradycardia can result, especially during suction of the mouth or airways, and during exertion. Cardiac monitoring is required for the first 2 weeks, and oximetry should be continued at night. A complete cervical injury is equivalent to a sympathectomy, reducing tone in blood vessels, denervating the cardiac sympathetic nerve supply and leaving parasympathetic tone unopposed. Vasopressors can cause complications (Inoue et al. 2014).

Therapeutic hypothermia may be applied in the early stages for neuroprotection. High lesions require MV, often for lengthy periods, and early tracheostomy is recommended (Ganuza 2011). Ventilator adjustments may be required during active exercise to maintain oxygenation. Most patients with a lesion at or below C4 can be weaned, and an initial vital capacity of more than 1 L indicates the likelihood of success, but a compromised hypercapnic respiratory drive complicates weaning for some patients (Raurich 2014). For those unable to wean, phrenic nerve pacing can coax the diaphragm to life and gain freedom from the ventilator, along with reduced pulmonary complications, along with better venous return, normal speech and eating, and improved mobility (Dalal & DiMarco 2014), or the patient may prefer NIV.

Environmental temperature must be controlled because impaired sympathetic outflow hinders thermoregulation. Bronchodilators may be required to reduce parasympathetic-induced bronchospasm. Deep vein thrombosis is a significant risk, requiring ultrasonography for diagnosis and intermittent pneumatic compression and/or elastic stockings for prevention (Matsumoto et al. 2015).

## Physiotherapy

*Aggressive management of atelectasis and secretions are the cornerstones of early treatment [and have] been shown to improve outcomes.*

***Berlly 2007***

The 3rd to 5th days after injury are when associated damage or aspiration may cause cardiorespiratory problems such as hypoxia or hypotension, leading to secondary harm to the spinal cord.

---

**PRACTICE TIP**

From day 1, all the team members need to be clear about taking care of the shoulder joints.

---

*Respiratory care.* Physiotherapy in the acute stage should take place little and often to avoid fatigue. Regular position change helps prevent atelectasis, which is the most common respiratory complication, while manual techniques and assisted coughing help clear secretions. Excess mucus may be created by loss of sympathetic control and unopposed vagal activity in the days to weeks after injury. The head-down position is best avoided, but if essential for postural drainage, care is needed to ensure that tipping is done slowly and not fully, cervical traction is maintained, suction is on hand in case of sudden sputum mobilization, and arterial and venous pressures are monitored because of impaired cardiovascular reflexes.

If MV is not required, hourly incentive spirometry and, if necessary, intermittent positive pressure breathing help prevent atelectasis, and early minitracheostomy is advisable if there is a hint of sputum retention, especially as the neck cannot be extended for effective nasopharyngeal suction. If suction is required, whether for an intubated or spontaneously breathing patient, it should be accompanied by close monitoring of $SpO_2$, HR and BP, with intravenous IV atropine or another suitable drug on hand in case of bradycardia.

Respiratory rehabilitation includes respiratory muscle training, which can increase lung volumes, cough strength and ability to use voice-activated equipment and hands-free phones (Ross 2005), and, in later stages, improve BP regulation (Aslan et al. 2016). However, it may increase spasticity in some patients (Van Houtte et al. 2008). Methods are by using a mouth trainer, a connector to the tracheal tube, weights on the abdomen (Casha & Christie 2011) or assisted treadmill walking (Iscoe & DiMarco 2014). Functional magnetic stimulation can improve inspiratory and expiratory function (Zhang et al. 2016f), and phrenic nerve stimulation may assist independence from MV (Sieg et al. 2016).

Coughing is assisted by:
- mechanical assistance with an insufflator–exsufflator, ending with insufflation to restore lung volume;
- breath-synchronized electrical stimulation of the abdominal muscles, which reduces the risk of pneumonia (Liebscher et al. 2016);
- if there is no paralytic ileus, manual assistance using a hand on each side of the lower ribs and one forearm exerting strong pressure upwards and inwards against the abdomen, in synchrony with any expiratory force that the patient can muster (some patients require two physiotherapists for this); care should be taken to avoid disturbing neck traction, jarring the fracture site, exacerbating associated injuries, or pushing towards the spine instead of the diaphragm (Fig. 22.9);
- self assistance by maximal-depth glossopharyngeal breathing (p. 112) followed by an abdominal thrust against the edge of a table (Bianchi et al. 2014);
- expiratory muscle training (Iscoe & DiMarco 2014).

*Musculoskeletal care.* Treatment of the limbs involves close attention to positioning and range of movement. A high proportion of patients develop rotator cuff tears, biceps tendon ruptures and shoulder arthrosis, and regular magnetic resonance imaging checks have been recommended (Eriks-Hoogland 2013). Prevention of shoulder problems is by early and frequent full-range movement, scapular stretches and extreme care with positioning, especially if there is cervical traction or use of a rotating bed. Passive movements are required for all joints, and in the lower limb may help prevent some of the vascular consequences of spinal cord injury (Venturelli et al. 2014). Close attention should be paid to pain prevention, which becomes chronic in an average 78% of patients (Ataoglu 2012).

Patients with complete lesions are best mobilized as soon as possible after surgery. Those with incomplete lesions are usually on bed rest for 6 weeks to ensure optimum perfusion to the spinal cord. Mobilization takes the form of gradual elevation with a tilt table, monitoring BP with every 10-degree rise. Standing is less comfortable than supine because the floppy abdominal muscles allow bulging of the abdomen. An abdominal binder for standing, sitting and coughing helps counteract this and also reduces postural hypotension (Cornwell et al. 2014). Impaired venous return and interrupted sympathetic outflow blunt the heart's response to exercise, which can limit exercise capacity. Wheelchair seats positioned parallel to the ground

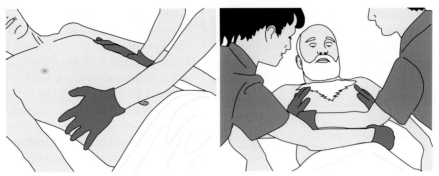

**FIGURE 22.9** Manual cough support.

may be a risk factor for shoulder pain (Giner-Pascual et al. 2011) and the footrest should be low enough to minimize ischial tuberosity pressure (Tederko et al. 2015).

Muscle spasticity and flaccidity have a complicated relationship. After the 'spinal shock' period of flaccidity, which varies from a few days to several weeks, the spinal cord below the lesion begins to transmit reflexes. The ensuing spasticity can reduce muscle wasting and risk of osteoporosis, and lung function may improve if spasticity and stiffening thoracic joints provide some compensation for loss of intercostal muscle function. However, if spasms cause pain, breathlessness, contractures or impaired mobility, they can be reduced by baclofen or TENS (Chung & Cheng 2010).

Exercise training should be initiated early in the rehabilitation process to improve breathlessness (Garshick et al. 2016), bone density, neuronal plasticity, coordination and neurological performance (Cristante et al. 2012). This should be paced to avoid fatigue, and ongoing to prevent continuing decline in lung function (Postma et al. 2013) and cardiovascular disease, which is the leading cause of mortality in later years (Chopra et al. 2016). Screening is required for autonomic dysreflexia, orthostatic hypotension, exercise-induced hypotension, thermoregulatory dysfunction, pressure sores, spasticity, pain (Tweedy et al. 2016) and depression, which hinders motivation and affects approximately 30% of inpatients but is undertreated (Bombardier et al. 2016).

Readmissions are reduced by follow-up physiotherapy (DeJong et al. 2013), and, for some patients, glossopharyngeal breathing which can provide up to 1900 mL maximum insufflation capacity (Toki et al. 2008). Patients with malignant lesions also benefit from rehabilitation (New 2017).

ICF categories can provide a structural base for evaluation in early rehabilitation (Nam et al. 2012):
- impaired body function and structure, e.g. musculoskeletal pain, lost sensation and motor function;
- activity limitation, e.g. deficits in activities of daily living or propelling a wheelchair;
- limited participation, e.g. obstacles to homemaking or social activities;

Singing therapy can aid all three, improving respiratory function, muscle strength, speech intensity, mood and social participation (Tamplin et al. 2013).

In the ensuing years, patients should aim at supported standing for 30–60 min a day (Paleg & Livingstone 2015). Annual re-hospitalization rates of 25%–40% have been reported, with cardiopulmonary causes being strongly related to modifiable risk factors rather than neurological impairment (Waddimba et al. 2009).

Patients need as much control over their environment and treatment as feasible, and support and encouragement in the early stages enable most patients to find the determination to rebuild their lives, including the ability to enjoy sex and have children (Linsenmeyer 2000). Many patients report that their initial response was that death was better than living with such a disability, but one study found 92% of patients glad to be alive later (DeLateur 1997), though acceptance can take 10 years (Reid 2017). People with tetraplegia place the highest priority on regaining upper limb function while those with paraplegia rank return of sexual function as their main priority (Harvey 2016). Outcomes are best measured by questionnaires (Lindberg et al. 2013, Fekete et al. 2013).

*It is a tribute to the human spirit that those who have a WHY to live will put up with almost any HOW.*

**DeLateur 1997**

## Other Neurological Conditions

*'I heard a lot more than I think they think I heard'.*
**Jablonski 1994**

Neurological conditions may lead to respiratory complications as a result of immobility, respiratory muscle weakness, aspiration pneumonia or neurogenic pulmonary oedema. Weaning can be hindered by reduced respiratory drive (Rialp et al. 2013) and rehabilitation by neuropathic pain (Jones et al. 2016c). Patients may benefit from neurophysiological facilitation of respiration (p. 187) or cough assistance (p. 217).

### ICU-acquired weakness

Over half of patients ventilated for more than 8 days develop systemic muscle weakness beyond disuse atrophy, leading to increased morbidity and mortality (McWilliams et al. 2017). **Critical illness polyneuropathy** is a motor and sensory neuropathy, and **critical illness myopathy** is a primary muscle disease. Triggers include immobility, sepsis, steroids, neuromuscular blocking agents (Zorowitz 2016), inadequate protein intake (Ökrös 2014), intravenous nutrition, sedatives and 'mechanical silence', i.e. lack of the stimulus to muscle that is normally provided by weight bearing or muscle stretch (Renaud et al. 2013). Compromised muscle regrowth leads to impaired regenerative capacity (Santos et al. 2016) and few patients regain functional independence (Walsh 2016).

Failure to recognize the condition is common (Koo et al. 2016) and leads to delay in reducing risk factors and misjudgement of weaning ability. It can be identified by electroneuromyography, histology, ultrasound, nonvolitional strength measurements (Hough et al. 2011) or simply hand grip strength (O'Brien et al. 2008). The physiotherapist may be the first to suspect the condition when a patient is unable to maintain trunk or head control during rehabilitation. If the patient is too weak to move their limbs against gravity, the diaphragm is also likely to be affected (Santos 2012).

| TABLE 22.2 | Barriers to early mobility |
|---|---|
| Institution problems | Insufficient staff |
| | Inadequate training |
| | Insufficient equipment or space |
| | Expense |
| | Not perceived as a priority by some team members |
| | Communication problems |
| | Delayed recognition of suitable patients |
| Patient problems | Medical instability or other safety concern |
| | Excessive sedation |
| | Fragile devices or lines |
| | Cognitive impairment |
| | Inadequate analgesia |
| | Inadequate nutrition |

From Koo et al. 2016.

Prevention is by passive movements and/or functional electrical stimulation (Parry et al. 2012), optimal nutrition, drug review, activating ventilatory modes and early mobility (Farhan et al. 2016), which may meet some barriers (Table 22.2). Short sessions are required to avoid exhaustion (Novak 2011) and a combined tilt table and stretcher chair reduces the time to mobilize (Fig. 22.10). Sensory neuropathy requires attention to skin integrity and limb positioning.

### Guillain-Barré syndrome

*'I felt as if every tissue in my spine had been superglued together'.*

**Savinson 2012**

Guillain-Barré syndrome is an autoimmune inflammatory demyelinating polyneuropathy and the most frequent cause of acute flaccid paralysis worldwide. It can occur in children (Spagnoli et al. 2015) but mainly affects young adults, 20% of whom are left disabled and 5% of whom die (Yuki & Hartung 2012). It often follows infection, with two-thirds of patients presenting with respiratory or gastrointestinal infection before onset (Yang & Jia 2015). It causes a predominantly motor deficit with some autonomic and sensory components.

Presenting features include fatigue and pain, which may both persist for some years after the illness (Merkies 2016), backache, paraesthesia and weakness.

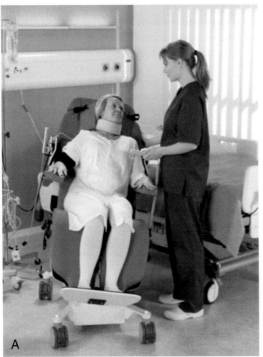 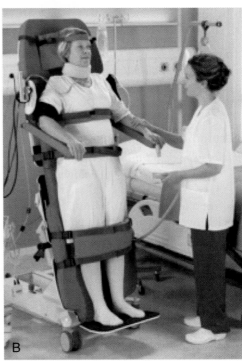

**FIGURE 22.10** Sara Combilizer. (From McWilliams et al. 2016b.)

Weakness progresses for up to a month, and ventilatory failure develops in 20%–30% of patients (Willison et al. 2016), sometimes with alarming speed. This can be predicted by difficulties with speech or swallowing, but reduced vital capacity is the most reliable warning sign. The decision to ventilate should be semielective to avoid emergency intubation (Mangera et al. 2012).

Medical treatment is mainly supportive, but patients may benefit from plasma exchange in which the patient's plasma is replaced by that of a donor, plasmapheresis in which albumin or other fluids are used for replacement, or intravenous antibodies purified from donated blood. Use of IV corticosteroids is a risk factor for poor short-term prognosis in patients requiring MV (Wu et al. 2015b).

### Physiotherapy

*'The physiotherapist was a most welcome person, as, despite the discomfort endured to have 'dead' limbs stretched and repositioned, this left me comfortable for several more hours'.*

***Clark 1985***

Physiotherapy at the beginning is aimed at avoiding the contractures that can become major components of disability. Muscle pain is exacerbated at initiation of movement but eased after a few moments of mobility exercises. Exercise should therefore be:

- regular and frequent
- preceded if necessary by anti-inflammatory drugs or accompanied by Entonox
- gentle at the start
- precise, to ensure full range without risking the damage that can occur with hypotonia
- brief to avoid fatigue

Spinal movements should be included, e.g. double knee-and-hip flexion, knee rolling, and neck movements with due care of the tracheal tube. Relatives can assist with some routine exercises and be shown the benefits of relaxation (Sendhilkumar 2016). Extremities may be hypersensitive.

Autonomic involvement leads to unstable BP and heart rate, and sustained hypertension may alternate with sudden hypotension. The risk of hypotension is reduced by ensuring that turning is gentle, by avoiding any intervention if central venous pressure is below 5 cmH$_2$O, and by slow acclimatization to the upright posture with a tilt table. Risk of bradycardia is reduced by oxygenation before and after suction.

Rehabilitation is hindered by fatigue, pain, anxiety, depression (Merkies 2016) and poor sleep (Karkare et al. 2013), all of which require teamwork. Physiotherapy can incorporate trips outside the ICU and, later, hydrotherapy. Recovery is prolonged but assisted by high-intensity rehabilitation (Khan et al. 2011). Long-term quality of life is often compromised by immobility and chronic pain (Witsch et al. 2013), and outcome measures are best based on activity and participation (Khan & Ng 2009). Self-help groups provide support from the ICU stage onwards (Appendix B, Links for patients).

---

### PRACTICE TIP

Next Sunday morning, on waking, have a cup of tea, go to the toilet, turn on the radio, smooth out the bottom sheet, get back into bed and make yourself comfortable and warm. Then see how long you can remain totally motionless.

Variations are to use an unfamiliar radio station at an unfamiliar volume, leave a crease in the sheet or lie on a damp pad.

---

### Myasthenia gravis

This progressive autoimmune disorder affects the neuromuscular junction and weakens muscles in proportion to their use. MV may be required after thymectomy and sometimes in a myasthenic crisis, which may present as ventilatory failure (Seung et al. 2015). Physiotherapy includes clearance of the excess bronchial secretions stimulated by the drug anticholinesterase, as well as the musculoskeletal care required for what may be prolonged MV (Lu et al. 2015).

## TRAUMA

Severe trauma can set off a catecholamine surge that affects systemic organs. A third of bleeding trauma patients present with a coagulopathy on admission (Shahn et al. 2013) and a quarter of trauma patients develop pneumonia (Hyllienmark et al. 2013), sometimes evolving into ARDS. Other complications of trauma are thromboembolism (Allen et al. 2016) or persistent immunosuppression (Vanzant 2014). Up to

25% of deaths caused by trauma is related to chest injuries (Richter & Ragaller 2011) and intensive physiotherapy may be required (Calthorpe et al. 2014), the outcome of which can be partly evaluated by the Quality of Trauma Care Patient-Reported Experience Measure (Bobrovitz et al. 2016). Acute brain trauma is described on p. 520.

### Rib Fracture

*Medical providers tend to underestimate the presence and severity of pain from rib fractures.*

***Azzam & Alam 2013***

Pain from rib fractures causes a restrictive defect, exacerbated if there is chest wall derangement, pneumothorax, subcutaneous emphysema or haemothorax. Poorly managed pain can lead to prolonged disability (Fabricant et al. 2013) and early pain control should be by thoracic epidural analgesia (Krupp & Balas 2016), sometimes with an added lignocaine patch (Cheng 2016). If chest drains are used for pneumothorax or haemothorax, local anaesthetic can be administered through the drain. A protocol to facilitate early analgesia and effective physiotherapy leads to a reduced incidence of pneumonia (Fig. 22.11).

The most common locations are the third to tenth ribs, often laterally where there is no muscle protection. Fractures of the well-protected first three ribs indicate prodigious force and are often accompanied by intrathoracic injury, although first-rib stress fractures can occur in adolescent athletes (Low et al. 2015). Lower rib fractures may be accompanied by intraabdominal injury. A flail chest results when two or more adjacent ribs are fractured at two different points, causing paradoxical breathing due to an incompetent segment of chest wall (Fig. 22.12). It may not be apparent in the first day or two, if muscle spasm stabilizes the chest wall.

Imaging can underestimate the presence and extent of rib fractures, especially anteriorly, but assessment should not include palpation, which elicits exquisite pain. A line of fractures suggests single trauma, while a transverse sternal fracture may be caused by hyperflexion over a seat belt. CT can help predict pulmonary complications (Chapman et al. 2016).

Trauma may lead to exsanguination into the thorax, each adult pleural space having the ability to hold 40% of blood volume (Craig 2017). Haemothorax requires early tube drainage if empyema is to be avoided (DuBose

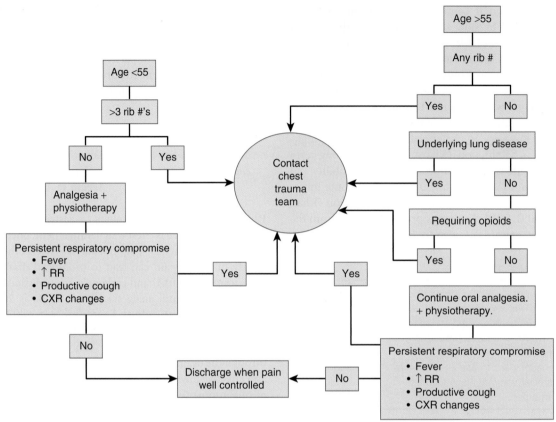

**FIGURE 22.11** Decision tool for fractured ribs. #, Fracture; *CXR*, chest X-ray; *RR*, respiratory rate. (Adapted from Curtis et al. 2016.)

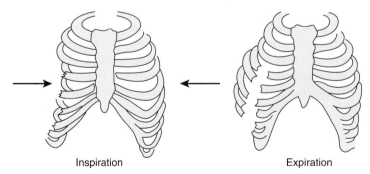

Inspiration                                    Expiration

**FIGURE 22.12** Flail chest caused by fractured ribs. The unstable segment is sucked in on inspiration and pushed out on expiration.

et al. 2012). Surgical stabilization may benefit patients with severe multiple fractures (Pieracci et al. 2017).

Physiotherapy usually requires liaison with the pain team because intensive treatment may be required to avoid pneumonia, a major complication (Jensen et al. 2016). If there is no pneumothorax, Entonox may be used (Ducassé et al. 2013). Once pain is controlled, regular incentive spirometry is advisable. If gas exchange is impaired, continuous positive airway pressure (CPAP) provides the added benefit of pneumatic stabilization of

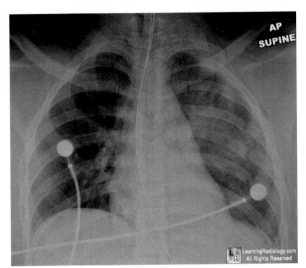

**FIGURE 22.13** Left lung contusion and posterior fractured ribs.

the rib cage without impairing cardiovascular function (Schweiger et al. 2003).

Before mobilizing patients who have a haemothorax, they can first be asked to clear some of the blood from their pleural space by lying with the chest drain dependent, so long as it is not uncomfortable and does not block the drain. A cough belt or towel can support coughing.

## Lung Contusion

Shearing or crushing forces to the chest can lead to pulmonary laceration and a form of 'blood pneumonia' known as contusion. Blood-filled alveoli cause a shunt, ventilation/perfusion mismatch, hypoxaemia and X-ray signs of nonlobular opacification (Fig. 22.13), followed by absorption of the infiltrate over 3–5 days or progression to ARDS (Daurat et al. 2016). Patients are breathless and produce bloody secretions. MV is needed if hypoxaemia is refractory to oxygen therapy or CPAP. If secretions are present, neither patient nor their bruised lungs take kindly to percussion or vibrations, but humidification and breathing techniques may be beneficial. If frank bleeding is present, suction is contraindicated.

## Diaphragmatic Rupture

Blunt injuries may rupture the diaphragm. Abdominal viscera herniate into the chest, requiring immediate surgical repair. The diagnosis may be missed clinically but can be confirmed by ultrasound, CT scan (Gao et al. 2015) or X-ray (see Fig. 1.3).

## Burns and Smoke Inhalation

Immediate management of burns is to:
- remove any clothing that is burning, constricting or covered with chemicals, but not clothing that is stuck to the skin;
- cool any burns less than 3 h old with cold water, but avoid hypothermia, especially in young or old people;
- cover the patient with something clean and dry;
- attend to other trauma such as bleeding, monitor perfusion to burn wounds and remove rings;
- if available, apply oxygen if there are major burns and 100% oxygen if carbon monoxide has been inhaled.

The patient will be intubated if there is stridor, hoarseness, facial injury, sooty sputum or burns to the face or neck. Airway swelling may develop within hours or after a delay (Dries & Endorf 2013). Electrical burns require extra fluid resuscitation and may bring hidden musculoskeletal damage (Sanford & Gamelli 2014).

### Pathology and clinical features

**Burns** set off an inflammatory cascade which can double energy needs (Chang 2014, p. 42) and leach skeletal muscle for fuel, just when a sustained supply of amino acids is required for wound healing (Porter 2013). This may lead to marked muscle wasting and delayed mobilization (Williams et al. 2011). Inflammation also inhibits hypoxic vasoconstriction, leading to alveolar ventilation to perfusion ($\dot{V}_A/\dot{Q}$) mismatch, and oxygen delivery may be further reduced by vascular permeability (Sio et al. 2010), shock and sometimes inhaled carbon monoxide.

The effects of burns can be prolonged:
1. Increased cardiac work lasts into the rehabilitation stage.
2. Catecholamine and corticosteroid levels increase 10- to 50-fold for up to 12 months.
3. Glucose metabolism is impaired for up to 3 years (Williams et al. 2011).

Other complications include restricted expansion due to a tight armour of scarring around the chest.

The heat from **smoke inhalation** is filtered by the upper airways at the expense of bronchospasm, mucosal swelling, paralysis of cilia and ulceration. Steam, crack cocaine and some other toxins can overwhelm these filtering properties, penetrating to alveoli and burning lung tissue. Of particular concern to the physiotherapist is atelectasis due to loss of surfactant, and destroyed mucociliary transport (Dries & Endorf 2013).

The stages of lung injury from smoke inhalation are:
- bronchospasm (first 12 h)
- pulmonary oedema (6–12 h postburn)
- bronchopneumonia (>60 h postburn)

Wheeze and black sputum may not appear for 24 h, and X-ray signs of pulmonary oedema are not apparent for some days. Infection is readily transmitted to the denuded airways from the hospital environment, infected burns or endogenous sepsis, and if pneumonia sets in, burn mortality increases by 40% (Mlcak et al. 2007). Epithelial damage can cause long-term hyperreactivity, tracheal stenosis and fibrin-based casts, which can further block airways.

### Medical management

Medical treatment is by:
- pain management, including opioids, lignocaine (Wasiak et al. 2012) or, for dressing changes, Entonox (Yuxiang et al. 2012);
- fluid resuscitation with Ringer's lactate or normal saline;
- humidified oxygen, CPAP if the face is not burned, or mechanical ventilation;
- modulation of the hypermetabolic response with early excision and grafting of burn wounds, environmental thermoregulation, and drugs to stimulate anabolism and oppose catabolism (Williams et al. 2011);
- meticulous wound care;
- early and continuous specialized feeding to counteract hypermetabolism, promote wound healing, increase resistance to infection and prevent persistent loss of muscle protein (Hsieh et al. 2016).

Medication may include:
- nebulizers for smoke inhalation, e.g. heparin diluted with 3 mL 0.9% saline 4-hourly for 5–7 days, or nebulized 20% acetylcysteine 3 mL every 4 h; these are irritants and should be discontinued if bronchospasm develops or worsens;
- nebulized adrenaline if bronchodilation is required (Lopez et al. 2016);
- antithrombin to attenuate inflammation and vascular leakage (Rehberg et al. 2013).

Prophylactic antibiotics may be given and a sputum specimen should be obtained at the earliest signs of infection.

Large mucous casts may need bronchoscopy or lavage. Ventilated patients require extubation over a fibreoptic bronchoscope in case of oedema.

### Physiotherapy

Respiratory care is aimed at maintaining lung volume and clearing the thick and prolific secretions caused by airway damage. Lavish humidification is needed. Bronchoscopy may have been performed for diagnosis and washout, but can only remove secretions to the second airway generation. Patients may not be productive immediately if soot has adhered to the respiratory epithelium, in which case the soot, along with necrotic airway mucosa, may slough at 24–72 h, necessitating 4-hourly physiotherapy day and night to prevent plugging of airways, sometimes using intrapulmonary percussive ventilation (Reper & Looy 2013).

Precautions are:
- treatment little and often because of the importance of prophylaxis and the inevitable fatigue;
- avoidance of percussion and vibrations over chest burns, whether dressed or not; if manual techniques are essential, a vibrator is reasonably comfortable over a sterile towel;
- for burns near the head or neck, avoidance of head-down postural drainage;
- suction, if it is necessary, to be gentle and scrupulously aseptic, and minimal to prevent further mucosal damage;
- nasopharyngeal suction to be avoided if there is voice change or stridor, which should be reported because intubation will be required;
- attention to communication if facial oedema affects vision or speech.

Oximetry may be falsely normal because the device cannot distinguish oxyhaemoglobin from carboxyhaemoglobin.

Two-hourly exercises are needed for burned limbs, especially the hands, using Entonox or other analgesia. Early mobility is recommended (Gille et al. 2016) and provision of a clean 'burn intensive care gym' encourages self management. Somatosensory rehabilitation may help neuropathic pain (Nedelec et al. 2016).

### Fat Embolism Syndrome

Fat emboli occur when fats are released from bone marrow into the circulation. This follows all long-bone fractures and many orthopaedic operations (Kwiatt 2013). Capillary inflammation and the multisystem disorder 'fat embolism syndrome' may develop, which affects organs with high blood flow such as lungs, brain and skin. Respiratory signs are dyspnoea, agitation, tachycardia, pyrexia and cyanosis within 72 h of trauma, sometimes leading to ARDS. CT may show gravity-dependent consolidation, scattered ground glass opacities or areas of crazy paving (Piolanti et al. 2016). The risk is increased if fractures are not immobilized because movement precipitates intravascular entry of the fat embolus.

## Non-fatal Drowning

Near drowning or non-fatal drowning can lead to aspiration, bronchospasm, inactivation of surfactant, blood-stained pulmonary oedema, atelectasis and hypoxaemia, especially with polymicrobial infections such as the 'tsunami lung' experienced after the Japanese 2011 earthquake (Kawakami et al. 2012). If water is swallowed, there is a high incidence of vomiting, sometimes followed by further aspiration.

Resuscitation attempts should be prolonged, with emphasis on the ventilation component because the main cause of cardiac arrhythmias is hypoxia (Mott 2016). Nobody should be considered dead until they are 'warm and dead', i.e. until they have been rewarmed to 35°C (Kjaergaard et al. 2008). Profound hypothermia may require extracorporeal rewarming (Jarosz et al. 2017).

Intensive chest clearance may be needed for at least 48 h to prevent atelectasis. Physiotherapy is not required after 'dry drowning', which accounts for 10% of admissions, caused by laryngospasm in a panicking victim, leading to apnoea and hypoxaemia.

## Poisoning and Parasuicide

Complications of poisoning include arrhythmias due to the toxin, fluid depletion due to vomiting or diarrhoea, and respiratory compromise due to ventilatory depression, upper airway obstruction or pulmonary oedema. Gastric lavage may cause aspiration or laryngeal spasm.

Carbon monoxide is the most common cause of fatal poisoning worldwide and has 220 times greater affinity for haemoglobin than oxygen, shifting the oxygen dissociation curve to the left, hindering the loading of oxygen from the lungs, interfering with its unloading to the tissues, sometimes causing brain injury (Wolf et al. 2017). $PaO_2$ is normal but $SpO_2$ is falsely high, and the presentation can mimic common illnesses or exacerbate

established disease. Symptoms vary from headache and dizziness to coma and death, with a mortality of 1%–3% (Rose et al. 2016). Apparent recovery may be followed 2 weeks later by neurological deterioration, which can be permanent. Monitoring is by pulse carbon-monoxide-oximetry (Sebbane 2013) and treatment is with 100% or hyperbaric oxygen (Wolf et al. 2017).

With self-inflicted poisoning, some health staff may show negative attitudes to parasuicide patients, including judgements about attention-seeking. However, these patients are often at the extremes of depression or desperation and the professional approach is to withhold personal judgement and care for the patient in such a way that they may believe that life is worth living after all. Following a successful suicide, bereaved relatives find recovery more difficult than after a normal death, and the care that they receive in the first hours can significantly ease their grief (Odell 1997).

# SYSTEMS FAILURE

## Disseminated Intravascular Coagulation

The normal response to tissue damage is a contained explosion of thrombin to stimulate coagulation and limit blood loss. This may become uncontained after severe damage, e.g. with sepsis, trauma, malignancy, brain injury, fat embolism syndrome, shock, haemorrhage, burns (Midura et al. 2016) or after major surgery. This deranged coagulopathy is called disseminated intravascular coagulation (DIC), in which liberated thromboplastin activates unrestrained clotting and blocks vessels with clumps of platelets and fibrin, causing ischaemia and organ damage. Once clotting factors have been depleted, bleeding can occur from the slightest trauma, including suction (Fig. 22.14).

Coagulation therapy and treatment of the underlying disorder are required, and comprehensive guidelines are available (Shahn et al. 2013). Suction is not contraindicated but should be minimized. DIC is not necessarily written in the notes or charts because it is not the primary diagnosis.

## Acute Kidney Injury

The kidney is central to BP and fluid regulation but its sensitivity to impaired perfusion means that acute kidney injury (AKI) develops in 50% of ICU patients (Golden et al. 2016), often precipitated by hypovolaemia or sepsis and increasing mortality two to six times

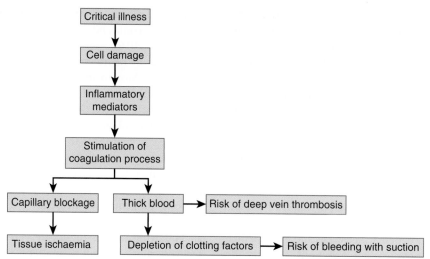

**FIGURE 22.14** Development of disseminated intravascular coagulation.

(Regner 2016). Multisystem failure may be either cause or effect, and AKI is the most common cause of organ dysfunction in critically ill adults (Doyle & Forni 2016), the organs most relevant to the physiotherapist being the lungs (Faubel 2016), muscles (Pomidori et al. 2016) and even the sturdy bones, which become vulnerable to fracture (Shiao et al. 2015).

Prevention includes automated alerts (Prendecki et al. 2016) and management is by accurate fluid management and renal replacement therapy:

1. Intermittent haemodialysis circulates the patient's blood outside their body and through a semipermeable membrane, allowing toxins and excess fluid to be removed. Complications include unstable BP, inflammation, wheeze, hypoxaemia due to capillary blockage, and bleeding due to anticoagulation. Vascular access is commonly by arteriovenous fistula.
2. Continuous haemofiltration and haemodiafiltration work more slowly and allow control of BP, electrolytes, medication and nutrition. Moderate anticoagulation is required.
3. Sustained low efficiency daily dialysis is a hybrid therapy combining both options.
4. Peritoneal dialysis uses the patient's own semipermeable peritoneal membrane but risks infection, impairs basal ventilation and is becoming a rarity. Physiotherapy should coincide with the end of the emptying cycle to ensure free diaphragmatic movement.

Exercise is thought to increase the anabolic effects of nutritional intervention, which would attenuate the muscle wasting characteristic in this group (Magnard et al. 2013). Physiotherapists need to develop a healthy respect for the renal vascular catheter or 'vascath' because it is highly sensitive to position change and disconnection leads to major blood loss, but transfers and walking on the spot are feasible (Toonstra et al. 2016). Other precautions are to be watchful of fluid volume changes, acid–base disturbance or hypertension, and to be aware of the risk of bleeding because of anticoagulation drugs.

Mortality is 40%–60% (Shiao et al. 2015) and survivors of severe AKI require surveillance because of long-term damage to cardiovascular and other systems (Shiao et al. 2015).

## Acute Liver Injury

Liver cells are also vulnerable to hypoxia. Acute liver injury can occur abruptly after viral, metabolic, vascular or autoimmune insult. Respiratory and cardiovascular complications are common, as are coagulopathy, encephalopathy and sepsis, and up to 80% of patients develop AKI (Regner 2016). Respiratory complications include $\dot{V}_A/\dot{Q}$ mismatch caused by intrapulmonary vascular dilation, hydrothorax caused by portal hypertension, leading to cough and dyspnoea, and pulmonary artery hypertension caused by portal hypertension (Ramalingam 2016).

Handling and suction should be minimal, and encephalopathy is a warning to take precautions similar to those for acute brain injury. The lungs may suffer a restrictive defect from ascites or pleural effusion.

Support of failing systems may allow the liver to recover or permit survival until a donor organ is available for transplant. Some patients are so poisoned by their own liver that it is removed even if no donor is immediately available. Liver resection can now be done by laparoscope, but transplantation needs a 'Mercedes-Benz' double subcostal incision and laparotomy, requiring intensive postoperative pain relief and bringing a 50% incidence of lung complications (Jiang et al. 2012). For survivors, posttransplant recovery is surprisingly rapid once the toxic liver has been removed, but rehabilitation may be slow due to deconditioning.

Cirrhosis is the final phase of chronic liver disease and may obstruct the portal vein, transmit back pressure throughout the portal system and cause oesophageal varices. These contraindicate most forms of physiotherapy because of the risk of bleeding.

More safeguards for treating patients with liver disease are detailed on p. 124.

## Acute Pancreatitis

*Acute pancreatitis presents a high mortality of up to 30% and is one of the most common diseases requiring multidisciplinary management.*

***Wei 2016***

The incidence of inflammation of the pancreas is increasing (Bollen 2016) and has a variety of causes including gallstones, alcoholism, drug reaction and eating disorder. Dissemination of inflammation leads to one-third of patients developing ARDS (Litmathe et al. 2013).

The disease activates enzymes that autodigest pancreatic tissue and set off a cascade of ischaemia, vasodilation, increased capillary permeability and DIC. Progressive liquefaction of the pancreas may cause abscesses and sepsis. Patients suffer paralytic ileus, which increases the risk of aspiration, and a rigidly distended abdomen and continuous epigastric pain, worse in supine. Complications are diaphragmatic splinting, atelectasis, pleural effusion and pneumonia, and respiratory failure is the main contributing factor to mortality in the early stages (Fig. 22.15).

Medical treatment aims to eliminate the cause, manage complications and prevent progression, using

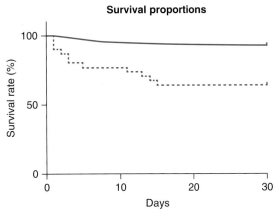

**Survival proportions**

**FIGURE 22.15** Correlation between respiratory failure and mortality in the first 3 weeks of hospitalization in acute pancreatitis. Solid line: patients without respiratory failure; dotted line: patients with respiratory failure. (From Dombernowsky et al. 2016.)

hydration, early enteral nutrition (Márta et al. 2016), MV if required and surgery if there is infection. A thoracic epidural limits pain and induces splanchnic vasodilatation, improving pancreatic perfusion and enhancing lung and liver function (Windisch et al. 2016).

Physiotherapy is aimed at preserving lung volume, and includes positioning, preferably with the whole bed tilted head-up about 15 degrees, use of auscultation and patient comfort for guidance.

## Abdominal Compartment Syndrome

*The abdominal compartment is a technical masterpiece.*

***Malbrain et al. 2016***

The abdomen houses 8.5 m of intestines and is bounded by the costal arch, the rigid spine and pelvis, and the partly flexible abdominal wall and diaphragm. Its size varies with respiration and intra-abdominal pressure. Abdominal hypertension is present if abdominal pressure exceeds 12 mmHg, and abdominal compartment syndrome is present if this exceeds 20 mmHg. Causes include either near-exsanguination or large volume fluid resuscitation (Luckianow et al. 2012). The gut is already precariously perfused, and excess pressure may effectively strangle it, leading to intra-abdominal organ failure.

Management is by thoracic epidural to reduce intraabdominal pressure and tilting the whole bed head-up; raising just the head of the bed should be avoided because at 45 degrees intraabdominal pressure increases by 5–15 mmHg (Malbrain et al. 2016). After decompressive laparotomy, the wound may be left open temporarily to prevent pressure buildup, especially with sepsis (Beckman et al. 2016).

# MULTISYSTEM FAILURE

**Colonization**: presence of microorganisms
**Infection**: invasion and multiplication of microorganisms
**Bacteraemia**: bacteria in blood
**Septicaemia**: systemic infection in which pathogen is present in blood
**Endotoxin**: toxin released by gram-negative bacteria as they disintegrate
**Sepsis**: life-threatening organ dysfunction caused by dysregulated host response to infection, carrying 10% mortality (Pickkers 2017)
**Multisystem failure**: systems failure caused by direct insult or sepsis, in which homeostasis cannot be maintained without intervention; also known as multiple organ failure or multiple organ dysfunction syndrome
**Shock**: tissue hypoxia due to failure of oxygen supply to meet oxygen demand

## Sepsis

Respiratory tract infections are the most common source of sepsis (Suárez et al. 2016). Clinical features include fever (or occasionally hypothermia), tachypnoea, and skin that is initially warm from peripheral vasodilation but may become cold if shock supervenes. Tachycardia and decreased systemic vascular resistance lead to increased cardiac output, which along with over-zealous fluid therapy may lead to a hyperdynamic state, i.e. increased circulatory volume, but because of widespread vasodilation, decreased BP. Elevated lactate leads to metabolic acidosis, and deranged coagulation is inevitable, with a 35% incidence of DIC (Kohji et al. 2016).

Impaired cerebrovascular autoregulation means that falls in BP are transferred directly to the vascular bed, risking brain and eye dysfunction (Erikson 2017). Muscle loss occurs at up to 15% in the first week (Corner & Brett

2014), the protein being broken down to provide amino acids for the inflammatory response. The diaphragm struggles for its share of oxygen and the process may lead to respiratory failure, circulatory collapse and multisystem failure (MSF), each new failing organ adding 15%–20% to the risk of death (Martin 2009).

Medical management is based on a 'sepsis bundle' of timely circulatory and ventilatory support. Aggressive fluid resuscitation is not advisable because much of the fluid escapes from the dilated vasculature and into the tissues, and vasopressors may be required to maintain a mean arterial pressure greater than 65 mmHg (Head 2016). MV should start as soon as rapid shallow breathing is apparent and not await hypercapnia (Magder 2009). Accurate antibiotics may control the infection source but do not reverse inflammatory and clotting cascades, which can sometimes be dampened by protection against oxidative stress (McCreath et al. 2016) and a thoracic epidural block to help preserve the anti-inflammatory response (Tyagi et al. 2016).

Sepsis-induced delirium occurs in up to 70% of patients (Donnelly et al. 2016), and prevention of delirium is considered a marker of the quality of care (Fig. 22.16). Delirium is reduced by nutrition and mobilization, which also bring earlier extubation and improved functional status at discharge (Gelinas 2016).

### Shock

In contrast to the layperson's shock-horror understanding of the term, shock in medicine occurs when the reserve capacity of tissue respiration is exhausted and hypoxia ensues. If prolonged, this leads to irreversible cellular injury. Once oxygen delivery ($DO_2$) can no longer satisfy $\dot{V}O_2$, a cascade of events supervenes:

Inadequate tissue perfusion
↓
Anaerobic metabolism
↓
Lactic acidosis
↓
Metabolic acidosis
↓
Cellular damage
↓
Organ failure

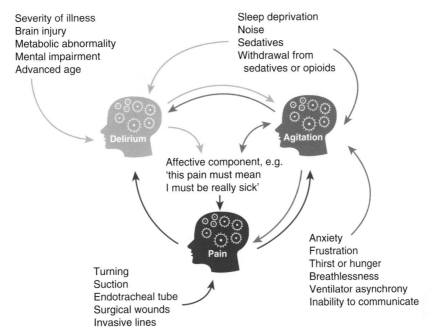

**FIGURE 22.16** Contributors to pain, anxiety and depression, and their interactions. (From Gelinas 2016.)

Shock is defined in terms of the cardiovascular component of $DO_2$, i.e. MAP <60 mmHg or systolic BP <90 mmHg, or a decrease in systolic BP greater than 40 mmHg (Nebout & Pirracchio 2012).

**Hypovolaemic** shock is caused by a 15% loss in intravascular volume. Reasons may be haemorrhage, burns, severe diarrhoea or diuresis. Early physiological compensation is by redistribution of fluid from extravascular to intravascular space, and selective vasoconstriction to nonvital systems.

**Cardiogenic** shock is caused by sudden heart failure, as in severe myocardial infarction, and brings 50% mortality (Diehl 2017). It is characterized by high CVP, low cardiac output (CO) and pulmonary oedema.

**Septic** shock is caused by dysregulation of the innate immune response to infection and brings a mortality of up to 50% (Huet & Chin 2014). Sepsis-induced hypotension and peripheral vasodilation deplete perfusion to the viscera; damaged organs release endotoxins, which stimulate nitric oxide to augment uncontrolled vasodilation, leading to a 'functional haemorrhage'. High CO cannot sustain an adequate BP, and hypoxic tissues cannot extract sufficient oxygen, as shown by a rise in mixed venous saturation ($S\overline{v}O_2$) above 85% and

loss of muscle tissue (Poulsen et al. 2011). Patients are pyrexial, flushed, tachypnoeic, hypotensive and have a bounding pulse, often with lactic acidosis. Skin mottling indicates microcirculatory impairment. Treatment is by vasopressors, 100% $O_2$ in the first 24 h (Calzia et al. 2010) and avoidance of inotropes (Wilkman et al. 2013).

Other types of shock are **anaphylactic** shock, an allergic reaction by more than one system, and **neurogenic** shock, loss of sympathetic tone following nervous system damage. Both are characterized by disordered vascular control and hypotension.

Hypovolaemic and cardiogenic shock lead to reduced CO. Other forms of shock lead to maldistribution of $DO_2$ between and within organs. Prompt treatment with fluids and vasopressors (Brown et al. 2013) during the first hour may prevent progression to MSF.

## Multisystem Failure
### Causes
MSF may follow sepsis, shock or any process that makes excessive demands on $\dot{V}O_2$, e.g.:
- aspiration
- burns, smoke inhalation or lung contusion

- multiple transfusions, especially of colloid or blood, or cardiopulmonary bypass
- complications of trauma or surgery
- brain injury
- non-fatal drowning and/or hypothermia
- pulmonary embolism or fat embolism syndrome
- neurogenic pulmonary oedema
- prolonged hypotension
- poisoning or drug abuse
- peritonitis or acute pancreatitis
- immunosuppression, e.g. neutropaenic or post-operative states
- DIC

Interaction of these predisposing factors can blur cause and effect, e.g. the inflammatory response can activate coagulation, leading to DIC, and shock can set off immunochaos, whereby homeostasis is lost.

## Pathophysiology

If a limb is amputated and then is sewn back on after a delay, the dying tissue releases endotoxins that invade the body and set off an inflammatory domino effect. Re-amputation is then required to prevent the rest of the body becoming poisoned. This is similar to MSF, except the whole body cannot be re-amputated. Circulating inflammatory products cause reperfusion injury, i.e. widespread capillary leak, hypovolaemic shock and multisystem damage. This 'rogue inflammation' subverts the normal healing process, a deadly cascade of inflammation escaping the usual control mechanisms and exacerbating rather than repairing injury.

The main culprit is the gut, whose vulnerability to hypoperfusion has earned it a reputation as the 'engine of MSF' by leaking its bacteria into the rest of the body. The main victim is the lung because of its large vascular component, now permeable, poisoned and vulnerable to ventilator-induced lung injury.

Circulating catecholamines increase CO and blood flow, but deranged autoregulation sends the circulating blood to robust tissues such as the skin, at the expense of needy systems such as the brain, gut and kidney. Patients are in effect poisoning themselves, which explains why some patients have no identifiable septic focus.

The resulting hypoxia is due to:
- refractory hypoxaemia;
- reduced gas diffusion at tissue level because of interstitial oedema and impaired oxygen extraction due to damaged microvasculature;

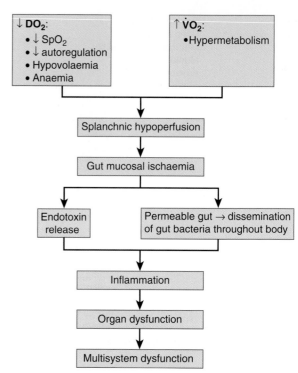

**FIGURE 22.17** Effect of imbalance in oxygen delivery and consumption, leading to multisystem failure. *CO*, Cardiac output; *DO₂*, oxygen delivery; *VO₂*, oxygen consumption.

- excess oxygen consumption due to hypermetabolism (Fig. 22.17).

The failing systems most relevant to the physiotherapist are the haematological, respiratory and muscular systems, leading to DIC, ARDS and muscle weakness (Solverson et al. 2016).

## Medical management

Any septic focus needs treatment to prevent further stimulation of the inflammatory response, e.g. excision of dead bowel or stabilization of fractures. The aims are then to restore homeostasis and sustain tissue perfusion rather than focus on a single system.

Glycaemic control and antibiotics are required within 1 h of diagnosis, and fluid resuscitation within 6 h (Dellinger et al. 2013), although too much fluid tends to escape into the leaky lung. Renal impairment complicates the picture, leading to the dilemma of whether to sacrifice the kidneys to keep the lungs dry, or increase fluids to restore urine output and risk the complications of more intense respiratory support. On balance, the aims are for a CVP of 10–12 $cmH_2O$ and a pulmonary artery wedge pressure (PAWP) of 18 $cmH_2O$.

$DO_2$ is supported by oxygen therapy, inotropes and vasodilators, with the aim of MAP of at least 65 mmHg, but this brings a similar dilemma of lower values risking AKI and higher values risking fluid overload (Corrêa et al. 2013). $\dot{V}O_2$ is reduced by respiratory support and avoidance of stress or pyrexia. Packed red cell transfusion or haemofiltration may be used to wash out circulating inflammatory mediators. Lactate-induced metabolic acidosis can usually be corrected by manipulation of MV to influence $PaCO_2$, but a pH below 7.2 requires haemofiltration. Neuromuscular electrical stimulation, normally used to stimulate weak muscles, may restore some endothelial function in patients who are not taking steroids at the same time (Stefanou et al. 2016).

Enteral nutrition helps stabilize the gut lining, but the septic response hinders the utilization of nutrition, as shown by high nitrogen excretion and relentless muscle wasting. Steroids may be helpful in sepsis because of their anti-inflammatory properties, but they suppress the patient's own adrenal function, and the outcome of much scientific deliberation is to follow a 'suck it and see' policy (Grover & Handy 2012). Cognitive impairment following sepsis may be treated by modulation of the adrenergic system (Tuon et al. 2008).

### Physiotherapy

Treatment should keep $\dot{V}O_2$ to a minimum, but preventive respiratory care is required as well as judicious exercise to manage the myopathy that is likely to arise from inactivity and inflammation.

Meningococcal septicaemia can cause hypoperfusion to the peripheries, leading to severe musculoskeletal and neurological consequences, including necrosis and gangrene. Passive movements require extreme care to safeguard the skin, and if fingers are affected, the hands may need to be splinted, with much padding, in a functional position to optimize circulation and prevent contractures. Teamwork requires a splinting specialist (occupational therapist or physiotherapist) and tissue viability nurse. Ultrasound-guided stellate ganglion blockade may restore perfusion to the extremities before necrosis sets in (Bataille et al. 2016).

# ACUTE RESPIRATORY DISTRESS SYNDROME

> **Atelectrauma**: alveolar damage caused by alveoli repeatedly collapsing and reopening during the respiratory cycle
>
> **Biotrauma**: inflammation caused by atelectrauma
>
> **Alveolar recruitment**: maintenance of open alveoli to (1) prevent atelectrauma and (2) promote gas exchange
>
> **Alveolar derecruitment**: collapse of alveoli

ARDS occurs in over 10% of ICU admissions and nearly 25% of ventilated patients (Cannon 2017). It is characterized by acute diffuse inflammatory lung injury invoked by a variety of systemic or pulmonary insults, leading to alveolar–capillary leak and noncardiogenic pulmonary oedema. It has also been called leaky lung syndrome, white lung due to its radiological appearance, or Nam lung due to its first description in badly injured US soldiers salvaged from Vietnam battlefields. Hospital mortality averages 40% (Confalonieri 2017), being highest for patients with septic shock or pneumonia, and lowest after trauma (Chiumello & Brioni 2016).

Lungs can be injured directly, e.g. by aspiration, contusion or smoke inhalation (Craig 2017), or indirectly by toxins let loose from MSF. Either way, patients who die usually succumb to MSF rather than respiratory failure (Kreyer et al. 2014). Severity is classified according to gas exchange at PEEP >5 $cmH_2O$:

| ARDS severity | PaO$_2$/FiO$_2$ on PEEP >5 | Mortality |
|---|---|---|
| Mild | 27–40 kPa (200–300 mmHg) | 27% |
| Moderate | 13.3–27 kPa (100–200 mmHg) | 32% |
| Severe | <13.3 kPa (<100 mmHg) | 45% |

### Pathophysiology

Both alveolar and vascular functions of the parenchyma are ravaged by inflammatory mediators, and the resulting sievelike alveolar–capillary membrane floods the alveoli with fluid containing protein and blood, leading to massive pulmonary oedema so that the patient feels as if they are drowning from the inside. The waterlogged lungs weigh nearly twice normal (Dirkes et al. 2012) and alveoli begin to collapse under their own weight, leading to compression atelectasis in dependent regions. Surfactant is washed out and hypoxic vasoconstriction (p. 13) is lost in the metabolic disarray, leading to a widened alveolar–arterial oxygen ($PAO_2$–$PaO_2$) gradient, a shunt that may exceed 25% and work of breathing averaging 50% of total oxygen consumption (Martin 2001). Vascular injury leads to pulmonary hypertension and sometimes right heart failure, which can be mitigated by protective ventilation and the prone position (Paternot 2016).

Only a proportion of alveoli can take part in gas exchange, leading to the term 'baby lung' to express their vulnerability. The restrictive defect worsens as the architecture of the lung, which has been intact during the florid **exudative phase** (days 1–5), is remodelled and weakened by the inflammatory process. The lungs may then recover or, over the next week, move into the **proliferative phase** when the alveolar exudate organizes. The **fibrotic phase** then dominates for the next few weeks, shown radiologically as cysts and honeycombing.

The alveoli that are still functioning are vulnerable to barotrauma, especially as the nonhomogenous loss of compliance causes alveoli to empty at different speeds, contributing to an uneven distribution of ventilation (Cressoni 2014):

1. Dependent alveoli are either consolidated with a proteinaceous fluid and inflammatory cells, or collapsed. Consolidated alveoli are nondistensible and therefore protected from atelectrauma, but are not contributing to gas exchange. Collapsed alveoli are recruitable in the early stages by prone positioning to place them uppermost, but later become fibrosed and nonrecruitable.
2. Alveoli in the middle are closed at end-expiration but recruitable and therefore susceptible to atelectrauma, becoming more vulnerable than dependent alveoli.
3. Nondependent alveoli stay open throughout the respiratory cycle but are overstretched and liable to succumb to barotrauma.

When $DO_2$ decreases to a critical level, oxygen extraction cannot increase to compensate, and $\dot{V}O_2$ becomes dependent on $DO_2$, thus reducing linearly with it instead of increasing according to need.

## Clinical Features

Signs begin 1–3 days from the provoking insult. Respiratory failure develops over the next 48 h as patients struggle to breathe through lungs that feel like a wet sponge. Both $PaO_2$ and $PaCO_2$ drop due to hypoxaemia and hyperventilation. Diagnosis is usually when virulent hypoxaemia develops and, in the spontaneously breathing patient, $PaCO_2$ rises as the patient tires. Development of the syndrome is less obvious if MV is already up and running, and the condition is not necessarily identified at the handover, unless specifically queried, because it is not the primary diagnosis. The physiotherapist picks it up by the history, intractable hypoxaemia, ventilator manipulations aimed at optimizing gas exchange without further damaging the lungs, and imaging, then checks with the team.

X-ray signs lag behind clinical signs by 24–48 h. Bilateral opacification is at first indistinguishable radiologically from pulmonary oedema, then increasingly dense 'snowstorm' consolidation fills the air spaces, often sparing the costophrenic angles (Fig. 22.18). If the patient remains supine, CT scanning shows dense consolidation in dependent regions (Fig. 22.19). Later a coarse reticular pattern of multiple interlacing line shadows indicate the development of fibrosis.

Breath sounds have a harsh edge to them, probably due to improved sound transmission through consolidated tissue (Räsänen et al. 2014). Pulmonary artery catheterization shows high pulmonary artery pressure,

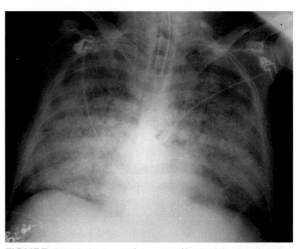

**FIGURE 22.18** Image of lungs affected by acute respiratory distress syndrome showing diffuse opacification and air bronchograms where airways show up against the white background. The endotracheal tube and electrocardiogram leads are apparent.

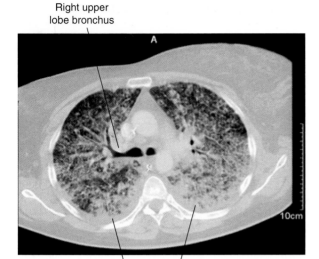

Right upper
lobe bronchus

Density of consolidation

**FIGURE 22.19** Computed tomography scan of ARDS lungs just below the carina, showing widespread opacities, most dense in dependent areas.

reflecting pulmonary hypertension. PAWP is <18 mmHg, in contrast to the high PAWP of cardiogenic pulmonary oedema, because ARDS is not a condition of generalized overhydration. A decision tool is available to distinguish ARDS from pulmonary oedema (Schmickl et al. 2012). $S\overline{v}O_2$ is usually reduced because of hypermetabolism, but may be increased if hypoxic cells are unable to extract oxygen.

## Medical Management

Early identification in at-risk populations aids prevention (Gong et al. 2016). Automated screening with electronic alerts from the laboratory and radiology department help early detection (Barbas et al. 2012). The cornerstone of treatment is then meticulous supportive care. Fluid management is aimed at zero fluid balance if there is no shock or renal failure (Roch et al. 2013), using ultrasound to guard against excessive fluid loading (Caltabeloti et al. 2014). A high fat, low carbohydrate diet minimizes $CO_2$ production, and immunonutrition helps reduce inflammation (Hecker et al. 2013). Enteral nutrition is feasible and safe even in prone patients (Fuente et al. 2016).

Pharmacotherapy includes pulmonary vasodilators, surfactant, hypertonic saline, and sometimes muscle relaxants. Instillation of vitamin D may reduce neutrophil recruitment, and aspirin may prevent microthrombi. More controversial are $\beta_2$-agonists, because of potentially harmful cardiac effects, and steroids (Boyle et al. 2013).

### Mechanical ventilation

MV worsens lung injury (Cereda et al. 2016) but is usually a necessary evil, high tidal volumes maintaining gas exchange but squeezing the bulk of inspiratory gas into the fragile baby lung, and low tidal volumes protecting lung tissue but risking further hypoxaemia. There is no safe driving pressure (Ochiai 2015) and the same strategies may be beneficial in certain stages of ARDS and harmful at other stages (Rittayamai 2015). Therefore in the early stages, or with less severe disease, high-flow nasal oxygen therapy (Messika et al. 2015) or NIV may be used (Huang et al. 2017). With MV, target $SpO_2$ is 88%–95% (Blakeman 2013) and after an initial period of controlled mechanical ventilation (Güldner et al. 2014), the following strategies attempt a balancing act:

1. **'Open lung' ventilation** uses recruitment manoeuvres (p. 493), e.g. high but judiciously applied PEEP, to stabilize alveoli, reduce intrinsic PEEP, distribute inspired gas more evenly and limit dissemination of inflammatory material (Graf & Marini 2008). High PEEP under CT or ultrasound guidance, and with early extubation to NIV, can quadruple aerated tissue but may cause barotrauma (De Matos et al. 2012), whereas decremental PEEP can improve oxygenation without barotrauma (Kacmarek et al. 2016). Other recruitment manoeuvres are 2-hourly CPAP at 30 cmH$_2$O for 40 s (Li et al. 2015d), sustained inspiratory pauses (Fig. 22.20A), increased inflation pressures (Fig. 22.20B) and inverse-ratio ventilation, which may themselves aggravate ventilator-induced lung injury (Müller-Redetzky et al. 2015). Recruitment manoeuvres show most benefit in the early stages before fibrosis sets in (Lapinsky 2003), and damage can be minimized by accurate positioning (as discussed later in the section/p. 547) (Marini 2016).

2. **Lung-protective ventilation** prevents over-distension of compliant lung by reducing high-pressure, high-volume MV. This can be achieved with pressure control ventilation to limit peak pressure to <30 cmH$_2$O (Koulouras et al. 2016) and lower tidal volume to temper alveolar stretch and possibly limit the spread of infectious material (Graf & Marini

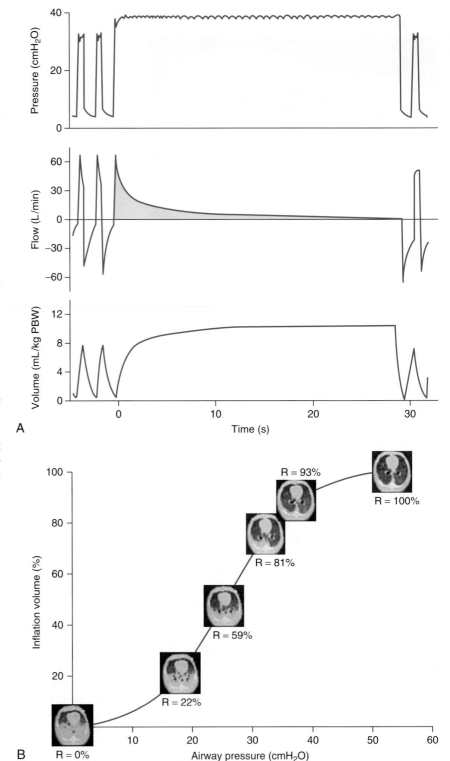

**FIGURE 22.20** (A) Recruitment manoeuvre comprising a 30-s breath-hold at 40 cmH$_2$O airway pressure, represented by pressure, flow and volume curves. (From Beitler et al. 2016.) (B) Recruitment in ARDS lungs as a function of applied airway pressure, shown by the opening up of alveoli along the volume–pressure curve. *R*, Percentage of recruitment occurring at the corresponding airway pressure. (From Gattinoni et al. 2001.)

2008), or by extracorporeal gas exchange or airway pressure release ventilation (p. 444), which draws gas into dependent lung during the time-cycled release phase.

Disadvantages of lung-protective strategies include retention of secretions (Volpe et al. 2008) and loss of volume (Kallet et al. 2001), the two core areas of physiotherapy. Disadvantages of recruitment manoeuvres are:

- a tendency to distend already overinflated alveoli (Smetkin 2012);
- risks of ventilator-induced lung injury (Cressoni 2017), barotrauma, hypotension, ventilator asynchrony and discomfort (Meade et al. 2008);
- ineffectiveness once fibrosis has set in (Mols 2006).

The benefits of recruitment manoeuvres are thought to last no longer than an hour (Benfield et al. 2007), or seconds if not stabilized with sufficient PEEP (Mols 2006). The potential for recruitment is low if ARDS is caused by a lung condition but higher if it is secondary to MSF (Gattinoni 2002). If these open lung strategies are used, lung damage may be reduced by slow inspirations (Silva et al. 2012) or prone positioning so that ventral lung tissue is cocooned against high volume/pressure. The limited survival benefit of open lung strategies may relate to atelectrauma being less damaging than volutrauma (Wakabayashi 2014).

*Maintaining adequate post-recruitment manoeuvre levels of PEEP is crucial in avoiding cliff-edge re-collapse of alveoli.*

**Das et al. 2015**

## Physiotherapy

> **KEY POINT**
>
> Physiotherapy aims to maximize oxygen delivery while causing the least harm.

Gratuitous increase in stress and energy expenditure must be avoided because the linear association between $DO_2$ and $\dot{V}O_2$ indicates lack of reserve. Unnecessary tension may be reflected in abdominal muscle activity, which can increase lung injury (Zhang et al. 2016g). The main respiratory problem is reduced functioning lung volume. Sputum retention is less of a problem: excess upper airway secretions caused by intubation should be cleared, but the excess fluids caused by ARDS are not accessible. Waterlogged alveoli do not respond to physical intervention, and inflammatory biofluids lurking in the deeper airways are best left undisturbed in the early stages (Ntoumenopoulos et al. 2013).

## Positioning

*Prone should be applied as early as possible when oedema, lung recruitability, and absence of structural alterations of the lung are most represented.*

**Koulouras et al. 2016**

Dependent lung is congested, heavy and collapsed. Prone positioning acts as a form of recruitment manoeuvre by opening up dorsal lung regions. It improves survival so long as it is instigated early enough, i.e. within 48 h (Bein et al. 2016), and for long enough, e.g. 12–36 h sessions, with brief daily periods in supine for nursing care (Koulouras et al. 2016) and for the passive movements that cannot be done in prone. It should be the first option before more complex interventions are attempted (Harcombe 2004), not as a rescue manoeuvre or last-ditch effort (Koulouras et al. 2016).

The rationale relates to the geometric reconfiguration of the lungs inside the chest wall. There are more alveoli in the posterior chest, partly due to the heart taking up space anteriorly and partly due to the shape of the chest creating greater volume posteriorly. In prone, more lung units are therefore freed from the weight of the dense lungs, with the bonus of the heart being supported by the sternum (Fig. 22.21) and causing less parenchymal distortion, leading to greater lung homogeneity (Gattinoni et al. 2013).

Benefits are:

- ↑ $\dot{V}_A/\dot{Q}$ match and basal lung volume, (Kallet 2015);
- ↑ drainage of secretions, ↓ ventilator-associated pneumonia (Dirkes et al. 2012);
- more uniform distribution of positive pressure, leading to improved $SpO_2$, chest wall mechanics, haemodynamics and lung protection (Koulouras et al. 2016);
- ↑ survival (Scholten et al. 2017).

Oxygenation may be greater if pressure against the abdomen is minimized by using an air-fluidized bed, a Respicair bed or support for the chest and pelvis with pillows.

There are few patients who show no improvement (Koulouras et al. 2016) but lack of response can be identified by ultrasound (Prat et al. 2016) or electrical impedance tomography (Liu et al. 2016d) and may relate to variations in chest shape or redistribution of blood flow to more-diseased lung. Delay reduces success

Supine position                    Prone position

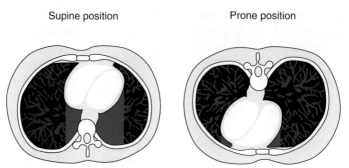

**FIGURE 22.21** Prone allows the heart to lay on the sternum so that its compressive force on dorsal lung regions is eliminated. (From Koulouras et al. 2016.)

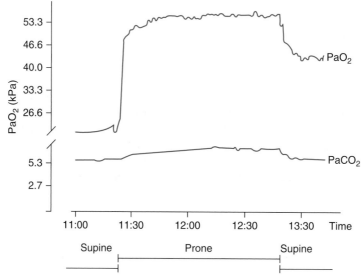

**FIGURE 22.22** Oxygenation over 3 h showing improvement during prone positioning. The dip during the turn reflects the effort of the manoeuvre. Some improvement is maintained on returning to supine, suggesting that recruitment of alveoli is sufficiently robust to partially withstand the mass of the lung that is now weighing down on it. (From Pappert et al. 1994.)

because fibrosis may set in. For patients who respond, saturation usually improves within 15 min, after an initial wobble (Fig. 22.22), but if it does not, patients should be left prone to allow them to respond, so long as there is no deterioration. Maximal oxygenation occurs after several hours to several days (Kallet 2015). For patients who do not respond, proning may or may not be beneficial if tried again later (Rowe 2004).

Contraindications are in Table 22.3. Proning has been used successfully, with care, following abdominal surgery (Gaudry et al. 2017), subarachnoid haemorrhage and with morbid obesity (Reinprecht et al. 2002).

Returning to supine may be required for various procedures, or overnight if a sufficiently skilled night staff is not available to return the patient rapidly to supine in case of cardiac arrest. During periods in supine, the physiotherapist can make a full assessment and maintain range of movement for all joints, including elbows, hips and shoulders, which can develop contractures if prone is prolonged.

Three to five staff members are required for the turn, including an intensivist or experienced nurse at the head of the bed to protect the airway and neck lines. A suggested procedure is described below.

**TABLE 22.3 Contraindications to proning**

| Absolute | Unmonitored intracranial hypertension |
| | Unstable spinal fractures |
| Relative | Increased intraocular pressure |
| | Difficult airway |
| | New tracheostomy |
| | Serious recent facial/chest/abdominal trauma |
| | Single anterior chest drain with air leak |
| | Massive haemoptysis |
| | Multiple trauma, unstable or pelvic fracture |
| | Kyphoscoliosis or advanced arthritis |
| | Seizures |
| | Ventricular assist device or intraaortic balloon pump |
| | Haemodynamic instability, recent cardiopulmonary arrest |
| | MAP <60 (Dirkes et al. 2012) |
| | Gestational ARDS (Schwaiberger et al. 2016) |

*ARDS*, Acute respiratory distress syndrome; *MAP*, mean arterial pressure.
Adapted from Koulouras et al. 2016.

1. Explain the procedure to the patient, with reassurance that they will be safe and turned towards the ventilator; obtain consent if they are able to communicate.
2. Ensure that mouth care, eye care and, if required, a chest X-ray have been done before the turn.
3. Stop enteral feed.
4. Close the eyes and protect with gel or a pad, with explanations to the patient.
5. Ensure reintubation equipment and staff are on hand.
6. Select direction of turn according to position of lines and ventilator.
7. Disconnect or plug lines as appropriate, redirect others in the axis of the body and track them during the turn.
8. Increase oxygen to 100%.
9. Suction, and prepare equipment for rapid suction after the turn.
10. Place the patient's palms against their thighs, thumbs upwards, elbows straight and shoulders neutral, ensuring protection of any arterial lines.
11. Place a clean sheet on top, wrap edges together with the underneath sheet to create a tight sandwich.
12. Slide the patient opposite to the direction of the turn, using the underneath sheet or glide sheet, according to hospital protocol.
13. Check that team members understand the vulnerability of the shoulders.
14. Roll patient into the lateral position using the underneath sheet.
15. Position two pillows on the bed, one for shoulder/chest support and the other for hip support, close enough to avoid lordosis. With a Respicair bed, deflate abdominal area.
16. Remove ECG leads, roll patient gingerly into prone while monitoring safety of lines and drains, relocate ECG leads to the back.
17. Suction.
18. Reconnect lines, remove eye cover if indicated.
19. Ensure that no joint is at end-range. Slight neck flexion can be facilitated by sliding the patient beyond the top of the bed and supporting their head on a cushioned table placed slightly below bed level. A pillow or horseshoe head support allows the tracheal tube to be unrestricted but secure.
20. Elevate the shoulder girdles slightly to ensure that the brachial plexus is not stretched.
21. Shoulder joints and neck should be near neutral. If the 'swimmers position' is used (Fig. 22.23), the elbow to which the head is semirotated should be flexed to no more than 90 degrees to avoid ulnar nerve stretch, and the other arm internally rotated by the side. If the neck is neutral and the head is on a cushioned table (No. 19, above) the arms can be either in the swimmers position or by the patient's side, shoulders internally rotated and palms upwards.
22. Ensure that women's breasts or men's genitals are not compressed, and that any lines or drains under the patient are padded.
23. Place two pillows under each shin to prevent peroneal nerve stretch, positioning them to avoid knee or toe pressure from the mattress.
24. Tilt the entire bed head-up 10 degrees (Ahota et al. 2014) and/or use a face-contoured device (Fig. 22.24) to prevent facial oedema or eye damage (O'Driscoll & White 2017). One case of blindness has been reported after 22 days in prone (Panchabhai et al. 2016).
25. Place gel cushions or silicone foam dressings on pressure areas, including between the tracheal tube

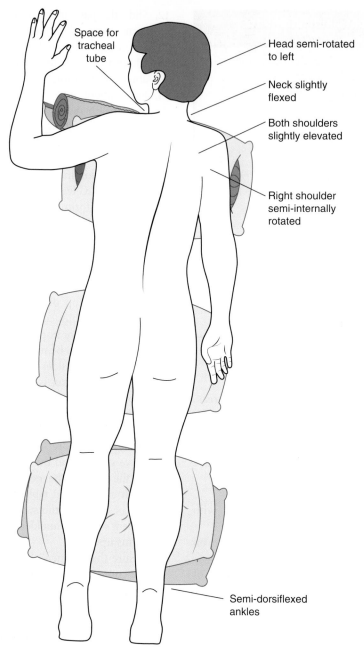

Space for
tracheal
tube

Head semi-rotated
to left

Neck slightly
flexed

Both shoulders
slightly elevated

Right shoulder
semi-internally
rotated

Semi-dorsiflexed
ankles

**FIGURE 22.23** Suggested position for a proned patient.

and skin to prevent injury (Fig. 22.25), reinstitute feed cautiously, return $FiO_2$ to original level once $SpO_2$ has settled, and liaise with intensivist to readjust PEEP (Beitler et al. 2015).

Head and arm positions are alternated 2-hourly. Pressure areas now include ears, cheeks, knees, toes, anterior superior iliac crests and any skin in contact with the tracheal tube. Potential cardiac arrest must be planned for and a protocol prepared for rapid return to supine.

Some clinicians find that placing 5 kg sandbags or a 5 L bag of fluid on the chest of a supine patient may have similar effects. It is thought that chest compression

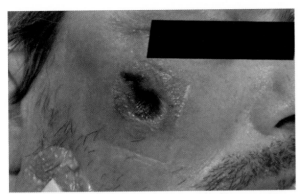

FIGURE 22.24 Pressure ulcer on the right cheek of a patient after 1 week of prone positioning using a commercially available endotracheal tube holder. (From Branson 2014.)

reduces the risk of barotrauma to nondependent lung regions while directing ventilation to dependent lung.

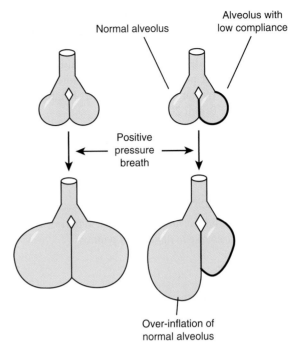

FIGURE 22.25 Effect of manual hyperinflation on *(left)* normal alveoli and *(right)* unevenly damaged alveoli. (From Cairo 2012.)

## MINI CLINICAL REASONING

*'Turning can be a frightening experience if the patient is not sedated adequately'.*

Dirkes et al. 2012

**Response**
Sedation may well be appropriate, but primarily the patient must be given explanations and talked through the procedure, otherwise sedation may leave the patient with a distorted and fearful memory.

## Hyperinflation

Manual hyperinflation is normally avoided, especially in the later stages, because barotrauma is a risk due to low lung compliance and heterogeneity of alveolar damage (Fig. 22.25). For ventilator hyperinflation, studies on recruitment manoeuvres are suspect if they do not check for complications such as immediate or delayed barotrauma, but the following benefits have been identified:

- 95% recruitment by means of PEEP at 35 cmH₂O above a driving pressure of 15 cmH₂O, followed by maintenance PEEP of 16 cmH₂O (Das et al. 2015);
- improved $PaO_2/FiO_2$ in half of subjects, by means of 2 min of 20 cmH₂O PEEP above driving pressure of 20 cmH₂O (Yun et al. 2016).

Computer simulations may assist in this delicate risk–benefit balancing act (Das et al. 2015).

## Manual techniques

ARDS itself is not a hypersecretory disease, but low tidal volume ventilation may increase sputum retention (Sharma et al. 2016) in which case manual techniques may be required.

## Suction

Damaged alveoli are vulnerable to derecruitment during suction, lung volume often falling to below functional residual capacity. Ventilator recruitment manoeuvres have been suggested after suction, such as pressure support at 40 cmH₂O (Maggiore 2003) or CPAP at 45 cmH₂O for 20 s (Dyhr 2002). However, these pressures could cause barotrauma, and many physiotherapists would prefer lower pressures, or simply ensure that closed-circuit catheters are used to avoid loss of PEEP, and FiO₂ increased until SpO₂ returns to normal.

## Rehabilitation

ICU-acquired weakness is ubiquitous and recovery may be incomplete 5 years after discharge, so rehabilitation should be continuous from admission to follow-up. Cognitive impairment has been found in 70%–100% of patients at discharge, 46%–80% at 1 year and 20% at 5 years (Herridge et al. 2016). One study found a 28% incidence of posttraumatic stress disorder, which was reduced by family support and rehabilitation (Chiumello & Brioni 2016).

An outcome measure that has been validated for ARDS survivors is the 4-metre gait speed test (Chan et al. 2016).

## CASE STUDY: MR AP

*Mr AP was admitted to the emergency department after inability to sleep due to abdominal pain.*

### Social history
- Unemployed
- 15 cigarettes/day
- 80 units alcohol/day

### On admission
- Distended tender abdomen
- ABG levels when self-ventilating on $FiO_2$ of 0.6: pH 7.26, $PaO_2$ 12.3 kPa, $PaCO_2$ 8.4 kPa, BE 1.5, $HCO_3^-$ 23.2
- ↑ White cell count
- Diagnosis: acute pancreatitis

### Medical treatment
- Nasogastric tube, analgesia, fluid resuscitation

### Progression
- $SpO_2$ deteriorated → intubation and ventilation → gradual increase in airway pressure
- Changed to pressure control → gradual reduction in tidal volume

### On examination
- ABG levels on IRV, $FiO_2$ of 0.85 and PEEP of 10: pH 7.20, $PaO_2$ 7.9 kPa, $PaCO_2$ 7.5 kPa, BE 1.0, $HCO_3^-$ 25.2
- Breath sounds absent bibasally

### Questions
1. What is causing the high airway pressure and then low tidal volume?
2. What is obliterating the breath sounds?
3. What syndrome is probably developing?
4. How is the ventilator set to enhance gas exchange?
5. How is the ventilator set to protect Mr P's lungs?
6. Problems?
7. Goals?
8. Plan?

*ABGs*, arterial blood gases; *BE*, base excess; *IRV*, inverse-ratio ventilation; *WCC*, white blood cell count.

### CLINICAL REASONING

*Comment on the rationale and evidence for 'chest physical therapy' in a group of mechanically ventilated patients:*

'The indications [for chest physical therapy] included … lung contusion.'
'Treatment times … averaged 67 min … [followed by increased] Qs/Qt in [50%] of the contusion patients.'
'The long-term clinical effect of these changes is unknown'.
**Crit Care Med** (1985) 13: 483–486

$Qs/Q_t$ = shunt fraction.

### Response to Case Study
1 & 2. Pressure against diaphragm from distended abdomen plus answer to question 3.
3. ARDS.
4. $FiO_2$ 0.6 then 0.85, IRV, high PEEP.
5. Pressure control ventilation, lung protection with permissive hypercapnia and PEEP maintaining open lungs.
6. Progressive compression atelectasis, with deteriorating gas exchange.
7. Reverse and prevent further atelectasis, rehabilitate.
8. Plan:
   - reverse Trendelenberg positioning (whole bed head-up)
   - if this does not improve gas exchange, prone after cutting hole in mattress for abdomen
   - hot water humidification
   - suction as required
   - musculoskeletal care

The prone position opened up the lung bases. Mr P survived and the experience motivated him to address his alcohol dependency.

## RESPONSE TO CLINICAL REASONING

Over an hour of postural drainage, percussion, vibration and suction is unlikely to be indicated for any condition, let alone lung contusion, i.e. bruising. Indeed, manual techniques are contraindicated with lung contusion because of the risk of further bleeding.

Blood in alveoli is not cleared by techniques aimed at airways.

Objectively this technique appeared damaging by increasing the shunt in half the patients with contusion.

Subjectively, one can only guess.

## RECOMMENDED READING

Athota, K.P., Millar, D., Branson, R.D., et al., 2014. A practical approach to the use of prone therapy in acute respiratory distress syndrome. Expert Rev. Respir. Med. 8 (4), 453–463.

Donnelly, J., 2016. Regulation of the cerebral circulation: bedside assessment and clinical implications. Crit. Care 20, 129.

Dunham, C.M., Hileman, B.M., Ransom, K.J., 2015. Trauma patient adverse outcomes are independently associated with rib cage fracture burden and severity of lung, head, and abdominal injuries. Int. J. Burns Trauma 5 (1), 46–55.

Giannoni-Pastor, A., 2016. Prevalence and predictors of posttraumatic stress symptomatology among burn survivors. J. Burn Care Res. 37 (1), e79–e89.

Girotra, S., Chan, P.S., Bradley, S.M., 2015. Post-resuscitation care following out-of-hospital and in-hospital cardiac arrest. Heart 101 (24), 1943–1949. doi:10.1136/heartjnl-2015-307450.

Go, L., Budinger, G.R., Kwasny, M.J., et al., 2016. Failure to improve the oxygenation index is a useful predictor of therapy failure in acute respiratory distress syndrome clinical trials. Crit. Care Med. 44 (1), e40–e44.

Goodwin, M., Ito, K., Gupta, A.H., et al., 2016. Protocolized care for early shock resuscitation. Curr. Opin. Crit. Care 22 (5), 416–423.

Hannawi, Y., Abers, M., Geocadin, R., et al., 2016. Abnormal movements in critical care patients with brain injury. Crit. Care 20, 60.

Horie, S., Masterson, C., Devaney, J., et al., 2016. Stem cell therapy for acute respiratory distress syndrome: a promising future? Curr. Opin. Crit. Care 22 (1), 14–20.

Jain, U., McCunn, M., Smith, C.E., et al., 2016. Management of the traumatized airway. Anesthesiology 124 (1), 199–206.

Kaml, G.J., Davis, K.A., 2016. Surgical critical care for the patient with sepsis and multiple organ dysfunction. Anesthesiol. Clin. 34 (4), 681–696.

Kangelaris, K.N., Ware, L.B., Wang, C.Y., et al., 2016. Timing of intubation and clinical outcomes in adults with acute respiratory distress syndrome. Crit. Care Med. 44 (1), 120–129.

Kaur, R., Prabhakar, A., Kochhar, S., et al., 2015. Blunt traumatic diaphragmatic hernia: Pictorial review of CT signs. Indian J. Radiol. Imaging 25 (3), 226–232.

Kellum, J.A., Bellomo, R., Ronco, C., 2016. Does this patient have acute kidney injury? Intensive Care Med. 42 (1), 96–99.

Khademi, S., Frye, M.A., Jeckel, K.M., et al., 2017. Hypoxia mediated pulmonary edema: potential influence of oxidative stress, sympathetic activation and cerebral blood flow. BMC Physiol. 15, 4.

Kim, R.S., Mullins, K., 2016. Preventing facial pressure ulcers in acute respiratory distress syndrome (ARDS). J. Wound Ostomy Continence Nurs. 43 (4), 427–429.

Klouwenberg, P.M.C.K., 2017. Incidence, predictors, and outcomes of new-onset atrial fibrillation in critically ill patients with sepsis. Am. J. Respir. Crit. Care Med. 195 (2), 205–211.

Leatherman, J., 2015. Mechanical ventilation for severe asthma. Chest 147 (6), 1671–1680. doi:10.1378/chest.14-1733.

Lelubre, C., Bouzat, P., Crippa, I.A., 2016. Anemia management after acute brain injury. Crit. Care 20, 152.

Li, X., Chen, C., Yang, X., et al., 2017. Acupuncture improved neurological recovery after traumatic brain injury by activating BDNF/TrkB pathway. Evid. Based Complement. Alternat. Med. 2017, 8460145.

Lipinska-Gediga, M., 2016. Sepsis and septic shock-is a microcirculation a main player? Anaesthesiol. Intensive Ther. 48 (4), 261–265.

Montanaro, N., 2016. Sepsis resuscitation: consensus and controversies. Crit. Care Nurs. Q. 39 (1), 58–63.

NICE, 2016. Sepsis: recognition, diagnosis and early management [NG51].

Reith, F.C.M., Van den Brande, R., Synnot, A., et al., 2016. The reliability of the Glasgow Coma Scale: a systematic review. Intensive Care Med. 42 (1), 3–15.

Rezende-Neto, J.B., 2013. Abdominal catastrophes in the intensive care unit setting. Crit. Care Clin. 29 (4), 1017–1044.

Rittenberger, J.C., 2015. Postcardiac arrest management. Emerg. Med. Clin. North Am. 33 (3), 691–712. doi:10.1016/j.emc.2015.04.011.

Shankar-Hari, M., Bertolini, G., Brunkhorst, F., et al., 2015. Judging quality of current septic shock definitions and criteria. Crit. Care 19, 445.

Simon, M., Braune, S., Lagmani, A., et al., 2016. Value of computed tomography of the chest in subjects with ARDS. Respir. Care 61 (3), 316–323.

Sottile, P.D., Nordon-Craft, A., Malone, D., et al., 2015. Physical therapist treatment of patients in the neurological intensive care unit. Phys. Ther. 95 (7), 1006–1014.

Spaite, D.W., Hu, C., Bobrow, H.J., 2017. The effect of combined out-of-hospital hypotension and hypoxia on mortality in major traumatic brain injury. Ann. Emerg. Med. 69 (1), 62–72.

Walker, P., Buehner, M., Wood, L., et al., 2015. Diagnosis and management of inhalation injury: an updated review. Crit. Care 19, 351.

Whyte, J., 2013. Disorders of consciousness. Arch. Phys. Med. Rehabil. 94 (10), 1851–1854.

Xu, X.D., Wang, Z.Y., Zhang, L.Y., et al., 2015. Acute pancreatitis classifications: basis and key goals. Medicine (Baltimore) 94 (48), e2182.

Zanata, I.L., Santos, R.S., Hirata, G.C., 2014. Tracheal decannulation protocol in patients affected by traumatic brain injury. Int. Arch. Otorhinolaryngol. 18 (2), 108–114.

# Evaluation of Cardiorespiratory Physiotherapy

## LEARNING OBJECTIVES

*On completion of this chapter the reader should be able to:*
- summarize the concepts behind outcomes, standards and cardiorespiratory audit;
- critically analyse the literature to identify valid research;
- supervise students and junior staff to ensure that they work effectively as part of the multidisciplinary team;
- apply evidence-based physiotherapy and clinical reasoning in the management of cardiorespiratory patients.

## INTRODUCTION

*Practice should not be based on tradition but on proven benefit and safety.*

***Cabello et al. 2013***

If a patient who is having physiotherapy gets better, is this due to the physiotherapy, the physiotherapist, the placebo effect or divine intervention? The credibility of cardiorespiratory physiotherapy is being challenged (Rubin et al. 2012), which is to be welcomed.

An evidence-based approach is facilitated by clinical reasoning, using the hierarchy of evidence on p. 180, but its components can be hampered by several factors:

1. Research is scarce and ambiguous, 'chest physiotherapy' is poorly defined, and variables such as simultaneous medical input can skew results.
2. There is evidence that:
   - one-third of patients adhere to therapy
   - one-third reject it outright
   - one-third accept it but get it wrong (Lloyd 1998).
3. There is lack of recognition of the need for physiotherapists to have time for reflection, which leads to frustration and a lower standard of care, according to Toft (2000), who goes on to quote Huxley: 'fear casts out intelligence, casts out goodness … in the end fear casts out even a man's humanity'. This could

be one explanation for the lack of humanity that we sometimes see when time seems ever shorter and fear of not keeping to targets can detach health staff from the reason that they chose to work in the health system.

Clinical reasoning incorporates the ability to:

*   access an organized knowledge base related to clinical problems
*   generate and test hypotheses
*   evaluate and use clinical data
*   use reflection to self-evaluate
*   generate knowledge from the reasoning process (Christensen et al. 2008)

Communicating this knowledge involves the multidisciplinary team and the patient.

> **KEY POINT**
>
> *The goal of clinical reasoning is wise action.*
> Jones et al. 2008

This chapter uses clinical reasoning to identify how critical evaluation of the research can inform practice, how continuous audit helps ensure that this is acted on, and how education can be used so that evaluation of cardiorespiratory physiotherapy does not become a luxury to be tagged on at the end if there is time.

> *Clinical expertise is reflected in the more thoughtful identification and compassionate use of individual patients' predicaments, rights, and preferences.*
> ***Gray et al. 1996***

## DEFINITIONS

> *Only about 15% of all contemporary clinical interventions are supported by objective scientific evidence that they do more good than harm.*
> ***White 1988***

**Benchmark** is an agreed criterion by which a practice can be judged.

**Clinical governance** is a framework to improve patient care using evidence-based guidelines. It includes audit, accountability and patient satisfaction (DoH 2011b).

**Clinical pathways** are locally developed, consensus-driven, evidence-based multidisciplinary steps that incorporate national guidelines into the care of patients with a specific clinical problem to increase efficiency and timeliness (Rotter et al. 2010).

**Clinical practice guidelines** are systematically developed recommendations on the effective management of different conditions or problems. They are consensus-driven, but accuracy may be elusive if 'various professional organizations fight over the same meta-analyses and come to different conclusions' (Stern 2013).

**Consensus statements** are syntheses of research with implications for re-evaluation of practice.

**Criteria** identify what should happen for a standard to be achieved.

**Evidence-based practice (EBP)** involves clinical decision-making based on the systematic search for, appraisal of and use of current evidence. Where there is lack of objective evidence, clinical expertise is used, but as a tool to be nurtured mindfully, not used as anecdotal justification.

**Guidelines** are sets of recommendations that identify management strategies based on the evidence, e.g. BTS/ACPRC (2009). They require references, explanation of reasoning and grading of both recommendations and quality of the evidence. For patients with multimorbidity, guidelines may drive polypharmacy (Hughes et al. 2013).

**Outcome measures** are subjective or objective changes due to physiotherapy input. They must be appropriate, reliable, valid and responsive.

**Peer review** is a review of the work of an individual by those who are equal in grade and speciality.

**Protocols** are precise instructions for a specific clinical problem, developed from a guideline. They are stricter, more explicit and usually shorter than guidelines.

**Standards**: see p. 559.

## RESEARCH

> *Some of the knowledge that we hold dear today will become the mythology of tomorrow.*
> ***Rubin 2015***

The above may or may not be ironic, but Kerry et al. (2012) claim that the majority of clinical reviews in rehabilitation medicine are not actually true. Other hurdles are:

- the lag between evidence and change in practice, usually due to lack of time and training, e.g. Lin and Murphy (2010) found an example of a 17-year gap between research and action;
- publication bias, which favours trials with positive results (Costa et al. 2013) while negative results, if they do get published, emerge more slowly;
- mechanistic reasoning, which led one researcher to discover that more patients had died as a result of anti-arrhythmic drugs than died throughout the Vietnam war, because normalizing the electrocardiogram was used as a surrogate endpoint in the research (Howick et al. 2010).

On the positive side, Hurley et al. (2012) identified ClinicalTrials.gov as a database of ongoing clinical trials to help bridge the gap, and Gehanno et al. (2013) acknowledged PubMed and Google Scholar as adequate general databases. Cochrane is useful but can be depressing with its usual conclusion '…there is insufficient evidence' for a physiotherapy technique. This is because many cardiorespiratory techniques have not been subject to the purifying heat of randomized controlled trials.

The paucity of research should not hinder the identification of other components of evidence-based practice (EBP). Stolper et al. (2009) state that results should be tempered by the richness and variety of different patients' needs and that even intuition can be included. Condon et al. (2016) said that 'A positive impact of EBP on patient outcomes is lacking … the use of professional networks may offer a better means to identify knowledge gaps and translate acquired knowledge into practice'.

'Bundles' of care have improved the management of patients with complex cardiorespiratory problems, but they have complicated the search for the active ingredient (Wakefield et al. 2013), and the physiotherapy component may sink from view.

The placebo effect is a constant presence in physiotherapy and cannot be ignored. Indeed it has been described as 'arguably more powerful than any physiotherapy technique has been' (Stack 2006). This can be harnessed, but selectively and honestly, and not as a substitute for research. The placebo effect in animal research suggests that its main driver is the relationship with the health professional (Haselen 2013). The more experienced the physiotherapist, the more the relationship with the patient is understood as the bedrock of effective treatment.

## LITERATURE APPRAISAL

*Why do kamikaze pilots wear helmets?*

A questioning and indeed a suspicious mind is necessary when reading the literature because research can prove or disprove almost anything and may be published in the most prestigious journals.

An assessment tool is available to reduce the risk of investigator bias (Farmer et al. 2012), which tends to occur in favour of sponsors who fund studies (Rubin & Haynes 2012), especially as disclosures are considered 'very rare' (Bindslev et al. 2013). Government guidelines are often funded by drug companies (Enright 2014), and in asthma research, 95% of studies report pharmaceutical involvement (Bond et al. 2012). In the US, pharmaceutical companies have had to pay billions in fines to settle investigations into fraudulent practice related to research (Braillon et al. 2012).

Beware of literature that contains:

- limited sample sizes, which lean towards reporting greater benefits (Zhang et al. 2013);
- extrapolation of results from healthy young volunteers, e.g. dynamic hyperinflation simulated by using continuous positive airway pressure (CPAP) with normal subjects;
- extrapolation of results from animals; dogs, for example, have a different chest shape and their pleural space communicates bilaterally;
- assessment of more than one technique in one study;
- ambiguous definitions; 'conventional chest physiotherapy', or even 'chest physiotherapy' traditionally refers to postural drainage and/or manual techniques, but (a) these techniques have not been conventional for some decades in the UK and (b) these techniques are often lumped together;
- lack of distinction between correlation and causation;
- interpretation without consideration of alternative explanations;
- uncontrolled variables;
- physiotherapists used as handmaidens to collect data rather than as designers of the study;
- extrapolation of results from medical research, e.g. the manual ventilation used by anaesthetists is not the same as the manual hyperinflation used by physiotherapists;
- lack of precision, e.g. 'chest physiotherapy was of no value', instead of the cumbersome but more accurate

'postural drainage with percussion in this way for this amount of time with these patients showed no evidence of faster mucociliary clearance/greater quantity of sputum/reduced airflow resistance/ improved quality of life';

- physiological illiteracy, e.g. one study attempted to evaluate respiratory muscle activity during 'unilateral' chest expansion, but did not distinguish inspiratory and expiratory muscles and used 'subjective observation' to judge the notoriously ambiguous 'unilateral' chest expansion (Ng & Stokes 1992);
- wasted time due to the conclusion being obvious from the start, e.g. a study described by Decramer (2009) concluded that inspiratory muscle training gave better results in patients with inspiratory muscle weakness than those without inspiratory muscle weakness;
- procedures carried out by different clinicians who would inevitably have varied levels of skill, as warned against by McSwain et al. (2015);
- procedures that do not describe, or even mention, the complications of a technique, e.g. recruitment manoeuvres (p. 493), or subjects with bronchiectasis, who are already at high risk of fatigue and stress incontinence, being asked to cough continuously for 20 min (Ramos et al. 2015).

## Examples

*Example 1.* From Bach et al. (2015):
'Insufflation and exsufflation pressures of 60–70 cmH$_2$O were used via the [tracheal] tubes ... we observed no clinically apparent barotrauma.'

- Response: the only form of barotrauma that is (sometimes) clinically apparent is subcutaneous emphysema. Others are only radiologically apparent.

*Example 2.* From Aquino et al. (2012):
Title: 'CPAP has no effect on clearance, sputum properties, or expectorated volume in cystic fibrosis.'

- Response: CPAP is not aimed at chest clearance.

*Example 3.* From José and Dal Corso (2016):
1. For patients with pneumonia, 'improvement in functional outcomes after an inpatient rehabilitation program was greater than the improvement after standard respiratory physiotherapy', the latter being manual techniques, diaphragmatic breathing, deep breathing and 10 min walking.
   - Response: comparing a technique aimed at improving functional capacity is likely to improve

functional capacity more than a technique aimed at clearing secretions.
2. The study also stated 'there is no evidence to support the routine use of standard respiratory physiotherapy in patients who are hospitalized for community-acquired pneumonia'.
   - Response: physiotherapy techniques should not be used routinely.

And there was no information on whether the patients had secretions.

*Example 4.* Weissman et al. (1984) did not define chest physical therapy in a paper associating it with major haemodynamic and metabolic stress.

*Example 5.* Leech et al. (2015) decided to do positioning and nasopharyngeal suction on a patient with 'complete opacification of the left hemithorax on chest X-ray'.

- Question 1 – can you see secretions on X-ray?
- Question 2 – would you do nasopharyngeal suction without any other technique to mobilize the secretions first, apart from positioning?
- Answer 1 – no, except in neglected bronchiectasis, in which case they do not appear as 'complete opacification'.
- Answer 2 – no!

The unfortunate patient actually had a pleural effusion, which would be suspected with opacification and could be confirmed with a percussion note.

*Example 6.* From Cross et al. (2012b):
1. The authors evaluated whether percussion, vibrations and shaking during an exacerbation of chronic obstructive pulmonary disease affected quality of life 6 months later.
   - Manual techniques are unlikely to affect quality of life 6 months later; immediate subjective and objective measures, and length of stay, might be more logical endpoints.
2. The background stated that 'although airway clearance techniques may improve sputum expectoration, there is no high quality evidence of either short- or long-term value'.
   - The study is investigating manual techniques, not airway clearance techniques.
   - See Chapter 7 for evidence.
3. 'The protocol included the active cycle of breathing technique.'
   - This is not 'percussion, vibration, and shaking'.
4. The procedure combined active cycle of breathing techniques with manual techniques.

- Active cycle of breath techniques cannot be done accurately at the same time as receiving manual techniques.
5. Sputum volume was collected to measure outcome.
   - This does not control for swallowing or saliva.
6. 'The results … do not lend support to the routine use of [manual techniques].'
   - Routine…?
7. Adverse events included increased shortness of breath, bronchospasm, arrhythmias, pain and thoracic haematoma.
   - Either some patients were unsuited to this technique or the technique was unsuitable (haematoma…?!)
   - Forty-one percent of patients (who were hospitalized with acute COPD) suffered oxygen desaturation, but this was not classed as an adverse event.

***Example 7.*** Torrington et al. (1984) imposed 4-hourly intermittent positive pressure breathing, 4-hourly incentive spirometry, 2-hourly deep breathing and 2-hourly nebulization on their hapless postoperative patients. The authors expressed surprise that additional 4-hourly postural drainage and percussion increased cost, discomfort and fever in one (presumably exhausted) group of patients, and without reducing atelectasis.

Worse, the study has been much quoted to claim that postoperative physiotherapy is ineffective.

On the positive side, the British Thoracic Society guideline on acute oxygen therapy is about as good as it gets (BTS 2017).

*All who drink of this remedy recover in a short time, except those whom it does not help, who all die. Therefore it is obvious that it fails only in incurable cases.*

**Galen, 2nd century**

## STANDARDS

*The perception is, if chest physiotherapy doesn't help, it won't hurt.*

**Eid 1991**

The above is, hopefully, tongue in cheek, but the concept still hovers over the profession. Evaluation of cardiorespiratory physiotherapy therefore needs standards against which outcomes are measured. Standards define the expected level of performance and must be

> ### BOX 23.1 Standards of Mobility for All Inpatients
>
> 1. All patients mobilize daily, independently or with assistance, unless:
>    - it is unsafe, e.g. haemodynamic or orthopaedic instability;
>    - it is impossible, e.g. coma.
> 2. For patients who do not mobilize, the reason and action taken are documented, e.g. pain, contraindication, patient unwilling, staff shortage.
> 3. The daily exercise programme is documented:
>    - in the patient notes, if given verbally to the patient, or
>    - as a handout for the patient, copied in the notes.
> 4. Documentation demonstrates progress, or reason for lack of progress.

measurable, understandable, desirable and achievable. They are usually subject to staffing levels. Standards are only useful if audited and if audit leads to change in practice. Box 23.1 gives an example for mobility.

Other standards could include identification of which surgical patients are assessed, time between referral and assessment for acute and nonacute medical patients, agreement with patients of goals and plans, explanation to patients about limitations and risks of treatment, provision for patient self-management and liaison with the multidisciplinary team.

## OUTCOMES

*The most important outcomes in clinical trials are patient-centred outcomes.*

**Alifano et al. 2010**

Economic austerity renders areas of physiotherapy vulnerable to closure unless outcome is documented (Duncan & Murray 2012). Outcome measures also motivate patients by providing tangible proof of their progress even if it is slow.

Both subjective and objective measures should show, when possible:
- how effective one outcome measure is compared with others (validity)
- the extent to which they yield repeatable results on the same person over time (reliability)

- how well they detect a change in an individual (responsiveness)

Unlike research, outcomes can include the complete package of treatment as well as individual components. Herbert et al. (2005) provide a thoughtful perspective on outcomes.

## Subjective Measurement

The patient experience is positively associated with clinical effectiveness and patient safety (Doyle 2013) and is included in quality of life scales and questionnaires.

## Objective Measurement

Obstacles to measuring cardiorespiratory outcomes include:

- arterial oxygen saturation ($SpO_2$) and other measurements varying with factors other than physiotherapy
- quality not equating with the number and length of treatments
- postoperative atelectasis sometimes being self-limiting
- mouthpieces interfering with measurement
- cardiorespiratory disease often complicated by multipathology

Some outcome measures are suitable if taken in the context of the full clinical picture:

- ↑ oxygenation: e.g. $SpO_2$
- ↑ oxygen delivery: e.g. mixed venous saturation
- ↑ ventilation: ↓ $PaCO_2$
- in the case of hyperventilation syndrome: ↓ minute ventilation, as reflected by ↑ $PaCO_2$
- increase or maintenance of exercise tolerance
- ↑ independence e.g. with activities of daily living
- increase or maintenance of lung volume (p. 195)
- clearance of secretions (p. 224)
- ↓ work of breathing (p. 244)
- lack of deterioration

Measurements currently used for research may become bedside outcome measures in the future, e.g. vibration energy computed before and after treatment to monitor secretion clearance (Fig. 23.1).

Data collection requires training, administrative support and time. It is best that the choice of outcome measures is not organizationally imposed (Duncan & Murray 2012).

On-call criteria (Appendix A, Chapter 21) provide guidance for on-call staff, an indication of the adequacy

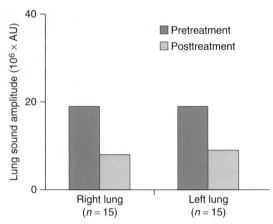

**FIGURE 23.1** Reduced vibration energy after secretion clearance in the right and left lungs of 15 mechanically ventilated patients. (From Ntoumenopoulos & Glickman 2012.)

of training and a means of monitoring the appropriateness of the call. Lack of improvement in the patient does not necessarily mean an inappropriate call-out.

## Successes Folder

To help compensate for the dearth of research, it is wise to build up a record of objective markers of success, e.g. before-and-after auscultation, $SpO_2$ or X-rays (Fig. 23.2). This is a crude measure which does not reflect the effects of education and prevention on a patient's quality of life, but is useful for continuing professional development, comes in handy if challenged by budget holders and helps towards outcomes becoming embedded in practice.

## COST EFFECTIVENESS

*Do no harm – cheaply.*

***Hughes 1980***

Efficiency is allied to effectiveness because time is freed up for other input. Measures to save time include:

- avoiding treatment that is not evidence-based;
- virtual journal clubs (Chetlen et al. 2017);
- assistants supported and valued;
- for inpatients: handouts to reinforce education, mobility tick charts to involve nursing staff with

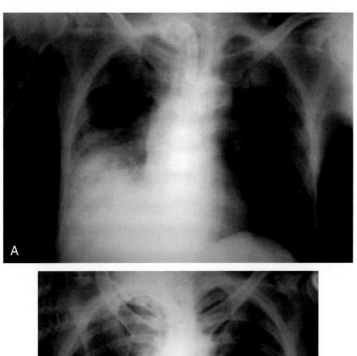

**FIGURE 23.2** Before (A) and after (B) physiotherapy for a tracheostomied patient showing clearance of right lower lobe atelectasis.

| BOX 23.2 | **Referrals for Physiotherapy** | | | |
|---|---|---|---|---|
| **Week:** _____ | **Ward:** _____ | **Physiotherapist:** _____ | | **Bleep:** _____ |
| Date: | Name of patient: | Referrer (print name and designation): | Physiotherapy problem for which assessment is requested: | |
| | | | | |

Suzanne Roberts, Whittington Hospital, London.

rehabilitation, and a written weekly referral sheet to assist the ward report, pinned up in a confidential area at the nurses' station, to be filled out by referring staff and checked daily by the physiotherapist (e.g. Box 23.2);

- for outpatients: information sent out before the first appointment, follow-up phone calls for motivation and support when face-to-face contact is not essential;
- for ICU patients, early rehabilitation, which in one hospital trust cut almost 8 days from the

average length of stay and saved over £2 million (Frontline 2014);

- information for nursing and medical staff about appropriate referrals, by problem or condition (Appendix A).

Extended scope physiotherapists improve efficiency by training in skills such as taking arterial or capillary blood gases, supervising weaning, heading up ICU outreach or tracheostomy teams and sometimes performing bronchoscopies or minitracheostomies, thus being able to progress treatment without waiting for medical input. Physiotherapists do not improve efficiency by learning techniques which do not save physiotherapy time or improve effectiveness.

It is cost-effective to spend time individualizing pre-written daily exercise programmes if this motivates the patient. It is cost-effective to reduce a patient's need for medication. It is cost-effective to increase a patient's independence and reduce their need for other services.

An on-call service is cost effective if it prevents deterioration or avoids the need for more time-consuming interventions. It is not cost effective if nonrespiratory physiotherapists have not developed the competencies to deal with critically ill patients.

The credibility of respiratory physiotherapy has been clearly extolled: 'We cannot claim to offer 24-h care for patients while working only eight of them' (Nicholls 1996).

Short-termism must not intrude on cost effectiveness. Prevention and rehabilitation are central to efficient respiratory care.

*If you go for cost, you will lose quality.*
*If you go for quality, you will save money.*

                                              ***Taylor & Odell 2011***

## THE AUDIT CYCLE

*People do not resist change. They resist being changed.*

                                              ***Lloyd 1998***

Research and patient feedback tell us the right thing to do. Audit tells us if we are doing the right thing right. It entails clinically-led peer review, which systematically analyses practice and outcome against agreed standards, then modifies practice where indicated.

Protected time, simple topics and minimal documentation are advised. Liaison with the clinical audit department is a useful first step. The topic chosen should have the potential for improvement and be responsive to physiotherapy, e.g.:

- percentage of problems resolved
- percentage of referrals or call-outs considered appropriate
- percentage of medical patients receiving discharge advice
- percentage of surgical patients discharged with preoperative function

An audit process can also be used as part of clinical education (Ivers et al. 2012). If the full audit cycle (Fig. 23.3) is not completed, the exercise is wasted.

Box 23.3 is an example of a biannual audit to monitor the efficacy of postoperative physiotherapy.

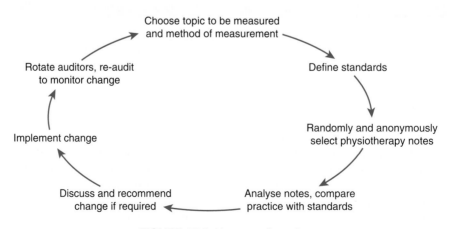

**FIGURE 23.3** Notes audit cycle.

## BOX 23.3    Postoperative Audit

| | |
|---|---|
| **Standard** | Patients will be able to climb one flight of stairs on their third postoperative day. |
| **Patients** | Patients admitted for open surgery in March and September who were able to climb one flight of stairs preoperatively. |
| **Method** | Stairs assessment on third postoperative day. |
| **Audit meeting** | Assess notes, identify cause of any shortfall, recommend change, and agree who is to be next auditor and date of the next meeting to monitor change. |

## BOX 23.4    Inpatient Delayed Discharges

**Patient label:**          **Ward:**

Date due for discharge:

Cause(s) of delayed discharge:    Social services/home circumstances ☐
If yes, details:

Staff shortage ☐
If yes, which discipline:

Other ☐
If yes, details:

Date discharged:

If it is felt that staff shortage is slowing patient discharges, this could be audited in association with the hospital discharge officer. Box 23.4 shows a method of collecting information for a delayed discharge audit.

We are the most available and abiding judges of our own work, e.g.:

- Am I allowing myself to get swamped with acute cardiorespiratory work and not tackling prevention or rehabilitation?
- Do I favour patients who are appreciative and cooperative rather than those who are demanding or depressed?
- Have I achieved the appropriate balance between patients' needs and my professional development?
- How do I handle my mistakes?

*There's nothing quite as frightening as someone who knows they are right.*

**Michael Faraday, 19th Century**

# EDUCATION AND CONTINUING EDUCATION

*Why is evidence … so hard to transform into daily routines?*

**Flaatten 2012**

## Needs of Students and Junior Staff

It is the human qualities of supervisors that are often considered equal to, or more important than, clinical skills (Neville & French 1991), e.g.:

- enthusiasm, honesty and commitment;
- respect for juniors and students so that they in turn respect their patients;
- tolerance of a range of normality;
- avoidance of labelling patients as difficult;
- constructive relationships with medical and other staff;
- willingness to say 'I don't know';
- ability to coax the nervous patient, soothe the fearful and encourage the weary.

Clinical placements play a major role in fostering motivation (Brindley 2013), and our finest clinicians should analyse their intuitive process so that they can pass on how they recognize subtle changes in a breathing pattern, sense a patient's motivation or adjust their treatment in response to barely perceptible clues.

Junior staff and students also need:

- clarification of expectations;
- assistance in setting feasible objectives and assessing whether these are met;
- encouragement to work creatively and not become a clone of their senior;
- regular feedback, case discussions and troubleshooting, while aiming at a balance of guidance and responsibility;
- praise when due;
- enjoyment in their work;
- correction in a way that does not undermine confidence, especially in front of patients;
- for junior staff and senior students, consultation on how closely they want to be supervised;
- for staff after their first on-calls, debriefing to encourage reflective practice;
- for students, reinforcement of the curriculum emphasis on involvement of carers, expansion of community care and patient self-management (Roskell 2012);

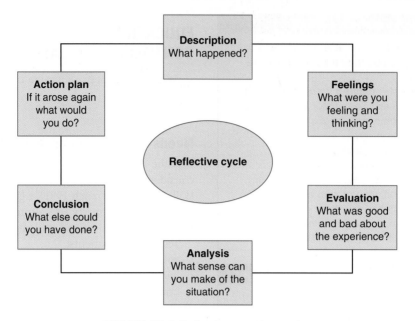

**FIGURE 23.4** Reflective practice cycle.

- when possible, a simulated critical care experience, which can increase students' confidence and interest in the specialty (Ohtake et al. 2013);
- encouragement to learn from patients, e.g. Appendix D, or structured feedback sessions with patients (Thomson & Hilton 2013);
- when available, a mentor who is not their manager or supervisor;
- guided journal writing (Constantinou & Kuys 2013);
- time for reflection, using Fig. 23.4 or social media (Rowe 2012);
- an information folder (Appendix A).

Imaginative ways of increasing confidence have been developed, e.g. interactive case-based educational sessions for clinical decision-making in ICU rehabilitation (Toonstra et al. 2016), suction task training systems (Khan et al. 2015) and case-based learning (Bennal et al. 2016).

When asking a patient's permission for a student to be present, the student should be outside so that the patient feels free to refuse. Permission should also be sought for the student to read the medical notes (Wilkie 1997), and the patient advised, when appropriate, of the student's gender.

Patients often appreciate the extra time that students have to spend with them. As one supervisor said: 'It seems to me the patients really enjoy the interaction of having students around' (Davies et al. 2011).

For qualified staff, a questionnaire is available to measure EBP (Bernhardsson & Larsson 2013). UK physiotherapists are granted 6 days a year minimum for education, on top of mandatory training (Dimond 2009, p. 58).

> **PRACTICE TIP**
>
> Students can draw the lung and heart surface markings on a T-shirt as an aid to learning.

Clinical practice on its own does not necessarily develop empathy (Thomson et al. 1997), which needs to be facilitated rather than blunted by the casual insensitivities of the health system. For example, if there has been a ward round in which a patient's needs have been ignored, debriefing is required for the student afterwards. Supervisors should maintain awareness lest students feel obliged to conform to what may be 'normal' but is not acceptable. Box 23.5 is the experience of a student who would have benefitted from a debrief.

## Competencies for On-Calls and Weekends

The attributes required for competent practice have been itemized by Thomas et al. (2008):

*'The patient was looking beautiful. He'd been washed and his hair was combed. He looked a bit stony-faced, eyes gazing across the room. He's better today, I thought. I put my hands round his chest. "Just take a nice deep breath," I said. I chatted away to him. I kept waiting for his next breath. "You're looking well," I said. He still hadn't taken a breath. Unease grew. I finished a long sentence. My hands were glued to his chest. My eyes were glued to his eyes. Physios don't see dead patients do they? But I couldn't keep up the charade. Had I killed him? I backed away. I forgot everything except thinking "I must leave the ward". I found my supervisor and said "I went to see Mr Jones but he was dead". She said "Oh fine". I couldn't tell anyone about it for a year.'*

AI 1990

- practical assessment and treatment skills;
- cognitive skills: theory, application of knowledge, interpretation of findings and reasoning;
- attitude: empathy, professionalism and ethical awareness;
- independent learning skills: learning methods, reflection, awareness of limitations;
- critical thinking;
- communication skills: verbal and written, including record keeping.

Staff numbers may allow weekend teams to contain a mix of experienced and inexperienced staff, but evidence-based protocols have been used successfully by nonspecialist physiotherapists working in the ICU (Hanekom et al. 2013). A no-blame culture allows errors to be reported and reflected upon (Kiekkas 2011).

## Clinical Reasoning – Learnt or Taught?

*To prepare students for clinical practice, education should foster ethical wisdom and emotional curiosity.*

***Jensen & Greenfield 2012***

Clinical reasoning refers to the thinking and decision-making processes associated with clinical practice. This can be learnt by examining different clinical reasoning models, exploring the differences in reasoning between novices and experts, and discussion with peers. For students, a case study may be discussed or role-played,

followed by questions on clinical reasoning by educators and their peers.

Continuing education lays the foundation for life-long self-evaluation. It also provides the opportunity for supervisors to show that compassion is fundamental for effective cardiorespiratory care, not just an old-fashioned unscientific luxury.

*When educators are humanistic in their training of students, the students become more humanistic in their care of patients.*

***Williams & Deci 1998***

## CASE STUDY: MR FF

*What has happened to this 33-year-old man who was admitted after eating a spicy Mexican meal?*

### History of present complaint

Vomiting → back pain → collapse

### Subjective

Breathless

### Phase 1 questions (Fig. 23.5A)

1. Auscultation?
2. Percussion note?

**CLINICAL REASONING**

*How helpful is this study which reported, in an uncontrolled trial, that people with an exacerbation of cystic fibrosis benefitted from 'rest, intravenous antibiotics, physical therapy, high-calorie diet and regular medical review'?*

*Phys Ther* (1994) 74: 583–593

### Response to Case Study Phase 1

1. Auscultation: breath sounds ↓ on the left.
2. Percussion note: hyperresonant left upper zone, stony dull left lower zone.

### What happened

Vomiting → ruptured oesophagus → empyema → development of gas-forming organism → pneumothorax.

### Management and progress

- Chest tube drained air and foul-smelling liquid from pleura.

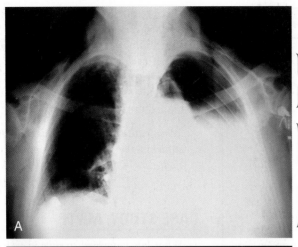

Blackness indicates air.
Lack of lung
markings
indicates that the
air is in the pleura,
not the lung

Density of opacity,
and lack of its
location to a lobe,
suggests pleural
rather than lung
pathology

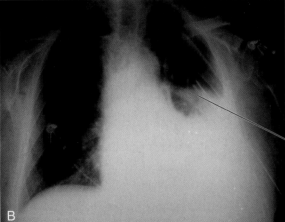

Lung markings
now present,
indicating
some lung
expansion

Chest drain

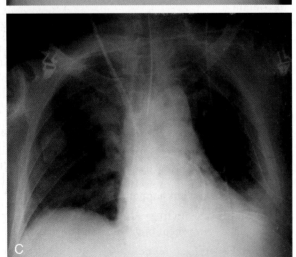

Lung
mostly
expanded

**FIGURE 23.5** Mr FF. (Courtesy Claude Pierre-Jerome.)

- Fig. 23.5B shows opacity still present in left lower zone, suggesting continuing empyema, confirmed by stony dull percussion note.
- Deterioration in arterial blood gases → intubation, mechanical ventilation on volume control → increasing airway pressure (indicating ↓ lung compliance) → pressure control initiated.

## Phase 2 questions

1. What might be developing?
2. Physiotherapy?

### RESPONSE TO CLINICAL REASONING

This is all very nice but the plethora of interventions does not allow identification of which was helpful. Maybe it was the rest that was beneficial, maybe the physical therapy, maybe natural recovery from an exacerbation.

## Response to Case Study Phase 2

1. Acute respiratory distress syndrome, demonstrated by deteriorating blood gases, increasing airway pressure and initiation of pressure control ventilation.
2. Prone positioning, preventive respiratory care, musculoskeletal care.

## Outcome

Patient improved (Fig. 23.5C), recovered, decided to avoid spicy restaurants.

## RECOMMENDED READING

Ahn, R., 2017. Financial ties of principal investigators and randomized controlled trial outcomes: cross sectional study. Br. Med. J. 356, i6770.

Armijo-Olivo, S., Fuentes, J., da Costa, B.R., et al., 2017. Blinding in physical therapy trials and its association with treatment effects: a meta-epidemiological study. Am. J. Phys. Med. Rehabil. 96 (1), 34–44.

Barrett, F.H., 2013. Supporting the case for qualitative research in physical therapy. Phys. Ther. Rev. 18 (2), 144–145.

Betit, P., 2015. Guidelines, pathways, bundles, and protocols: clinical recipes for success. Respir. Care 60 (3), 469–470.

Bruton, A., Garrod, R., Thomas, M., 2011. Respiratory physiotherapy: towards a clearer definition of the terminology. Physiotherapy 97, 345–349.

Busari, J.O., 2013. Clinical reasoning: reflecting on the decision-making process in respiratory medicine. Breathe 10, 413–417.

Connors, G.R., Siner, J.M., 2015. Clinical reasoning and risk in the intensive care unit. Clin. Chest Med. 36 (3), 449–459.

Dannapfel, P., Peolsson, A., Ståhl, C., et al., 2014. Applying self-determination theory for improved understanding of physiotherapists' rationale for using research in clinical practice: a qualitative study in Sweden. Physiother. Theory Pract. 30 (1), 20–28.

Dean, M., Levis, A., 2016. Does the use of a university lecturer as a visiting tutor support learning and assessment during physiotherapy students' clinical placements? Physiotherapy 102 (4), 365–370.

Debray, T.P.A., 2017. A guide to systematic review and meta-analysis of prediction model performance. Br. Med. J. 356, i6460.

Fuller, J., 2013. Rhetoric and argumentation: how clinical practice guidelines think. J. Eval. Clin. Pract. 19 (3), 433–441.

Hammon, R., Cross, V., Moore, A., 2016. The construction of professional identity by physiotherapists. Physiotherapy 102 (1), 71–77.

Holdar, U., Wallin, L., Heiwe, S., 2013. Why do we do as we do? Factors influencing clinical reasoning and decision-making among physiotherapists in an acute setting. Physiother. Res. Int. 18 (4), 220–229.

Jones, P.W., Beeh, K.M., Chapman, K.R., et al., 2014. Minimal clinically important differences in pharmacological trials. Am. J. Respir. Crit. Care Med. 189 (3), 250–255.

Macleod, M., 2014. Minimal clinically important differences in pharmacological trials. Some salt with your statin, professor? PLoS Biol. 12 (1), e1001768.

Mishoe, S.C., Welch, M.A., 2002. Critical Thinking in Respiratory Care. McGraw Hill, New York.

Nasters, D., Burns, L., Range, A., 2016. An innovative use of respiratory students to gain experience in high stakes neonatal simulations. Respir. Care 61 (10), 2529769.

Ottenbacher, K.J., Jette, A.M., Fuhrer, M.J., et al., 2012. Looking back and thinking forward: 20 years of disability and rehabilitation research. Arch. Phys. Med. Rehab. 93 (8), 1392–1394.

Rosner, A.L., 2012. Evidence-based medicine: revisiting the pyramid of priorities. J. Bodywork Movement Ther. 16 (1), 42–49.

Rye, K.J., 2011. Critical thinking in respiratory therapy. Respir. Care 56 (3), 364–365.

Stoller, J.K., 2010. Implementing change in respiratory care. Respir. Care 55 (6), 749–757.

# GLOSSARY OF ABBREVIATIONS, DEFINITIONS, SYMBOLS AND VALUES

If a definition is not here, see the index. Values in [square brackets] are American. Most values are approximate.

**N** normal

**Δ** change, e.g. $\Delta V/\Delta P$ = change in volume in response to change in pressure, i.e. compliance

**μ** micro-, prefix indicating $10^{-6}$, i.e. 0.000001

**μm** micrometre or micron, i.e. one millionth of a metre, or $1\times10^{-6}$ of a metre

**μmol** micromole, i.e. one millionth of a mole

**>** more than

**<** less than

**±** 'and/or' or 'with/without'

**~** approximately

**Dot over symbol** value per unit time, e.g. $\dot{V}O_2$: oxygen consumption

**Line over symbol** mean value, e.g. $\bar{v}$: mixed venous

**Conversion of mmHg to kPa** multiply the value by 0.1333, or google

**1RM** one repetition maximum, i.e. the maximum load that can be moved once over full range of motion without compensatory movements

**6MWT** six-minute walk test

**A** alveolar, e.g. $PAO_2$

**a** arterial, e.g. $PaO_2$

**AAA** abdominal aortic aneurysm

**AAT** alpha$_1$-antitrypsin

**ABGs** arterial blood gases

**ACBT** active cycle of breathing techniques

**ACBT/AD** active cycle of breathing techniques ± autogenic drainage

**ACE inhibitors** angiotensin-converting enzyme inhibitor drugs

**ACPRC** Association of Chartered Physiotherapists in Respiratory Care (UK)

**ACS** acute coronary syndrome

**AD** autogenic drainage

**ADL** activities of daily living

**Adult respiratory distress syndrome** old terminology for acute respiratory distress syndrome

**Adventitious sounds** added sounds on auscultation

**AF** atrial fibrillation

**Aggressive treatment** intensive treatment

**AIDS** acquired immune deficiency syndrome

**Air bronchogram** visibility of airways on X-ray due to opacification of surrounding alveoli

**Airway** (1) natural passageway for air to travel from atmosphere to alveoli, or (2) artificial device to hold open upper airway for relief of obstruction or to allow suction or mechanical ventilation

**Airway closure** closure of small airways, common in dependent lung regions at end-expiration

**Albumin** N, 40–60 g/L, [4.0–6.0 g/100 mL]

**Albuterol** US terminology for salbutamol

**Alkalaemia** alkalosis of blood

**Alveolar–arterial oxygen gradient** see: $PAO_2$–$PaO_2$

**Ambulating** US terminology for walking

**Ambulatory surgery** day surgery (not surgery while walking about!)

**Angioplasty** invasive but nonsurgical dilation of coronary artery stenosis, using catheter via femoral puncture, or laser; now called percutaneous coronary intervention

**Anoxia** complete lack of oxygen

**Antigen** allergen, i.e. irritant that elicits an immune response

**Antioxidant** substance which counteracts the effects of free radicals such as tobacco smoke

**AP** anteroposterior

**Apneustic breathing** prolonged inspiration, usually due to brain damage

**Apnoea** absence of breathing for >10 s

**APTT** see: clotting studies

**ARDS** acute respiratory distress syndrome

**ARF** (1) acute respiratory failure, or (2) acute renal failure

**Arnold's nerve** auricular branch of vagus nerve, responsible for the cough reflex in a proportion of the population, whereby a cough can be facilitated by ear stimulation; also responsible for ear pain being an occasional early presentation of laryngeal cancer

**Arteriovenous oxygen difference** difference between $O_2$ delivered to and returning from the tissues:
- calculated from arterial and mixed venous blood samples
- related to metabolic rate

**Ascites** fluid in the abdominal cavity

**Aspiration** (1) inhalation of unwanted substances (e.g. gastric acid or sea water) beyond the vocal cords, or (2) therapeutic removal of fluid or gas from a cavity such as the pleural space

**Atelectasis** collapse of alveoli

**Atelectrauma** damage to alveoli due to repetitive opening and closing

**Atopy** allergic hypersensitivity

**Auscultation** use of stethoscope to hear sounds from a body cavity

**Auto PEEP** intrinsic PEEP

**Automatic tube compensation** facility on some ventilators to eliminate the excess work of breathing through the tubing

**Autoregulation** ability of an organ to maintain constant blood flow despite changes in perfusion pressure

**BAL** bronchoalveolar lavage: bronchoscopic washing out of bronchioles and alveoli with sterile saline for diagnosis or treatment

**Barotrauma** air in the wrong place, e.g. pneumothorax or subcutaneous emphysema

**b.d.**  twice a day

**BE**  base excess

**Biofilm**  cluster of bacteria enclosed in a matrix

**BiPAP**  bilevel positive airway pressure

**BIPAP**  biphasic positive airway pressure

**Bleb**  collection of air under the visceral pleura (see also: bulla)

**Blood pressure**  pressure exerted by the blood on the arteries (see also: mean arterial pressure)

**Blood sugar**  3.5–5.5 mmol/L before meals, rising after meals by a few mmol/L; $\uparrow$ in stress, $\uparrow\uparrow$ in diabetes mellitus, $\downarrow$ in liver failure or starvation

**bpm**  breaths per minute or heart beats per minute

**Bradyarrythmia**  slow and abnormal heart beat

**Bradycardia**  resting HR <60/min in adults

**Bronchiole**  small airway unsupported by cartilage

**Bronchitis**  acute or chronic inflammation of mucous membranes of tracheobronchial tree

**Bronchopleural fistula**  communication between lung and pleura, caused by thoracic surgery, trauma or pulmonary disease

**Bronchospasm**  abnormal contraction of smooth bronchial muscle, causing narrowing of airway

**BTS**  British Thoracic Society

**Bulla**  collection of air in lung tissue which is more than 1 cm in diameter, usually caused by alveolar destruction or occasionally by barotrauma

**BUN**  blood urea nitrogen: US terminology for urea

**CABG**  coronary artery bypass graft

**Calcium**  N, 2.2–2.6 mmol/L

**CaO$_2$**  see: oxygen content

**Capnography**  measurement of expired $\pm$ inspired $CO_2$ concentration and its graphical display

**Cardiac enzymes**  enzymes released from damaged heart muscle after myocardial infarction

**Cardiac index**  cardiac output / body surface area: N, 2.5–3.5 L/min/m$^2$; highest at age 10, then decreasing with age

**Cardiac output (CO or Q)**  blood ejected by left ventricle per minute, i.e. HR × stroke volume; N, 4–8 L/min at rest, up to 25 L/min on exercise

**Catecholamine**  compound having sympathomimetic action, e.g. adrenaline

**Caudad**  towards the feet

**CCF**  congestive cardiac failure

**Centers for Disease Control and Prevention**  includes page on measuring physical activity: http://www.cdc.gov/physicalactivity/basics/measuring/index.html

**Central line**  catheter inserted into a large vein such as the internal jugular, subclavian or femoral for monitoring or the administration of thick fluids

**Central venous oxygen saturation (ScvO$_2$)**  oxygen saturation of haemoglobin (Hb) in large central veins, reflecting gas exchange in lungs, cardiac output, metabolic rate, Hb levels and tissue oxygen uptake; N, 73%–82%

**Centrilobular emphysema**  emphysema affecting mainly the respiratory bronchioles

**Cephalad**  towards the head

**CF**  cystic fibrosis

**CFA**  cryptogenic fibrosing alveolitis

**CHD**  coronary heart disease

**Cheyne-Stokes breathing**  episodes of rapid breathing, slow breathing and apnoea

**Chloride (Cl$^-$)**  chief anion in extracellular fluid: $\downarrow$ in plasma indicates acidosis, some kidney problems, prolonged vomiting; $\uparrow$ in sweat can be diagnostic of cystic fibrosis

**Churg-Strauss syndrome**  multiorgan necrotizing arteritis that occurs occasionally in people with severe asthma

**Closing capacity**  lung volume at which airway closure begins due to narrowing of dependent airways as lung deflates, i.e. sum of closing volume and residual volume; reduced by obesity or the supine position

**Closing volume**  closing capacity minus residual volume, which increases (becomes a greater proportion of FRC) with small airways disease, smoking, obesity and young or old age. Young person: 10% of VC. Age 65: 40% of VC

**Clotting studies**

- ACT (activated clotting time): monitors high-dose heparin therapy, e.g. during cardiopulmonary bypass. N, 100–140 s
- APTT (activated partial thromboplastin time): monitors low-dose heparin therapy. N, 30–40 s

- bleeding time. N, 3–9 min
- FDPs (fibrinogen degradation products). N, <10 mg/mL
- fibrinogen level. N, >150 mg/dL
- INR (international normalized ratio): ratio of time blood normally takes to clot compared to increased time it takes to clot, e.g. for monitoring warfarin or detecting bleeding disorders. N, 1–3. Higher means increased clotting time and risk of bleeding, e.g. 2–4 for a patient on warfarin, 10 in a patient at severe risk of bleeding
- KPTT (kaolin partial thromboplastin time). N, <7 s above control
- platelet count. N, 140,000–450,000 mm$^{-3}$. Risk of bleeding with suction: <50,000 mm$^{-3}$. Spontaneous bleeding: <20,000 mm$^{-3}$
- PT (prothrombin time). N, 11–15 s
- PTT (partial thromboplastin time). N, 12–30 s

**CMV**  (1) controlled mandatory ventilation or conventional mechanical ventilation, (2) cytomegalovirus

**CNS**  central nervous system

**CO**  (1) cardiac output, (2) carbon monoxide

**CO$_2$**  carbon dioxide

**Coagulation**  see: clotting studies

**Cognition**  mental activities involved in acquiring and processing information

**Collagen vascular disease**  connective tissue disease, with a predilection for the lungs

**Collateral channels**  airways between adjacent lung units which allow inspired gas to bypass normal airways if these are obstructed: pores of Kohn between alveoli, channels of Lambert between bronchioles and alveoli, channels of Martin between bronchioles

**Collateral ventilation**  ventilation through collateral channels when normal airways are obstructed

**Compliance of lung**  change in volume in response to change in transpulmonary pressure, i.e. $\Delta V/\Delta P$

- static compliance: compliance with zero gas flow, N, 200 mL/cmH$_2$O, measurement on MV: $V_T / P_{plat}$ – PEEP
- dynamic compliance: compliance during gas flow (less than or equal to static lung compliance), N, 180 mL/cmH$_2$O, measurement on MV: $V_T$ / PIP – PEEP

**Concordance**  negotiated agreement between professional and patient

**Consolidation**   replacement of alveolar air by substance of greater density, e.g. the inflammatory exudate of pneumonia

**Contralateral**   opposite side

**COPD**   chronic obstructive pulmonary disease

**Cough peak flow**   see: peak cough flow

**Cough syncope**   loss of consciousness for a few seconds following cough (benign unless while driving)

**CPAP**   continuous positive airway pressure

**CPET**   cardiopulmonary exercise test

**CPT**   chest physiotherapy comprising postural drainage, percussion and vibrations

**Creatinine**   electrolyte in plasma or urine, formed from muscle breakdown (end-product of normal muscle metabolism) and excreted by kidneys, the most common biomarker used to evaluate kidney function
- N in plasma: 50–100 $\mu$mol/L [0.6–1.2 mg/100 mL]
- $\uparrow$ in hypovolaemia or kidney failure, $\uparrow\uparrow$ in septic shock

**Cryptogenic**   of unknown cause

**CSF**   cerebrospinal fluid

**CT**   computed tomography

**CVP**   central venous pressure N, 0–8 mmHg or 5–12 cmH$_2$O

**CVS**   cardiovascular system

**CXR**   chest X-ray

**Cytokine**   inflammatory product

**Decubitus**   side-lying
- right decubitus: lying on R side
- left decubitus: lying on L side

**Dependent**   underneath

**Derecruitment**   collapse of alveoli

**Desaturation**   $\downarrow$ oxygen saturation of haemoglobin in arterial blood

**Diastole**   ventricular relaxation

**DIC**   disseminated intravascular coagulation (see: clotting)

**DNAR**   do not attempt resuscitation

**DO$_2$**   see: oxygen delivery

**Downstream**   towards the mouth

**Driving pressure**   of ventilator – inspiratory plateau pressure minus PEEP

**Duty cycle**   see: tension-time index

**DVT**   deep vein thrombosis

**Dysarthria**   difficulty speaking due to weak muscles

**Dysphagia**   difficulty swallowing

**Dyspnoea**   distressing breathlessness

**ECCO$_2$R**   extracorporeal CO$_2$ removal

**ECG**   electrocardiogram

**ECMO**   extracorporeal membrane oxygenation

**-ectomy**   removal

**EKC**   US terminology for ECG

**Elastance**   opposite of compliance

**EMLA**   eutectic mixture of local anaesthetics: cream for numbing skin before skin puncture

**Endotoxin**   toxin inside bacterial cell, released after destruction of bacterial cell wall

**End-tidal CO$_2$ concentration**   CO$_2$ levels measured by capnography, which monitors exhaled CO$_2$ at the mouth at the end of a quiet exhalation
- N, 4%–6%

**Endurance**   capacity of muscle to sustain contraction

**Enteral**   via the gut

**Entonox**   analgesic gas mixture comprising 50% nitrous oxide and 50% oxygen, also known as laughing gas

**Entrainment**   dilution of gas stream or aerosol with external gas such as room air

**Eosinophilia**   excess eosinophils, indicating allergic state

**Eosinophils**   inflammatory cells associated with hypersensitivity reaction
- $\uparrow$ in allergy, e.g. extrinsic asthma

**Epiglottis**   cartilage which diverts food to oesophagus by closing over trachea

**Epinephrine**   US terminology for adrenaline

**ERCP**   endoscopic retrograde cholangiopancreatography: procedure for detection and treatment of gallstones

**Erythrocytosis**   polycythaemia

**ETCO$_2$**   see: end-tidal CO$_2$

**ETT**   endotracheal tube

**Extracorporeal**   outside the body

**Fatigue**
- central: reduced force generation due to events proximal to neuromuscular junction
- peripheral: failure at or beyond neuromuscular junction

**FBC**   full blood count

**FDP**   see: clotting studies

**FEF$_{25-75}$**   mid forced expiratory flow

**FEF$_{50}$**   mid forced expiratory flow

**FET**   forced expiration technique

**FEV$_1$**   forced expiratory volume in 1 second

**FFP**   fresh frozen plasma, contains all clotting factors at normal concentration

**FG**   size of catheter or tube defined as the outside diameter in units of $\frac{1}{3}$ mm, e.g. 12 French Gauge catheter has outer diameter of 4 mm

**FiO$_2$**   fraction of inspired oxygen, expressed as decimal, e.g. FiO$_2$ of 0.6 = 60% inspired oxygen, FiO$_2$ of 0.21 = room air

**Fluid bolus**   between 100 mL and >1000 mL intravenous fluids delivered from immediately to 60 min

**Fluid overload**   10% or greater increase in weight due to excess fluid

**Frailty**   multidimensional syndrome of vulnerability, characterized by loss of physiologic and cognitive reserve

**FRC**   functional residual capacity

**Fremitus**   vibratory tremors palpable through the chest wall

**FVC**   forced vital capacity

**GCS**   Glasgow coma scale

**Glottis**   vocal folds and space between them

**Glucose**   see: blood sugar

**GOR**   gastroesophageal reflux

**GORD**   gastroesophageal reflux disease

**H$^+$**   hydrogen ion

**Haematocrit**   concentration of red blood cells in blood
- N, 36%–46% in women, 40%–50% in men,
- anaemia: <36%; polycythaemia: >55%

**Haemoglobin**   respiratory pigment in red blood cells which combines reversibly with oxygen
- N, 11.5–15 g/100 mL in women, 14–17 g/100 mL in men
- $\downarrow$ in anaemia, $\uparrow$ in polycythaemia

**Haemoptysis**   coughing up blood ('frank haemoptysis' is coughing up pure blood)

**Haldane effect**   decreased affinity of haemoglobin for CO$_2$ in hyperoxic conditions

**Harrison's sulcus**   permanent indentation of the chest wall along the costal margins where the diaphragm inserts, caused by pull of diaphragm on ribs which are either not yet calcified or weakened by rickets

**Hb**   see: haemoglobin

**HCO$_3^-$**   bicarbonate ion concentration

**Hepatomegaly**   enlarged liver

**HF**   heart failure

**Hiccup**   involuntary clonic spasm of intercostals and diaphragm followed by abrupt glottic closure, of unknown aetiology

**HIV**  human immunodeficiency virus

**HME**  heat–moisture exchanger

**HR**  heart rate, N, 60–100 bpm

**HRCT**  high resolution computed tomography

**HRR**  heart rate reserve: difference between maximum HR and resting HR

**HVS**  hyperventilation syndrome

**Hyaline membrane disease**  respiratory distress syndrome in neonates

**Hypercapnia**  $\uparrow PaCO_2$

**Hyperdynamic**  status signalling onset of septic shock: galloping pulse, pyrexia, shaking chill, flushing of skin, high cardiac output, unstable BP

**Hyperkalaemia**  $\uparrow$ serum potassium

**Hypermetabolism**  $\uparrow$ energy expenditure by >10%

**Hypernatraemia**  $\uparrow$ serum sodium

**Hyperosmolar**  $\uparrow$ concentration of osmotically active ingredients

**Hyperoxia**  abnormally high oxygen tension in blood

**Hyperreactivity**  $\uparrow$ sensitivity to variety of stimuli

- present in asthma airways, sometimes present with COPD, bronchiectasis, CF, sarcoidosis and LVF

**Hyperthermia**  core temperature >40.5°C

**Hyperventilation**  exhaled $CO_2$ in excess of $CO_2$ production, causing $PaCO_2$ <4.7 kPa (35 mmHg)

**Hypervolaemia**  fluid overload

**Hypoalbuminaemia**  $\downarrow$ albumin

**Hypocalcaemia**  $\downarrow$ calcium in blood

**Hypocapnia**  $\downarrow CO_2$ in arterial blood

**Hypocarbia**  as previous entry

**Hypokalaemia**  $\downarrow$ potassium in blood

**Hyponatraemia**  $\downarrow$ sodium in blood

**Hypopnoea**  shallow slow breathing

**Hypoventilation**  $CO_2$ production in excess of $CO_2$ removal, leading to $PaCO_2$ >6.0 kPa (45 mmHg)

**Hypovolaemia**  $\downarrow$ blood volume due to, e.g. dehydration or haemorrhage

**Hypoxaemia**  $\downarrow$ oxygen in arterial blood

**Hypoxia**  $\downarrow$ oxygen in tissues

**Hysteresis**  difference in compliance between inspiration and expiration, due to extra energy required during inspiration to recruit additional alveoli

**IABP**  intraaortic balloon pump

**Iatrogenic**  harm caused by medical intervention

**ICF framework**  International Classification of Functioning, Disability and Health

**ICP**  intracranial pressure

**ICU**  intensive care unit

**I:E ratio**  see: inspiratory:expiratory ratio

**Ileus**  gut obstruction, e.g. due to paralytic ileus, as indicated by lack of bowel sounds

**Immotile cilia syndrome**  primary ciliary dyskinesia

**Immunoglobulin**  antibody,

- examples in respiratory secretions: IgA, IgE, IgG, IgM

**Infection**  presence of microorganisms or their products in normally sterile tissue

**Infiltrate**  fluid, cells or other substance in tissue space, e.g. pulmonary interstitial infiltrate = fluid between capillary and alveolus, showing on X-ray as diffuse shadowing

**Inotropes**  drugs which $\uparrow$ force of cardiac contraction

**INR**  see: clotting studies

**Inspiratory capacity**  volume inspired during maximum inspiration from resting end-expiratory position

**Inspiratory:expiratory ratio**  duration of inspiration relative to expiration

**Inspiratory force**  see: MIP

**Insufflation**  blowing air into the lungs

**Intracranial hypertension**  $\uparrow$ intracranial pressure

**Intrapleural pressure**  pressure in pleural space

**Intrapulmonary pressure**  alveolar pressure

**Intrathoracic pressure**  pleural pressure

**Intrinsic PEEP**  trapped gas left in lungs at end-exhalation due to obstructed airways ± breathing through artificial airways

**IPPB**  intermittent positive pressure breathing

**IPPV**  intermittent positive pressure ventilation, i.e. mechanical ventilation

**IRV**  (1) inspiratory reserve volume or (2) inverse ratio ventilation

**IS**  incentive spirometry

**Isotonic**  same osmotic pressure as body fluids, e.g. isotonic saline contains salt equal to that in body

**ISWT**  incremental shuttle walk test

**IV**  intravenous

**JVP**  jugular venous pressure

**K**  potassium

**Kerley B lines**  thin radiological 2 cm horizontal lines, perpendicular to visceral pleural surface, representing engorged lymphatics and thickened interlobular septa

- become visible when pulmonary artery wedge pressure exceeds 25 mmHg, indicating pulmonary oedema

**kPa**  kilopascal (unit of pressure)

**KTPP**  see: clotting studies

**Kussmaul breathing**  deep sighing breathing often seen in patients with metabolic acidosis

**L**  (1) litre, or (2) left

**Lactate**  (in blood, i.e. serum lactate) marker of ischaemia and a waste product of anaerobic glycolysis, reflecting disease severity

- N, <1 mmol/L, anaerobic metabolism: >2 mmol/L, poor prognosis: >3 mmol/L

**Laparoscopy**  minimal access incision through abdominal wall

**Laparotomy**  full surgical incision through abdominal wall

**Larynx**  section of airway connecting pharynx and trachea and containing vocal cords

**LFT**  (1) lung function test, or (2) liver function test

**Loculated pleural effusion**  pleural effusion in which fluid is trapped in pockets

**LTOT**  long-term oxygen therapy

**Lung clearance index**  a measure of ventilation inhomogeneity derived from multiple breath washout tests

**LVEDP**  left ventricular end-diastolic pressure

**LVEDV**  left ventricular end-diastolic volume

- determinant of preload
- depends on venous return to L ventricle, circulating blood volume and efficiency of L atrial contraction
- measured, by assumption, from PAWP, which relates to LVEDP

**LVF**  left ventricular failure

**Lymphadenopathy**  enlarged lymph nodes

**MAP**  see: mean arterial pressure

**Mast cell**  connective tissue cell involved in hypersensitivity reactions, releasing histamine in response to specific stimuli

- increased in asthma

**Maximal HR**  220 − age (years)

**Maximum expiratory flow rate**  US terminology for peak expiratory flow rate (peak flow)

**Maximum oxygen consumption ($\dot{V}O_2$max)**  maximal rate at which

oxygen can be used by an individual during maximal work, i.e. aerobic capacity, reflecting neural, cardiopulmonary and metabolic components of aerobic fitness and requiring $\dot{V}O_2$ to attain a plateau
- ↑ with fitness, ↓ with advancing age but rate of decline slower in physically active people
- N, 2 L/min or >25 mL/kg/min or 25 times resting level
- COPD: typically 1 L/min
- see also: anaerobic threshold

**MDI** metered dose inhaler

**Mean arterial pressure** average pressure pushing blood through systemic circulation, i.e. cardiac output × peripheral vascular resistance
- N, 80–100 mmHg
- compromised circulation to vital organs: <60 mmHg
- compromised circulation to injured brain: <80 mmHg

**MEF$_{50}$** maximum expiratory flow in mid-expiration

**MEP** maximum expiratory pressure
- N, 100 cmH$_2$O, inadequate cough: <40 cmH$_2$O

**mEq** milliequivalent, i.e. one thousandth of molecular weight of substance

**mEq/L** milliequivalents per litre of solution, e.g. of electrolyte concentration
- also expressed as mmol/L

**MH** manual hyperinflation

**MI** see: myocardial infarction

**Micro** one millionth

**Microatelectasis** collapse of lung units smaller than a segment, not detectable clinically or radiologically

**Micrometre or micron (μm)** one millionth of a metre

**Minute ventilation** see next entry

**Minute volume or minute ventilation ($\dot{V}_E$)** amount of gas expelled from lungs per minute, i.e. tidal volume × RR
- N, 5–9 L

**MIP** maximum inspiratory pressure: assessment of respiratory muscle strength
- N, minus 100–130 cmH$_2$O (men), minus 70–100 (women)
- typical value for hypercapnic COPD: minus 55 (men), minus 40 (women)

**Mixed venous blood** blood in pulmonary artery

**Mixed venous oxygen content** (Hb × S$\bar{\text{v}}$O$_2$ × 1.39) + (PvO$_2$ × 0.023)

**Mixed venous oxygen saturation (S$\bar{\text{v}}$O$_2$)** oxygen saturation of Hb in pulmonary artery, reflecting gas exchange in lungs, cardiac output, metabolic rate, Hb levels and tissue oxygen uptake
- N, 75%

**MMEF** maximum mid-expiratory flow

**mmHg** millimetres of mercury (unit of pressure)

**MRI** magnetic resonance imaging

**MRSA** methicillin-resistant staphylococcus aureus

**Mucoactive** affecting quality or quantity of mucus

**Mucokinetic** accelerating mucus transport

**Mucolytic** substance which degrades mucin in mucus gel

**Mucoviscidosis** cystic fibrosis

**Multimorbidity** coexistence of two or more chronic conditions, without reference to a primary condition

**Multiorgan failure** multisystem failure

**MV** mechanical ventilation

**MVA** motor vehicle accident (US)

**Mycoplasma pneumonia** atypical pneumonia which affects otherwise healthy people

**Myocardial infarction** death of portion of heart muscle due to myocardial ischaemia

**Na** see: sodium

**NBM** nil by mouth (NPO in US)

**Neuromuscular blockade** chemical paralysis by neuromuscular blocking agents

**Neutropaenia** ↓ neutrophils, i.e. <1.5 × 10$^9$, leaving patient vulnerable to infection

**Neutrophil** white blood cell used for phagocytosis of bacteria but which in excess releases tissue-damaging enzymes as part of uncontrolled inflammation

**NICE** National Institute for Health and Care Excellence: UK body established to reduce the postcode lottery in provision of health services

**NICU** neonatal intensive care unit

**NIPPV** nasal (or noninvasive) intermittent positive pressure ventilation, i.e. noninvasive ventilation

**NIV** noninvasive ventilation

**NO** nitric oxide

**Normocapnia** normal PaCO$_2$

**Normoxaemia** normal blood oxygenation

**Normovolaemia** normal blood volume

**NPO** nil per os, i.e. nil by mouth

**NSAIDs** nonsteroidal antiinflammatory drugs

**NSTEMI** non ST-segment elevation MI

**O$_2$** oxygen

**Occult PEEP** intrinsic PEEP

**Oesophageal varices** dilated veins in lower third of the oesophagus, at junction of portal and systemic venous systems, due to raised portal pressure

**Oliguria** ↓ urine output, i.e. <20 mL/h (normal 50–60 mL/h)

**Oncotic pressure** osmotic pressure exerted by colloids

**Orthopnoea** dyspnoea on lying flat

**Orthostatic hypotension/intolerance** drop of >20 mmHg in systolic ± drop of >10 mmHg in diastolic BP on standing up

**Osmolality** number of osmotically active particles per kg of solvent, the most significant factor in the distribution of water between intracellular and extracellular fluid

**Osmolarity** number of osmotically active particles per L of solution

**-ostomy** formation of artificial opening to skin surface

**-otomy** incision

**OT** occupational therapy/therapist

**Oxidants** substances which occur naturally in the body but can damage the immune system if not neutralized by antioxidants

**Oxidative stress** imbalance between generation and breakdown of oxygen free radicals (reactive oxygen species), accelerated by smoking, inflammation, air pollution, hyperoxia and hypoxia, which results in net gain of oxygen free radicals and potential for harm, including respiratory disease

**Oxygen consumption** amount of oxygen consumed by tissues each minute, i.e. CI × (CaO$_2$–CvO$_2$) × 10 mL/min/m$^2$
- N at rest: 150–300 mL/min/m$^2$ (if contributing values normal, i.e. CO 5 L/min, Hb 15 g/100 mL, SaO$_2$ 97%, S$\bar{\text{v}}$O$_2$ 75%),
- critical illness: >600 mL/min/m$^2$

**Oxygen content (CaO$_2$)** total amount of oxygen in blood, i.e. (Hb × SaO$_2$ × 1.39) + (PaO$_2$ × 0.023)
- N in arterial blood: 16–20 mL/100 mL or mL/dL

**Oxygen cost of breathing**  energy requirements of respiratory muscles and indirect measure of work of breathing
- N, 1 mL/L of ventilation

**Oxygen delivery ($DO_2$)**  volume of oxygen presented to tissues, i.e. CI × $CaO_2$
- N, 600–1000 mL/min, i.e. ~25% of oxygen the tissues receive

**Oxygen demand**  oxygen needed by cells for aerobic metabolism, estimated by $\dot{V}O_2$

**Oxygen extraction**  oxygen transferred from blood to tissues, i.e. $CaO_2$ difference between arterial and mixed venous blood, equivalent to $\dot{V}O_2/DO_2$
- N, 20%–30%
- 32% indicates ↑ oxygen demand or occasionally ↓ $DO_2$
- <22% indicates damaged tissues unable to extract $O_2$, or hyperdynamic circulation, e.g. early sepsis

**Oxygen extraction ratio ($\dot{V}O_2/DO_2$)**  ratio of oxygen consumption to oxygen delivery, indicating efficiency of tissues in extracting oxygen
- calculation: $CaO_2 - C\bar{v}O_2/CaO_2$,
- N, 25%
- high oxygen extraction to meet excess metabolic needs: >35%
- maximum for most tissues: 60%–70%

**Oxygen flux**  % oxygen that reaches tissues

**Oxygen transport**  transport of oxygen from lungs to mitochondria

**Oxygen uptake**  oxygen consumption

**Ozone**  gas that provides protective layer to the Earth's atmosphere, but at ground level causes inflammation in hyperreactive airways

**$P_{50}$**  $PO_2$ at which 50% of haemoglobin is saturated with oxygen
- N, 27–28 mmHg

**PA**  posteroanterior

**Pack years**  average number of packs smoked daily × years smoked, e.g. smoking one pack/day for 30 years = 30 pack-year history

**Packed cell volume**
- equivalent to haematocrit
- N, 0.36–0.46 (women), 0.40–0.50 (men)
- ↑ in polycythaemia, ↓ in anaemia

**$PaCO_2$**  partial pressure of $CO_2$ in arterial blood
- N, 4.7–6.0 kPa (35–45 mmHg)

**Palliation**  alleviation of symptoms

**Panic attack**  rapid onset of fear accompanied by somatic symptoms

**Panacinar or panlobular emphysema**  emphysema affecting mainly alveoli

**$PAO_2$**  partial pressure of oxygen in alveoli

**$PaO_2$**  partial pressure of oxygen in arterial blood
- N, 11–14 kPa (80–100 mmHg), declining by 0.55 kPa (4 mmHg) per 10 years

**$PaO_2/FiO_2$**  ratio of $PaO_2$ to inspired oxygen, more relevant than $PaO_2$ alone, estimates shunt
- N, 40 kPa (300 mmHg),
- e.g. $PaO_2$:$FiO_2$ of 27 could mean $PaO_2$ of 10.7 kPa at $FiO_2$ of 0.40 or $PaO_2$ of 16 kPa at $FiO_2$ of 0.60

**$PAO_2$–$PaO_2$ or $PA$-$aO_2$ or A–a gradient**  alveolar–arterial oxygen gradient or A–a gradient: difference in oxygen tension across alveolar membrane, i.e. $PAO_2$ minus $PaO_2$
- indicates efficiency of gas transfer, varies with $FiO_2$
- N on room air: 0.7–2.7 kPa (5–20 mmHg), reflecting normal anatomical shunt
- ↑ on exercise, ↑ in the elderly, ↑ on supplemental oxygen, ↑ with diffusion impairment, e.g. pulmonary oedema, fibrosis or ARDS

**PAOP**  pulmonary artery occlusion pressure (= PAWP)

**PAP**  (1) peak airway pressure (peak inspiratory pressure) or (2) pulmonary artery pressure

**Paralytic ileus**  decrease or absence of peristalsis

**Parenchyma**  foamlike substance comprising gas exchanging part of lung, made up of alveoli, tiniest airways, capillaries and supporting tissue

**Parenchymal lung disease**  disease affecting parenchyma, e.g. interstitial lung disease, pneumonia, TB, ARDS

**Parenteral**  other than through the gut, usually relates to intravenous feeding

**$P_{aw}$**  mean airway pressure

**PAWP**  pulmonary artery wedge pressure
- N, 2–15 mmHg
- pulmonary congestion: 20 mmHg
- pulmonary oedema: 25 mmHg

**PC**  pressure control ventilation

**PCA**  patient controlled analgesia

**PCV**  (1) pressure control ventilation or (2) packed cell volume

**PCWP**  pulmonary capillary wedge pressure (= PAWP)

**PD**  (1) postural drainage or (2) peritoneal dialysis

**PE**  pulmonary embolus

**Peak cough flow**  N, 720 L/min

**Peak $\dot{V}O_2$**  oxygen consumption averaged over a 20- to 30-s period of maximal effort, may or may not equal $\dot{V}O_2$max

**PEEP**  positive end-expiratory pressure

**PEEPi**  intrinsic positive end-expiratory pressure

**PEFR**  peak expiratory flow rate

**PEG**  percutaneous endoscopic gastrostomy: surgical opening into gut for enteral feeding

**$P_E$max**  maximum expiratory pressure at mouth, see: MEP

**PEP**  positive expiratory pressure

**Percussion**  (1) (therapeutic) clapping the chest wall to loosen airway secretions, or (2) (diagnostic) tapping chest wall to identify density of underlying tissue

**Percutaneous**  through the skin

**PF**  peak flow, i.e. peak expiratory flow rate

**pH**  measure of hydrogen ions in solution, i.e. inverse of log of hydrogen ion concentration
- N, 7.35–7.45

**Pharmacodynamics**  what a drug does to the body

**Pharmacokinetics**  what the body does to a drug

**Phrenic**  relating to the diaphragm

**PICC line**  catheter inserted into a central vein for long-term intravenous antibiotics, nutrition or drugs

**PiCCO**  pulse index continuous cardiac output

**PICU**  paediatric intensive care unit

**PIF**  peak inspiratory flow
- N, 40–50 L/min
- when breathless or with exercise: up to 200 L/min

**PIFR**  peak inspiratory flow rate (peak inspiratory flow)

**$P_I$max**  maximum inspiratory pressure at the mouth, see: MIP

**PIP**  peak inspiratory pressure

**Plasma colloid osmotic pressure**
- N, 3.4 kPa (26 mmHg)
- risk of pulmonary oedema: 1.45 kPa (11 mmHg)

**Plate atelectasis**  subsegmental atelectasis

**Platelet count**   see: clotting studies

**Platelets**   cell fragments in blood which assist in clotting

**Plethoric**   florid complexion due to excess red blood cells

**Pleural pressure**   pressure in pleural space

**Pleural tap**   see: thoracentesis

**PN**   percussion note

**PND**   paroxysmal nocturnal dyspnoea

**Pneumectomy**   lung volume reduction surgery (cf. pneumonectomy: removal of a lung)

**Pneumococcal disease**   infection caused by *Streptococcus pneumoniae*, resulting in pneumonia, sepsis or meningitis, the bacteria being spread through direct contact, coughing or sneezing

**PO₂**   partial pressure or tension of oxygen

**Polycythaemia**   excess red blood cells due to late-stage lung disease, cyanotic congenital heart disease, high-altitude living or sleep apnoea

**Polypharmacy**   multiple medications or more medications than clinically indicated

**Polysomnography**   recording of physiological parameters during sleep

**Polyuria**   ↑ urine output, i.e. >100 mL/h

**Post-pneumonectomy syndrome**   tracheobronchial stenosis and severe dyspnoea, treated surgically using a saline-filled tissue expander

**Postural hypotension**   ↓ BP of >5 mmHg on moving to upright position

**Potassium (K)**   electrolyte in plasma or urine
- N in plasma: 3.5–5.0 mmol/L

**P$_{plat}$**   plateau pressure on MV

**PR**   pulmonary rehabilitation

**Pressure–time product**   pressure generated by respiratory muscles during inspiration
- average: 90 cmH₂O/s/min

**p.r.n.**   'as required', i.e. when the patient requests; usually relates to drug administration

**PSV**   pressure support ventilation

**PT**   see: clotting studies

**PTCA**   percutaneous transluminal coronary angioplasty

**PtcCO₂**   transcutaneous CO₂ tension

**PtcO₂**   transcutaneous oxygen tension

**PTSD**   post traumatic stress disorder

**PTT**   see: clotting studies

**Pulmonary artery pressure**
- N, 10–20 mmHg (systolic 22, diastolic 10, mean 15)
- pulmonary hypertension: >15 mmHg

**Pulmonary infarction**   death of area of lung, usually due to pulmonary embolus

**Pulmonary osteoarthropathy**   pain and swelling of joints associated with lung, liver or congenital heart disease

**Pulmonary vascular resistance**
- N, 25–125 dyn.s.cm$^{-5}$

**Pulse pressure**   difference between systolic and diastolic pressures: indicates blood flow
- N, 40 mmHg
- ↑ with hypertension, ↓ with poor stroke volume
- dangerously low tissue perfusion: 20 mmHg.

**Pulsus paradoxus**   weaker pulse on inspiration than expiration caused by expansion of pulmonary vascular bed on inspiration, i.e. excess negative pressure in chest
- occurs with severe acute asthma, hypovolaemic patient on MV, cardiac tamponade
- N, 10 mmHg, higher value indicating laboured breathing

**Purulent**   containing pus

**P$\bar{v}$CO₂**   mixed venous CO₂ tension
- N, 6.1 kPa (46 mmHg)

**PVD**   peripheral vascular disease (= peripheral arterial disease)

**P$\bar{v}$O₂**   mixed venous oxygen tension
- N, 4.7–5.3 kPa
- minimum acceptable: 3.7 kPa (28 mmHg)

**Pyothorax**   large empyema

**Q**   blood flow

**q.d.s.**   four times a day

**QoL**   see: quality of life

**Qs**   shunted blood

**Q$_T$**   alternative abbreviation for cardiac output

**Qs/Q$_T$**   shunt fraction

**Quality of life**   encompasses physical, psychological and social dimensions, to include independence, finance, functioning ability including ADL, individuals' perception of their situation and symptoms

**R**   right

**Radiolabelling**   monitoring radiolabelled aerosol, which, for estimating mucous clearance, is inhaled and its clearance followed by gamma camera

**RAP**   right atrial pressure

**Rapid shallow breathing index**   ratio of RR to V$_T$, e.g. patient with RR of 25/min and V$_T$ of 250 mL/breath has rapid shallow breathing index of (25/0.25) = 100 breaths/min/L
- used to judge if patients have the strength to wean from mechanical ventilation

**Raynaud phenomenon of the lung**   vasospasm in the lungs associated with Raynaud syndrome

**Reactive oxygen species**   natural byproduct of the normal metabolism of oxygen, increased during inflammation or environmental stress, leading to oxidative stress

**Rebreathing**   inspired breath containing the CO₂ and the reduced oxygen content from the previous exhaled breath

**Recruitment**   opening up of alveoli

**Relative humidity**   water in gas expressed as a percentage of that which would fully saturate the volume of gas at a given temperature (%). See also: absolute humidity
- N in ambient air: 25–50%
- N in upper trachea: 95%

**REM**   rapid-eye-movement phase of sleep cycle

**Resistance to gas flow through the airways**
- spontaneous ventilation: 0.5–5.0 cmH₂O/L/s
- mechanical ventilation: (peak inspiratory pressure – plateau pressure)/mean flow
- COPD: 13–18 cmH₂O/L/s

**Respiratory inductive plethysmography**   spirometry for ventilated patients, including measurement of lung volume to detect intrinsic PEEP

**Respiratory pump**   components that deliver oxygen to alveolar–capillary membrane and remove CO₂, i.e. respiratory centres, nerves, muscles, chest wall (thoracic cage + thoracoabdominal interface)

**Respiratory quotient (RQ)**   ratio of CO₂ produced to O₂ consumed, providing a measure of energy consumption
- N, <1.0, expired $\dot{V}_E$ being less than inspired $\dot{V}_E$, because CO₂ is used for other purposes and less is excreted than O₂ absorbed
- RQ of carbohydrate oxidation: 1.0
- RQ of fat oxidation: 0.7

**Respiratory therapist (US)** Respiratory physiotherapist (UK) combined with respiratory technician.

**Resuscitation**
- cardiopulmonary (CPR) – manual attempt to restart circulation and breathing
- fluid – replacement of intravascular fluids after dehydration, diarrhoea, vomiting, surgery, trauma or shock

**Reverse Trendelenburg** positioning the whole bed head up

**RFT** respiratory function test

**Rhinitis** inflammation of mucus membrane of nose, either seasonal (hayfever) or perennial

**Rhonchi** low-pitched snoring-like wheeze on auscultation, often related to airway secretions

**Right middle lobe syndrome** recurrent atelectasis, pneumonitis ± bronchiectasis of middle lobe in children due to poor collateral ventilation

**SaO$_2$** saturation of haemoglobin with oxygen in arterial blood
- N, 95%–98%

**Sarcopenia** loss of muscle cells

**SARS** severe acute respiratory syndrome: viral disease that may be contracted by exposure to coronavirus, causing fever and dry cough

**ScvO$_2$** see: central venous oxygen saturation

**SD** standard deviation

**Sengstaken tube** double-balloon tube inserted into the stomach, with oesophageal and gastric balloons which can be inflated to prevent bleeding

**Shunt** blood passing from right to left side of the heart without seeing alveolar gas, due to heart or lung disease
- N, 2% of cardiac output

**Silent lung zone** small airways where airflow resistance is difficult to measure so that damage may not be detectable in early obstructive airways disease

**SIRS** systemic inflammatory response syndrome: generalized inflammatory response, caused by infection or other insult such as trauma or pancreatitis

**Situs inversus** transposition of organs in chest and abdomen to the opposite side, e.g. heart on right side

**SLE** systemic lupus erythematosus

**SOB** shortness of breath

**SOBOE** shortness of breath on exertion

**Sodium (Na)** electrolyte in plasma or urine
- N in plasma: 134–148 mmol/L [135–147 mEq/L]

**Somatization** distress expressed as a physical symptom

**SOOB** sit out of bed

**Speech pathologist** US terminology for speech language therapist

**SpO$_2$** oxygen saturation by pulse oximetry, usually equivalent to SaO$_2$

**Sputum** expectorated secretions

**STEMI** ST-segment elevation MI

**Stokes Adams attack** transient but pulseless loss of consciousness, often associated with complete heart block

**Stridor** high-pitched sound produced by turbulent airflow through partially obstructed upper airway, heard on inspiration, expiration or both

**Stroke volume** volume ejected from ventricle with each beat
- dependent on preload, afterload and contractility, normally the same for each ventricle
- N, 60–130 mL

**Subcutaneous emphysema** collection of air under the skin

**Surgical emphysema** subcutaneous emphysema

**SVR** see: systemic vascular resistance

**S$\bar{\text{v}}$O$_2$** see: mixed venous oxygen saturation.

**Syncope** transient loss of consciousness, e.g. faint

**Systemic vascular resistance** (MAP–CVP / cardiac output) × 79.9
- N, 800–1400 dyn.s.cm$^{-5}$
- septic shock: <300

**Tamponade** fluid in pericardium

**t.d.s.** three times a day

**TED stockings** thromboembolus deterrent stockings

**Tension time index (TT)** or **diaphragmatic tension time index (TTdi)** or **duty cycle (T$_I$/T$_{TOT}$)**
- ratio of inspiratory time to total respiratory cycle time
- indicates proportion of muscle's maximum capacity that can be sustained indefinitely
- quantifies relationship between load and capacity.

**Thoracentesis** withdrawal of fluid from pleural cavity

**Thoracocentesis** alternative term for thoracentesis

**Thoracoscopy** minimal access incision through chest wall

**Thoracotomy** full incision through chest wall

**Thrombolysis** dissolution of thrombus

**TIA** transient ischaemic attack

**Tidal breathing** breathing at tidal volume

**Tidal volume** volume of air inhaled and exhaled at each normal sized breath
- N, 7 mL/kg with spontaneous breathing, 7–10 mL/kg with MV, up to 12 mL/kg in acute respiratory failure

**T$_I$/T$_{TOT}$** see: tension time index

**TLC** total lung capacity

**TLCO** total lung transfer capacity for carbon monoxide

**Tonicity** osmotic equivalence of fluids: isotonic fluids have same osmolality as plasma, hypotonic fluids have less, hypertonic fluids have more

**Torr** measurement of pressure (US), equivalent to mmHg

**Toxic shock syndrome** shock caused by a storm of inflammatory mediators, leading to respiratory failure and vascular leakage

**TPN** total parenteral nutrition, i.e. food administered intravenously

**Tracheal sounds** sounds heard on auscultation at suprasternal notch

**Tracheal tube** endotracheal or tracheostomy tube

**Transdiaphragmatic pressure** diaphragmatic strength, measured by comparing oesophageal and gastric pressures using swallowed balloons. See also: twitch diaphragmatic pressure

**Transmural (transpulmonary) pressure** pressure difference inside and outside lung, i.e. difference between alveolar and pleural pressures, representing driving pressure responsible for inflating lungs

**Transpulmonary pressure** as previous entry

**Trendelenburg position** head-down tilt

**TTdi** diaphragmatic tension-time index

**T$_{TOT}$** total respiratory cycle

**Tussive** related to cough

**Twitch diaphragmatic pressure** measurement of diaphragmatic strength by bilateral phrenic nerve stimulation

- N, 35 cmH$_2$O
- weakness: typically 20 cmH$_2$O in patients with respiratory muscle weakness secondary to COPD
- weak enough to require MV: 15 cmH$_2$O or less

**U & Es**   urea and electrolytes

**Upper respiratory tract**   nose (or mouth), pharynx and larynx

**Upstream**   away from the mouth

**Urea**   electrolyte in plasma or urine, formed from protein breakdown and excreted by kidneys, levels affected by kidney function, diet, hypercatabolism, tissue necrosis, volume depletion and steroids
- N in plasma: 2.5–10 mmol/L
- dehydration: >8, hypovolaemia: >18, kidney injury: 55

**Urine output**
- normal: 1 mL/h/kg, average 50–60 mL/h
- renal failure: <half normal

**V**   volume of gas

**v**   venous

**Valsalva manoeuvre**   forced expiratory effort against a closed airway

**VAP**   ventilator-associated pneumonia

**VAS**   visual analogue scale

**Vascath**   vascular catheter, i.e. specialized central venous catheter used in dialysis

**Vasoactive drugs**   vasodilators and vasopressors

**Vasodilator**   drug which relaxes smooth muscle in blood vessels.

**Vasopressor**   drug that constricts blood vessels

**VATS**   video-assisted thoracoscopic surgery

**VC**   (1) vital capacity, or (2) volume controlled ventilation

**VCIRV**   volume control inverse-ratio ventilation

**VCO$_2$**   CO$_2$ production
- N, 200 mL/min at rest, increasing by 7% for each 1°C rise in body temperature

**V$_D$**   volume of dead space gas
- N, for anatomical V$_D$: 2 mL/kg body weight

**V$_D$/V$_T$**   dead space in relation to tidal volume
- N, 0.3, i.e. 30%, depending on body position
- critical increase: 0.6

**Venous admixture**   mixing of shunted venous blood with oxygenated blood, i.e. mixture of 'true' shunt which bypasses pulmonary capillary bed, and 'effective' shunt due to $\dot{V}_A/\dot{Q}$ mismatch
- N, 5% of cardiac output

**Venous return**   blood returning to heart

**Ventilatory pump**   see: respiratory pump

**Venturi effect**   reduction in pressure of air or liquid when a it flows through narrow tubing

**VF**   ventricular fibrillation

**VILI**   ventilator-induced lung injury

**Vital capacity**   maximum volume of gas that can be exhaled after a full inspiration

**Volutrauma**   damage to alveoli due to overstretch

**V$_T$**   see: tidal volume.

**$\bar{v}$**   mixed venous

**$\dot{V}$**   volume of gas per unit time, i.e. flow

**$\dot{V}_A/\dot{Q}$**   ratio of alveolar ventilation to perfusion,
- N, 0.8 (4 L/min for alveolar ventilation, 5 L/min for perfusion)

**$\dot{V}_E$**   see: minute volume

**$\dot{V}O_2$**   see: oxygen consumption

**$\dot{V}O_2/DO_2$**   see: oxygen extraction ratio

**$\dot{V}O_2$max**   see: maximum oxygen consumption

**$\dot{V}O_2$peak**   highest value of $\dot{V}O_2$ attained on a particular exercise test (compared to $\dot{V}O_2$max, which is the highest value attained by an individual)

**WCC**   see next entry

**White blood cell count**   4–10 10$^9$ cells/L [4000–10,000/mm$^{-3}$]
- bacterial infection: >10,000/mm$^3$
- vulnerability to infection: <4000/mm$^3$

**WHO**   World Health Organization

**WOB**   see next entry

**Work of breathing**
- N, 0.3–0.5 kg m/min or joules/L